Biochemistry and the
Central Nervous System

Biochemistry and the Central Nervous System

Henry McIlwain Ph.D. D.Sc.

Professor of Biochemistry in the University of London at the Institute of Psychiatry (British Postgraduate Medical Federation); Honorary Biochemist, the Bethlem Royal Hospital and the Maudsley Hospital

H.S. Bachelard, M.Sc. Ph.D.

Senior Lecturer in Biochemistry in the University of London at the Institute of Psychiatry

Fourth Edition

1971

CHURCHILL LIVINGSTONE   Edinburgh and London

First Edition - 1955
  Spanish translation
  Japanese translation
Second Edition - 1959
  Russian translation
Third Edition - 1966
Fourth Edition - 1971

I.S.B.N. 0 7000 1522 1

© J. & A. Churchill Ltd. 1966
© Longman Group Ltd. 1971

Any correspondence relating to this volume should be directed to the publishers at 104 Gloucester Place, London, W1H 4AE.

Printed in Great Britain

Preface to the Fourth Edition

THIS new edition again bears witness to the rapid development of biochemical studies of the central nervous system. It is nearly half as large again as the third edition, and new material, plus regrouping of much previously written has given two new chapters: those concerned with metabolic regulation and with nucleic acids and proteins. The object of the book remains unchanged, in giving a reasoned exposition of the current status of its subject to students and research workers in medicine and science, especially to those concerned with biochemistry, neurophysiology, neurochemistry, neurology and psychiatry.

The present edition comes at a time when its subject is increasingly taught both at undergraduate and at postgraduate level. A decade ago the main formal teaching in the Department of Biochemistry of this Institute was for postgraduate diplomas in psychological medicine. One such diploma has now developed to become the M.Phil. degree in psychiatry, and in prospect are the qualifications of the newly-established Royal College of Psychiatrists. The replanning of biochemical teaching for such purposes is one factor which has given stimulus to the new edition. Another is the initiation of an M.Sc. in Neurochemistry in the University of London, in the organization of which biochemical teachers of this Department have collaborated with those of the Institutes of Neurology and Ophthalmology. Increasing also are the calls on members of this Department for neurochemical teaching in first degree courses in science and medicine; in recent years such teaching has been given at five schools of London University, with numerous special lectures elsewhere. This reflects in part the growth of psychiatry in medical curricula: an associated Department of Biochemistry is called on to give correspondingly increased time to the biochemistry of neural systems. Courses in biochemistry to meet the needs of students of pharmacology, physiology and other of the neurosciences have also involved much growth of neurochemical teaching.

In this rewriting we have been greatly helped by discussion in this and other Institutes, and with many workers who have come as students and colleagues and who have added expertise and variety to an already intriguing realm of research. Thanks are also due to the publishers for the care which has been given in producing the book.

H. McILWAIN
H. S. BACHELARD
Department of Biochemistry
Institute of Psychiatry
London

Preface to the First Edition

THIS book has developed from research and from teaching in faculties both of medicine and science. Its subject forms part of teaching in physiology and in psychological medicine, in the University of London. In addition, the story of chemical change and structure in the central nervous system presents to the biochemist a well developed branch of his own subject and one which has often been in the forefront of biochemical discovery. Attention has been paid to each of these aspects in the present book.

Biochemistry and the central nervous system overlaps and adjoins several other subjects, notably pharmacology and endocrinology; each year some 3,000 papers appear which concern chemical substances or processes and the central nervous system. It has therefore been a major problem to decide how much to include in the present book. The solution chosen has been to include sufficient reference to neighbouring subjects to illustrate where they are applicable to biochemistry and the central nervous system, and it to the neighbouring subjects. When several aspects of the action of a drug can be seen to be linked by known biochemical mechanisms, these are indicated. When hormonal interactions with the central nervous system have as yet little biochemical logic, mention is brief or absent.

Because the subject of the present book extends beyond the limits of biochemistry itself, I have been most grateful for comments on it from Professor Aubrey Lewis and Professor Alfred Meyer, as well as from Professor F. Dickens and from members of the Department of Biochemistry of this Institute. It also owes much to informal discussion in this and in other departments where I have worked, including the Department of Physiology of the University of Chicago, and the Medical School at Dunedin, New Zealand. The last chapter contains material from the Christian Herter Lecture given at New York University College of Medicine in 1954.

H. MCILWAIN

Contents

Contents

1 Biochemical Studies of the Brain

When chemical investigation of the organs of the animal body developed about 1800, the gross anatomy of the central nervous system was familiar but little was known of its physiology and pathology. These, and especially the histology of the brain, grew to be major subjects during the nineteenth century. Biochemical and electrophysiological studies of the brain remained rudimentary until after the first quarter of the present century. Berger's discovery of rhythmic potential changes from the brain measurable outside the head was made in 1929; reasonably accurate measurement of respiration of cerebral systems began about 1920 with separated tissue, was obtained in perfused animals in 1939 but in normal human subjects not until 1947. Until relatively recently, therefore, there has been much scope for speculation with respect to these most fundamental aspects of cerebral metabolism: the level of energy utilization in the brain and the manner of its adjustment to functional requirements.

Electrophysiological and biochemical exploration of the brain are akin not only in the time at which they developed but also in the velocity of the processes with which they are concerned. Typical changes in electrical potential seen with the electroencephalogram occupy periods of 1 to 1/50 of a second. Changes observed by ordinary biochemical techniques usually take some minutes, but early in the exact study of cerebral constituents it was found necessary to measure processes lasting a second or less. Now one can estimate that during the 1/10 second occupied by a ripple of potential change at alpha frequency appreciable proportions of many important cerebral metabolites are degraded or synthesized. Here one is dealing, not with the fastest cerebral processes in which voltage change and ion migration occupy only parts of a millisecond, but with processes occurring at speeds commensurate with ordinary impressions of the activities of the brain. Interrelations between biochemical and more overt aspects of cerebral functioning have played a large part in making this book. It remains, nevertheless, within a framework largely biochemical for in this manner can best be expressed the biochemical properties on which cerebral function is based and by which also it is characterized and restricted.

The Growth of Chemical Knowledge of the Brain

Metabolic studies of the brain though of recent development had notable precursors. During most of the past 150 years, investigation of neural systems

1

by chemical methods has attracted a reasonable proportion of the chemical resources of the times. It has passed through many phases, which will now be briefly summarized in a fashion which introduces the literature of the subject.

Fractionation of Cerebral Constituents

The first satisfactory application of chemical methods to the brain was made in studying its composition. This commenced before chemistry had fully emerged as a science; Hensing's notable account dates from 1719. Other eighteenth-century writers contributed knowledge of inorganic constituents of the brain, but the realization that it and other organs contained a multiplicity of organic constituents did not come until about 1800. Vauquelin (1811) developed a type of investigation which almost became the standard chemical approach of the nineteenth century. By systematic use of an organic solvent and a heavy metal precipitant (ethanol and lead salts) he separated cerebral constituents to fractions with the intention of accounting for all the brain in terms of materials of definite composition. Of the many workers who developed this theme, Couerbe (1833) is noteworthy in attempting to show differences in the composition of the brain in mental disorder and Thudichum in the comprehensiveness of his study: *The Chemical Constitution of the Brain* (1884; 1901; see McIlwain, 1958c) lists some 140 constituents and carries a comprehensive bibliography. Because of the large proportion of fatty materials in the brain, much of this study concerned lipids. Although succinic acid and proteins also featured, it was their "chemical statics" with which, in Thudichum's own phrase, he was concerned. Fractionation of cerebral constituents from this point of view is still in progress; it represents an important route to chemical understanding and features prominently in the *Symposia* (1956a, b; 1957b), *Colloquium* (1958) and *Handbook*.

Metabolic Studies

It is a mark of the distinctiveness of biochemistry as a discipline, that chemical fractionation of cerebral constituents gave a body of knowledge which did not in itself afford much understanding of cerebral functioning. To a much greater extent, this has come, as in physiology as a whole, by two main routes: by study of energy and of membrane relationships, and by the chemical characterization of substances which perform some specific role as substrate, intermediary metabolite, vitamin, enzyme or hormone. In the present account, as much quantitative information as possible has been collated about such substances and processes, specifically in the central nervous system. These aspects first received comprehensive treatment by Winterstein (1929) in his contributions on the *General Physiology of Nerve* and on the *Central Nervous System* to Bethe's *Handbook*. Peripheral nerve had then been studied in isolation, both biochemically and electrophysiologically, and such investigations were beginning also with the central nervous system. Winterstein's account of these investigations, to which his laboratory greatly contributed, is excellent in its description of relations between energy metabolism and functional activity. He could of necessity say little or nothing of intermediary metabolism.

This aspect was as far as possible supplied in Page's (1937) *Chemistry of the Brain* but, it is very significant, largely in terms of investigation with tissues from organs other than the brain. Several aspects of cerebral metabolism came to their own in Himwich's (1951) *Brain Metabolism and Cerebral Disorders*, especially those concerned with carbohydrate metabolism. They are also prominent in a Conference (1952) and in several Symposia (1952, 1955, 1956*a, b*; 1957*b*; 1959*a, b*) and Collected papers (1954, 1955): the subject, it will be noted, was expanding rapidly in the 1950s.

Study of Substances acting on the Brain

Chemical factors were first recognized as capable of a major role in cerebral activities not by the metabolic studies just described, but rather by the spectacular way in which defined substances modified the activities of the brain. Lack of oxygen or the administration of alcohol or morphine were among the earliest examples, followed around 1850 by synthetic drugs developed specifically for their central effects, as has been recounted in *Chemotherapy and the Central Nervous System* (McIlwain, 1957). Chemical induction of changed mental states by such substances gave important data to those who, in the past century, invoked chemical factors in normal mental functioning and in its derangement in disease (see McIlwain, 1955, 1958*a, b*). The subjects now often termed neuropharmacology and psychopharmacology have for some time formed a notable part of pharmacological texts, and have recently been the subject of separate publications as is indicated in Chapters 14 and 15.

Neurochemistry

These various applications of chemistry and biochemistry to the study of the brain have formed a large part of the now well-established subject of neurochemistry. The term *Nervenchemie* in the 1850s meant, more literally, the chemistry of the nervous system (see Schlossberger, 1856). To judge by present literature, for example, the *Handbook of Neurochemistry* (1969–70) and the *Journal of Neurochemistry* (1956 to date), the term is now envisaged to include a much wider application of chemical concepts, techniques and reagents in the many sciences which are concerned with neural structures. Collected papers entitled *Neurochemistry* appeared in 1955, 1956 (*Symposium*, 1956*b*), 1958 (*Colloquium*, 1958) and 1962. International Symposia in Neurochemistry commenced in 1954 and have to date concerned the development of the nervous system, its metabolism, chemical pathology and also comparative and regional aspects of its chemistry, physiology and pharmacology. The structural units to which these sciences are applied are primarily the neurons and their assemblies. In biochemical as in biological characteristics, neurons are highly complex and versatile cell-types with a long history of development as part of the organs and organisms to which they contribute. Among the most interesting aspects of current neurochemistry are the quantitative comparisons now being established between chemical concomitants of excitation in neural components as diverse as the giant axons of marine invertebrates and the finely-ramifying dendrites of the mammalian brain.

Reviews of neurochemistry first appeared in the *Annual Review of Biochemistry* in 1959, and in the Annual Reports of the Chemical Society for 1960; *Practical Neurochemistry* (McIlwain & Rodnight, 1962) is more immediately connected with laboratory work. The International Society for Neurochemistry held its first meetings in 1967 and 1969 and neurochemical societies or cognate associations have been formed in several countries (Bulletin, 1967). In Britain a Neurochemical Group of the *Biochemical Society* (1967 to date) has held meetings since 1967. The International Brain Research Organization (*IBRO Bulletin*, 1962 to date) includes a neurochemical panel, and national Brain Research associations have also been formed in several localities, often with major neurochemical representation. A Journal of Neurobiology commenced in 1969 and includes neurochemical subjects. The Neurosciences Research Program (1969) has published a Bulletin since 1964, and also includes biochemical subjects. The UCLA Brain Information Service issues bibliographies and a guide to neuroenzyme literature (Hoijer, 1969).

Metabolic Adaptation and Behavioural Studies

The present account of biochemistry and the central nervous system has a sphere of interest which includes the neurochemistry of the brain but extends beyond it to involve many phenomena of the living animal interacting with its environment. Input at the special senses is itself primarily chemical, as is indicated in brief accounts of taste, smell and vision in later chapters. An important aspect of subsequent events in the brain itself is the fashion in which incoming signals affect future responses of an animal to repetition of the same or of concomitant signals: phenomena which form part of the study of conditioning, learning and memory. Several recent approaches to these subjects have invoked chemical mechanisms, in which the change representing learning occurs primarily in nucleic acids, at special polypeptide messengers, or by growth of cell-contacts (John, 1967; Kandel & Spencer, 1968; Eccles, 1966).

A complementary approach (McIlwain, 1970, 1971) has been to see the brain as the main organ of adaptation in higher animals and to seek in cerebral systems the enzyme induction or metabolic adaptation which operates in other organs and organisms. The occurrence of such adaptation in the brain has long been evident: most of the substance of the brain is first synthesized or assembled while the animal concerned is receiving sensory signals. Synthesis and degradation of structural materials and metabolic machinery of the brain continues throughout life, and is open to the influence of hormones, substrates, activators and inhibitors which modify enzymes and other specific proteins in biological systems generally. Thus the cerebral utilization of β-hydroxybutyrate is observed to increase in parallel with supply of β-hydroxybutyrate to the brain (Fig. 2.2), and these increases can progress to the stage when β-hydroxybutyrate replaces glucose as the major source of metabolically derived energy for the brain of man or the rat.

More complex is a specialized reaction to visual signals. Noradrenaline released from sympathetic terminals of an optic pathway by light signals can increase the pineal synthesis of melatonin, and by this route impose a circadean rhythm on production of the hormone melatonin. This proceeds (Fig. 14.9) by increase in the cerebral hydroxyindole-O-methyltransferase which catalyses the final step in melatonin formation, the enzyme induction being catalysed by noradrenaline and inhibited by puromycin or by denervation. Certain aspects of drug-tolerance and dependence also constitute adaptive cerebral changes.

Adaptation which shows features in common with that of the preceding paragraphs can also occur to purely electrical input to the brain. Displacement of the normal standing potential at the mammalian neocortex by surface-positive polarization, increases cell-firing, and the resultant increase persists when after a few minutes the polarizing current is discontinued. The persistent change in cell-firing is inhibited by prior application to the cortex, of inhibitors of protein-synthesis in concentrations which do not affect the increase in cell-firing during application of the polarizing current.

These examples show the brain adapting to changed chemical milieu, to changed sensory input and to intracerebrally-generated alterations in neural activity by adaptive changes familiar from the study of metabolic or enzymic adaptation and regulation in other parts of the body and in other organisms. Such changes may thus give a basis for the adaptation of cerebral function which is manifest as changed behaviour or performance, and is ascribed to conditioned reflexes or to learning.

Biochemistry and Psychiatry

Problems of mental illness have given important stimulus to chemical as to other studies of the brain. As psychiatry is much concerned with adaptation and interactions among individuals and groups, the adaptive processes of the previous section may well represent an important approach of which exploration is just commencing. Current methods employ analysis or enzyme assay of the brain and of other parts of the body (Sourkes, 1962) and also orthodox chemotherapeutic processes which constitute a major application of chemistry to diseases of the central nervous system (McIlwain, 1957; Gordon, 1967). Programmed synthesis of organic compounds, guided by assays which include behavioural tests have afforded compounds which disturb normal cerebral functioning as well as others which restore such function when it is abnormal.

Comments on psychoactive compounds of these various categories will be found widely distributed among the chapters of the present book; conversely, substances or processes which may afford starting-points for future therapeutic applications are also likely to be widely dispersed. Thus journals of neurology and psychiatry have in recent years contained up to 40% of papers with pronounced chemical or pharmacological interests. The bibliographies of the present book will be noted to contain many references to such journals, and year books in these subjects which also carry chemical aspects include *Recent Progress in Psychiatry*, *Progress in Neurology and Psychiatry* and the Research Publications of the *Association for Research in Nervous and Mental Disease*. Literature quoted in the present book is necessarily selected but is intended to cover or to lead to information on the greater part of the subject especially in its quantitative aspects. It has also been considered important to indicate clearly the type of neural system and preparation which afforded the information recorded. The following references include a few general publications related to biochemistry and the nervous system as well as those which received specific mention above.

REFERENCES

Association for Research in Nervous and Mental Disease (1920 to date). Research Publications. Baltimore: Williams & Wilkins.

Biochemical Society (1967 to date). *Yearbook and Annual Reports*. London: The Biochemical Society.

Bulletin (1967). Japanese Neurochemical Society. Tokyo: Ogata Shoten.

BUNIATIAN, H. C. (1966 to date). Problems of Brain Biochemistry. Erevan: Academy of Sciences of the Armenian S.S.R.

Collected papers (1954). Biochemistry of the Nervous System. Ed. A. V. Palladin. Kiev.

Collected papers (1955, 1962). Neurochemistry. Ed. K. A. C. Elliott, I. H. Page & J. H. Quastel, Springfield: Thomas.

Collected papers (1964). Problems of the Biochemistry of the Nervous System. Ed. A. V. Palladin. Transl. Freisinger, Hillman & Woodman. Oxford: Pergamon.

Colloquium (1958). Neurochemistry. *Neurology*, **8**, suppl. 1.

Conference (1952). The Biology of Mental Health and Disease. New York: Hoeber.

COUERBE, J. P. (1833). *Ann. Chim. Phys.* **56**, 160.

CUMINGS, J. N. & KREMER, M. (1959, 1965). Biochemical Aspects of Neurological Disorders, Blackwell: Oxford.

ECCLES, J. C. (1966). Brain and Conscious Experience, p. 314, 335. Berlin: Springer.

EIDUSON, S., GELLER, E., YUWILER, A. & EIDUSON, B. T. (1964). Biochemistry and Behaviour. Princeton, N.J.: Van Nostrand.

GORDON, M. (1967). Psychopharmacological Agents. New York: Academic Press.

Handbook of Neurochemistry (1969–70). Ed. A. Lajtha. New York: Plenum Press.

HENSING, J. T. (1719). Cerebri Examen Chemicum, etc. Giessen, See Tower, *Colloquium* (1958).

HIMWICH, H. E. (1951). Brain Metabolism and Cerebral Disorders. Baltimore: Williams and Wilkins.

HOIJER, D. J. (1969). A Bibliographic Guide to Neuroenzyme Literature. University of California, Los Angeles; New York: Plenum.

IBRO Bulletin (1962). International Brain Research Organization. Paris: UNESCO.

International Society for Neurochemistry (1967, 1969). Programmes of meetings in Strasbourg and in Milan.

JOHN, E. R. (1967). Mechanisms of Memory. New York: Academic Press.

KANDEL, E. R. & SPENCER, W. A. (1968). *Physiol. Rev.* **48**, 65.

McILWAIN, H. (1955). Maudsley, Mott & Mann on the Chemical Physiology and Pathology of the Mind. London: Lewis.

McILWAIN, H. (1957). Chemotherapy and the Central Nervous System. London: Churchill.

McILWAIN, H. (1958*a*). Neurochemistry. In Lectures on the Scientific Basis of Medicine. London: Athlone Press.

McILWAIN, H. (1958*b*). Chemical Contributions, especially from the 19th century, to knowledge of the Brain and its Functioning. In Symposium (1958).

McILWAIN, H. (1958*c*). Thudichum and the Medical Chemistry of the 1860s to 1880s. *Proc. R. Soc. Med.* **51**, 127.

McILWAIN, H. (1970). *Nature, Lond.* **226**, 803.

McILWAIN, H. (1971). *Essays in Biochemistry*, **7**. London: The Biochemical Society.

McILWAIN, H. & RODNIGHT, R. (1962). Practical Neurochemistry. London: Churchill.

Neurosciences Research Program Bulletin (1969) Brookline: Massachusetts Institute of Technology.

PAGE, I. H. (1937). The Chemistry of the Brain, Springfield: Thomas.

Progress in Brain Research (1963 to date). Amsterdam: Elsevier.

Progress in Neurology and Psychiatry (1946 to date). Ed. A. Spiegel. New York: Grune & Stratton.

Recent Progress in Psychiatry (1944, 1950). Ed. G. W. T. H. Fleming. London: Churchill.

SCHLOSSBERGER, J. E. (1856). Erster Versuch einer Allgemeine und Vergleichenden Thier-Chemie. Leipzig: Winter.

SOURKES, T. L. (1962). Biochemistry of Mental Disease. New York: Hoeber.

Symposium (1952). *Biochem. Soc. Sympos.* **8**. Cambridge: University Press.

Symposium (1955). Biochemistry of the Developing Nervous System. *Proc. Internat. Neurochem. Sympos.* **1**. Ed. H. Waelsch. New York: Academic Press.

Symposium (1956a). Aspects of the anatomy, biochemistry, and pathology of the nervous system. *Guy's Hospital Reports*, **105**, 1–150.

Symposium (1956b). Neurochemistry. *Progress in Neurobiology*, **1**. Ed. S. R. Korey & J. I. Nurnberger. Cassell: London (Hoeber: New York).

Symposium (1956c). Psychopharmacology. Washington: American Association for the Advancement of Science.

Symposium (1957a). The Pharmacology of Psychotomimetic and Psychotherapeutic Drugs. *Ann. N.Y. Acad. Sci.* **66**, 417.

Symposium (1957b). Metabolism of the Nervous System. *Proc. Internat. Neurochem. Sympos.* **2**. Ed. D. Richter. London: Pergamon.

Symposium (1958). The History and Philosophy of Knowledge of the Brain and its Functions. Oxford: Blackwell.

Symposium (1959a). Biochemie des Zentralnervensystems. *Sympos III, IV Internationaler Kongress für Biochem.* Ed. F. Brücke.

Symposium (1959b). Chemical Pathology of the Nervous System. *Proc. Internat. Neurochem. Sympos.* **3**. Ed. J. Folch-Pi. Oxford: Pergamon.

Symposium (1961b). Regional Neurochemistry. *Proc. Internat. Neurochem. Sympos.* **4**. Ed. S. S. Kety & J. Elkes. Oxford: Pergamon.

Symposium (1964). Comparative Neurochemistry. *Proc. Internat. Neurochem. Sympos.* **5**. Ed. D. Richter. Oxford: Pergamon.

THUDICHUM, J. L. W. (1884). A Treatise on the Chemical Constitution of the Brain. London: Baillière, Tindall & Cox.

THUDICHUM, J. L. W. (1901). Die Chemische Konstitution des Gehirns des Menschen und der Tiere. Tubingen: Pietzker.

VAUQUELIN, N. L. (1811). *Ann. du Mus. d'Hist. nat.*, **18**, 212; *Annals of Philosophy*, 1813, **1**, 332.

WINTERSTEIN, H. (1929). In Handbuch der Normalen und Pathologischen Physiologie, **9**. Ed. A. Bethe. Berlin: Springer.

2   Metabolism of the Brain *In Situ*

The brain is continually active, as is evident from ordinary experience and from the continuously fluctuating electrical potentials which can be detected in the head. No means are available for supporting such activity other than a continuous supply of substances to the brain by the bloodstream. The nature of these substances can be determined by analysing the blood which enters the brain from the heart. The substances taken from or added to the blood by the brain can be determined by comparing the composition of the blood entering the brain with the composition of that leaving it.

Many such determinations have now been carried out especially in man, so that information is available on cerebral metabolism in a variety of circumstances, and such information constitutes the larger part of this chapter. Blood from the heart can be sampled at any convenient artery, for example in man at the arm or the thigh; but there are relatively few points which afford a representative sample of venous blood from the brain when, as in the present account, it is being considered as a single organ. Among the most suitable in man is the internal jugular vein, especially at its superior bulb. When arterial and cerebral venous blood are analysed it is found that the greatest differences between them are in substances concerned in carbohydrate metabolism (Table 2.1). Blood constituents such as water, protein, total base or inorganic phosphate, show little change. The change in oxygen content is outstanding. It falls by about 6.7 ml./100 ml. of blood, which is a somewhat greater fall than is found to take place in oxygen when the blood traverses most of the other organs of the body. This is reflected in the relatively low value of 62% for the oxygen saturation level of the cerebral venous blood.

Substances exchanged between Blood and Brain

The briskness of normal cerebral respiration leads to enquiry as to the substrate oxidized. Its nature in the normal subjects who afforded the data of Table 2.1 is indicated by the concomitant change in carbon dioxide which at 6·6 ml./100 ml. of blood is almost exactly equivalent to the oxygen absorbed; that is, the normal cerebral respiratory quotient is almost unity. This leads to the conclusion that, of blood constituents, glucose is most likely to be the main substance oxidized, and indeed the arteriovenous difference in glucose is found to be large. At 9·8 mg./100 ml. it is somewhat larger than is required to account

8

for the oxygen used in respiration, so that even if all the respiratory carbon dioxide is derived from glucose, other substances requiring less oxygen for their formation must also be produced. One likely product is the lactic acid of Table 2.1, and a further product is pyruvic acid.

These three substances, carbon dioxide, lactic acid and pyruvic acid, account remarkably completely for the glucose utilized by the human brain under normal conditions. In an instance (Himwich & Himwich, 1946) in which the arteriovenous difference in glucose was 10·2 mg./100 ml. of blood the carbon

Table 2.1

Changes in blood on its passing through the brain

The blood content of the brain is relatively low at about 3–3·5% of the total volume compared with a CSF content of some 9% (Ponten, 1963; Everett, Simmons & Lasher, 1956; Rosomoff, 1961) and is renewed rapidly. In the adult human, with a total-body blood-volume of 5500 ml., the blood flows through the 1300-g. brain at a rate of 750 ml./min. (Dobbing, 1961).

Constituent	Blood levels		Venous—Arterial levels (±standard deviation)
	Arterial	Venous	
Oxygen:			
Content (ml./100 ml.)	19·6	12·9	− 6·7 ±0·8
Capacity (ml./100 ml.)	20·9	20·8	− 0·1
Saturation (%)	93·9	61·8	−31·7 ±3·9
Carbon dioxide:			
Content (ml./100 ml.)	48·2	54·8	+ 6·6 ±0·8
Tension (mm. Hg)	39·9	49·9	+10·0 ±1·2
Glucose (mg./100 ml)	92·0	82·0	− 9·8 ±1·7
Lactic acid (mg./100 ml.)	9·9	11·5	+ 1·6 ±0·9
Free amino acids* (mg. α-amino-N/100 ml. plasma)	6·16	6·02	− 0·14 —
pH at 38°C	7·42	7·37	− 0·05
Inorganic phosphate (mg./100 ml.)	3·4	3·4	0
Total base (mequiv./1. serum)	152·9	154·1	+ 1·2 ±1·2

The values are the mean results obtained by Gibbs *et al.* (1942) for 50 healthy men of 18–29 years of age, at rest. Blood was sampled at the internal jugular vein and femoral artery. The respiratory quotient was 0·99 ± 0·03.

* Sacks (1969).

dioxide found was equivalent to 8·9 mg. of glucose/100 ml.; the lactic acid to 1·2 and the pyruvic acid to 0·2, a total 10·3 mg/100 ml. Several subsequent studies have confirmed such equivalence (see Sokoloff, 1960) though the change in lactate and pyruvate can be variable. Thus, immediately after a carbohydrate-rich meal when blood concentrations of lactate and pyruvate were above average, they diminished on passing the brain (Rowe *et al.*, 1959). The brain, also, can display new properties towards ketone bodies when these are present at high levels during starvation (see p. 19).

The prompt oxidation of glucose to carbon dioxide at the brain has been shown also by isotopically-labelled glucose, administered systemically to

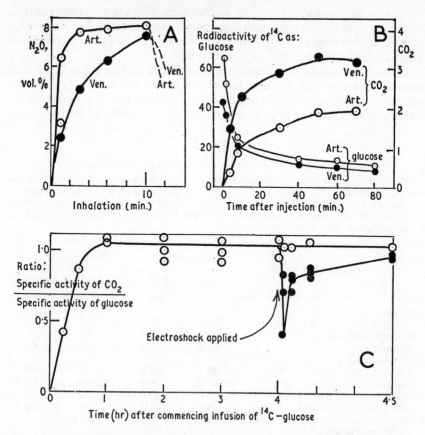

FIG. 2.1. Interchange of substances at the brain, as measured by analysis
of arterial and cerebral venous blood.

A. *Redistribution without metabolic change:* nitrous oxide is not
altered chemically in the brain but diffuses from the arterial blood to
cerebral tissues. The data come from its use in man to measure the rate
of blood flow. The gas is inhaled for 10 min., at which time its concentrations in arterial and venous blood have become nearly equal. The dotted
lines show the loss of N_2O from the brain during subsequent inhalation
of air only.

B. *Metabolic change:* using ^{14}C and reflecting a process operating at
steady rate. ^{14}C-Glucose, after a single injection is yielding [14]CO_2 in
human subjects. The ^{14}C-glucose of cerebral venous blood is throughout
lower than that of arterial samples, while [14]CO_2 shows the reverse
relationship.

C. *Metabolic change,* with alteration in the rate of metabolism. The
processes measured in **B** are here observed in anaesthetized dogs
during a constant infusion of ^{14}C-glucose. Some animals were subjected
to electroshock at the time indicated; note the change in time-scale at
this point. The data in this case are expressed as the ratio of the specific
activities of glucose utilized and CO_2 produced, calculated from
analyses of arterial and cerebral venous blood.
(Kety, 1948; Sacks, 1957; Coxon & Robinson, 1959; Gainer *et al.*,
1963.)

man (Fig. 2.1). Cerebral venous blood consistently contained less of the isotope as glucose, and more as CO_2, than did arterial blood. In these experiments the organs of the body competed for the labelled glucose, and values indicated that between 7 and 20% of the glucose injected was oxidized to CO_2 at the brain. Although under normal conditions glucose forms the main oxidizable substrate for other organs of the body as well as for the brain, the brain is unusual among the larger organs in its dependence on glucose. When blood glucose falls, muscle, liver, or kidney oxidize other substrates and their level of functioning does not immediately change. The contrast in this respect between cerebral and muscular tissues is shown well in the experiment with dogs, fasted and rendered hypoglycaemic with insulin, which is quoted in Table 2.2. It is instructive to see that in the brain the fall in arteriovenous

Table 2.2

Hypoglycaemia on oxidations in brain and muscle

Measurement	Arterial blood glucose (mg./100 ml.)	Arteriovenous difference	
		glucose (mg./100 ml.)	oxygen (ml.O₂/100 ml.)
Brain:			
Before experiment	90	13·1	9·3
Moderate hypoglycaemia	30	12·5	8·0
Intense hypoglycaemia	12	3·0	3·8
Muscle:			
Before experiment	90	7·6	6·9
Hypoglycaemia	20	1·7	6·0

Dogs were fasted and rendered hypoglycaemic with insulin (Himwich & Fazekas, 1937).

difference in oxygen paralleled that in glucose as blood glucose was lowered. Reduction of arterial glucose to 30 mg./100 ml. was associated with a small fall in each arteriovenous difference, while at 12 mg./100 ml. both had fallen considerably. Changes in blood on its passing through skeletal muscle reacted differently to hypoglycaemia: at 20 mg. glucose/100 ml. arterial blood, the arteriovenous difference in glucose was less than one-quarter of its normal value while oxygen uptake was little changed. Muscle therefore oxidizes substances other than glucose when glucose is lacking; the brain has only a limited ability to do so. This makes it understandable that it is cerebral function which fails in hypoglycaemia rather than, for example, muscular function: coma ensues with the heart still beating. These matters are examined more fully below.

Of the two isomeric forms of glucose, α and β, which are normally circulating in the bloodstream, the brain removes more of the β compound (Sacks & Sacks, 1969). Preference of the brain for β-glucose is indicated also by the presence of mutarotase which has similar activity and kinetic properties to the kidney enzyme (Keston, 1954; 1957).

^{14}C-Glucose and $^{14}CO_2$

Experiments with isotopically-labelled substrates in dogs have confirmed the dependence of the brain on glucose. Infusing ^{14}C-glucose intravenously to the anaesthetized animals and measuring the $^{14}CO_2$ in blood from the brain, it was found to reach a specific activity equal to that of the glucose within an hour (C, Fig. 2.1). The accuracy of the data was sufficient to indicate that 90–100% of the CO_2 was derived from glucose and substances which equilibrated relatively quickly with glucose; after displacement by electrical stimulation (see below) equilibrium was re-established in some 30 min.

The output of CO_2 from the brain, which has been described above, is a net process and can be accompanied by processes which lead to uptake of CO_2. Inhaled $^{14}CO_2$, or ^{14}C-bicarbonate by intracarotid injection, yields a number of ^{14}C-metabolites in the brain, and associated evidence indicates that they are formed in the brain itself (Waelsch *et al.*, 1964). Such processes of CO_2-fixation in cat brain yielded in greatest abundance ^{14}C-aspartate and glutamine (q.v.). Understandably, these compounds are among the cerebral metabolites found after administering ^{14}C-glucose (Gaitonde *et al.*, 1964) as is described more fully in subsequent Chapters. Other instances of the formation of $^{14}CO_2$ from substrates supplied to the brain *in situ* are described later in this Chapter.

Measurement of Cerebral Metabolic Rates

The level of metabolic activity exhibited by an organ or by a tissue with respect to a particular substance is often best expressed as a metabolic rate. This gives the quantity of substance caused to react in unit time by unit weight of the organ or tissue. Measurements of metabolic rate of the brain have usually been expressed in ml. or mg. of substance caused to react, per 100 g. fresh weight of brain per minute. Determination of change in concentration of a substance in the blood as it passes through the brain, gives one part of the data needed to express its activity as a metabolic rate. The other part of the data needed is the rate of flow of blood through the brain. Thus, when arterial blood loses 6·6 ml. of oxygen per 100 ml. on passing through the brain at the rate of 50 ml. per 100 g. of brain per minute, the cerebral respiratory rate is $6·6 \times 50/100$, or 3·3 ml. oxygen/100 g./min. This manner of expressing metabolic activity is valuable because, as will become evident later, the rate of blood flow through the brain varies greatly in different conditions and often in such a way that with decreased cerebral activity the flow slackens, while with increased activity it increases. Changed cerebral metabolism is thus only partly reflected in changed arteriovenous differences.

When comparing different cerebral metabolites, quantities of material are conveniently expressed in molar units. A cerebral respiratory rate of 3·3 ml. O_2/100 g. tissue/min. then becomes $3·3/22·4 = 0·147$ mmoles/100 g./min. or 88·5 µmoles/g. hr. The utilization of glucose of 10·2 mg./100 ml. blood or 5·1 mg/100 g. tissue/min. corresponds to $5·1 \times 60/180$ or 1·7 mmoles/100 g. hr. This is 17 µmoles/g. hr., requiring $6 \times 17 = 102$ µmoles O_2/g. hr. for complete oxidation ($C_6H_{12}O_6 + 6O_2$). This is equivalent to the complete oxidation of about 85% of the glucose removed by the brain, or some 20 µmoles/g. cerebral tissue/hr. in man. Similar rates obtain in the brain of the dog, but the rates of cerebral oxidation of glucose in small rodents, rats and mice, may be higher. Thus ^{14}C-glucose injected into these species was calculated to be consumed at the brain at rates between 30 and 40 μmoles/g. hr. (Lowry *et al.*, 1964; Gaitonde, 1965; Cremer, 1970).

Methods

These are described in more detail by McIlwain & Rodnight (1962), Lassen (1966), Sacks (1969) and Sokoloff (1966).

The measurements of cerebral blood flow on which most of the results quoted below depend, is a diffusion method devised by Kety (1948, 1960) and Schmidt (1950; Fig. 2.1, and see Sokoloff, 1959, 1960). The method has been applied largely to man and also to monkeys and to the dog. It depends on measuring the rate of entry to the brain of a foreign substance added to the blood. Hydrogen, nitrous oxide, and isotopes of krypton or xenon have been the most frequently-used foreign substances for they are freely diffusible, easily measured, and readily introduced to the bloodstream by inhalation. Nitrous oxide is used as a mixture of about 15% N_2O, 20% O_2 and 65% N_2 which does not affect the subjects breathing it (80% N_2O with 20% O_2 can be excitant or depressant). From the lungs the added gas passes to the heart and at uniform concentration to all parts of the body in arterial blood. During the first few minutes of inhalation, the blood flowing from an organ such as the brain contains less of the adduct than that entering it, because the gas is being lost to the substance of the brain (A, Fig. 2.1). The more sluggish the flow of the blood, the greater is the arteriovenous difference in the added substance, and the longer does it persist.

Four determinations of arterial and venous concentrations of the added substance in the first ten minutes after inhalation, are sufficient to give both the rate of approach to equilibrium and its final value, which are required for calculating the rate of flow. The necessary samples are taken to syringes previously connected through taps to needles in the femoral artery and the superior bulb of the internal jugular vein. As, throughout, it is concentrations of adduct which have been determined and not actual amounts, the rate of blood flow is obtained as a quantity per unit quantity of brain, and commonly expressed as ml. blood/100 g. brain/min.

Other procedures may be noted briefly. The regional peculiarities of cerebral circulation and metabolism make it difficult to apply thermocouple methods, or dye dilution methods, to the measurement of blood flow. These methods can, however, reveal regional differences in blood flow (Sokoloff, 1959), and have afforded some satisfactory values for cerebral respiratory rate. By using radioactive forms of the inert gases krypton and xenon, automatic recording of the blood concentrations of the added compound is facilitated (Kety, 1960; Lassen *et al.*, 1960). Electrode methods for hydrogen, oxygen, CO_2, and electrolytes have also been developed and applied to automatic recording in blood from different areas of the brain (Meyer *et al.*, 1962). Analytical methods applicable to further cerebral metabolites have been described elsewhere (McIlwain & Rodnight, 1962; Sacks, 1969).

The most detailed estimates of regional blood flow have been made by measuring the arrival of isotopically-labelled trifluoroiodomethane, $^{131}ICF_3$, at different parts of the brain of cats (Kety, *Symposium*, 1963). The compound was infused intravenously at constant rate; at chosen times after a few minutes' infusion, prompt decapitation and freezing of the head followed. Sections and autoradiographs were made in the still-frozen preparations. In the 25 areas evaluated, blood flow in ml./min. ranged from 0·14 of spinal white matter to 1·8 of the inferior colliculus. The cerebral cortex gave 0·8–1·4 ml/min. and the cerebellar cortex, 0·7; flow in several of the grey-matter areas was depressed by thiopentone, as noted in Chapter 15.

Normal Values for Cerebral Respiratory Rate

The volume of blood flowing through the human brain is normally a considerable proportion of the total which the heart supplies to the body as a whole: about 15% in adults under basal metabolic conditions, although the weight of their brain is only 2·5% of that of the body.

As noted above, blood flowing through the brain suffers a reduction in its oxygen content which is somewhat greater than that occurring in the blood in the rest of the body, and assessments of the ratio of oxygen absorbed cerebrally to that breathed show that up to 20–25% is removed by the brain. This is a surprisingly large proportion for an organ which performs no obvious external mechanical, osmotic or chemical work. It reflects the importance of the brain in higher animals and consideration is given below to how the respiration of the brain supports its activities. It is of course under resting metabolic conditions that cerebral respiration accounts for such a large proportion of the oxygen breathed: that is, when the oxygen consumption of the body as a whole is equivalent to some 1800 Kcals/day. When with considerable physical work this is raised five-fold, cerebral oxygen consumption would be some 5% of the total.

Conversely, under other conditions an even greater proportion of the oxygen of the blood has been estimated to be consumed cerebrally: in infants and children up to four years of age, cerebral respiration can account for half the oxygen consumed by the resting body as a whole. This is understandable when it is realized that the weight of the brain at these ages approximates to the sum of those of the liver, kidneys, heart and spleen, organs which with the brain contribute largely to basal metabolism. It appears to be part of normal growth in man for cerebral respiratory rate to fall after childhood, becoming relatively stable in the adult (Table 2.3; Dastur *et al.*, 1963).

It is a normal impression that moderate changes in posture, exercise or breathing do not greatly affect activities of the brain. They can, however, lead to appreciable changes in cerebral circulation and arteriovenous difference in oxygen. Thus, on changing from a prone to an upright position, the flow of blood through the brain falls at least temporarily (Table 2.3); but arteriovenous difference in oxygen increases reciprocally and cerebral respiratory rate remains unchanged. Over-breathing, or breathing air rich in oxygen, increases arterial oxygen levels and decreases blood flow. Breathing air high in carbon dioxide or somewhat low in oxygen (Table 2.3) can greatly increase

Table 2.3

Cerebral blood flow and respiratory rate in man

Condition (adult subjects except as specified)	Cerebral blood flow (ml./100 g. tissue/min.)	Cerebral respiratory rate (ml. O_2/100 g. tissue/min.)
Children, mean age 6·2 years[9]	102	5·1
Normal resting subjects A[1]	54	3·3
Normal resting subjects B[2]	58	3·2
Normal subjects C, supine[6]	65	3·8
Normal subjects C, erect[6]	52	3·8
Hyperventilation[1]	34	3·7
Breathing 5–7% CO_2[1]	93	3·5
Breathing 85–100% O_2[1]	45	3·2
Breathing 10% O_2[1]	73	3·3
Insulin hypoglycaemia*[1] arterial glucose level 19 mg. %	61	2·6
Insulin coma*[1] arterial glucose level 9 mg. %	63	1·9
Irreversible insulin coma[8] arterial glucose, 360 mg. %	52	1·5
Natural sleep[10]	65	3·4
Thiopentone anaesthesia, subjects D[1,3]	52	1·9
Thiopentone; hyperventilation, subjects E[4]	28	1·5
Schizophrenics[1]	54	3·3
Uraemic subjects[2]	50	2·3
In diabetic acidosis[1]	45	2·7
In diabetic coma[1]	65	1·7
In myxedema[7]	40	2·8
Extreme apprehensiveness (occasionally; see text)[10]	–	5·0
Adrenaline perfusion (see text)[10]	61	4·2
In cerebral haemangioma[5]	164	3·3

* Carried out with schizophrenic subjects.
[1] Kety (1948); Lassen (1966); Sacks (1969). [2] Heyman *et al.* (1951). [3] Wechsler *et al.* (1951). [4] Pierce *et al.* (1962). [5] Schmidt (1950). [6] Scheinberg & Stead (1949); for comparison of these values with those for subjects A, see Kety (1955, 1957). [7] Scheinberg *et al.* (1950). [8] Fazekas *et al.* (1951). [9] Kennedy (1956). [10] Sokoloff (1956).
For data from cat, rat, dog and monkey: see Sacks (1969).

cerebral blood flow but under none of these circumstances does cerebral respiratory rate significantly change. Reference must be made elsewhere for accounts of the interesting subject of control of cerebral blood flow and its relationship to blood pressure, pharmacological agents and other factors (Kety, 1960; *Symposium*, 1963; Lassen, 1966; Scheinberg, 1966; Espagno, 1969).

Against this background of relative stability in cerebral respiratory rate must be judged the effects of various circumstances in which changed cerebral functioning is associated with changed cerebral respiration; these will now be described.

Changes in Cerebral Metabolism

Measurement of cerebral metabolism *in vivo* by the methods just described has been applied to a number of circumstances in which cerebral functioning has changed. Those in which the change has been induced experimentally and is therefore relatively well defined are described first. They afford a basis for comparison with results in pathological conditions. Of the metabolic characteristics measured, cerebral respiration has attracted most attention, and the majority of the studies show with considerable consistency that the functioning of the central nervous system is disturbed whenever cerebral respiration falls by 20–30 % from its normal value.

Cerebral Respiration in Hypoglycaemia

When the level of blood glucose in man and in other higher animals is lowered, for example by insulin or by hepatectomy, their behaviour changes in fashions which can be ascribed to disturbance of the central nervous system. Concomitant disturbance is seen in the electrical activity of the brain. Both types of disturbance are relieved by administration of glucose. In man during insulin hypoglycaemia, changes in sensation as judged by subjective reports, and in the electrical activity of the brain, may commence when blood glucose has fallen from its normal value of some 80–100 to 50–70 mg./100 ml. (Davis, 1941; Hill & Parr, 1963). In man and the cat the electroencephalogram shows a gradual change with glucose level over a much wider range of concentrations; the 4 per second voltage fluctuations (delta waves) increase gradually as blood glucose falls from 170 to 40 mg/100 ml. (Brazier *et al.*, 1944; Creutzfeldt & Meisch, 1962). Under these circumstances change has not been reported in the respiration or glucose consumption of the brain as a whole.

Clear indication of fall in cerebral respiratory rate is seen when blood glucose reaches about 20 mg/100 ml. (Table 2.3); the rate then falls 24 % below its normal value and the electroencephalogram is grossly disturbed or absent. The markedly lowered arteriovenous difference in oxygen is not made good by increased cerebral blood flow; though that increases, it remains 50 % below the value reached with high carbon dioxide. The increased blood flow with high CO_2 (or low O_2) occurs through cerebral vasodilatation; hypoglycaemia apparently does not induce such dilatation. With insulin sufficient to lower arterial glucose to 9 mg./100 ml. and to induce coma, cerebral respiration is reduced by 44 %. In other experiments of similar type the associated fall in arteriovenous difference in oxygen was even greater, suffering a reduction reaching 75 % and was accompanied by correspondingly reduced values for arteriovenous difference in glucose. Hypoglycaemia which terminated fatally was found to be associated with an even greater lowering of cerebral respiration, which did not recover after administering much glucose. As coma continued, respiratory rates became progressively smaller, in some cases remaining at 0·5–1 ml. O_2/100 g. tissue/min. for some days before death.

Whereas the general effects of insulin on cerebral metabolism are due to the lowered levels of blood glucose, there may be a direct effect of the hormone on the brain itself. Glucose uptake into human brain *in vivo* has been reported to be insulin-sensitive although the response was slower than in peripheral tissues (Butterfield *et al.*, 1966). Insulin, injected directly into rat brain, caused increased cerebral contents of glycogen and glucose 6-phosphate; the results were interpreted in terms of an effect on glucose uptake to the brain (Mellerup & Rafaelson, 1969; Strang & Bachelard, 1971). Hypoglycaemic symptoms are relatively difficult to produce in the sheep, but are produced unusually easily in the new-born pig; peculiarities probably to be ascribed to aspects of general bodily metabolism as well as cerebral metabolism. Thus the acetate present at relatively high level in sheep blood does not undergo change in concentration on passing the brain but adrenaline-like substances are released after insulin and can delay hypoglycaemic symptoms (Setchell & Waites, 1962). Adaptive changes which enable the brain to utilize substrates alternative to glucose, are described in a following section. The increase in secretion of adrenaline during insulin-induced hypoglycaemia in rats was found to occur when the glucose concentration fell to 40 mg/100 ml. 3-Methylglucose, which retards glucose uptake from the bloodstream, increased the rate of secretion of adrenaline presumably by action on a receptor which mediates in the adrenaline liberation. The effective stimulus was concluded to be a depressed rate of utilization of glucose by the receptor tissue (Himsworth, 1968).

Substrates Alternative to Glucose

When cerebral activity has failed temporarily in hypoglycaemia, with the associated fall in glucose catabolism and in respiration, administration of glucose can normally restore all three quite promptly. In man rendered hypoglycaemic with insulin, this occurs within three minutes of the intravenous injection of glucose, 4–25 g. according to the severity of the coma. In hepatectomized dogs and cats, Mann (1927) found 0·25 g. glucose/kg. body weight/hr. to be sufficient for maintenance of the animals. Hypoglycaemic subjects which respond in this way to glucose afford an excellent opportunity for seeing how specific is the relationship between the brain and glucose; for seeing whether other substances will replace blood glucose in maintaining cerebral functions and whether restoration of function is always associated with increased cerebral respiration. In general, positive association of this type is found and in acute experiments the specificity to glucose is high.

Mannose and maltose restored normal behaviour and cerebral electrical activity to hepatectomized animals (Mann & Magath, 1922; Maddock *et al.*, 1939) but were concluded to do so only after their conversion to glucose elsewhere in the body. Comparable or greater quantities of fructose, galactose, hexose diphosphate, of succinic, lactic, pyruvic and glutamic acids, and of glyceraldehyde and ethanol did not do so. These substances, therefore, are not converted to blood glucose at an adequate rate, nor do they themselves reach the brain in adequate quantity to support its activities. In some cases, with ethanol or succinate for example, this is probably due to the substances themselves being unsuitable as major energy-yielding substrates for cerebral tissues. Many of the others, as is discussed more fully below, are probably suitable but do not reach the brain in adequate concentrations. Limited penetration has been demonstrated on the part of fructose and lactic and pyruvic acids by analysis of cerebral tissues from animals to which the substances have been administered (Stone, 1938; Klein & Olson, 1946). Recent reexamination of comparable questions in man by administering ^{14}C-labelled galactose and ribose (Sacks, 1969) again showed little or no uptake of the two sugars by the brain. A quite limited cerebral output of $^{14}CO_2$ was observed and attributed to prior metabolic conversion of the ^{14}C-substrates, elsewhere in the body.

Several substances can be oxidized by the brain although they do not replace glucose in supporting normal cerebral activities. Lactic and pyruvic acids are of especial interest as potential substrates for they are normal blood constituents and cerebral products. Administration of 10–20 g. of sodium lactate, or 7·5 g. of sodium pyruvate, to human subjects in hypoglycaemic coma induced by insulin caused however only small increases in cerebral arteriovenous difference in oxygen, and also did not restore consciousness (Wortis *et al.*, 1941). Determination of arterial and venous levels of lactate after its administration did not show an increased utilization of lactate. Lactate was similarly ineffective in eviscerated dogs. Pyruvate permitted a small increase in arteriovenous difference in oxygen, but without recovery from hypoglycaemia (Goldfarb & Wortis, 1941). Ethanol was without effect in either respect after administration of solutions containing 50 g. orally or 5 g. intravenously. Several ^{14}C-labelled intermediates of the tricarboxylic cycle (q.v.), and ^{14}C-glucose-phosphates, can yield $^{14}CO_2$ at limited rates at the brain *in situ* (Sacks, 1969).

Oxidation of butyrate, fumarate, and aspartate has been shown to occur at the human brain after intravenous injection of the ^{14}C-labelled substrates. In experiments analogous to those of Fig. 2.1 (Sacks, 1957, 1958) cerebral venous $^{14}CO_2$ rose promptly above the arterial level, and examination of the blood for likely ^{14}C-intermediates demonstrated the directness of the cerebral oxidation of the administered substrates. They yielded at the brain some 1–4% of the total $^{14}CO_2$ formed in the body, whereas glucose in analogous experiments yielded 10–20% at the brain. It is noteworthy that although ^{14}C-glycerol by this technique afforded appreciable $^{14}CO_2$ at the brain, much of this was shown to be derived from ^{14}C-glucose produced elsewhere in the body. From studies of ^{14}C-labelled intermediates, the glycerol utilized at the brain was concluded to be metabolized mainly through serine (Seiler *et al.*, 1969). Also, ^{14}C-glucose 6-phosphate lowered the arteriovenous difference in glucose; the ^{14}C present in the glucose indicated dephosphorylation of the phosphate ester during its passage through the brain (Sacks & Sacks, 1968). A number of other substrates yielded negligible $^{14}CO_2$ at the brain. Tissues of sheep and other ruminants derive a major part of their energy from fatty acids, and in sheep ^{14}C from butyrate and propionate was found to appear very promptly in the free amino acids of the brain (O'Neal *et al.*, 1966); acetate was less active in this regard.

Several amino acids are oxidized by the mammalian brain *in vivo*, though, again, they do not replace glucose as substrates supporting cerebral activities. A small arteriovenous difference in amino-N at the brain in man, suggests utilization equivalent to 3 μmoles amino acid/g. brain/hr. (Sacks, 1969), which is comparable to the ability of the brain to synthesize urea (q.v.). Of individual amino acids, ^{14}C-alanine, -serine and -γ-aminobutyrate readily yielded $^{14}CO_2$, and some $^{14}CO_2$ was yielded also from labelled glutamate, phenylalanine and tyrosine (q.v.).

Adaptation to Substrates other than Glucose

The mammalian brain's normal use of glucose as only major energy-source, is a metabolic specialization which can be understood as advantageous under normal circumstances, but as hazardous when glucose is lacking. The body has only limited carbohydrate resources, stored or metabolically-available.

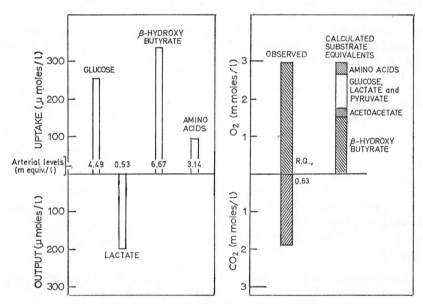

FIG. 2.2. Substrates oxidized by the brain during starvation (Cahill *et al.* 1968; Owen *et al.*, 1967). Data obtained by analysis of arterial and cerebral venous blood of 3 patients, weighing initially 123–147 kg., after 38–41 days' starvation during which they had lost 22–25% of their body weight.

Yet cerebral functioning in man continues during some weeks of starvation. This has been found to depend on the ability of the normal brain to utilize other metabolites in place of glucose: an ability not evident during the briefer experiments which were recounted above, and which lasted minutes or hours rather than days or weeks.

Men and women who were grossly overweight and who were being treated by total starvation, were examined metabolically after 5–6 weeks on a regimen of salt, water, vitamins and flavouring (Fig. 2.2). They were then in ketosis but were mentally alert, and analysis of arterial blood samples showed the major oxidizable substrate to be β-hydroxybutyrate, with acetoacetate also available and glucose a little diminished from its normal level. Cerebral venous blood taken from the internal jugular bulb simultaneously with the arterial sampling, enabled the values of Fig. 2.2 to be calculated. The O_2 and CO_2 data gave a cerebral respiratory quotient of 0·63, showing that the usual oxidation of glucose was not taking place. Removal of glucose at the brain was, indeed, less than the removal of β-hydroxybutyrate. Calculation of the oxygen utilization which corresponded to complete oxidation of the substrates removed from the arterial blood, showed that changes in glucose, lactate and pyruvate collectively accounted for only one-third of the oxygen uptake. β-Hydroxy-butyrate, amino acids and acetoacetate accounted for the remainder.

Blood flow and cerebral respiratory rates were obtained by blood analysis after inhaling [45]Kr (Cahill *et al.*, 1968) and showed rates of 45 ml. blood/100 g. brain/min., and utilization of 3·02 ml. O_2/100 g. brain/min.: values only slightly below those observed in normal adult subjects (Table 2.3). Oxidation of ketone bodies has thus, on starvation, replaced a considerable proportion of the brain's normal oxidation of glucose. It has been demonstrated also in the rat that ketone bodies are oxidized at the brain whenever they are present in the blood in adequate concentration (Hawkins, 1971; Page, Krebs & Williamson, 1971.) Thus acetoacetate was so utilized when it was infused to normal rats, and also when it occurred naturally in infant rats, which normally receive a fat-rich milk by suckling. These abilities of the brain depend on enzymic properties of the cerebral systems which utilize acetoacetate and β-hydroxybutyrate, as described subsequently. Oxidation of β-hydroxybutyrate by mitochondrial preparations from the brain has been demonstrated to give a normal yield of adenosine triphosphate (see Chapter 6).

Persons undergoing this dietary treatment for obesity required hospitalization, but were mentally alert and showed no untoward mental changes (Kollar & Atkinson, 1966).

Hypoxia

The oxygen content of air breathed by man can be reduced from 20 to 10% without appreciable change in cerebral respiration. The arteriovenous difference in oxygen falls but blood flow increases (Schmidt, 1950). Blood flow also increases in hypoxia in the monkey and cat (Schneider, 1957; Sokoloff, 1960); cerebral blood vessels are dilated in hypoxia (Scheinberg, 1966). Normally, the blood leaving the brain still carries oxygen at 60–65% of saturation but when this falls below 24%, through diminution in blood flow or in the oxygen of the air breathed, then consciousness is lost (Refsum, 1963; Sokoloff, 1960). When blood flow was gradually decreased in the isolated head of the cat, the first appearance of abnormal electrocorticograms occurred at the same point as the first reduction in oxygen uptake. Arteriovenous difference in oxygen in dogs was always very much lower than normal when they were caused to breathe air with less than 7% of oxygen, and other signs of changed cerebral metabolism appeared at about the same oxygen level: increased lactic acid, and marked changes in cerebral electrical potentials (Gurdjian *et al.*, 1944). Arteriovenous difference in oxygen, and cerebral respiration, can both be reduced to very low levels in dogs by the injection of cyanides (Fazekas *et al.*, 1939). With a near-lethal dose (20 mg. of KCN), arteriovenous difference was less than 10 % of its normal value for over 18 min. and was still depressed by 50 %, an hour and a half later.

Marked hypoxia thus depresses cerebral metabolism, but little indication of metabolic change is associated with the milder degrees of hypoxia at which signs of changed cerebral functioning are first evident. The head-ache, lassitude, and difficulty in concentrating which are encountered at altitudes of 10,000–16,000 ft. can be reproduced in experiments with correspondingly reduced oxygen tensions at ordinary pressures (14–11 % oxygen in the air breathed). Increasingly poor performances are given in tests of memory and word association; visual sensitivity also markedly falls (McFarland, 1952). Here it is important to note that deprivation of oxygen acts selectively on different parts of the central nervous system (Meyer, 1936; Himwich, 1951; *Symposium*, 1963). Thus cyanide or carbon monoxide poisoning results in degeneration of neurons more consistently in the globus pallidus and in certain parts of the cerebellum and cerebral white matter than elsewhere in the brain. Selective action of this type makes it possible that localized metabolic changes are induced in the central nervous system by mild degrees of hypoxia but are not seen in measuring the metabolism of the brain as a whole. Occlusion of particular blood vessels supplying the brain of monkeys, produced local cortical anoxia with minimal effect on cerebral venous oxygen (Meyer *et al.*, 1962). Metabolic and clinical questions raised by perinatal hypoxia and asphyxia have been reviewed (James & Myers, 1967); they are only in part open to examination by the methods now under discussion and receive further comment in Chapter 13.

Effects of hypoxia in experimental animals can to some extent be made good by administering agents which increase cerebral blood flow. Dimethylamino-ethyl-*p*-chlorophenoxyacetate has been developed for this purpose and is effective in increasing the penetration of ^{14}C-glucose to the cerebral tissues of mice (Nickel *et al.*, 1963).

Hypothermia and Hibernation

Techniques involving the lowering of body temperature are employed surgically, because they extend the time during which blood supply to an organ can be diminished or halted, and thus extend also the time available for surgical procedures. This extension depends on lowered metabolism of vulnerable organs, and especially of the brain, at the lowered temperatures employed. Histologically-observed damage developed in the brain of the dog when blood supply to it was occluded for more than 5 min. at 37°, while 15–20 min. occlusion was tolerated at a body temperature of 25° (Rosomoff, 1966). The oxygen consumption of the brain of the dog at 25° was found to be about one-third its normal value. Cerebral respiration has been studied also in monkeys at body temperatures of 19–38°: and in one instance an approximately linear relationship found between the logarithm of cerebral respiratory rate, and the reciprocal of the absolute temperature (Sokoloff, 1960; Rosomoff, 1966). Application of hypothermic techniques to intracranial surgery in man is described by MacCarty *et al.* (1966); temperatures down to 15° were employed, with circulatory arrest for up to 44 min.

When animals hibernate, the temperature of their brain falls to values slightly above ambient temperature (Hoffman, 1968). Metabolic rates, including those of the brain, fall; they rise during the periodic arousals which are characteristic of the hibernating state. Electroencephalographic measures of the electrical activity of the brain show major diminution during hibernation; the fall in activity differed in different cerebral regions.

Sleep, Depression and Excitation

Previous sections have shown how metabolic factors can limit the overt activities of the brain; the present data indicate how far cerebral metabolism is affected by changes in cerebral functioning.

1. During natural sleep, the cerebral respiratory rate of young adult subjects has been found to remain at the normal level observed during waking periods (Table 2.3). A small increase occurred in cerebral blood flow; the sleep was associated with the usual electroencephalographic pattern of slow waves of large amplitude. Increase in blood flow occurred, especially during periods of rapid eye-movement (Kety, 1967). Administration of barbiturates in doses causing only sedation, and of chlorpromazine and reserpine in the dosages employed as tranquillizing agents, also had no appreciable action on cerebral respiration (Sokoloff, 1959), though cerebral vascular effects were again found (Scheinberg, 1966). That sleep does not change cerebral respiration is discussed by Kety (*Symposium*, 1961) in relation to the balance of activities in different parts of the brain.

2. Depressant drugs used as in surgery to obtain general anaesthesia, do however markedly lower cerebral respiratory rate. Although during early stages of thiopentone narcosis, in which consciousness is clouded and reactions are impeded, no clear change in cerebral respiration was observed; yet with loss of contact with surroundings, and relatively light surgical anaesthesia, cerebral respiration fell to 2·1 ml./100 g./min., a loss of 35 % of the normal rate. Considerable changes in the electrical activity of the brain take place with concentrations of anaesthetics which have no effect on cerebral respiration. At the levels which depress respiration, the electrical activity as seen in the electro-encephalogram of a number of animal species is decreased, slowed, and may be absent from parts of the brain (Toman & Davis, 1949; Wikler, 1950). With halothane anaesthesia, cerebral respiration was just over half its normal value (McDowell *et al.*, 1963); this and other anesthetics are discussed further in Chapter 15.

3. Adrenaline, and extreme anxiety can probably increase cerebral respiratory rate (Table 2.3). An occasional instance in which measurement of cerebral blood flow caused apprehensiveness in the person being studied, was noted as associated with a high cerebral respiratory rate; and during investigation of possible effects of mental arithmetic on cerebral activity, increased cerebral respiratory rate was occasionally observed but considered to be associated with anxiety rather than with the mental work as such. The subjects showing the increase showed also, signs of sympathetic discharge. Moreover, when

adrenaline itself was perfused intravenously in small doses sufficient to raise the mean arterial blood pressure by some 20%, increased cerebral respiration was observed (Sokoloff, 1956, 1959, and see Fazekas *et al.*, 1960; Scheinberg, 1966). Noradrenaline was without effect on cerebral respiration, as also was amphetamine.

4. In animals, experimentally induced convulsions are associated with increased cerebral metabolic rates. This has been shown in monkeys, by the nitrous oxide technique, on administering convulsive drugs (Schmidt *et al.*, 1945). In monkeys and dogs artificially ventilated with O_2 after muscular paralysis, seizures induced by electroshock or by pentamethylene tetrazole (Plum *et al.*, 1969) greatly increased cerebral metabolic activity, a four-fold increase in energy metabolism being estimated. Increased respiration during brief periods has also been shown by potentiometric methods (Gurdjian *et al.*, 1946). Interestingly, pentamethylenetetrazole proved to increase both cerebral electrical activity and oxygen uptake, before the occurrence of the overt convulsion. This is seen in the following chapter to be one of a pattern of changes in cerebral constituents which are associated with the action of convulsive agents.

Cerebral Metabolism in some Pathological Conditions

Again, the aspect of cerebral metabolism about which most is known concerns respiratory exchange; notes on other processes follow.

Cerebral Respiration

Observation of the way in which behaviour and consciousness in man and animals change on depriving the brain of oxygen or of its oxidizable substrates, led to much speculation on the possible rate of cerebral respiration in pathological conditions affecting the central nervous system and gave impetus to development of the methods just described. Lowered cerebral respiration has now been demonstrated to be associated with the changed mental conditions of certain disorders; in other cases no change has been detected (Table 2.3).

1. Elderly persons with organic dementia, or with cerebral arteriosclerosis and senile psychoses showed rates of cerebral blood flow and respiration significantly below those of their normal contemporaries (Lassen *et al.*, 1960; Dastur *et al.*, 1963; Sokoloff, 1966). In a group of mean age 72 years and suffering a chronic brain syndrome with psychosis, respiration had fallen to 2·7 ml./100 g./min. Diminution in cerebral respiratory rate is not an inevitable accompaniment of old age, for normal rates were found in healthy men of 70 years. These were necessarily a selected group; Sokoloff (1966) discusses the clinical and selection problems in arriving at such conclusions and notes that cerebral vascular disease, when it occurs, sets the pace for other aging processes in the brain.

2. Subjects with cerebral tumours and in coma were found to have cerebral respiratory rates some 25% lower than normal; in others still conscious, the respiratory rate was more normal (Schmidt, 1950). The extent to which cerebral blood flow can be increased while leaving cerebral respiration relatively normal

is illustrated by the cerebral haemangioma of Table 2.3, when the short-circuiting of blood supply led to a three-fold increase in normal blood flow, accompanied however by an arteriovenous difference one-third of normal.

3. Diabetic coma. When diabetes had led to a confusional state or to coma, cerebral oxygen uptake was found to be diminished by 20 or 50% (Table 2.3). In these conditions, glucose was present in excess (perhaps 300 mg. %) and cerebral blood flow was changed only some 15% from normal; the decreased respiration is not therefore due to these factors, but to others of the metabolic disturbances characteristic of diabetes. Of these, the level of blood ketones appears to be most important, for Kety *et al.* (1948; see also Kety, 1950) found a significant correlation between fall in cerebral respiration and ketone level in a series of subjects. Injected acetoacetate induced coma. The lowered respiration was not as closely correlated with the concomitant acidosis. Diabetic coma resulting from lack of insulin is thus akin in its mechanism to surgical anaesthesia and markedly different from the hypoglycaemic coma caused by excess insulin.

4. Uraemia. Here also the drowsy or confused state associated with the disorder was found to be accompanied by marked lowering in cerebral respiration and not in general metabolism (Heyman *et al.*, 1951). Blood flow was little changed when cerebral respiration had fallen by 35%. The condition is presumably an intoxication by unusual blood constituents, although the degree of reduction in cerebral oxygen uptake was not correlated with change in blood urea or electrolytes caused by the disorder. Protein degradation products have been suggested as involved, including phenolic acids which accumulate in the blood in uraemia (Dastur, 1961; Hicks *et al.*, 1962).

5. Hepatic coma. Gross liver damage frequently causes neuropsychiatric disturbances which culminate in hepatic coma; cerebral respiratory rate is then found to have fallen by some 35% (Fazekas *et al.*, 1956). Much evidence indicates chemical intermediation between liver and brain; haemodialysis, or a diet low in protein, can each ameliorate the condition. More than one substance appears to be involved; in some instances ammonium salts may be preponderant factors: on administration they can precipitate coma. So also may methionine, the effects of which are antagonized by antibiotics which also ameliorate the syndrome itself: the intestinal flora is then involved (Dawson *et al.*, 1957). Bile salts and other circulating metabolites can depress the respiration of cerebral tissues and were examined in relation to hepatic coma by Lascelles & Taylor (1968).

6. Schizophrenia. Cerebral respiration in schizophrenia has often featured in discussion of the nature of the disorder. Schizophrenia has been considered to show some changes in thought similar to those induced by hypoxia, and to be associated with low basal metabolic rate, but neither of these suggestions is very specific or secure. Observations indicating that cerebral arteriovenous difference in oxygen was normal in schizophrenics (Wortis *et al.*, 1940) were at first doubted but later fully confirmed (Kety *et al.*, 1947; Kety, 1959). Moreover, cerebral blood flow and hence respiratory rates in schizophrenics were also indistinguishable from those of normal subjects, both in their average values and in their standard deviation from such values. Cerebral exchange in carbon dioxide and glucose was also normal, the respiratory quotient remain-

ing unity. Cerebral respiration in schizophrenics also responded normally to insulin and to thiopentone. In making these observations some 30 subjects affected with various types of schizophrenia for various periods were examined both collectively and in groups according to their age or the type and duration of illness and the length of their hospitalization, but no group differed significantly from normal. A subsequent investigation has suggested that certain chronic schizophrenics show lowered cerebral respiratory rate, but without indicating the change to be characteristic of or important to the illness.

7. Other conditions. Cerebral respiration has been examined in *epileptics* who suffered from frequent seizures, determining arteriovenous difference and blood flow during interseizure periods (Gibbs *et al.*, 1947; Jasper *et al.*, 1969). No difference from normal subjects was found. It would of course be especially interesting and relevant to obtain such data during seizures, but the period of excitation during these is normally brief and the experimental difficulties considerable. A transitory increase in respiration is to be expected as is observed during induced seizures (see above and Plum *et al.*, 1969).

In *hyperthyroidism*, mental activities are frequently disturbed, but cerebral respiration in hyperthyroid subjects was found to be little if at all different from normal (Scheinberg, 1950). In *myxoedema*, however, cerebral respiration has been reported to share in the fall of metabolic rate found in the body as a whole. This would give direct basis for the alteration of mental status which occurs in the disease but contrary evidence has also been given. The change is clearest in young animals during development (q.v.) when maturation, including its metabolic aspects, can be accelerated by thyroxine (Ford, 1968). Under these circumstances it is suggested that increased respiration is related to an increase in synthetic processes, and especially to protein synthesis.

Other Aspects of Cerebral Metabolism

Measurement of cerebral respiration has thus provided important evidence of defects in the brain itself in association with changes in cerebral functioning. Appreciably more information could probably come by comparably detailed study of other cerebral metabolites, though processes revealed are likely to remain smaller in metabolic rate than those of glucose breakdown; respiratory quotient has in most studies remained close to unity but a notable exception was found in the adaptive changes during ketosis. Substrate utilization by the brain can clearly depend on the composition of the blood supplied to the brain.

In normal men, determination of cerebral arteriovenous difference in glucose, lactate, and pyruvate showed that when blood concentrations of the latter substances increased on eating a meal after 14 hr. without food, their uptake by the brain increased while cerebral respiration remained unchanged (Rowe *et al.*, 1959). Oxidation of butyrate, fumarate, and aspartate at the brain when they were at unusually high concentrations in the blood, was noted above. Studies employing ^{14}C-labelled glucose in normal human subjects have shown the CO_2 added to the blood by the brain to derive in part from other substrates, and here the glucose, glycogen, and amino acids already present in the brain made a major contribution (Sacks, 1957). Some additional substrates, possibly

2

glycogen or amino acids, were also oxidized by the brain of the dog on electrical stimulation in the experiments of C, Fig. 2.1. These findings do not demonstrate that other substrates supplied by the blood are themselves oxidized at the brain, but emphasize the metabolic interchanges within the brain which are the subject of subsequent Chapters.

Metabolism and Maintenance of the Partly Isolated and Perfused Central Nervous System

Values for respiratory rate of the intact mammalian brain which are now recognized as the first dependable ones were obtained not by the methods of the previous section, but by those of perfusion. This is understandable when it is recalled that the difficulty in determining respiratory rate of the brain *in situ* lay not in analysis of the blood entering and leaving the organ, but in its sampling and in determining its rate of flow. These difficulties can be obviated by artificially causing the blood to flow at a defined rate through a route chosen by suitable cannulation. In this way, Chute & Smyth (1939) led the defibrinated blood of cats through the brain at 60–90 ml./min. and found an arteriovenous difference in oxygen which gave respiratory rates of 3·3–5 ml. O_2/100 g./min. Utilization of glucose and lactate was also observed in the perfused brain; lactate oxidation increased when blood glucose was low. An important aspect of this investigation lay in its being the first determination of the respiratory rate of the brain *in situ* which approximated in its value to those found using the separated tissue in simple glucose–saline solutions. Earlier estimates of natural cerebral blood flow had placed its value, and hence that of cerebral respiratory rate, about twice as high as is now recognized as correct. Perfusion of the isolated head of the cat has shown that blood flow could be diminished to half its normal value without affecting cerebral respiration but that further retardation, which brought cerebral venous oxygen tension below 29 mm., lowered respiration and disturbed the electrical activity of the brain (Hirsch *et al.*, 1955).

Though many aspects of the functioning of several organs have been successfully maintained by perfusing them with saline solutions while they are completely separated from the rest of the body, great success has not so far been achieved in this respect with the mammalian brain. It is impressive to see the heart beating for many hours, isolated from the body and perfused with an oxygenated salt–glucose mixture. Peripheral nerve is also relatively hardy in this respect. The spinal cord must be handled more carefully, and can then respond electrically as *in vivo* (Rudin & Eisenman, 1954). The closest approach with cerebral tissues has been observed with part of the brain of the goldfish or of the frog. If the frog brain is separated carefully from the rest of the animal, the olfactory bulb continues to show rhythmic fluctuations in potential which are somewhat similar to those *in vivo* and which are modified in various ways by brief immersion in solutions of substrates, salts and inhibitors; some concomitant changes in respiration have also been observed (Adrian & Buytendijk, 1931; Brooks *et al.*, 1949).

The mammalian brain, however, demands a greater or more continuous exchange of materials with the bloodstream. Some success has been obtained in perfusing the cat's brain with ox blood or a suspension of blood corpuscles in saline or in protein-containing solutions (Geiger, 1958). Continued EEG-like activity has been achieved by this procedure. The further addition of a liver extract or derived substances appear to be necessary for the maintenance of cerebral respiration and electrical activity, especially after momentary hypoglycaemia. The brain so maintained differs from normal in some aspects of its composition, but its utilization of ^{14}C-labelled substrates has been extensively studied (see Gombos et al., 1963; Sacks, 1969). The rat spinal cord has been perfused also with washed erythrocytes suspended in protein-containing salines (Tschirgi et al., 1949). Glucose was then utilized and electrical responses to stimulation could be maintained not only by glucose but also by pyruvate, isocitrate, α-oxoglutarate, glutamate and glutamine. Lactate, fumarate, succinate and certain other substances were ineffective in this respect. Glutamate also was ineffective in maintaining respiration in the cerebral preparation.

Parts of the Brain examined in situ

Localized areas of the brain have also been the subject of perfusion studies. A block of the cat's cerebral cortex a few sq. cm. in area, separated from adjoining portions but with its normal blood supply intact, does not show spontaneous changes in electrical potential corresponding to the electrocorticogram seen in vivo. It will, however, transmit potential changes in response to applied electrical impulses (Burns, 1958; Burns & Smith, 1962) and constitutes an excellent experimental arrangement for studying such transmission. Action of some added agents (not substrates) on the conduction has been examined and the fluid and electrolyte contents of the neuronally-isolated slab have been determined (Reiffenstein & Robinson, 1969). Localized perfusion of small areas of the cerebral cortex has been carried out by cannulating a superficial cerebral arteriole and permitting venous return by normal routes (Grenell & Davies, 1950). This does not appear likely to yield quantitative data for metabolic rates but can be a valuable means of observing the effect of added substances on the electrical activity of cortical areas a few millimeters in diameter. Also, by using minute push–pull cannulae in cerebral extracellular spaces, quite local regions can be sampled (De Feudis, Delgado & Roth, 1969). Quantitative values were obtained in this way for the output of amino acids and catecholamines (q.v.) from the amygdala and putamen of monkeys while the animals were awake and normally active.

Superfusion of parts of the brain has been carried out by causing solutions to flow over the outer cerebral surfaces or within the cerebral ventricles. Metabolic exchanges with the limited layer of tissue accessible by diffusion can then be observed. An application of the technique in demonstrating potassium movements, using $^{42}K^+$, is shown in C, Fig. 2.2; output of amino acids from the cerebral cortex of rabbits is described by van Harreveld & Kooiman (1965). Use of superfusion methods in study of neural transmitters is exemplified in Chapter 14; by carefully planning the cannulation of the cerebral ventricles, much specificity can be obtained in the regions exposed to a superfusing fluid (Feldberg & Fleischhauer, 1965). Penetration of added substances through the brain may on occasion be more limited after intracisternal or intracerebral injections than if the substances were administered systemically; this is the case with ^{14}C-sucrose, ^{125}I-iodide, ^{32}P-phosphate and ^3H-nucleotide bases (Altman & Chorover, 1963; Bakay, 1964; Shimada & Nakamura, 1966; Korobkin, Lorenzo and Cutler, 1968).

Oxygen tension measured electrometrically at the exposed cerebral cortex of experimental animals has emphasized the considerable local variations which normally occur in oxygen tension in the tissue. The tension close to a venule was half that near an arteriole; 30 μ from a venule, tension was still lower (Davies & Bronk, 1957). Near a small pial vein a value of 25 mm. Hg. was found; on occluding the vessel, the oxygen tension fell nearly to zero in about 1 sec.

Appraisal of Arteriovenous Techniques

The experiments described above afford ample metabolic basis for the extreme minute-to-minute dependence of the mammalian brain on its blood supply. The normal respiratory rate of the brain is such that the oxygen of the blood in the brain at any one time, plus the oxygen dissolved in the brain itself, could be expected to be consumed in 10 sec. It is important to note that the majority of the methods described above for measuring cerebral respiration have the advantages and disadvantages of giving results in relation to the brain as a whole, without specific relationship to the activities of its different parts. Anatomically and functionally these parts are very diverse, so that some have described the brain as a hierarchy of organs rather than a single organ. Biochemically also, the brain is markedly heterogeneous. For this reason the positive findings given above carry greater significance than the negative ones. That cerebral respiration falls in hypoglycaemia, anoxia, diabetic coma or uremia indicates it to be important in the loss of cerebral functioning in these conditions. The lack of change observed in light anaesthesia or in schizophrenia does not exclude changes in small areas.

It is especially to be noted that only certain aspects of cerebral metabolism are open to study by analysis of the blood flowing to and from the brain. The two main reasons for this are: (1) changes which concern a small proportion only of a substance supplied to the brain, are obscured by natural fluctuations in blood composition. Thus many compounds including vitamins are undoubtedly assimilated by the brain from the bloodstream but without marked arteriovenous difference as the small quantities concerned are normally obtained over periods which are very long in comparison with the few seconds in which want of oxygen can be evident. Further, (2), substances of which relatively large quantities undergo extremely rapid change within the brain may nevertheless be exchanged with the bloodstream only slowly; such is inorganic phosphate and several of its esters. Some of the complementary methods adopted to study such substances are the subject of the next chapter.

REFERENCES

ADRIAN, E. D. & BUYTENDIJK, F. J. J. (1931). *J. Physiol.* **71**, 121.
ALTMAN, J. & CHOROVER, S. L. (1963). *J. Physiol.* **169**, 770.
BAKAY, L. (1964). *Arch. Neurol. Psychiat.* **71**, 673.

BRAZIER, M. A. B., FINESINGER, J. E. & SCHWAB, R. S. (1944). *J. clin. Invest*, **23**, 313, 319.
BROOKS, V. B., RANSMEIER, R. E. & GERARD, R. W. (1949). *Amer. J. Physiol.* **157**, 299.
BURNS, B. D. (1958). The Mammalian Cerebral Cortex. London: Arnold.
BURNS, B. D. & SMITH, G. K. (1962). *J. Physiol.* **164**, 238.
BUTTERFIELD, W. J. H., ABRAMS, M. E., SELLS, R. A., STERKY, G. & WHICHELOW, M. J. (1966). *Lancet*, **i**, 557.
CAHILL, G. F., OWEN, O. E. & MORGAN, A. P. (1968). *Advances in Enzyme Regulation*, **6**, 143.
CHUTE, A. L. & SMYTH, D. H. (1939). *Quart. J. exp. Physiol.* **29**, 379.
COXON, R. V. & ROBINSON, R. J. (1959). *J. Physiol.* **147**, 487.
CREMER, J. E. (1970) *Biochem. J.* **119**, 95.
CREUTZFELDT, O. D. & MEISCH, J. J. (1962). *Electroenceph. clin. Neurophysiol.* **14**, 420.
DASTUR, D. K. (1961). *Arch. intern. Med.* **108**, 136.
DASTUR, D. K., LANE, M. H., HANSEN, D. B., KETY, S. S., BUTLER, R. N., PERLIN, S. & SOKOLOFF, L. (1963). In Human Aging. Ed. J. E. Birren. Washington, D.C.: U.S. Public Health Service.
DAWSON, A. M., MCLAREN, J. & SHERLOCK, S. (1957). *Lancet*, **ii**, 1263.
DAVIES, P. W. & BRONK, D. W. (1957). *Fed. Proc.* **16**, 689.
DAVIS, P. A. (1941). *Amer. J. Physiol.* **113**, 259.
DEFEUDIS, F. V., DELGADO, J. M. R. & ROTH, R. H. (1969). *Nature, Lond.* **223**, 74.
DOBBING, J. (1961). *Physiol. Revs.* **41**, 130.
ESPAGNO, J. (1969). *Neurochirurgie*, **15**, 1.
EVERETT, N. B., SIMMONS, B. & LASHER, E. P. (1956). *Circulation Res.* **4**, 419.
FAZEKAS, J. F., ALMAN, R. W. & PARRISH, A. E. (1951). *Amer. J. med. Sci.* **222**, 640.
FAZEKAS, J. F., COLYER, H. & HIMWICH, H. E. (1939). *Proc. Soc. exp. Biol. N.Y.* **42**, 496.
FAZEKAS, J. F., TICKTIN, H. E., EHRMANTRAUT, W. R. & ALMAN, R. W. (1956). *Amer. J. Med.* **2**, 843.
FAZEKAS, J. F., THOMAS, A., JOHNSON, J. V. V. & YOUNG, W. K. (1960). *A.M.A. Arch. Neurol.* **2**, 435.
FELDBERG, W. & FLEISCHHAUER, K. (1965). *Brit. med. Bull.* **21**, 36.
FORD, D. H. (1968). *Brain Research*, **7**, 329.
GAINER, H., ALLWEIS, C. L. & CHAIKOFF, I. L. (1963). *J. Neurochem.* **10**, 903.
GAITONDE, M. K. (1965). *Biochem. J.* **95**, 803.
GAITONDE, M. K., MARCHI, S. A. & RICHTER, D. (1964). *Proc. Roy. Soc. B*, **160**, 124.
GEIGER, A. (1958). *Physiol. Rev.* **38**, 1.
GIBBS, E. L., GIBBS, F. A., HAYNE, R. & MAXWELL, H. (1947). *Res. Publ. Ass. nerv. ment. Dis.* **26**, 131.
GIBBS, E. L., LENNOX, W. G., NIMS, L. F. & GIBBS, F. A. (1942). *J. biol. Chem.* **144**, 325.
GOLDFARB, W. & WORTIS, J. (1941). *Proc. Soc. exp. Biol. N.Y.* **46**, 121.
GOMBOS, G., GEIGER, A. & OTSUKI, S. (1963). *J. Neurochem.* **10**, 405.
GRENELL, R. G. & DAVIES, P. W. (1950). *Trans. Amer. Neurol. Ass.* **75**, 105.
GURDJIAN, E. S., STONE, W. E. & WEBSTER, J. E. (1944). *Arch. Neurol. Pyschiat.* **51**, 472.
GURDJIAN, E. S., WEBSTER, J. E. & STONE, W. E. (1946). *Res. Publ. Ass. nerv. ment. Dis.* **26**, 184.
HAWKINS, R. A. (1971). *Biochem. J.* **171**, 17P.
HEYMAN, A., PATTERSON, J. L. & JONES, R. W. (1951). *Circulation*, **3**, 558.
HICKS, J. M., WOOTTON, I. D. P. & YOUNG, D. S. (1962). *Biochem. J.* **82**, 29P.
HILL, D. & PARR, G. (1963). Electroencephalography. London: Macdonald.
HIMSWORTH, R. L. (1968). *J. Physiol.* **198**, 451, 467.
HIMWICH, H. E. (1951). Brain Metabolism and Cerebral Disorders. Baltimore: Williams & Wilkins.
HIMWICH, H. E. & FAZEKAS, J. F. (1937). *Endocrinology*, **21**, 800.
HIMWICH, W. A. & HIMWICH, H. E. (1946). *J. Neurophysiol.* **9**, 133.
HIRSCH, H., KRENKEL, W., SCHNEIDER, M. & SNELLENBACKER, F. (1955). *Pflug. Arch. ges. Physiol.* **261**, 392, 402.
HOFFMAN, R. A. (1968). *Fed. Proc.* **27**, 999.

JAMES, L. S. & MYERS, R. E. (1967) (Ed.). Brain Damage in the Fetus and Newborn from Hypoxia or Asphyxia. Columbus, Ohio: Ross Laboratories.

JASPER, H. H., WARD, A. A. & POPE, A. (1969). Edit. Basic Mechanisms of the Epilepsies. Boston: Little, Brown.

KENNEDY, C. (1956). *Progr. Neurobiol.* 1, 230.

KESTON, A. S. (1954). *Science*, 120, 355.

KESTON, A. S. (1957). *Fed. Proc.* 16, 203.

KETY, S. S. (1948). *Meth. med. Res.* 1, 204.

KETY, S. S. (1950). *Amer. J. Med.* 8, 205.

KETY, S. S. (1955, 1957). *Proc. Internat. Neurochem. Sympos.* 1, 208; 2, 221.

KETY, S. S. (1959). *Science*, 29, 1528.

KETY, S. S. (1960). In *Neurophysiology* Sect. 1, 3, 1751. Washington, D.C.: Amer. Physiol. Soc.

KETY, S. S. (1967). *Proc. Assoc. Res. nerv. ment. Dis.* 45, 39.

KETY, S. S., POLIS, B. D., NADLER, C. S. & SCHMIDT, C. F. (1948). *J. clin. Invest.* 27, 500.

KETY, S. S., WOODFORD, R. B., HARMEL, M. H., FREYHAN, F. A., APPEL, K. E. & SCHMIDT, C. F. (1947). *Amer. J. Psychiat.* 104, 765.

KLEIN, J. R. & OLSEN, N. S. (1946). *J. biol. Chem.* 167, 1.

KOLLAR, E. J. & ATKINSON, R. M. (1966). *Psychosom. Med.* 28, 227.

KOROBKIN, R. K., LORENZO, A. V. & CUTLER, R. W. P. (1968). *J. Pharmacol. Exp. Therap.* 164, 412.

LASCELLES, P. T. & TAYLOR, W. H. (1968). *Clin. Sci.* 35, 63.

LASSEN, N. A. (1966). *Proc. Assoc. Res. nerv. ment. Dis.* 41, 205.

LASSEN, N. A., FEINBERG, I. & LANE, M. H. (1960). *J. clin. Invest.* 39, 491.

LOWRY, O. H., PASSONNEAU, J. V., HASSELBERGER, F. X. & SCHULZ, D. W. (1964). *J. biol. Chem.* 239, 18.

MacCARTY, C. F., KIRKLIN, J. W. & UIHLEIN, A. (1966). *Proc. Assoc. Res. nerv. ment. Dis.* 41, 127.

MADDOCK, S., HAWKINS, J. E. & HOLMES, E. (1939). *Amer. J. Physiol.* 125, 551.

MANN, F. C. (1927). *Medicine*, 6, 419.

MANN, F. C. & MAGATH, T. B. (1922). *Arch. Int. Med.* 30, 171.

McDOWELL, D. G., HARPER, A. M. & JACOBSON, I. (1963). *Brit. J. Anaesthesia*, 35, 394.

McFARLAND, R. A. (1952). In The Biology of Mental Health and Disease. London: Cassell.

McILWAIN, H. & RODNIGHT, R. (1962). Practical Neurochemistry. London: Churchill.

MELLERUP, E. T. & RAFAELSON, O. J. (1969). *J. Neurochem.* 16, 777.

MEYER, A. (1936). *Proc. R. Soc. Med.* 29, 49.

MEYER, J. S., GOTOH, F., TAZAKI, Y., HAMAGUCHI, K., ISHIKAWA, S., NOUAILHAT, F. & SYMON, L. (1962). *Arch. Neurol.* 7, 560.

NICKEL, J., BREYER, U., CLAVER, B. & QUADBECK, G. (1963). *ArzneimittelForsch.* 13, 881.

O'NEAL, R. M., KOEPP, R. E. & WILLIAMS, E. I. (1966). *Biochem. J.* 101, 591.

OWEN, O. E., MORGAN, A. P., KEMP, H. G., SULLIVAN, J. M., HERRERA, M. G. & CAHILL, G. F. (1967). *J. clin. Invest.* 46, 1589.

PAGE, M. A., KREBS, H. A. & WILLIAMSON, D. H. (1971). *Biochem. J.* 121, 49.

PIERCE, E. C., LAMBERTSEN, C. J., DEUTSCH, S., CHASE, P. E., LINDE, H. W., DRIPPS, R. D. & PRICE, H. L. (1962). *J. clin. Invest.* 41, 1664.

PLUM, F., POSNER, J. B. & COLLINS, R. C. (1969). *Second Internat. Neurochem. Meeting*, p. 57. Milan: Tamburini.

PONTEN, U. (1963). *Experientia*, 19, 312.

REFSUM, H. E. (1963). *Clin. Sci.* 25, 361.

REIFFENSTEIN, R. J. & ROBINSON, K. (1969). *J. Neurochem.* 16, 1551.

ROSOMOFF, H. L. (1961). *J. appl. Physiol.* 16, 395.

ROSOMOFF, H. L. (1966). *Proc. Assoc. Res. nerv. ment. Dis.* 41, 116.

ROWE, G. G., MAXWELL, G. M., CASTILLO, C. A., FREEMAN, D. J. & CRUMPTON, C. W. (1959). *J. clin. Invest.* 38, 2154.

RUDIN, D. O. & EISENMAN, G. (1954). *J. gen. Physiol.* **37**, 505.

SACKS, W. (1957). *J. appl. Physiol.* **10**, 37.

SACKS, W. (1958). *J. appl. Physiol.* **12**, 311.

SACKS, W. (1969). *Handbook of Neurochemistry*, **1**, 301.

SACKS, W. & SACKS, S. (1968). *J. appl. Physiol.* **24**, 817.

SACKS, W. & SACKS, S. (1969). *Second Internat. Neurochem. Meeting*, p. 349. Milan: Tamburini.

SCHEINBERG, P. (1950). *J. clin. Invest.* **29**, 1010.

SCHEINBERG, P. (1966). *Proc. Assoc. Res. nerv. ment. Dis.* **41**, 216.

SCHEINBERG, P. & STEAD, E. A. Jr. (1949). *J. clin. Invest.* **28**, 1163.

SCHEINBERG, P., STEAD, E. A., BRANNON, E. S. & WARREN, J. V. (1950). *J. clin. Invest.* **29**, 1139.

SCHMIDT, C. F. (1950). The Cerebral Circulation in Health and Disease. Springfield, Illinois: Thomas.

SCHMIDT, C. F., KETY, S. S. & PENNES, H. H. (1945). *Amer. J. Physiol.* **143**, 33.

SCHNEIDER, M. (1957). *Proc. Internat. Neurochem. Sympos.* **2**, 238.

SEILER, N., MOLLER, H. & WERNER, G. (1969). *Hoppe-Seyl. Z.* **350**, 815.

SETCHELL, B. P. & WAITES, G. M. H. (1962). *J. Physiol.* **164**, 200.

SHIMADA, M. & NAKAMURA, T. (1966). *J. Neurochem.* **13**, 391.

SOKOLOFF, L. (1956). *Progr. Neurobiol.* **1**, 216.

SOKOLOFF, L. (1959). *Pharmacol. Rev.* **11**, 1.

SOKOLOFF, L. (1960). In *Neurophysiology* Sect. 1, **3**, 1843. Washington, D.C.: Amer. Physiol. Soc.

SOKOLOFF, L. (1966). *Proc. Assoc. Res. nerv. ment. Dis.* **41**, 237.

STONE, W. E. (1938). *Biochem. J.* **32**, 1908.

STRANG, R. H. C. & BACHELARD, H. S. (1971). *J. Neurochem.* **18**.

Symposium (1961). The Nature of Sleep. CIBA Foundation Symposium. Ed. Wolstenholme & O'Connor. London: Churchill.

Symposium (1963). Selective Vulnerability of the Brain in Hypoxaemia. Ed. Schade & McMenemey. Oxford: Blackwell.

TOMAN, J. E. P. & DAVIS, J. P. (1949). *J. Pharmacol.* **97**, 425.

TSCHIRGI, R. D., GERARD, R. W., JENERICK, H., BOYARSKY, L. L. & HEARON, J. Z. (1949). *Fed. Proc.* **8**, 166.

VAN HARREVELD, A. & KOOIMAN, M. (1965). *J. Neurochem.* **12**, 431.

WAELSCH, H., BERL, S., ROSSI, C. A., CLARK, D. D. & PURPURA, D. P. (1964). *J. Neurochem.* **11**, 717.

WECHSLER, R. L., DRIPPS, R. D. & KETY, S. S. (1951). *Anaesthesiology*, **12**, 308.

WIKLER, A. (1950). *Pharmacol. Rev.* **2**, 435.

WORTIS, J., BOWMAN, K. M. & GOLDFARB, W. (1940). *Amer. J. Psychiat.* **97**, 552.

WORTIS, J., BOWMAN, K. M., GOLDFARB, W., FAZEKAS, J. F. & HIMWICH, H. E. (1941). *J. Neurophysiol.* **4**, 243.

3   The Chemical Composition of the Brain

In the foregoing chapter the brain has been considered, chemically speaking, from the outside; knowledge has been gained of substances entering and leaving it but not of the interconnexion between substrate and product, and the interaction of substrate with material of the brain itself. For such information the brain must be studied by more direct means and one of these—analysis of the brain itself—is the subject of the present chapter. Following a brief account only of the main categories of cerebral constituents, several of which concern later sections of the book, most attention is given to constituents which undergo rapid change in association with changes in cerebral functioning.

The Main Categories of Cerebral Constituents

Analysis of mammalian brain into its major components is given in Table 3.1 together with comparable values for muscle. Water constitutes three-quarters to four-fifths of each. In the brain its proportion in grey matter (about 85%) is markedly greater than in the white. The levels of most substances in the

Table 3.1

Approximate composition of muscle and brain

Component	Skeletal muscle %	Whole brain %	Human brain (%) Grey matter	Human brain (%) White matter
Water	75	77 to 78	83	70
Inorganic salts	1	1·1	1·0	1·3
Soluble organic substances	3 to 5	2	–	–
Carbohydrate	1	1	–	–
Protein	18 to 20	8	7·5	8·5
Lipids: Simple fats	1	1	–	–
Cholesterol	1	2 to 3	1·0	3·9
Phosphatides	2	5 to 6	3·9	6·5
Cerebrosides	1	2	0·9	4·4

Further data are given in this book under the individual substances concerned; and also in the *Handbook* (1969, especially vol. 1).

white matter of the brain, where myelinated fibres preponderate, are appreciably different from their levels in grey matter, where cell bodies and unmyelinated fibres and dendrites are the main histological components. This is illustrated in the human brain by the data in Table 3.1 and is recorded in more detail by Hess *et al.* (1965) and in Chapter 12.

The lipids of the brain are outstanding for they are components which by their amount and nature can be said to characterize the organ. They are described in Chapter 11. Here it may be noted that in whole brain they average two to three times the quantity in muscle, constituting over half the total dry weight of the tissue. Nevertheless, their availability for general metabolism is more limited than is that of the lipids of most organs. Their quantity in the brain is little affected by extreme starvation in adult animals. Proteins and simple organic substances make up much of the metabolic and contractile machinery in muscle. Although their concentrations in the brain as a whole are only half those of muscle they constitute about the same proportion of the fat-free dry weight of the tissue, and they have comparable importance in representing the means by which the brain carries out much of its functional activity. The chemical basis for this is best appreciated by considering first the simple electrolytes of the brain and its fluid environment.

Cerebral Fluids and Electrolytes

Any appraisal of the composition of the brain must be made in relation to that of the fluids which bathe it. This is especially so in relation to simple

Table 3.2

Constituents of human brain, blood plasma, and cerebrospinal fluid

Constituent	μequiv./g. or ml.			Ratios C_i/C_e
	Brain	Plasma	Cerebrospinal fluid	
Na^+	57	141	141	0·15
K^+	96	5	2·5	45
Ca^{2+}	2	5	2·5	1·2
Total cations	166	153	148	–
Cl^-	37	101	127	–
HCO_3^-	12	27	18	0·65
Phosphates	16	2	1	–
N-Acetyl-L-aspartic acid	12	*c.* 0·1	–	100
Other simple organic acids	10	2	2	–
Total anions in above categories	87	132	148	–
Probable contribution to anions by:				
Proteins	(40)	20	0	–
Lipids	(40)	0	0	–

See Davson (1960), Katzman (1961), Manery (1952), and Tschirgi (1960). The ratios of the last column are between the computed intracellular concentrations of the ions, C_i and those of the cerebrospinal fluid, C_e; see text and McIlwain (1963); Gibson & McIlwain (1965).

electrolytes, for electrical activity in all neural systems depends on differential ion concentrations between cellular components and the fluids which surround them. Such concentration differences are very evident in the mammalian brain, as is shown in Table 3.2.

Extracellular Fluids

The immediate environment of cerebral cells is an interstitial fluid. This is separated from the blood by the capillary walls, and from the cerebrospinal fluid at the ventricles and outer surfaces of the brain. It occupies a proportion of the cerebral volume estimated at 20–25%. These values, which are important in conditioning the ratios quoted in Table 3.2, derive from the following data (see Tschirgi, 1960; Katzman, 1961; McIlwain, 1963; Brinley, 1963; Reed & Woodbury, 1963).

Intravenous administration of inulin or of isotopically labelled sulphate, followed by analysis of the brain and the blood, shows that 3–5% of the water of the brain is more accessible to these substances than is the remainder. Extracellular spaces seen in cerebral tissues after fixation for electron microscopy in buffered aqueous osmium tetroxide also corresponded to about 5% of the tissue. However the application of more adequate fixation techniques resulted in observation of much larger extracellular spaces. Before fixation with osmium tetroxide, the tissues were rapidly frozen within 30 sec. of circulatory arrest and then treated either by drying at $-79°$ or by substitution of the tissue water with acetone at $-85°$. These techniques gave values for extracellular space which corresponded to some 20% of the original volume of the fresh tissues which had been sampled. If the rapid freezing of the tissues was delayed until 5–6 min. after circulatory arrest, the extracellular space decreased to below 5%; anoxia was therefore considered to produce the low extracellular spaces reported earlier (van Harreveld et al., 1965; van Harreveld & Malhotra 1966, 1967). Conductimetric measurements, applied in vivo, also gave values equivalent to 25% of the cerebral cortex being occupied by a continuous aqueous phase, presumably representing extracellular fluid. This method also shows this phase to be labile; anoxia promptly increased the impedance of the cerebral cortex, slowly during the first 2 min. and sharply after 3 min. This was concluded to be due to entry to the cellular phase of fluid and electrolytes previously extracellular; histochemical methods showed chloride to enter neurons during anoxia and other situations when energy-yielding reactions are inadequate (Van Harreveld & Schadé, 1960; Ochs, 1962). Chloride normally diffuses readily into cells and gave an apparent chloride space of 23–40% in experiments in which the inulin or sucrose space was 15–30% of the tissue volume (Bourke et al., 1965; values are given for several mammalian species).

In appraising such data, two factors to be taken into account are: (i) the glial cells are relatively permeable to ions and so contribute to the electrical conductivity of the brain; (ii) the blood-brain barrier (see below) limits access of ions from the blood. This is a property of the brain as an organ and due to special cellular arrangements at the cerebral capillaries. These are evident microscopically and are such that much of the materials entering the brain from the blood probably pass through (rather than between) cellular processes from the astrocytes, which line the capillaries. Much easier access is given to many substances, including Na, K and Cl, when cerebral tissue is examined *in vitro* (see Chapter 4); the cerebral capillaries are not then involved. The *in vitro* data (Gibson & McIlwain, 1965) also give support to a value of 20–25% for extra-cellular space in the original tissue, and this value is adopted in Table 3.2.

Much of this extracellular space is not, or is only with difficulty, accessible to substances coming from the blood or from the cerebrospinal fluid. Thus cellular structures at the capillaries and at the outer surfaces of the brain play an active role, especially in relation to Na, K and Cl. In addition, all differential distribution of substances between blood and brain is not to be ascribed to structures adjacent to the capillaries; much depends on exclusion or assimilation by the cerebral cells themselves. Slow equilibration of urea with glial cells is suggested as basis for the shrinkage of cerebral volume, with lowering of the pressure of the cerebrospinal fluid, which can be brought about by hypertonic urea solutions given intravenously (Reed & Woodbury, 1963; Buckell, 1964). This has been applied in neurosurgery. Much of the exclusion or assimilation by cerebral cells themselves is still manifested in isolated cerebral tissues, as is indicated in Chapter 4.

Cerebrospinal Fluid and Cerebral Solutes

The *cerebrospinal fluid* originates from the blood largely at the choroid plexus, though some comes from the cerebral capillaries and in transit has presumably formed part of the interstitial fluid of the brain itself. Extraventri-cular sources of the fluid have been concluded to contribute some 20–45% of the total formed (Bering, 1965). It is similar to blood plasma in its content of substances of small molecular weight (Table 3.2), but increased chlorides in the cerebrospinal fluid replace the proteins of the plasma, in partial compliance with Gibbs-Donnan equilibria. The cerebrospinal fluid is also at a slightly greater hydrostatic pressure and is negative in electrical potential in relation to general body fluids. Equilibrium of several substances between cerebrospinal fluid and the blood is only slowly established. Some hours are required before administered bromide reaches its peak concentration in the cerebrospinal fluid, or before change in Na^+ or Cl^- in the bloodstream is fully reflected in the cerebrospinal fluid. Changes in concentration, or the appearance of radio-active Na^+ or Cl^-, then occur in the brain and cerebrospinal fluid approxim-ately in parallel. For these reasons the composition of the cerebrospinal fluid has been taken as the best guide available to the probable composition of the interstitial fluid of the brain though the two fluids originate from the blood largely by different routes. The slowness with which equilibrium is established between blood and cerebrospinal fluid has been ascribed to a *cerebrospinal fluid-blood barrier*, largely at the choroid plexus; here passage through cells, with specific secretory properties towards different substances, again appears to occur. In particular, the active transport of sodium ions and of fluid involve an ouabain-sensitive adenosine triphosphatase (see Chapter 12 and Bonting, 1964). This enzyme in the choroid plexus of cats was inhibited when $0 \cdot 1$–$10 \, \mu M$ solutions of ouabain were perfused intraventricularly, and the degree of its inhibition closely paralleled that of the concomitant inhibition of c.s.f. flow.

The fluids of the brain, intracellular and extracellular, are almost exactly isoosmotic with blood-plasma, as shown by melting-point methods. In the brain, the sum of simple anions and cations accounts for some 250 μequiv. of the 300 μequiv. involved (Table 3.2), but the distribution between anions and cations is unusual. The total cerebral cations—mainly Na^+ and K^+—are in somewhat greater concentration in the brain than in plasma or cerebrospinal fluid, but whereas in these fluids the chloride ion accounts for 65–85% of the balancing anions, this is not the case in the brain. Bicarbonate here is also lower. Inorganic phosphate in the brain is only a little higher than in plasma, but organic phosphates and simple organic acids contribute much more; especially notable is the contribution by N-acetyl-L-aspartic acid. Isethionic acid (hydroxyethane sulphonic acid) has been detected in neural tissues and is the major anion in squid axon where it occurs at concentrations of 28 mg/g. fresh tissue (Koechlin, 1955). Formed enzymically by deamination of taurine in rat cerebral cortex in vitro (Peck & Awapura, 1967), it has been used as the replacement anion for Cl in experiments in vitro (Bourke & Tower, 1966). These compounds, listed in Table 3.2, leave some 80 μequiv. of cerebral anions/ g. of tissue to be accounted for. In plasma, a corresponding deficit of some 20 μequiv. is accounted for by protein, and it has been estimated that the cerebral proteins might contribute twice that amount in the brain. The bulk of the remainder—and here the brain is unusual among tissues—is contributed by the lipids.

When the lipids are extracted from cerebral tissues by organic solvents, they carry inorganic salts with them to the solvents in quantities up to some 50 μequiv./g. of brain. Folch et al. (1957) found that the sulphuric ester fraction carried with it 12% of the K^+ of the tissue; the phosphatidyl serine 16% of the K^+ and 20% of the Na^+; and the diphosphoinositide, about 50% of the Ca^{2+} and Mg^{2+}. The association of particular cations with particular lipids may partly depend on the methods of extraction and fractionation employed, but the contribution of the lipids as a whole to ion balance is considerable. The fixed anions have significance in relation to Donnan equilibria.

Access of Organic Substances to the Brain

The majority of cerebral organic constituents are synthesized in the brain itself from simpler compounds supplied by the bloodstream. The removal of specified products of cerebral metabolism from the brain is also mainly by the blood. Movement of substrates and products between the brain and the body as a whole is subject to multiple controls, of which some, capable of study in vivo, are now described. Others will be recounted subsequently in considering the metabolism of individual substances; mechanisms which are best investigated in isolated cerebral tissues are described in the following chapter.

Observations with administered dyestuffs, e.g. Trypan blue, and with naturally-occurring coloured compounds, first led to suggestions of special relationships in movement of substances between the brain and circulating fluids, and prompted the term blood-brain barrier. The relative slowness of equilibration of small ions such as thiocyanate between blood and the intracellular fluids of the brain was also ascribed to the existence of such a barrier, noted above to be due to special cellular arrangements at cerebral capillaries. 'Tight' junctions were seen by electron microscopy between pericapillary cells (Symposium, 1970); at such junctions the cells were not separated by the usual 200 Å intercellular distance, but by a smaller space about the size sufficient for a monosaccharide to pass. Much of the material which enters the brain from the blood thus passes through cells which line the capillaries. Capillary permeability factors were concluded for example to form the basis for restricted uptake of urea (Kleeman et al., 1962). Impairment of cerebral permeability occurs in various pathological states, such as brain tumours or kernicterus, when alterations in cellular structure ensue (Bakay, 1968). Limitations on entry of small molecules are not likely to be due necessarily to the properties of cerebral capillaries; limited uptake of a variety of compounds, including sugars

Table 3.3

Factors conditioning the entry of substances from the bloodstream to the brain

Substance	Entry promoted by	Cerebral concentration limited by
Glucose	Carrier-mediated transport mechanism	Capacity of influx mechanism
Amino acids	Carrier-mediated active transport	Capacity of influx mechanism; active extrusion
Anions (carboxylic acids, thiocyanate, chloride)	Concentration gradient	Electrochemical gradient; membrane permeability
Cholesterol	Concentration gradient	Membrane permeability
Uncharged non-metabolized compounds (e.g. sucrose)	–	Membrane permeability
Large molecules (e.g. proteins, inulin)	–	Membrane permeability

and amino acids has been shown to occur in cell-containing cerebral preparations *in vitro*, where the capillary blood supply has been replaced by incubation media (see Chapters 4, 5 and 8).

Active uptake of many substances by the normal brain is as prominent a process as is the exclusion of others; the extent of net uptake depends on the balance of inward and outward flow as discussed below. The variety of relationships which may serve to condition movements between the blood and the brain is exemplified in Table 3.3. As more information on transport phenomena emerges, the more evident does it appear that these are related to metabolic activities of the tissue. It should therefore be emphasized that the "barrier" is not due to any one single phenomenon; as pointed out by Hertin (1956) it should be regarded as embracing a number of unrelated or heterogeneous phenomena. These act by various mechanisms to restrict the entry of some materials and facilitate the entry of others into the brain and include osmosis, ultrafiltration, chemical factors such as net charge or lipid solubility, affinity of transport carrier systems and specific aspects of tissue metabolism. The different processes which contribute to the "barrier" play also a homeo-static role.

Mechanisms underlying the selectivity of processes contributing to "barrier" phenomena have been the subject of much study, often by measuring differences in the behaviour of chemically closely-related substances. Thus the cerebral concentrations of many solutes, as glutamate, are not elevated by greatly increasing their plasma levels. This contrasts with other solutes often structurally-related (as glutamine) which do accumulate in the brain when plasma levels are raised. Use of radio-isotopes has demonstrated that many solutes which do not accumulate, do in fact equilibrate rapidly between blood and brain. Thus many observations of an apparent barrier to transport of specified compounds into the tissue, have been concluded to be due partly to transport systems oriented towards efflux of solutes from the brain to the surrounding fluids. The ease of access may be conditioned by the chemical properties of the solute; an instance in which access is conditioned by lipo-philic properties (Davson, 1955) is given in A, Fig. 3.1. Thiourea is concentrated less rapidly in the brain and the cerebrospinal fluid than is the more lipophilic ethyl thiourea when the plasma concentration of these substances is maintained constant.

Other "barrier" properties illustrated in Fig. 3.1 relate to stereospecificity. The preference for the (−) isomer of D-arabinose in movement of the isomers from the bloodstream into the perfused brain is shown (B, Fig. 3.1). Amino acids also exhibit stereospecificity in affinity for cerebral transport mechanisms (C, Fig. 3.1); the uptake of the L-form of tyrosine is more rapid than that of the D-form when the amino acids are administered by the bloodstream. The brain content of the L-isomer after 2 hr. was similar to the plasma level whereas D-tyrosine did not equilibrate to the same extent. D, Fig. 3.1 illustrates the importance of the efflux of solutes from the brain. After subarachnoid injection, efflux of various isotopically-labelled amino acids occurred at different rates. L-Leucine levels were decreased by over 90% within the first hour, whereas the efflux of lysine, proline and phenylalanine was considerably slower. Differences were also observed in rates of efflux of these amino acids over the second hour. The amino acids of this and similar studies were selected for their relatively slow metabolism in the brain; their disappearance from the tissue is therefore likely to reflect efflux rather than catabolism.

A further fashion in which barrier phenomena or restricted movements are manifested between blood and brain, relates to the retention of solutes within the brain. This occurs with potassium ions, as noted below. Extracellular space may also be a return route necessary as counterpart to the axoplasmic flow which takes materials preponderantly from cell body to cell extremities. The importance of this in relation to extracellular amino acids has been noted (McIlwain, 1971 and in Symposium, 1970); it may be of wider significance. Also, the extracellular or cerebrospinal fluids have been emphasized as consti-tuting routes for the transport of neurohumoural agents (Norman, 1969). For further discussion of cerebral tissue-fluid barriers see Davson (1963), Dobbing (1961, 1968) and Lajtha & Ford (1968).

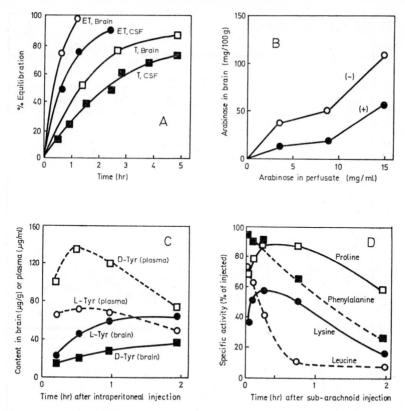

FIG. 3.1. Movement of substances between blood, cerebrospinal fluid
and brain.

A. Entry to rabbit brain and to cerebrospinal fluid, of thiourea (T) and
ethylthiourea (ET). The compounds were maintained at constant levels
in blood plasma during the experiment.

B. Uptake of D(−)arabinose, which is more rapid than that of the
D(+) compound, into the perfused cat brain.

C. Uptake of D- and L-tyrosine from the blood to rat brain.

D. Efflux of ^{14}C-labelled amino acids from the brain of the rat after the
subarachnoid administration.

Data from Chirigos *et al.* (1960), Lajtha & Mela (1961), Davson (1963)
and Eidelberg *et al.* (1967).

Electrolytes and Membrane Potentials

When the brain or spinal cord is penetrated by electrodes small enough to
enter individual cells, potentials negative to surrounding fluids are recorded
from regions about the size of the neurons present (Fig. 3.2). The regions are
identified as neurons by stimulation along known tracts. The potentials
recorded are between −50 and −90 mv and on stimulation, the resulting
impulse normally reaches a small positive potential of 10–20 mv before approaching the original resting potential. Chemical interpretation of such
phenomena owes much to investigations of simpler neural systems (Hodgkin,

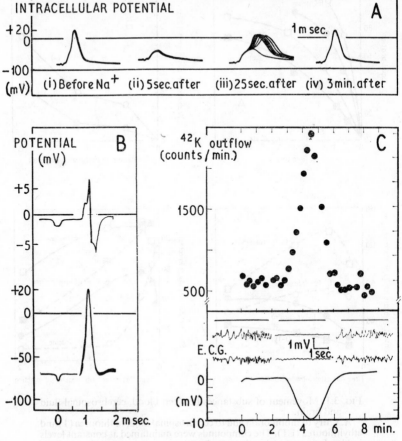

FIG. 3.2. Electrical potentials and ion relationships in the central
nervous system.

A. In motoneurons of the lower lumbar region of the cat spinal cord
(Coombs, Eccles & Fatt, 1955). The first discharge was obtained by
antidromic stimulation under normal conditions, and the others after
injecting 50 p equiv. Na^+; it was estimated that this diminished the cell
content of K^+ from 35 to about 15 p equiv. For properties of cortical
pyramidal cells see Eccles (1966).

B. Discharge of Betz cells of the motor cortex of the cat, stimulated
by an electrode (Ag wire 80 μ diam.) at the cortical surface. The upper
record was obtained extracellularly and the lower record intracellularly
(note its much greater amplitude, and the change of ordinate scale;
Phillips, 1956).

C. Measurements during the progress of spreading depression initiated in the rabbit cerebral cortex previously irrigated with a ^{42}K salt
(Brinley, Kandel & Marshall, 1960; Brinley, 1963). Above: outflow of
^{42}K; below: concomitant change in d.c. potential; centre, electrocorticogram in a comparable experiment.

1958, 1965; Woodbury, 1969); in judging its applicability to the central
nervous system, the following data are to be noted.

The potentials observed (Fig. 3.2) correspond, to a first approximation, to values which would be established across semipermeable membranes by the differential concentrations of sodium and potassium salts found in the brain. The concentration gradients of these two ions are opposed, and at different phases of the nerve action potential the effects of first K^+ and then Na^+ preponderate. This can be expressed by equation (i), derived from the Nernst relationship (see Hodgkin, 1958; Ochs, 1965):

$$E_m = 62 \log \frac{[K^+]_e + b[Na^+]_e}{[K^+]_i + b[Na^+]_i} \qquad (i)$$

(Here E_m is membrane potential in mv at $37°$; suffixes e and i indicate extra-cellular and intracellular concentrations, here taken as proportional to activities; and b is the apparent permeability of sodium relative to that of potassium. For further quantitative details and consideration of circumstances in which the relationship is applicable, see Gibson & McIlwain, 1965; Casteels, 1969.)

Resting cells before stimulation behave as though their permeability to Na^+ is relatively small ($b = 0·01–0·08$); the negative potential of the cell interior is a manifestation of the tendency of K^+ to flow from its high internal to its low external concentration. Increased extracellular K^+ added to fluids surrounding the tissue, diminished (brought towards zero) the negative resting potential. On stimulation, however, permeability alters and the potential at the peak of the action potential approaches that of the sodium gradient, which with the ratio Na_i/Na_e of $0·15$ (Table 3.2) is $+20$ mv. When the sodium of a spinal neurone is increased by causing Na^+ to enter from a micropipette, so that this ratio increases, the positive peak of the cell discharge is diminished or lost (**A**, Fig. 3.2). It is, therefore, concluded that the rising phase of the cell discharge is accompanied by increasing sodium permeability. When the Na^+ thus permitted to enter has diminished or reversed the negative potential of the cell, a further change is concluded to leave the membrane more permeable to K^+, whose outflow restores the original polarity.

Cation Movements *in vivo*

Much in these fundamental aspects of neural activity is thus ascribed to the outer membrane of cerebral cells, as an agent controlling the movement of ions. Investigation of membrane properties in cerebral tissues is described further in Chapter 12; returning to their significance in relation to cerebral composition, it will be noted that the flow of Na^+ and K^+ during the nerve impulse is in each case from a region of high to one of lower concentration. A nerve impulse thus utilizes some of the potential energy represented by the relatively high K and low Na content of the brain. This energy ultimately is supplied by the utilization of glucose and oxygen described in the previous chapter, and the cerebral content of Na and K remains remarkably constant during the continuous electrical activity of the normal brain. The central nervous systems of lower animals have provided valuable opportunities for studying changes in Na or K resulting from neural activity (Baylor & Nicholls, 1969; Kerkut & York, 1969). Also with gross change in functional state, change in ion composition is demonstrable in the mammalian brain: exchange of $^{42}K^+$

from the cerebral cortex of rabbits with K^+ of a bathing fluid was accelerated during spreading depression (**C**, Fig. 3.2; see below). Again, in association with convulsions produced by electrical stimulation of the brain of rats, cerebral Na increased at 1–2 μequiv./g. min. and subsequently returned to normal values (Woodbury, 1955; see McIlwain, 1963). After addition of Na^+ to an individual nerve cell by micropipette in the experiment of **A**, Fig. 3.2 recovery of membrane potential during the succeeding few minutes is pictured to be associated with extrusion of Na^+; indeed from isolated cerebral tissues Na^+ has been shown by direct measurement to be extruded at comparable speed (see Chapter 4).

These relationships are illustrated in Fig. 3.3. The "downhill" ion movements (ii) of Fig. 3.3, are thus pictured as continuously occurring in the normal brain, and accentuated on excitation. They must, therefore, be balanced by restoring

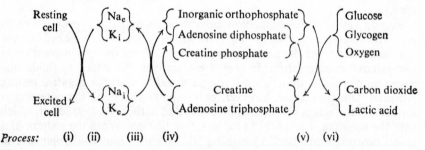

| *Process:* | (i) | (ii) | (iii) | (iv) | | (v) | (vi) |

FIG. 3.3. Linkage between neural excitation, ion movements, and metabolism (McIlwain, 1963). Reference is made in the text to the numbered sequence (i)–(vi) in interpreting the actions of several agents which modify cerebral functioning. Suffixes *e* and *i*: extracellularly and intracellularly sited ions (see Table 3.2).

energy-consuming processes (iii) which link them to the main cerebral substrates (vi). Recognition of intermediates involved in stages between (iii) and (vi) is described in a following section. Continuous occurrence of both active and passive cation movements in the brain *in vivo* is demonstrated also by the disrupting actions of agents which block these processes. The highly poisonous tetrodotoxin includes central with its other effects (Kao, 1966) and acts by inhibiting the entry of Na^+ during excitation: process (ii), Fig. 3.3. Applied intraventricularly or iontophoretically to the neocortex, tetrodotoxin lowered body temperature and depressed firing in the pyramidal tract (Phillis *et al.*, 1968). The lithium ion, Li^+, enters as does Na^+ on stimulation of some excitable cells but is not comparably extruded. Administration of Li^+ salts in man diminished cortical somatosensory responses observed electrically, and has been applied in depressive psychoses and other disorders of mood (Gartside *et al.*, 1966; Report, 1970).

Glial Cells as Buffering Agents

Microelectrodes in exploring the brain penetrate not only neurons, recognizable by their action potentials, but also glial cells which are recognizable subsequently by histochemical techniques. Cells so characterized in the cat cerebral cortex were of high resting potential, -71 ± 12 mv but of low resistance, 20–500 ohms/cm^2 (Trachtenberg & Pollen, 1970). Calculation showed the values to be compatible with equilibration of K$^+$ across cell membranes which were highly permeable to K$^+$.

Prompt uptake of K$^+$ has indeed been proposed as a major function of glial cells during neuronal activity (Kuffler, 1967). Cell firing can readily release sufficient K$^+$ to the limited extracellular spaces of the brain, for the membrane potential of adjacent cells to be altered. During 10/sec. bursts of neuronal firing, the potential difference observed across glial cell membranes fell by 5 mv; increase of intercellular K$^+$ by 1 mM was calculated to diminish the potential difference by 7·6 mv. By taking up K$^+$ from extracellular regions adjacent to cells which are firing, glial cells thus protect or buffer these regions from cation changes which would disturb the behaviour of adjacent neurons. The glia may, indeed, perform this function more widely in relation to other substances released or consumed during neuronal activity.

Labile Organic Constituents of the Brain

The processes of excitation and depression already noted as altering the respiration and electrolyte content of the brain, alter also the cerebral content of a number of intermediary metabolites. These include phosphocreatine, adenine nucleotides, glycogen, and lactic acid, which were examined in the brain shortly after their importance had been recognized in other excitable tissues: in muscle and peripheral nerve. Determination of these substances in the brain at first gave extremely erratic results and this was concluded to be due to adventitious stimulation or to disturbance of cerebral blood supply during the process of removing the brain for sampling. Techniques for rapidly fixing the composition of the brain *in situ*, especially by freezing with liquid nitrogen at about $-180°C$, were accordingly developed, and receive comment now.

Techniques

It is by rapid-freezing methods that information has been obtained about many metabolic processes of functional importance in the brain *in vivo*. The following data about the technique itself are, therefore, relevant; for practical details, see McIlwain & Rodnight (1962). Thermo-couples, inserted to different depths in the cerebral tissue of living rats of about 40 g. enabled the time-course of changes in cerebral temperature to be followed (Richter & Dawson, 1948). When such rats were immersed whole in liquid air, the temperature of the surface of the cerebral cortex fell to 0°C in 4–5 sec. In deeper parts of the brain 9–20 sec. were required for freezing, but it was noted that the temperature remained almost at the initial 37°C, until it suddenly fell to below zero. This suggests that the circulation in successively deeper layers may be maintained until almost immediately before they are frozen. Other observations may be taken as confirming this. Thus Kerr (1935) determined phosphocreatine in the brain of the cat or dog after pouring liquid air around the exposed skull of the animals. His values were close to those found for animals such as mice or small rats cooled by immersion in liquid air, even though cooling of the depths of the brain of the cat or dog must have been much slower, requiring some 30 sec. for freezing to a depth of 1 cm. A further point concerns cerebral lactic acid. The brain fixed in liquid air, as distinct from that excised by ordinary methods, contains little lactate. Comparably low values are obtained by an independent method of fixation, namely by injecting sodium iodoacetate. A further re-examination (Thorn et al., 1958) has again shown freezing in situ to be more satisfactory than other methods; rapid cooling just short of freezing may also be effective. Rapid freezing of the brain immediately following decapitation was shown recently to be less satisfactory than freezing in situ; in rats, freezing of the brain and cessation of glycolysis in the decapitated head required 30 sec. to 2 min., depending on the size of the animal (Jongkind & Bruntink, 1970).

The immersion of small animals in liquid nitrogen causes the nitrogen to boil; the gas formed at the body surface may insulate the tissue against rapid temperature change. Isopentane or Freon-12 (CF_2Cl_2), chilled to $-150°$ with liquid nitrogen, have been used to achieve rapid freezing without the concomitant formation of a vapour phase (see, for example, Folbergrova et al., 1969). An alternative procedure is the "near-freezing" technique of Takahashi & Aprison (1964) in which the animal is immersed in coolant for predetermined and accurately-measured short time intervals. The conditions are chosen so that the brain temperature decreases rapidly to $0°$ but the brain does not freeze. The levels of acetylcholine were similar to those obtained by rapid-freezing; the technique offers advantages if dissection of discrete brain areas at $0°$ is desired. A further modification is the technique of Granham et al. (1968) in which rapid freezing of the brains of anaesthetized cats and rats was effected by pouring liquid nitrogen into a plastic funnel fitted into a skin incision over the craniotomy. While freezing took place, lung ventilation and the blood circulation were upheld. The technique produced lower values for ADP and lactate and higher values for creatine phosphate (Table 3.4) than those reported when anaesthetized animals were immersed in the coolant.

Rapid-freezing techniques have been applied by Lowry and his co-workers in the course of examining the brain at defined brief times after decapitation (see Chapter 5). The rates of change of labile constituents (Fig. 3.4) were obtained during the first seconds or minutes after isolating the brain in this way, and while it continued to metabolize endogenous substrates (Lowry et al., 1964; Folbergrova et al., 1970).

Discussion of the cerebral content of lactic acid, glucose, glycogen, phosphates and nucleotides now follows; many other important labile constituents are described in succeeding chapters: e.g. transmitters in Chapter 14.

Lactic Acid and Glycogen

Consistent results have been obtained on estimating the cerebral content of lactic acid in trichloroacetic acid or perchloric acid extracts of the brain using colourimetric or specific enzymatic methods (McIlwain & Rodnight, 1962; Lowry et al., 1964). By rapid-freezing methods the normal cerebral content of lactic acid was found to be about 1–2 μmoles/g., one-half to one-fifth that previously found. The origin of the additional lactate in unfixed brain post-mortem was soon found in examining other carbohydrate constituents of the brain.

Rapid fixation yielded values for cerebral *glycogen* much higher than those previously found (Kerr, 1936). Again, seconds sufficed for breakdown of a large part of cerebral glycogen in mammalian brain although it was more stable in other tissues or in the brain of lower animals. The glycogen was later isolated and found to be indistinguishable from liver glycogen in its elementary composition, specific rotation, precipitation with alcohol, and behaviour to

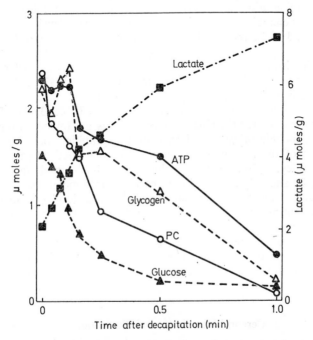

Fig. 3.4. Concentrations of phosphocreatine (PC), adenosine triphosphate (ATP), glucose, glycogen and lactate in the brains of adult mice rapidly frozen at different intervals within the first minute after decapitation. The zero time levels are from the brains of whole mice rapidly frozen (from Lowry *et al.*, 1964).

iodine or on hydrolysis (Kerr, 1938). Glycogen from the brain fixed in liquid air after decapitation was reported as more highly-branched than liver glycogen (Goncharova, 1963; Khaikina & Goncharova, 1964; see also Chapter 5). The possibility that brain glycogen is more highly-branched should be viewed with caution; the rapid breakdown of glycogen during post mortem autolysis (Lowry *et al.*, 1964) would be expected to result in the glycogen which survives having a higher degree of branching since it is the peripheral ends of the chains which are first removed during catabolism (Stetton & Stetton, 1960). However, as noted in Chapter 5, the cerebral glycogen synthesized *in vitro* appears also to be more highly branched than liver glycogen. The most commonly-used methods for extracting glycogen from the brain, where it occurs both free and bound to lipids and proteins, are based on extraction into trichloroacetic acid or perchloric acid, techniques which have recently been reported as resulting in partial degradation. Extraction of animal tissues with dimethyl sulphoxide (Whistler & BeMiller, 1962) or cold water (Orrell & Bueding, 1964) have been concluded to produce glycogen in a more native state.

The normal cerebral content of glycogen ranges in different species from 0·6 to 1·6 mg./g. and about half is bound in the sense that it is not easily extracted by cold 0·6 M-trichloroacetic acid (Carter & Stone, 1961; Merrick, 1961). Levels of bound glycogen are lowered by physostigmine, insulin or by deprivation of paradoxical sleep (Karadzic & Mrsulja, 1969; Rakic & Mrsulja, 1969) without changing the content of free glycogen; the levels of bound glycogen are stated to be increased by amphetamine (Khaikina & Goncharova, 1964).

The brain also contains free and phosphorylated glucose which contributes to the lactic acid found post-mortem (Kerr & Ghantus, 1937). Values for lactic acid, glycogen, and glucose are included in Tables 3.5 and 5.3; for phosphorylated intermediates, totalling about 2 μmoles/g., see Tables 3.4 and 5.3. Values ordinarily obtained for the glucose of cerebral tissues by measuring reducing substances, include other materials. Chromatographic separation suggested the glucose of the rapidly fixed brain of unanaesthetized rats to be 0·45 μmoles/g. (Gey, 1956). In mice, values of 0·75–1·5 μmoles/g. were found (Fig. 7.2). Presumably the rapidity of carbohydrate metabolism in the brain contributes to these values being so much below the blood glucose of 4·5 mM.

This account of cerebral constituents considers next the group of phosphorylated intermediates whose connection with cerebral activities is adumbrated in Fig. 3.3. This scheme depends much on investigations of isolated cerebral preparations to be described in subsequent chapters, as well as on the findings, now to be recounted, of their occurrence and change in the mammalian brain *in situ*.

Cerebral Phosphates and Nucleotides

The brain is rich in phosphate derivatives (Table 3.4; see Brady & Tower, 1960; Heald, 1960), many of which concern subsequent chapters. The substances now to be discussed form categories (4), (5) and (6) of Table 3.4 and include about one-quarter of the total cerebral phosphorus. They are of relatively small molecular size and are readily extracted by cold dilute acids, for example by grinding frozen samples of the brain in 0·5 M-trichloroacetic acid or 5% perchloric acid at 0°. Substances of categories (2) and (3) are described in Chapters 10, 11 and 12; they are insoluble in the acid, but those of categories (7) and (8) are also extracted, and feature in Chapters 5 and 11.

Inorganic Phosphate and Phosphocreatine

Phosphates are exchanged only slowly between the brain and the blood, in contrast to their rapid metabolism within the brain itself. Arteriovenous methods detect no net loss or gain, but after administering inorganic orthophosphate enriched in ^{32}P to a number of mammalian species including man, cerebral ^{32}P increases slowly and persists for several days or weeks (Fig. 3.5). The penetration is much slower than to skeletal muscles or to most other organs of the body. The ^{32}P of the cerebrospinal fluid also rises only slowly after

Table 3.4

Phosphate derivatives of the normal mammalian brain

Category	Content (μmoles P/g. fresh tissue)		
	Mouse or rat	Guinea pig	Cat or dog
(1) *Total phosphorus*	98	97	96
(2) *Phospholipids*	72	62 ± 4	60 ± 4
(3) *Other acid-insoluble compounds*	–	–	10·5
Ribonucleic acid	2·5	–	2·5
Deoxyribonucleic acid	2·1	–	1·9
Phosphoprotein	–	–	1·1
(4) *Inorganic orthophosphate*	5	3·5	3·5
(5) *Phosphocreatine*	3·2; 5·0[a]	3	3·5; 4·8[a]
(6) *Nucleotides*			
Adenosine triphosphate (3P/mole)	9	12	8·5
Adenosine diphosphate (2P/mole)	0·8	–	–
Adenylic acid	0·2	–	–
Guanine nucleotides (total, as P)	2·4	1·7	1·5
Uridine nucleotides (total, as P)	2·4	–	–
Cytidine nucleotides (total, as P)	0·8	–	–
Nicotinamide-adenine dinucleotide (2P/mole)	0·7	0·7	–
Nicotinamide-adenine dinucleotide phosphate (3P/mole)	0·03	–	–
(7) *Carbohydrate derivates*			
Hexose monophosphates	0·1	1·3	1·35
Hexose diphosphates (2P/mole)	0·3	–	–
Triose phosphates	0·03	–	–
3-Phosphoglyceric acid	1·0	–	–
(8) *Other esters*			
Phosphorylethanolamine	–	–	1·5
Phosphorylserine	0·3	–	–
Phosphorylcholine	0·5	–	–

With mice, rats, and guinea-pigs the intact unanaesthetized animals were fixed and the whole brain used for analysis. In other species the cerebral cortex was exposed under anaesthesia, fixed, and used for analysis.

Data from McIlwain (1957), Heald (1960), Nyman & Whittaker (1963), Goldberg *et al.* (1966) and sources quoted in the text.

[a] Animals were anaesthetized with phenobarbitone; the exposed brain was rapidly frozen while ventilation and circulation were upheld (Granham *et al.*, 1968).

systemic administration, and for studying cerebral phosphate incorporation, intracisternal injection is advantageous.

After administering ^{32}P-orthophosphate and fractionating cerebral extracts, orthophosphate itself proves to be the compound of highest specific activity, but increasingly with time the specific activities of other phosphates rise and the ^{32}P becomes widely distributed among tissue constituents (Fig. 3.5). Phosphocreatine and nucleotides collectively are much more rapidly labelled than are phospholipids or nucleic acids. These findings, with associated data, show a variety of processes of phosphorylation and transphosphorylation to to be in progress in the brain, as will be detailed later.

Phosphocreatine merits description first among the organic phosphates of the mammalian brain, for following its characterization as the major phosphagen of muscle it was found to be of similar status in the brain (Kerr, 1935). It was isolated as the crystalline calcium salt from the rapidly-frozen brain of

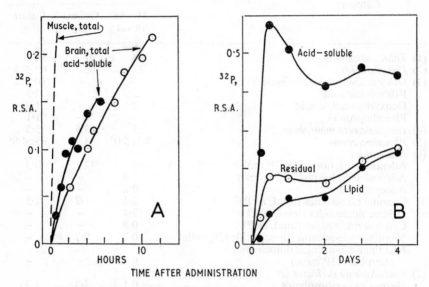

FIG. 3.5. Incorporation of ^{32}P injected into mice as inorganic orthophosphate.
  A. Relative specific activity (RSA) values give the ^{32}P counts per unit weight of tissue in muscle and brain, relative to those found in blood at the same time-period.
  B. RSA values give the ^{32}P counts per unit of weight of brain, relative to those of the inorganic orthophosphate in the same samples.
  "Acid-soluble" phosphates include groups (4) to (8) of Table 3.4, and "residual", group (3). (Dziewiatkowski & Bodian, 1950; Locksley *et al.*, 1954).

dogs and occurred also in the frog and turtle, being more stable in these species. Its hydrolysis in aqueous solution was catalysed by molybdate and was at the same rate as that of the synthetic compound. Cerebral phosphocreatine has been characterized chromatographically and determined by its yield of creatine as well as of phosphate. Its lability in the mammalian brain exceeds that in muscle; if rapid freezing techniques are not applied, 70% is lost in 3 sec.

The total creatine of the brain is about 7–10 μmoles/g. (Klein & Olsen, 1947) and of this about one-third is normally phosphorylated. By intracisternal injection of ^{14}C-arginine to rats, the arginine has been shown to act within the brain itself as a precursor of creatine (Defalco & Davies, 1961). The cerebral content of creatine, phosphocreatine, and inorganic phosphate can change rapidly on excitation or anoxia, as will shortly be described.

Nucleotides

Adenine nucleotides preponderate in the brain as in other organs, and adenosine triphosphate itself contributes much more than any other compound to the cerebral phosphates extracted by cold dilute acids (Table 3.4). Its consistent determination in such extracts by a variety of methods: enzymatic, spectrophotometric, chromatographic and by hydrolysis, contribute to its secure characterization (see McIlwain & Rodnight, 1962). On injecting ^{32}P-orthophosphates intracisternally to rats, the acid-labile phosphate of the cerebral adenosine triphosphate became labelled extremely rapidly, reaching in 2 min. half the activity of the orthophosphate in the same samples (Lindberg & Ernster, 1950); the ^{32}P of phosphocreatine closely followed. Not only exchange, but also rapid loss and resynthesis of cerebral adenosine triphosphate have been demonstrated (Fig. 3.4 and 3.7). Adenosine diphosphate, the immediate product from the triphosphate, is thus also a labile cerebral constituent; under normal conditions its quantity is about one-fifth to one-tenth that of the concomitant triphosphate.

Guanine nucleotides were recognized in the brain by Kerr (1942), in quantity about one-quarter that of the adenosine phosphates: a proportion greater than in most tissues. Chromatographic methods now show mono-, di-, and tri-phosphates of guanosine, the latter preponderating (0·8 μequiv./g. rat brain: Tarr et al., 1962). Collectively, the uridine nucleotides also contribute about 1 μmole/g. with the triphosphate preponderating and including not only the mono- and di-phosphates, but also uridine diphosphate glucose, important in the synthesis of glycogen (q.v.; Schmitz et al., 1954; Tarr et al., 1962). Cytidine mono-, di-, and tri-phosphates, and inosine phosphates, were also demonstrated. The content and metabolism of cerebral nucleotides receive detailed attention in Chapter 9.

Patterns of Changes in Labile Cerebral Constituents

Co-ordination between the changes in labile constituents can already be recognized in those which take place during the first few seconds after death. With loss of labile phosphates, inorganic phosphate and phosphorylated hexoses accumulate; glycogen and glucose are lost with formation of the hexose phosphates and of lactic acid. The operative factor in this period is probably the cessation of blood supply, for Kerr found the same changes to commence even when fixation of the brain was rapid, if circulation was not maintained during the fixation. The post-mortem changes thus emphasize again that the cerebral composition is the result of a balance: between energy-yielding processes which maintain the high-energy phosphates, and energy-consuming processes which utilize them (Fig. 3.3). Already it has been seen that the main energy-yielding process is normally oxidation of glucose, and that at any one time the brain has no more than 1–10 sec. reserve of oxygen. When this fails, then prominent among the energy-yielding processes still available are the formation of lactic acid from glucose or glycogen, and of inorganic phosphate from phosphocreatine and adenosine triphosphate.

Following sections describe changes in labile cerebral constituents which are observed under different conditions of cerebral activity. In such studies it is important to establish the degree to which the changes observed are a reflection of events in the central nervous system rather than in other parts of the body. For this purpose, several of the constituents named have been determined in the brain after periods of considerable muscular activity or after injecting into the bloodstream excess of the substance being determined, and these experiments have shown much smaller changes in the constituents concerned (Richter & Dawson, 1948; Stone, 1938).

Hypoxia, Cyanide and Anaemia

When hypoxia is deliberately induced by causing animals to breathe air low in oxygen, a pattern of changes can be recognized which is similar to that occurring post-mortem but which shows interesting variations in the degree of change in the different constituents (Table 3.5). When the gas breathed contains 5–10% O_2, glycogen and glucose can remain normal while lactic acid and inorganic phosphate increase and creatine phosphate falls. This presumably follows because the blood-stream is still providing adequate carbohydrate though not oxygen. Results are influenced by the concomitant levels of carbon dioxide in the lungs of the animals being studied, higher carbon dioxide minimizing the effect of hypoxia probably because it can cause increased ventilation and cerebral vasodilatation. Little change in adenosine triphosphate was reported in some instances in which cerebral phosphocreatine had fallen, and this is consistent with maintenance of the triphosphate by phosphocreatine, for phosphocreatine though lowered was always present. When, however, the gas breathed carried less than 1·2% O_2, and blood flow was blocked, all phosphocreatine and most adenosine triphosphate were lost.

The effects of administered cyanides are seen to be very similar to those of hypoxia (Table 3.5). The dose which was examined in rats resulted in increased breathing, agitation, incoordination, and convulsions. It was found to inhibit cytochrome oxidase of the brain itself by about 50% when this was studied in tissue separated at the end of convulsive activity (Albaum *et al.*, 1946). It is presumably this inhibition of aerobic processes which leads to the other changes in cerebral constituents. These include breakdown of glycogen and of the energy-rich compounds of the tissue and accumulation of inorganic phosphate and of the anaerobic product lactic acid.

Comparable studies in cats (Fig. 3.6) were coupled with observation of the electrical activity of the brain. The subconvulsive dose of sodium cyanide of 0·4 g./kg. (not quoted in Table 3.5) led to a period of a few minutes' disturbance in electrical signs without change in phosphates but with additional lactic acid formation. Possibly here the increased glycolysis was nearly adequate to maintain normal cerebral activities. The convulsive doses greatly changed the electrical activity of the brain and samples of cerebral tissues were taken after these changes had been in progress for different lengths of time. These showed a fall in phosphocreatine which at its maximum left only 40% of the normal amount in the brain. Lactic acid and inorganic phosphate were then high. Fig. 3.6 shows the regular development of these changes which increased with increasing duration of electrical abnormality; then, more slowly, the substances reverted to their normal levels with the resumption of normal cerebral potentials.

It is valuable to know how quickly the energy-rich phosphates, phosphocreatine and adenosine triphosphate, can be utilized in the brain when re-

TABLE 3.5

Changes in labile constituents of mammalian brain

Changes are given in percentage of the normal values quoted in the text or in Table 3.4.

Experimental conditions	Species; author reference	Phospho-creatine	Adenosine triphos-phate[10]	In-organic phos-phate	Gly-cogen	Glucose	Lactic acid
Hypoxia:							
Breathing 5–10% O_2	Dog[1]	None to −60	None	None to +125	−50 to +30	None	+100 to 900
Breathing N_2–CO_2, and aeschemia	Rabbit[2]	−100	−90	+175	–	–	+800
Sodium cyanide, 0·8 mg./kg.	Cat[3]	−24	−45	+36	–	–	+290
,, ,, 1·2 ,,	Cat[3]	−46	−30	+57	–	–	+195
,, ,, 5·0 ,,	Rat[4]	−39	−60	+173	−35	–	+320
Insulin hypoglycaemia:							
Moderate	Cat[5]	−40	−25	+30	−20	−90	None
Severe (coma)	Cat[5]	−75	−100	+110	−80	−95	−40
Intracerebral insulin	Rat[12]	–	–	–	+100	–	–
Depressants:							
Allobarbitone	Mouse[7]	+35	+3	−21	None	–	−73
Pentobarbitone	Mouse[7]	+36	+10	−26	–	–	−49
Phenobarbitone	Mouse[11]	–	–	–	+200	+150	−60
Chlorpromazine	Mouse[11]	–	–	–	–	+400	−35
Sleep	Rat[8]	–	–	–	–	–	−35
Excitation:							
Various convulsant states	Cat[6]	−50	−62	+40	−31	−40	+150
Pentamethylene tetrazole	Dog[9] Mouse[7]	−25	−8	+31	−32	–	+271
Methionine sulphoximine (before onset of seizures)	Mouse[13]	–	–	–	+62	+95	None
Electrical stimulation for 5 sec.	Rat[2]	−60	−25	+63	–	–	–

Author references: [1] Gurdjian *et al.* (1944). [2] Thorn *et al.* (1955); see also Samson *et al.* (1960). [3] Klein & Olsen (1947). [4] Albaum *et al.* (1946). [5] Kerr (1936); see also Tarr *et al.* (1962). [6] Kerr & Ghantus (1936). [7] Stone (1940); Carter & Stone (1961). [8] Richter & Dawson (1948). [9] Stone, Webster & Gurdjian (1945). [10] Including in some instances other compounds. [11] Mayman *et al.*, 1964; Nelson *et al.*, 1968. [12] Mellerup & Rafaelson, 1969. [13] Folbergrova *et al.*, 1969.

actions forming them are blocked. Fig. 3.6 shows an initial rate of loss of phosphocreatine at about 100 μmoles/g. hr., but during this experiment the anaerobic conversion of glucose or glycogen to lactic acid could still yield energy. When, however, such glycolysis was inhibited by prior injection of iodoacetic acid (see Chapter 5) replacement of O_2 by N_2 in the gas breathed caused a much more rapid change (A, Fig. 3.7). Here adenosine triphosphate is measured, and after an interval of 8 sec. falls at the rate of 900 μmoles/g. hr. During the 8 sec., adenosine triphosphate appears likely to be resynthesized from phosphocreatine. The normal brain can thus consume its content of

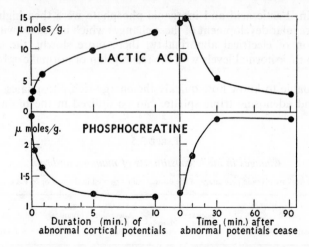

FIG. 3.6. Correlated changes in electrical activity, phosphocreatine and
     lactic acid in the brain following administration of sodium cyanide
     (16 μmoles/kg.) to rats. The graphs on the left hand show develop-
     ment of the abnormalities, and those on the right, recovery from
     them. (Data from Olsen & Klein, 1947).

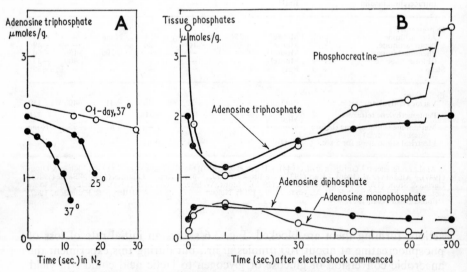

FIG. 3.7. Rapid changes in the labile phosphates of rat brain. From data
     of Samson et al., 1960, and Minard & Davis, 1962.
     A. With anoxia, in animals already treated with sodium iodoacetate
(1 μmole/g. intraperitoneally). Rats were 21 days old except when stated
otherwise.
     B. Adult rats with electroshock (60 cyc./sec. a.c., 95 mamp. for 1 sec.)
applied at zero time; animals transferred to liquid nitrogen at the time
indicated.

energy-rich phosphate in about 15 secs. The data of **B**, Fig. 3.7, are shown below to afford comparable values.

Studies made of cerebral constituents during brief periods after decapitation have been examined by Lowry *et al.* (1964), mainly in mice, with results shown in Fig. 3.4. The decapitation can be regarded as a drastic form of aeschemia, involving also however, a drainage of blood from the head and severance of neural connections. Lactate was formed at the expense of both glucose and glycogen, involving a seven-fold increase in glycolytic rate; phosphocreatine and adenosine triphosphate nevertheless fell. Regional differences are notable in the changes which follow hypoxia and were seen also in the mouse after decapitation (James & Myers, 1967; Gatfield *et al.*, 1966).

With changed Blood Glucose

Dietary changes, fasting, overfeeding, and glucose infusion caused no appreciable change in the glycogen, lactic acid or phosphocreatine of the brain (Kerr & Ghantus, 1936; Thorn *et al.*, 1958, 1961), but marked changes were seen during insulin hypoglycaemia (Table 3.5). Here again they concerned some constituents more than others. In animals in which hypoglycaemia was considerable but had not led to coma, cerebral glucose had fallen severely and glycogen less so. Labile phosphates had fallen and inorganic phosphate increased. Lactate changed little, its formation possibly tending to be decreased by lack of glucose and increased by the increased inorganic phosphate. With hypoglycaemia leading to coma, all the changes described were accentuated and lactic acid also fell.

Low blood glucose did not, however, lead to all these changes in very young rats (Tarr *et al.*, 1962); nor, in Kerr's study, did it do so when cerebral activity was depressed by amylobarbitone. The lowered glucose and glycogen persisted, but no change was found in phosphocreatine. This indicates how the cerebral content of phosphocreatine is conditioned by the balance between processes leading to its formation, and to its utilization in support of cerebral activities. These latter it will now be seen, are reduced by the depressant.

Depressant Drugs

A variety of agents which induce the unconsciousness of surgical anaesthesia are alike in the effects which they produce on cerebral constituents. The effects are different from all those described above, involving increase in creatine phosphate and adenosine polyphosphates, and fall in inorganic phosphate and lactic acid. Thus, although cerebral respiration is decreased during anaesthesia, energy-rich substances accumulate. Cerebral utilization of energy-rich substances thus appears to be decreased by depressants, a conclusion fully in accordance with the general impression of lesser activity on the part of the brain during anaesthesia; the action of the drugs is discussed further in Chapter 15. In one instance a similar change occurred during natural sleep.

Several of the changes produced in mice by barbiturates and quoted in Table 3.5 have been paralleled in rats (Richter & Dawson, 1948) and with pentobarbitone and with ether (Stone, 1938). One point necessary to their further interpretation concerns the physiological state corresponding to the values for untreated animals. The fixation by liquid air undoubtedly involves some cerebral stimulation during the brief period when the brain is in the course of being frozen (Kerr, 1935). The same procedure is applied to sleeping, anaesthetized and control animals but it remains possible that the changes induced by depressants are not on cerebral metabolism before fixing but occur during the second or so of stimulation by the fixing agent. Various experimental findings, however, limit this possibility, including the decrease in cerebral respiration caused by depressants. Stimulation by the fixing procedure when adequately applied cannot be great, for very much larger chemical changes occur during excitation by drugs. Also, changes in cerebral constituents during the terminal handling of the animals or on extraction can be differentiated from sustained action *in vivo*. Chlorpromazine was concluded to affect the former but not the latter (Weiner & Huls, 1961; Minard & Davis, 1962), and appraisal of results must note technical details, e.g. body weight of animals examined.

The conclusion that anaesthesia is associated with accumulation of energy-rich metabolites, has been extended by examining changes in the brain of the mouse on imposing aeschemia in presence and absence of phenobarbitone (Gatfield *et al.*, 1966). Glucose, glycogen, ATP and phosphocreatine increased; in several cerebral layers and regions, anaesthesia was concluded to diminish the rate at which energy-rich reserves were utilized. This occurred in white-matter regions as well as in grey.

Central Excitation

Changes in cerebral constituents on excitation of the central nervous system are in many instances the reverse of those which occur during its depression. During the great increase in cerebral activity associated with convulsions which originate in the brain, phosphocreatine and adenosine polyphosphates are lost with formation of inorganic phosphate. Lactic acid greatly increases at the expense of cerebral glucose and glycogen (Table 3.5). This pattern of change is characteristic of the state of convulsive activity rather than of the agent leading to convulsions; pentamethylenetetrazole, picrotoxin, bromocamphor, caffeine and electrical stimulation of the brain from large electrodes applied to the brain or to the head, each induced similar changes in the constituents of Table 3.5. In other respects, several convulsants can have divergent effects on cerebral constituents, which contribute to understanding their mechanism (see Stone *et al.*, 1960), e.g. anticholinesterases on acetylcholine (q.v.); fluoro-acetate (q.v.) on citrate, or agents combining with pyridoxal (q.v.) on pyridoxal-requiring enzymes. Of the latter agents, 1,1-dimethylhydrazine induced convulsive episodes in rats, and on fixation *in situ* the brain showed diminishing amounts of glycogen after successive episodes. Moreover, the glycogen remaining was shorter in side-chain length than that normal to the brain (Minard *et al.*, 1965; see also Khaikina & Goncharova, 1964). Excitation which is more specific than that of convulsive activity can also modify cerebral glycogen: thus stress diminished the glycogen content of the anterior pituitary, the median eminence and the hypothalamus (Jacobwitz & Marks, 1964). Phosphorylase (q.v., Chapter 5) is likely to be a critical factor in conditioning the changes in glycogen.

Metabolic Rates During Excitation

Among convulsive agents recently studied in individual detail are methionine sulphoximine and a hexafluoroether, $(CF_3.CH_2)_2O$ (Indoklon). The fluoroether (Sacktor et al., 1966) caused rapid fall in phosphocreatine and increased glycolytic flux about three-fold above basal rate. With methionine sulphoximine (q.v.; Folbergrova et al., 1969) large and varied metabolic changes were induced. Glucose and glycogen increased before the onset of seizures (Table 3.5) but the changes brought about by the seizure were different from those produced by other convulsants in that the levels of glucose and glycogen increased further; lactate levels, constant until the onset of seizures, fell as a result of the seizure. The difference between the effects of methionine sulphoximine and the other convulsants listed above may be linked with the observation that methionine sulphoximine caused an increase in brain glucose levels; levels of ammonia (q.v.) were also increased. Both these investigations receive further comment in discussing metabolic regulation (Chapter 7).

Electrocorticograms during the action of the convulsants of Table 3.5 showed great increase in the electrical activity of the brain. In instances when the brain was not fixed during the increased activity, this activity could be succeeded by intermittent periods of coma when electrical activity in the cerebral cortex was almost absent. Analysis showed cerebral constituents to be similar during the two phases (Olsen & Klein, 1947). In cases where the brain has been rapidly fixed seconds after electrical stimulation for 1 sec., rates of lactate formation increased greatly. These were calculated to be 720 μmoles/g. hr. in dog or cat brain and 1,000 μmoles/g. hr. in mouse cerebral cortex fixed 10 seconds after stimulation. In the mouse measurements over shorter time periods indicated that considerably higher initial rates of some 2,500 μmoles/g. hr. might be attained (Klein & Olsen, 1947; King et al., 1967).

The chemical data thus indicate greatly increased utilization of energy-rich substances during the increased electrical activity at the commencement of convulsive action, leading to exhaustion of a large part of the tissue's reserves; the subsequent absence of cerebral potentials gives an electrical picture of exhaustion which parallels the chemical one. In the case of electrical stimulation the time-course of change in chemical constituents can be related exactly to the time of application of the stimuli to the brain. Results of such an experiment are shown in **B**, Fig. 3.7. In animals transferred to liquid air within 1 sec. of applying electrical impulses, half the phosphocreatine of the brain had already been lost. Even supposing this change to take place partly during the few seconds before the cortex was entirely fixed, the change was extremely rapid and was complete before the outward signs of convulsive activity began. The major change in phosphorus derivatives thus corresponds to the period when rapid high-voltage electrical discharges are induced in the cortex and, in man, consciousness is lost. The overt convulsions themselves appear to represent an unorganized return of activity in the brain rather than a direct response to the applied potentials.

By regarding the change initiated by electroshock (**B**, Fig. 3.7) as continuing during the 5 sec. involved in fixing the cortex, the initial fall in phosphocreatine and adenosine triphosphate, together of 2·1 μmoles, can be seen to correspond to loss at 1250 μmoles/g. hr. In the second interval (1–10 sec.) the loss is at about 500 μmoles/g. hr. In an experiment with younger rats (Dawson & Richter, 1950), loss of phosphocreatine similarly computed corresponds to some 1,000 μmoles/g. hr. These rates will be noted as quite close to that of 900 μmoles/g. hr. deduced from A, Fig. 3.7 as occurring when synthesis of labile phosphates was stopped rather than its utilization being accelerated. Rates of formation of lactate in the first few seconds after electroshock were compatible with these rates of utilization of energy-rich substrates (King *et al.*, 1967; see also Chapter 5).

Spread of Excitation and Depression in the Cerebral Cortex

This is a major neurophysiological subject; of its chemical aspects, several which concern transmitter substances active in minute amounts are examined in Chapter 14. The firing of individual cerebral cells can be initiated or modified by local electrical stimuli from small electrodes, e.g. those of 80 μ diam. whose effects are shown in Fig. 3.2. The results of such stimulation are normally transmitted by discrete neural pathways; typical consequences within the cerebral cortex are the *direct cortical responses* in which potential changes are caused, up to a cm. away, transmitted at about 2 m./sec. Some components involve dendrites and others, subcortical fibres from cortical cells (Burns, 1958; Ochs, 1965).

The electrical stimulation which initiates the convulsive conditions just described is typically a massive one from electrodes large enough to bring a considerable part of the brain within the applied voltage-gradient. Attention is now directed to the consequences of intermediate stimuli, for example at wires less than 1 mm. in diam., 1·5 mm. apart on the rabbit cerebral cortex. These can initiate a distinctive phenomenon termed spreading depression (Leão, 1944; Ochs, 1962): recording electrodes near the area stimulated show first the normal electrical activity of the brain, then spike discharges, then loss of electrical activity. This sequence with associated changes in d.c. potential (C, Fig. 3.2), spreads out from the origin at the quite slow speed of 2–6 mm./min., followed by return to normal electrical activity.

Marked chemical changes are associated with the advancing wave of electrical disturbance: the increased potassium efflux of Fig. 3.2, altered fluid distribution, a diminution in phosphocreatine, glycogen and glucose, and an increase in lactate and orthophosphate (Bureš, 1964; Křivánek, 1958). These will be recognized as the changes accompanying convulsions, and indeed similarities have been pointed out between Leão's phenomenon and the march of Jacksonian epilepsy. In experimental animals, spreading depression can be initiated in presence and absence of anaesthesia, and in absence may be seen to be associated with an initial phase of excitation or of increased excitability. The rate of spread in each case remains a few mm./min., which is much too slow for ordinary neural conduction. It has, therefore, been suggested that certain of the chemical changes listed may stand in causal relationship to the spread of the disturbance, for it can be initiated not only electrically but also mechanically, by a light tap on the cortex, and by small localized applications of a number of substances: 80 mM-KCl, 35 mM-L-glutamic acid, and by

2,4-dinitrophenol, iodoacetic acid, fluorides and azides in concentrations in which they act as metabolic inhibitors (Grafstein, 1956, 1964; van Harreveld, 1959). Properties of K^+ in this regard have been examined by local ventricular perfusion with cerebrospinal fluid of increased K^+ concentration (Zuckermann & Glaser, 1968). Applied to the hippocampus this caused paroxysmal discharges, increasing in frequency as $[K^+]$ was increased to 16 mM.

Release from cortical cells of a substance which itself excites adjacent neurons affords a mechanism for spreading depression which, if the substance is readily diffusible, is compatible with the rate of spread of the disturbance. Potassium salts could immediately fill this role; NaF and the dinitrophenol which initiate the depression diminish tissue K (Joanny & Hillman, 1963) and properties of glutamic acid (q.v.) indicate it also a possible mediator. Such a mechanism requires the substances released to remain locally rather than be removed from the brain by the bloodstream. Net loss of K from brain to blood even in convulsions is barely if at all detectable (see McIlwain, 1963) reflecting a normally beneficent mechanism which may, however, contribute to both electroshock coma and spreading depression when the cortex is subjected to exceptional stimuli.

Comment

Results outlined in this chapter give a picture of cerebral composition which is entirely compatible with the large change which the brain makes in the oxygen and glucose of blood flowing through it. Between the fine ramifying processes of cerebral cells and the fluid which bathes them, large concentration gradients are maintained; substances requiring much energy for their formation disappear rapidly when the level of activity in the brain increases or when its substrates are not available. Yet normally, the cerebral content of energy-rich substances is remarkably constant and a changed level of activity is rapidly followed by a correspondingly changed rate of usage of glucose or oxygen.

To understand how this comes about, it is necessary to examine in much greater detail processes which are intermediate between the supply of oxygen and the maintenance of energy-rich substances. These processes form the subject of the following chapter.

REFERENCES

ALBAUM, H. G., TEPPERMAN, J. & BODANSKY, O. (1946). *J. biol. Chem.* **164**, 45.
BAKAY, L. (1968). *Progress in Brain Res.* **29**, 314.
BAYLOR, D. A. & NICHOLLS, J. G. (1969). *J. Physiol.* **203**, 555, 571.
BERING, E. A. (1965). In Cerebrospinal fluid and the Regulation of Ventilation, p. 396. Ed. C. McC. Brooks, F. F. Kao & B. B. Lloyd. Oxford: Blackwell.
BONTING, S. L. (1964) In Water and Electrolyte Metabolism. Ed. de Graeff & Leijnse. Amsterdam: Elsevier.
BOURKE, R. S. & TOWER, D. B. (1966) *J. Neurochem.* **13**, 1099.
BOURKE, R. S., GREENBERG, E. S. & TOWER, D. B. (1965) *Amer. J. Physiol.* **208**, 682.
BRADY, R. O. & TOWER, D. B. (1960), (Ed.). The Neurochemistry of Nucleotides and Amino Acids. New York: Wiley.
BRINLEY, F. J. (1963). *Internat. Rev. Neurobiol.* **5**, 183.
BRINLEY, F. J., KANDEL, E. R. & MARSHALL, W. H. (1960) *J. Neurophysiol.* **23**, 246.
BUCKELL, M. (1964). *Clin. Sci.* **27**, 223.

3

Bureš, J. (1964). In Animal Behaviour and Drug Action. Ciba Foundation Symposium. Ed. H. Steinberg, A. V. S. de Reuck & J. Knight. London: Churchill.
Burns, B. D. (1958). The Mammalian Cerebral Cortex. London: Arnold.
Carter, S. H. & Stone, W. E. (1961). J. Neurochem. 7, 16.
Casteels, R. (1969). J. Physiol. 205, 193.
Chirigos, M. A., Greengard, P. & Udenfriend, S. (1960). J. biol. Chem. 235, 2075.
Coombs, J. S., Eccles, J. C. & Fatt, P. (1955). J. Physiol. 130, 291, 326.
Davson, H. (1955). J. Physiol. 129, 111.
Davson, H. (1960). In Neurophysiology, 3, 1761. Washington, D.C.: American Physiological Society.
Davson, H. (1963). Ergebn. Physiol. 52, 20.
Dawson, R. M. C. & Richter, D. (1950). Amer. J. Physiol. 160, 203.
Defalco, A. J. & Davies, R. K. (1961). J. Neurochem. 7, 308.
Dobbing, J. (1961). Physiol. Revs. 41, 130.
Dobbing, J, (1968). In Applied Neurochemistry, p. 317. Ed. A. N. Davison & J. Dobbing. Oxford: Blackwell.
Dziewiatkowski, D. & Bodian, D. (1950) J. cell comp. Physiol. 35, 141, 155.
Eccles, J. C. (1957). The Physiology of Nerve Cells. London: Oxford University Press.
Eccles, J. C. (1966) (Ed.). Brain and Conscious Experience. Berlin: Springer.
Eidelberg, E., Fishman, J. & Hams, M. L. (1967). J. Physiol. 191, 47.
Folbergrova, J., Lowry, O. H. & Passonneau, J. V. (1970). J. Neurochem. 17, 1155.
Folbergrova, J., Passonneau, J. V., Lowry, O. H. & Schulz, D. W. (1969). J. Neurochem. 16, 191.
Folch, J., Lees, M. & Sloane-Stanley, G. H. (1957). Proc. Internat. Neurochem. Sympos. 2, 174.
Gartside, I. B., Lippold, O. C. J. & Meldrum, B. S. (1966). Electroenceph. clin. Neurophysiol. 20, 382.
Gatfield, P. D., Lowry, O. H., Schulz, D. W. & Passonneau, J. V. (1966). J. Neurochem. 13, 185.
Gey, K. F. (1956). Biochem. J. 64, 145.
Gibson, J. & McIlwain, H. (1965). J. Physiol. 176, 261.
Goldberg, N. D., Passonneau, J. V. & Lowry, O. H. (1966). J. biol. Chem. 241, 3997.
Goncharova, E. E. (1963). In Proc. All-Union Neurochem. Conf., Erevan, p. 455. Ed. A. V. Palladin & H. Ch. Buniatian. Acad. Sci. Armenian S.S.R.
Grafstein, B. (1956). J. Neurophysiol. 19, 154.
Grafstein, B. (1964). In Brain Function. Ed. Brazier. Berkeley: Univ. Calif. Press.
Granham, L., Kaasik, A. E., Nilsson, L. & Siesjö, B. K. (1968) Acta Physiol. Scand. 74, 398.
Gurdjian, E. S., Stone, W. E. & Webster, J. E. (1944). Arch. Neurol. Psychiat. 51, 472.
Handbook (1969) Handbook of Neurochemistry. Ed. A. Lajtha. New York: Plenum Press.
Heald, P. J. (1960). Phosphorus Metabolism of Brain. Oxford: Pergamon.
Hertin, L. (1956). Acta Physiol. Scand. 37, Suppl. 127.
Hess, H. H. & Lewin, E. (1965). J. Neurochem. 12, 205, 213.
Hess, H. H. & Thalheimer, C. (1965). J. Neurochem. 12, 193.
Hodgkin, A. L. (1958). Proc. Roy. Soc. B. 148, 1.
Hodgkin, A, L. (1965). The Conduction of the Nervous Impulse. Liverpool: University Press.
James, L. S. & Myers, R. E. (1967) (Ed.). Brain Damage in the Fetus and Newborn from Hypoxia or Asphyxia. Columbus: Ross Laboratories.
Joanny, P. & Hillman, H. H. (1963). J. Neurochem. 10, 655.
Jongkind, J. F. & Bruntink, R. (1970). J. Neurochem. 17, 1615.
Jacobwitz, D. & Marks, B. H. (1964). Endocrinol. 75, 86.
Kao, C. Y. (1966). Pharmacol. Rev. 18, 997.
Karadzic, V. & Mrsulja, B. (1969). J. Neurochem. 16, 29.
Katzman, R. (1961). Neurology, 11, 27.

KERKUT, G. A. & YORK, B. (1969). *Comp. Biochem. Physiol.* **28**, 1125.
KERR, S. E. (1935). *J. biol. Chem.* **110**, 625.
KERR, S. E. (1936). *J. biol. Chem.* **116**, 1.
KERR, S. E. (1938). *J. biol. Chem.* **123**, 443.
KERR, S. E. (1942). *J. biol. Chem.* **145**, 647.
KERR, S. E. & GHANTUS, M. (1936). *J. biol. Chem.* **116**, 9.
KERR, S. E. & GHANTUS, M. (1937). *J. biol. Chem.* **117**, 217.
KHAIKINA, B. I. & GONCHAROVA, E. E. (1964). In Problems of the Biochemistry of the Nervous System. Ed. A. V. Palladin. Transl. Freisinger, Hillman & Woodman. Oxford: Pergamon.
KING, L. J., LOWRY, O. H., PASSONNEAU, J. V. & VENSON, V. (1967). *J. Neurochem.* **14**, 599.
KLEEMAN, C. R., DAVSON, H. & LEVIN, E. (1962). *Amer. J. Physiol.* **203**, 739.
KLEIN, J. R. & OLSEN, N. S. (1947). *J. biol. Chem.* **167**, 747.
KOECHLIN, B. A. (1955). J. Biophys. Biochem. Cytol. **1**, 511.
KŘIVÁNEK, J. (1958). *J. Neurochem.* **2**, 337.
KUFFLER, S. W. (1967). *Proc. Roy. Soc.* **B168**, 1.
LAJTHA, A. & FORD, D. H. (1968). *Prog. Brain Res.* **29**, 135–172.
LAJTHA, A. & MELA, M. (1961). *J. Neurochem.* **7**, 210.
LEÃO, A. A. P. (1944). *J. Neurophysiol.* **7**, 359.
LINDBERG, O. & ERNSTER, L. (1950). *Biochem. J.* **46**, 43.
LOCKSLEY, H. B., SWEET, W. H., POWSNER, H. J. & DOW, E. (1954). *Arch. Neurol. Psychiat.* **71**, 684.
LOWRY, O. H., PASSONNEAU, J. V., HASSELBERGER, F. X. & SCHULZ, D. W. (1964). *J. biol. Chem.* **239**, 18.
MCILWAIN, H. (1957). *Proc. internat. neurochem. Sympos.* **2**, 341.
MCILWAIN, H. (1963). Chemical Exploration of the Brain: a Study of Cerebral Excitability and Ion Movement. Amsterdam: Elsevier.
MCILWAIN, H. (1971). In Cellular Organelles and Membranes in Mental Retardation. Ed. Benson. London: Churchill.
MCILWAIN, H. & RODNIGHT, R. (1962). Practical Neurochemistry. London: Churchill.
MANERY, J. F. (1952). In The Biology of Mental Health and Disease. London: Cassell.
MAYMAN, C. I., GATFIELD, P. D. & BRECKENRIDGE, B. M. (1964). *J. Neurochem.* **11**, 483.
MELLERUP, E. T. & RAFAELSON, O. J. (1969). *J. Neurochem.* **16**, 777.
MERRICK, A. W. (1961). *J. Physiol.* **158**, 476.
MINARD, F. N. & DAVIS, R. V. (1962a). *Nature*, **193**, 277.
MINARD, F. N. & DAVIS, R. V. (1962b). *J. biol. Chem.* **237**, 1283.
MINARD, F. N., KANG, C. H. & MUSHAHWAR, I. K. (1965). *J. Neurochem.* **12**, 279.
NELSON, S. R., SCHULZ, D. W., PASSONNEAU, J. V. & LOWRY, O. H. (1968). *J. Neurochem.* **15**, 1271.
NORMAN, N. (1969). In Adaptation Mechanisms. Ed. E. Bajusz. Oxford: Pergamon.
NYMAN, M. & WHITTAKER, V. P. (1963). *Biochem. J.* **87**, 248.
OCHS, S. (1962). *Internat. Rev. Neurobiol.* **4**, 1.
OCHS, S. (1965). Elements of Neurophysiology. New York: Wiley.
OLSEN, N. S. & KLEIN, J. R. (1946). *Res. Publ. Ass. nerv. ment. Dis.* **26**, 118.
OLSEN, N. S. & KLEIN, J. R. (1947). *J. biol. Chem.* **167**, 739.
ORRELL, S. A. & BUEDING, E. (1964). *J. biol. Chem.* **239**, 4021.
PECK, E. J. & AWAPURA, J. (1967). *Biochim. Biophys. Acta*, **141**, 499.
PHILLIPS, C. G. (1956). *Quart. J. exptl. Physiol.* **41**, 58.
PHILLIS, J. W., TEBECES, A. K. & YORK, D. H. (1968). *Nature, Lond.* **217**, 271.
POLLAY, M. & DAVSON, H. (1963). *Brain*, **86**, 137.
RAKIC, L. M. & MRSULJA, B. B. (1969). Abstr. 2nd Intern. Meeting, I.S.N., p. 333. Milan.
REED, D. J. & WOODBURY, D. M. (1963). *J. Physiol.* **169**, 816.
Report (1970). Lithium in the Treatment of Mood Disorders. NIMH Publ. 5033. Washington: U.S. Govt.

RICHTER, D. & DAWSON, R. M. C. (1948). *Amer. J. Physiol.* **154**, 73.
SACKTOR, B., WILSON, J. E. & TIEKERT, C. G. (1966). *J. biol. Chem.* **241**, 5071.
SAMSON, F. E., BALFOUR, W. M. & DAHL, N. A. (1960). *Amer. J. Physiol.* **198**, 213.
SCHMITZ, H., POTTER, V. R., HURLBERT, R. B. & WHITE, D. M. (1954). *Cancer Res.* **14**, 66.
STETTON, D. & STETTON, M. R. (1960). *Physiol. Revs.* **40**, 505.
STONE, W. E. (1938). *Biochem. J.* **32**, 1908.
STONE, W. E. (1940). *J. biol. Chem.* **135**, 43.
STONE, W. E., TEWS, J. K. & MITCHELL, E. N. (1960). *Neurology*, **10**, 241.
STONE, W. E., WEBSTER, J. E. & GURDJIAN, E. S. (1945). *J. Neurophysiol.* **8**, 233.
Symposium (1970). Wates Symposium on the Blood-Brain Barrier. Ed. R. V. Coxon. Oxford: Physiological Laboratory.
TAKAHASHI, R. & APRISON, M. H. (1964). *J. Neurochem.* **11**, 887.
TARR, M., BRADA, D. & SAMSON, F. E. (1962). *Amer. J. Physiol.* **203**, 690.
THORN, W., PFLEIDERER, G., FROWEIN, R. A. & ROSS, I. (1955). *Pflugers Archiv.* **261**, 334.
THORN, W., SCHOLL, H., PFLEIDERER, G. & MUELDENER, B. (1958). *J. Neurochem.* **2**, 150.
THORN, W. & SCHEITZA, H. (1961). *Pflugers Archiv. ges. Physiol.* **273**, 18.
TRACHTENBERG, M. C. & POLLEN, D. A. (1970). *Science*, **167**, 1248.
TSCHIRGI, R. D. (1960). In *Neurophysiology*, **3**, 1865. Washington, D.C.: American Physiological Society.
VAN HARREVELD, A. (1959). *J. Neurochem.* **3**, 300.
VAN HARREVELD, A., AHMED, N. & TANNER, D. J. (1966). *Amer. J. Physiol.* **210**, 777.
VAN HARREVELD, A., CROWEL, J. & MALHOTRA, S. K. (1965). *J. cell. Biol.* **25**, 117.
VAN HARREVELD, A. & MALHOTRA, S. K. (1966). *J. cell. Sci.* **1**, 223.
VAN HARREVELD, A. & MALHOTRA, S. K. (1967). *J. Anat.* **101**, 197.
VAN HARREVELD, A. & SCHADÉ, J. P. (1960). *Proc. 2nd Internat. Meeting Neurobiol.* p. 239. Amsterdam: Elsevier.
WEINER, N. & HULS, H. N. (1961). *J. Neurochem.* **7**, 180, 241.
WHISTLER, R. L. & BEMILLER, J. N. (1962). *Arch. Biochem. Biophys.* **98**, 120.
WOODBURY, D. M. (1955). *J. Pharmacol. exp. Therap.* **115**, 74.
WOODBURY, J. W. (1969). In Basic Mechanisms of the Epilepsies, p. 41. Ed. H. H. Jasper, A. A. Ward & A. Pope. Boston: Little, Brown.
ZUCKERMANN, E. C. & GLASER, G. H. (1968). *Exper. Neurol.* **20**, 87.

4 Metabolic, Ionic and Electrical Phenomena in Separated Cerebral Tissues

Interaction between the brain and the rest of the body can best be appreciated when information is available about the behaviour of the brain and of parts of it, not only *in situ* but also in isolation. Isolation yields systems which are artificial but in which a wide range of experimental studies are possible. In such systems the metabolic potentialities of cerebral tissues can be displayed; as will be seen below, the separated tissues prove to be remarkably autonomous. They maintain membrane potentials and susceptibility to suitable electrical stimulation. Samples of a few milligrams suspended in saline solutions, maintain defined concentrations of labile metabolites and of simple diffusible substances, which are often very different from those in the surrounding solutions. The samples may behave metabolically towards many substrates in salt solutions very much as does the brain *in vivo* towards substances in the bloodstream. With suitable substrates, the separated fragments restore and maintain a pattern of labile metabolites which is similar to that of the brain *in situ*, and different from that of other tissues suspended in similar fluids. Cerebral tissues could be recognized as such and differentiated from other tissues of the body, purely on the basis of metabolic characteristics of this type.

Parts of the brain can be prepared for metabolic studies in different ways, and with different modes of preparation characteristically different and often complementary information can be obtained. A major factor in this respect is cell structure: preparations retaining considerable cell structure are very different in their metabolic behaviour and requirements from those which are largely cell-free. In general, the cell-containing systems give information on the rate and balance of overall processes such as the formation of carbon dioxide or of lactic acid from glucose. Studies with cell-free systems show these processes to involve many distinct chemical stages and enable the characteristics of the individual stages to be investigated. The present account concerns cell-containing systems, whose behaviour is assessed in relation to that of the tissue *in situ*. Cell-containing systems are to be contrasted with the breis, ground suspensions, homogenates, or extracts of the tissue in which cell structure is partly or wholly broken and of which the metabolic properties will concern a later chapter.

61

Experimental Arrangements

Preparation of Tissue with Minimal Damage to Cell Structure

All methods of preparing the separated tissue for metabolic and electro-physiological studies are conditioned by the need to supply artificially the materials which normally reach it from the bloodstream. In particular, diffusion of glucose and oxygen to the separated specimen is no longer facilitated by the blood capillaries and must occur from artificially exposed surfaces, whose distance apart is conditioned by rates of diffusion of metabolites into the tissue, and the rates at which the metabolites are consumed by the tissue. These rates in mammalian tissues at 37°C are commonly such that in one direction the specimen should not be thicker than about 0·35 mm. (Warburg, 1930; Field, 1948). The simplest preparations are thus sheets of this thickness and of some convenient area between 0·1 and 3 cm.^{2}; weighing, therefore, 3–100 mg. Amphibian tissues are of lower metabolic rate especially at the lower temperatures normal to them, and this combined with its small size enables metabolic observations to be made with the intact brain of the frog.

In experiments with mammalian tissues, the thin sheets required are often cut from the cerebral hemispheres of laboratory animals, parallel to their outer surfaces, using a razor-like blade moistened with a physiological saline. A guide or template may be used so that slices of defined thickness are obtained. The blade may also be used with not a cutting but a chopping motion and slices of uniform thickness produced mechanically by cutting in directions chosen in relation to structural elements of the tissue (McIlwain & Rodnight, 1962). This is applicable not only to large and relatively uniform parts of the brain but also to small or intricately shaped parts or biopsy specimens, and to white matter which is soft and more difficult to slice by other means. Slicing methods have received detailed attention specifically in relation to mammalian neocortical tissues. It is best for the tissue to be cut without added saline, and to first meet experimental fluids when these are well oxygenated and at 37–38°. A quite narrow cutting blade is recommended (Harvey & McIlwain, 1969); a fine, oscillating, nylon thread has also been employed (Frank, Cornette & Schoffeniels, 1968).

Surface Relationships *in vivo* and *in vitro*

Any method of slicing obviously damages cell elements, especially in most parts of the central nervous system where cells are elongated and have processes running in several directions. The proportion of cells or of cell-processes damaged in cutting the cerebral cortex must be much higher than in tissues of more parenchymatous cell structure. On the other hand, the cerebral tissues when so cut lose a smaller proportion of their dry weight than do for example those of the liver. This can be understood as due to the high proportion of long and very narrow axons and dendritic processes from which leakage does not so readily occur. "Sealing" such cells by coagulation of cell constituents on contact with physiological salines has been described (Heilbrunn, 1952); the presence of Ca^{2+} salts in the salines is important in the resealing and enables cells to recover their original membrane resistance (Délèze, 1970). The cut surfaces remain an extremely small proportion of the total cell surface in the tissue. Thus Hill (1932) estimated the fibres, some 3–25 μ in diameter, in peripheral nerve to present a surface of some 2000 cm.^{2}/g. of tissue. Cerebral cortex, with fibres and dendrites of 1 to 5 μ in diameter, could present 10 times this area per unit weight and when estimates of fine cell-processes seen electron-microscopically are taken into account, the likely surface area is about 5×10^4 cm.^{2}/g. (see McIlwain, 1967; Harvey & McIlwain, 1968). In cutting a tissue specimen 0·35 mm. in thickness and weighing 100 mg., the surfaces disturbed (cut and resealed) are of about 30 cm.^{2}/g., or 0·06% of the estimated outer cell surfaces of the sample.

It is relevant to note that the external area of tissue samples prepared from the mammalian brain by sectioning as just described, approaches that of the blood capillaries which the samples carry. From the reported length and diameter of the capillaries of the rat brain, a value of 10 mm.^{2}/mm.^{3} may be obtained for the capillary area per unit tissue volume (McIlwain, 1967); the excised tissue sample has an external area of about 6 mm.^{2}/mm.^{3}. Thus the external areas which must form the route of supply of materials to the tissue sections after isolation, are quite similar to the area of the capillaries which constitute the route of supply to the tissue as it exists in the brain. Diffusion factors, indeed, condition both the biological structure *in vivo* and the choice of experimental arrangements *in vitro*.

Media replacing the Bloodstream

The frequent use of sliced tissues in studying cerebral metabolism has depended on the success with which many of their activities can be maintained by metabolites supplied in chemically defined media rather than as whole blood or blood serum. The present lack of comparable success with saline media as perfusion fluids for the mammalian brain was described above. The composition of media employed has been based on the inorganic constituents of blood plasma or cerebrospinal fluid, quoted in Table 3.2. A typical bicarbonate-buffered medium contains (Krebs, 1950; McIlwain & Rodnight, 1962) in μmoles/ml.: NaCl, 124; KCl, 5; KH$_2$PO$_4$, 1·2; MgSO$_4$, 1·3; CaCl$_2$, 0·75–2·8 (see below); NaHCO$_3$, 26 in equilibrium with a gas phase of 95% O$_2$–5% CO$_2$; and glucose, 10. A variety of other organic substances may replace or supplement glucose, as will be noted below; with O$_2$ as gas phase, 20 mM phosphate buffer or 30 mM glycylglycine may replace the bicarbonate and CO$_2$.

Most of the constituents of such media have specific metabolic and electro-physiological effects and a suitable medium for a particular study is selected experimentally. Several of the media deliberately depart from the composition of the bloodstream in some chosen respects. The main departures should be borne in mind; they are as follows. (1) The oxygen commonly used in place of air permits the use of thicker tissue slices than would otherwise be the case. Damage to structural elements is thus minimized; the higher oxygen tension to which the exterior of the tissue is exposed is not known to be deleterious, though higher pressures of oxygen can depress respiration. (2) The media are approximately *iso*osmotic with the bloodstream. For most but not all purposes it is not found necessary to replace the osmotic effects of the proteins of the blood by substances of comparably high molecular weight. (3) Plasma proteins may be replaced in their buffering capacity by a variety of agents: a simple peptide such as glycylglycine, by certain ammonium salts (20 or 30 mM-tris, *i.e.* 2-amino-2-hydroxymethylpropane-1:3-diol hydrochloride), or by inorganic phosphate. (4) Serum bicarbonate as a buffer is often similarly replaced. (5) Many constituents present in small amounts are commonly omitted but under specific circumstances, addition of limited amounts of the following substances has appeared advantageous (McIlwain & Rodnight, 1962): Mn^{2+}, Co^{2+}, creatine, adenosine, guanosine, nicotinamide, glutathione, plasma proteins, inulin, ganglioside components and salts of ascorbic, pyruvic, fumaric and glutamic acids.

Apparatus and Conditions for Studying Tissues

In vitro studies inevitably impose particular metabolic and electrical conditions on isolated neural tissues; as will be recounted below, these two sets of conditions interact in the tissue *in vitro* as well as in the brain *in situ*. Consequently, the experimental arrangements now noted briefly are designed to allow electrical measurements concomitantly with metabolic observations, or to provide facilities for applying electrical stimuli to the tissue. At least three markedly different types of arrangement should be noted.

(1) Superfusion. *In vivo* conditions are most closely simulated with a separated tissue when saline flows over it at a rate comparable to the flow of blood through the tissue *in vivo*. This arrangement has been applied to cerebral tissues using the apparatus of Fig. 4.1, to peripheral nerve, to the spinal cord of small animals and to ganglia (A, Fig. 4.2). The ganglion is shown in an apparatus which allows stimuli to be applied and their consequences seen, both as impulses in postganglionic fibres and as alterations in metabolic rate, e.g. by the O_2-tension of the flowing fluid. The cerebral tissue may also be examined in a slice-chamber (see below) which allows it to be explored by micropipette electrodes, which with stimulating electrodes can be manoeuvered to different parts of the tissue to record membrane potentials and examine their dependence on electrical stimuli and on fluid constituents. Also, the slice can be removed rapidly for analysis.

(2) Cerebral tissues may be provided with substrate sufficient for some minutes' or an hour's metabolism, in volumes of fluid about equal to that of the tissue itself (Rodnight & McIlwain, 1954): a volume of fluid, that is, which would flow through the tissue *in situ* in about 2 min. Such experiments must be brief, or substrates must be provided at concentrations greater than normal. Both substrate and oxygen may be very satisfactorily provided in non-aqueous fluids when the tissue is suitably supported.

(3) The majority of experiments with separated cerebral tissues has been carried out with the fragments of tissue suspended in glucose salines, of some 30 to 200 times the volume of the tissue. This is the quantity of fluid which would flow through the tissue *in vivo* in about 1–6 h., and within this range falls the duration of most such experiments. Ample buffer and substrate can thus be provided in fluids similar in composition to blood sera. The large fluid

volume to which the tissue is throughout exposed represents an artificial situation which may deplete the tissue and which also encourages the accumulation of metabolites. These factors are often advantageous in studying intermediary metabolism but they limit comparison with the behaviour of the

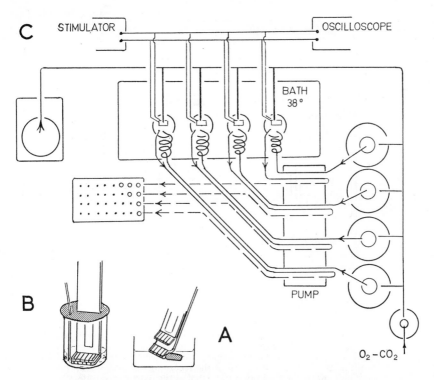

FIG. 4.1. A superfusion apparatus for cerebral samples (McIlwain & Snyder, 1970).

  A. The tissue sample is inserted in the apparatus by picking it from a dish of incubation fluid by the jaws of a tissue-holder. The holder may, as illustrated, carry electrodes.

  B. The tissue-holder is shown fitted to a small beaker which also receives tubes carrying O_2 or O_2—CO_2, and the inflow and outflow of the chosen incubation fluid (one only of these tubes is shown).

  C. Four tissue samples mounted as in B, and supplied with fluid during incubation. The associated apparatus is shown in plan. The incubating solution for each beaker comes oxygenated, from an individual reservoir through a heating-coil immersed in the incubating-bath. Inflow and outflow to each beaker are actuated by the same peristaltic pump, and the outflow is fed to a rack of sample-tubes.

  Results obtained with the apparatus are included in this Chapter and in Chapter 14.

tissue *in vivo*. The bathing medium can be regarded as an extension of the interstitial fluid of the brain, and active relationships are found to be maintained between tissue and fluid in exchange of soluble materials and metabolites (see McIlwain, 1970).

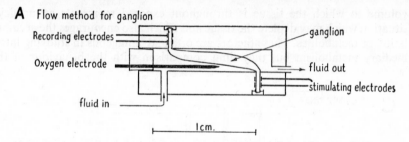

A   Flow method for ganglion

Recording electrodes

Oxygen electrode

ganglion

fluid out

stimulating electrodes

fluid in

1 cm.

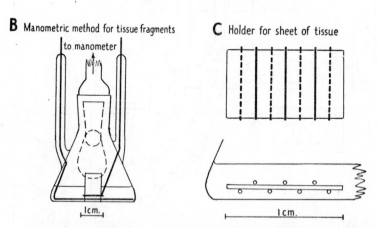

B   Manometric method for tissue fragments

to manometer

1cm.

C   Holder for sheet of tissue

1 cm.

Fig. 4.2. Apparatus for metabolic studies of parts of the nervous system.
   A. A small plastic chamber, volume about 15–50 µl., through which
oxygenated nutrient saline flows at about 200 µl./hr. over an isolated
ganglion or section of nerve (Larrabee & Bronk, 1952). Oxygen uptake
is measured by the current between electrodes sensitive to oxygen
tension. The ganglion so maintained can be electrically stimulated,
the conducted impulse observed at the recording electrodes, and concomitant effects on respiration measured at the oxygen electrode. (See
also Larrabee, 1958; Horowicz & Larrabee, 1962.)
   B. Conical electrode vessel of about 15 ml., taking 10–100 mg. of tissue
fragments in 2–5 ml. fluid. Respiration or acid formation can be
measured manometrically with or without the passage of electrical
impulses between electrodes. Electrodes are in the form of two concentric rings, between which lie the fluid and tissue (McIlwain, 1951;
Ayres & McIlwain, 1953).
   C. Relation between wires and a sheet of tissue, $10 \times 6 \times 0.35$ mm.,
in grid holders used for supporting and applying electrical pulses to the
tissue. The wires can be wound onto a small plastic frame and placed
as shown in the diagram in a vessel similar to B but without concentric
electrodes. The tissue in the frame in such a vessel can be studied with
or without added saline, or in oils. It may also be held in a beaker for
rapid transference and analysis of tissue constituents (Rodnight &
McIlwain, 1954; Heald & McIlwain, 1956; McIlwain, 1960; Gainer
et al., 1962).

   (4) Cerebral tissues may also be studied in an electrically excited condition
by applying electrical pulses to the separated, metabolizing tissue (Figs. 4.1
and 4.2). To do this the tissue may be held in a grid of wires between which
fluctuating potential gradients are established. Alternatively, the tissue may

be permitted to float freely in saline which is entirely within the field established by concentric electrodes. For experiments lasting from a few minutes to an hour or two the grid with its tissue may be held in a beaker of saline from which it can be rapidly transferred to fixing solutions. The tissue-holder of **B**, Fig. 4.1, is convenient for such experiments; it would then be used without the tubes for inflow and outflow of incubation fluid (McIlwain & Rodnight, 1962).

Respiration

Uptake of oxygen by sliced cerebral tissues has been measured more frequently and under a greater variety of conditions than has any other of their metabolic properties. This is understandable, as respiration is a prerequisite to many other of the tissues' activities.

Normal Rates with Glucose

The relative specialization of cerebral metabolism *in vivo* to glucose as substrate gives a criterion for judging the behaviour of the separated tissue. This, *in vitro*, actively metabolized added glucose and results of typical

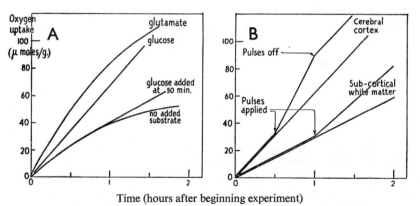

Time (hours after beginning experiment)

FIG. 4.3. The course of respiration of cerebral tissues (see McIlwain, 1956, 1968).
    A. Guinea pig cerebral cortex with different substrates in phosphate-buffered media.
    B. Human cerebral tissues in the phosphate saline with glucose, and electrically stimulated (by condenser pulses, 100/sec., time-constant 0·4 msec., peak potential gradient 3 v/mm.).
    Lines are drawn through points giving the volume of oxygen absorbed at each 5 min., calculated from manometric readings of oxygen pressure in vessels similar to that of **B**, Fig. 4.2.

respiratory experiments are shown in Fig. 4.3 and Table 4.1. From this it is seen that even without added substrate, oxygen is nevertheless absorbed. Also, carbon dioxide is evolved, evidently from endogenous substrates; their utilization is prominent in human cerebral tissues, and involves substances not fully characterized. Endogenous respiration markedly falls with time, being only about one-third of its initial value after 1 hr. at 37°C. Glucose prevents this fall, and moreover if present from the beginning of the experiment it provides a much higher and stable respiratory rate for several hours. Experiments with isotopically labelled glucose have shown the added glucose to be used in preference to endogenous substrates (Sutherland *et al.*, 1956).

This stable rate, in for example cerebral cortex, is largely independent of the degree to which the tissue has been cut, between particle sizes of 100 and 0·01 mg. The tissue/fluid ratio can be altered greatly, for example between 1 and 0·01, without appreciable change in respiratory rate. It is therefore valuable to compare the magnitude of respiration in the separated tissue with that *in vivo*, and an approximate computation for human cerebral tissues is given in Table 4.1. Here the respiratory rate, especially for cerebral cortex, is found to be quite high and comparable with those of other of the more metabolically

Table 4.1

Respiratory rate of the human brain in vivo *and of preparations from it* in vitro

Method of preparation	Part of the brain	Respiration (μmoles O_2/g. hr.)
IN VIVO		
Arterial-venous difference and blood flow	Whole	90
Estimate*	Grey matter	120
	White matter	60
IN VITRO		
Slice; glucose-phosphate saline, no electrical stimulation	Grey matter	60
	White matter	30
Slice; same saline, electrical stimulation	Grey matter	120
	White matter	50

* Estimate, regarding the brain as of equal volumes of white and grey matter, the grey of twice the respiratory rate of the white. Data from Kety *et al.* (1948), McIlwain (1953, 1969), Korey & Orchen (1959) and sources there quoted.

active tissues such as liver or kidney. Nevertheless, the rates of the cerebral tissues are only about half of those computed for respiration *in vivo*. A similar relationship is found in the other species examined.

Clearly the *in vitro* conditions are in some way unrepresentative of those *in vivo*. Several circumstances can in fact induce higher respiratory rates in the isolated tissue. These include the provision of additional substrates, the omission of calcium salts from the media or the addition of high—some 30–50 mM—concentrations of potassium salts, or addition of some dyestuffs such as phenosafranine (see Chapter 10). Most of these circumstances however depart further from, rather than restore, conditions normal to the environment of the tissue *in vivo*. Knowing the connection between cerebral metabolism and activity outlined in preceding chapters, the difference between a respiratory rate of, for instance, 120 μmoles/g. hr. for the cerebral cortex *in vivo* and 60 μmoles/g. hr. *in vitro*, may be considered to be related to the level of functional activity in the tissue under the two circumstances. The data of Table 4.1 and of the following section show this to be the case.

During Electrical Stimulation

Before observations were made with cerebral tissues, respiration of isolated muscle and peripheral nerve was known to increase when increased activity was induced electrically. Among the earliest comparable studies of the central nervous system were those of Winterstein on the frog spinal cord (**A**, Fig. 4.4).

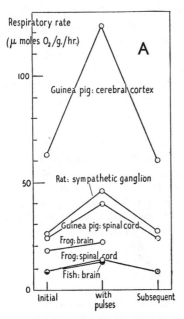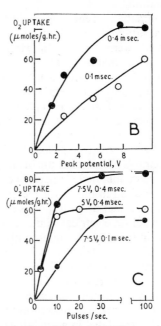

FIG. 4.4 Electrical stimulation of the respiration of preparations from the central nervous system.

A. Organs from the frog and fish (*Luciopenia sandra*) were examined at about 16° to 18° and respiration measured by a capillary respirometer; electrical pulses were from induction coils or mechanical interruptors. Rat and guinea pig tissues were examined at 37°, respiration of the ganglion potentiometrically in flowing salt-glucose solutions and of the brain and spinal cord, manometrically (see Winterstein, 1929; McIlwain, 1956).

B and **C**. Changes in the respiratory rate of guinea pig cerebral cortex during the application of electrical pulses of rectangular time–voltage relationships. **B** Dependence on potential; pulses were of the duration quoted, applied at 100/sec. **C** Dependence on frequency; pulses were of the potential and duration quoted: McIlwain & Joanny (1963).

The cord when kept in oxygen or in oxygen-saturated salt solutions in a closed vessel at room temperature retained its ability to transmit impulses, as could be shown by leaving outside the vessel its connections through the sciatic nerve to the leg. Respiration of the cord normally progressed steadily for many hours, but stimulation with an induction coil, sufficient to cause tetanus in the leg for some 50 minutes, led, during that time, to a marked increase in respiration of the cord itself. When applied impulses were stopped, respiration reverted to its previous value. The increase was greater with more intense stimulation and respiration could be nearly doubled. Some increase was found also by applying impulses to isolated frog brain under similar circumstances. Later studies showed that parts of the frog brain will continue to discharge rhythmically after careful removal of the brain from the frog, and that the pattern of discharge changes with applied electrical pulses (Libet & Gerard, 1939). Increased respiration has also been demonstrated in cerebral tissues from fish on electrical stimulation.

Mammalian cerebral tissues at first proved more refractory to such studies. Several attempts to show spontaneous electrical discharge in separated fragments were unsuccessful. However, applied electrical pulses were found to bring about major metabolic changes in the tissues. Respiration markedly increased (Figs. 4.3 and 4.4). Also, the changes so induced included ones which in muscle and peripheral nerve are associated with increased functional activity: loss of energy-rich phosphates, accumulation of inorganic phosphate and phosphate-acceptors, and increase in glycolysis. The increase in respiration with human cerebral tissues is 70–100 % and brings the respiratory rate of the excited separated tissue close to that normal to the brain *in vivo* (Table 4.1). Comparable increase occurs in all species examined and the higher respiratory rates are maintained for periods of an hour or more. The electrical characteristics required in pulses for metabolic effects are similar to those of pulses to which the intact brain responds *in vivo* (Fig. 4.4; see also Chapter 15). As will be seen below, electrical stimulation tends to make the tissue *in vitro* more akin to that in the intact brain not only in respiratory rate but also in respect to its susceptibility to change in substrate and to inhibitory agents.

In order that electrical stimulation should increase respiration, the main energy-yielding reaction of cerebral tissues, it will be noted that no additional provision of substrate or oxygen is needed: these are already present in excess. This emphasizes that respiration in unstimulated tissues is controlled; moreover, it is regulated in a quantitatively defined fashion. Each pulse of optimal characteristics in the experiments of **B**, Fig. 4.4, caused an increase in oxygen uptake of 1·6 nmoles/g. of cerebral cortex (McIlwain & Joanny, 1963). This and the knowledge that comparable regulation occurs *in vivo*, increase the significance of such control and prompt the study of its mechanism. The increased respiration is found again to be one of a group of associated changes, which will be encountered in the following sections, and which prove to be linked as shown previously in Fig. 3.3. Intermediates of the respiratory chain have been observed spectrophotometrically in cerebral tissues (see Chapter 6); prompt increase in NADH and in reduced cytochrome c were caused by electrical stimulation and blocked by tetrodotoxin (q.v.). Synaptosomal preparations are also susceptible to electrical stimulation, as described in Chapter 12.

Substances supporting Respiration of Cerebral Tissues

Most observations on the reactions of cerebral tissues to different substrates have been made with the cerebral cortex of the rat, mouse or guinea pig by incorporating the substance concerned in place of glucose in salines similar to media described above. Other data are derived from two more recent types of study: with human cerebral tissues (Elliott & Sutherland, 1952; Sutherland *et al.*, 1956; McIlwain, 1963) and with electrically stimulated tissues (McIlwain, 1953, 1956, 1968).

Consideration may be given first to glucose and to other hexoses. Hypoglycaemia following the administration of insulin to intact animals results in lowered cerebral respiration; comparable dependence of respiration on glucose concentration, is found *in vitro* under suitable conditions. Fig. 4.5 shows how the respiration of cerebral tissues increases with increasing glucose concentration between zero and 1–1·5 mM (about 20–30 mg./100 ml.). Thereafter, respiration alters only a little, if at all, while glucose is increased to 10 mM.

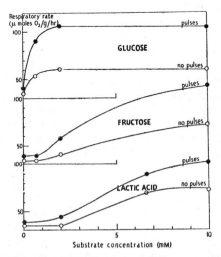

FIG. 4.5. Rate of respiration of guinea pig cerebral cortex in phosphate-salines with glucose, fructose or lactates as substrates, between 1 and 10 mM.

Rates plotted correspond to the slopes of lines such as those of FIG. 4.3 which record the course of oxygen uptake. Electrical pulses: alternating, exponential time-voltage relationships with time-constant of 0·4 msec., at 100/sec. and peak potential gradient of 2 v/mm. Results quoted are for the period 60–90 min. after commencing metabolism; other periods gave comparable values (McIlwain, 1953).

The dependence on glucose concentration is much greater in tissues subjected to electrical impulses, when respiration increases three-fold between 0 and 1·5 mM. Such sensitivity is adequate to afford a basis for severe hypoglycaemic coma with its associated fall in cerebral respiration; changes at higher glucose levels are referred to below, in discussing cerebral glycolysis. Moreover, electrical stimulation revealed defects in cerebral tissues taken from sheep in insulin coma (Setchell, 1959). When the tissues were examined in media with excess glucose, their respiration was normal but it failed to increase on stimulation.

Fructose, mannose, and galactose have been observed when provided in relatively high concentrations to increase the respiration of separated cerebral tissues. As shown in Fig. 4.5, fructose is required at levels approximately 10 times those of glucose to produce comparable effect. Rat cerebral cortex with ^{14}C-fructose yielded $^{14}CO_2$, but this was largely suppressed by adding an equal amount of glucose. On the other hand, formation of $^{14}CO_2$ from glucose was unaffected by fructose; this is in accord with the relative affinity of hexokinase (q.v.) for the two hexoses. This data (Dipietro & Weinhouse, 1959), and the limited access of fructose to the brain *in vivo*, appear adequate to explain the inability of fructose to rouse subjects from hypoglycaemic coma. It is probable that similar considerations apply to the other hexoses though comparably detailed study is not available.

Of carboxylic acids, lactic and pyruvic acids, both of which are produced by the brain *in vivo* and also by separated cerebral tissues, can in addition serve as oxidizable substrates when present in adequate concentrations. With pyruvate the level giving maximal respiration is quite low, about 0·5 mM, but of lactate appreciably higher concentrations are required (Fig. 4.5) especially to give maximal respiration during the application of electrical pulses. Oxaloacetic acid, 5 or 25 mM, affords high respiratory rates (Woodman & McIlwain, 1961). Fatty acids from octanoate to duodecanoate increased the respiration of cerebral tissues in presence of glucose by 20–30 μmoles O_2/g. hr., for a limited time only (Ahmed & Scholefield, 1961). This appeared to occur by modifying respiratory control in the tissue rather than by the compounds acting as oxidizable substrates; ^{14}C-octanoate yielded $^{14}CO_2$ at less than 1 μmole/g. hr. (Chapters 7 and 11).

Respiration of cerebral tissues in saline solutions is increased also by the following substances, though their limiting concentrations have not been studied in comparable detail: α-glycerophosphates, phosphoglycerates, succinates, fumarates, α-ketoglutarates, and citrates. It is noteworthy, however, that concentrations of these substances which support respiration of the cerebral cortex in saline mixtures under ordinary conditions, do not permit metabolic response by the tissue to applied electrical pulses. In this respect they do not replace glucose *in vitro*; nor, as noted above, do they do so *in vivo*. Glutamic acid and related compounds are important metabolites in cerebral tissues, and are described with other amino acids in Chapter 8.

Isolated cerebral tissues show specific *in vitro* relationships to acetoacetates and β-hydroxybutyrates (Krebs, 1961; Phillips, 1964): observations which parallel, though they do not fully interpret, the special relationship of the brain *in vivo* to these compounds. Sliced rat brain cortex incubated with acetoacetate as only added oxidizable substrate, removed the compound at some 30 μequiv./g. fresh tissue/hr., largely by oxidation; a minority was reduced to β-hydroxybutyrate. Acetoacetate, and especially the hydroxybutyrate when added as such, were the only substances of a number examined which increased the oxygen uptake of neocortical tissues respiring in glucose-containing solutions. The increase, of some 15–20%, was not large; these relationships are discussed further in Chapters 6 and 7.

Further details regarding the metabolism of cerebral tissues *in vitro*, with the effects of a number of variables, and data from a range of mammalian species and cerebral areas, are given by Woodman & McIlwain (1961), McIlwain & Rodnight (1962), Elliott & Wolfe (1962) and Ridge (1967).

Glycolysis

Separated, cell-containing cerebral tissues readily produce lactic acid from glucose in saline mixtures such as those of page 63. Thus the second major energy-yielding reaction occurring in the brain *in vivo* can be reproduced *in vitro*. Like respiration, it is a process of several stages which can be revealed by its study in cell-free systems (Chapter 5), where however the factors which govern it are different from those, now to be described, which condition its operation in the cell-containing tissue.

Aerobic Accumulation of Lactate in Normal Media

While cerebral tissues are respiring in glucose-containing media, lactic acid accumulates in the fluid. The accumulation often follows a course such as that of curve A, Fig. 4.6, which concerns cerebral cortex placed in 50 volumes of

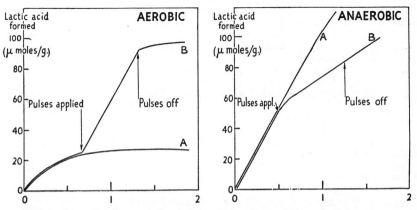

FIG. 4.6. The course of glycolysis by guinea pig or rabbit cerebral tissue in bicarbonate salines, as measured by CO_2 evolution and determination of lactic acid. Aerobic: in O_2 with 5% CO_2. Anaerobically: in N_2 with 5% CO_2. A, unmodified and B, with electrical pulses, as in Fig. 4.3, applied during the period indicated (McIlwain, 1956).

fluid. Increase in lactic acid is at first relatively rapid, at some 50 μmoles/g. hr., but falls after some minutes to rates about a quarter of this value. If the same quantity of tissue is incubated in a smaller volume of the same glucose-containing fluid, the formation of lactic acid is considerably less; in each case the rate of formation falls after the lactic acid produced has reached a given concentration. A reason for this is to be found in the fashion in which lactic acid itself serves as oxidizable substrate when its concentration is greater than about 3 mM (Fig. 4.5).

The normal rate of formation of lactic acid from glucose by human cerebral tissues in small volumes of fluid can be close to that determined by arteriovenous difference *in vivo* (Table 4.2). Under both these conditions the tissues convert to lactic acid about 15–20% of the glucose which they consume, nearly all the remainder being oxidized to carbon dioxide.

The increase in the lactic acid of the brain which accompanies increased cerebral activity in intact animals (Chapter 3) has its parallel *in vitro* in the increase in glycolysis which can be induced in the separated tissues by electrical stimulation. Table 4.2 and Fig. 4.6 show that the rate can be increased two- to ten-fold by this means. In experiments with cerebral cortex in several times its volume of glucose-containing fluids, rates of 100 μmoles lactic acid formed/g. of tissue/hr. can be maintained for periods of an hour or more. Glycolysis

Table 4.2

Lactic acid formation by the brain in vivo *and by sections of cerebral tissues* in vitro

Species	Conditions and method	Lactic acid formation (μmoles/g. hr.)	
		No pulses	With electrical pulses
Man	Normal whole brain; arteriovenous differ-ence and blood flow	6·0	–
,,	Normal separated cerebral cortex; equal vol. saline	5·0	–
,,	Normal separated cerebral cortex; 50 vol. saline	29	62
,,	Normal subcortical white matter; 50 vol. saline	21	39
,,	Surrounding an astrocytoma; 50 vol. saline	107	124
,,	Surrounding a glioma; 50 vol. saline	41	53
Cat, dog and mouse	Analysis of brain fixed rapidly *in vivo* after stimulation	–	340–1,000
Guinea pig	Analysis of tissue fixed rapidly *in vitro* after stimulation	–	400
,,	Incubation *in vitro*: sustained rate in 50 vol. saline	30	100
,,	Incubation *in vitro*: superfused at 3.5 ml. saline/min.	35	300

Data: see Table 4.1, and Klein & Olsen (1947); Rodnight & McIlwain (1954); McIlwain (1954); McIlwain & Tresize (1956). Tissues examined *in vitro* were in oxygenated phosphate salines with 10 mM glucose, and lactic acid was determined chemically after about 90 min. incubation. Tissues fixed *in vivo* were rapidly frozen 10 sec. after stimulation for 1 sec. (see Chapter 3).

Guinea pig tissues *in vitro* were incubated in bicarbonate glucose salines; superfusion was carried out with the apparatus of Fig. 4.1 (McIlwain & Snyder, 1970 and unpublished).

reverts to its unstimulated value within a minute or less when pulses cease. Stimulation does not maintain for these periods the high rates of some 400–1,000 μmoles/g. hr. which can be reached during convulsive activity *in vivo* and during brief periods of electrical stimulation *in vitro*. These persist for a few seconds only and concern the conversion to lactic acid of carbohydrate already existing intracellularly. In the sliced tissue, though initial rates are higher, the values of 100 μmoles/g. hr. are typical of sustained, stimulated glycolysis unless tissues are superfused when values of some 300 μequiv. lactate/g. hr. can be reached (Table 4.2).

The concentration of glucose provided to cerebral tissues greatly conditions their rate of glycolysis. For maximum rate with applied electrical pulses, concentrations are required beyond the 2 mM at which the tissues' respiration is maximal (Fig. 4.5). Suboptimal glycolysis may thus be suggested as basis for the development of hypoglycaemic symptoms in animals at blood glucose levels of 2–4 mM, when cerebral respiration is little if at all lower than at normal levels of 5 mM. A parallel situation is that of glycolysis in the retina, which is rapid, has specific control, and is believed to maintain components of the electroretinogram not maintained by respiration (Noell, 1951; Pirie & van Heyningen, 1956; Graymore, 1969). With cerebral tissues, fructose and fructose diphosphate also yield lactic acid but with these substrates at 10 mM the lactate formed is still less than that produced from 2 mM glucose. Lowered glycolysis may thus contribute to the inability of fructose to replace glucose in supporting cerebral function in eviscerated animals.

Glycolysis in Modified Media and Anaerobically

Circumstances other than applied electrical impulses also lead to high rates of glycolysis in cerebral tissues. Many of these circumstances at first sight appear to have little in common, but they are related in that each involves loss of the tissue's content in energy-rich phosphates, and probably depolarization of tissue cells (see below).

Aerobically, lactic acid formation is increased in several of the media in which concomitant respiration is high (Ashford & Dixon, 1935; Dickens, 1936; McIlwain et al., 1950, 1963; Wollenberger, 1955). This applies to the cerebral cortex of rat, guinea pig or rabbit in glucose-containing fluids which are high in potassium salts, which have added ammonium salts, or which are low in calcium salts. Glucose utilization is increased through the increased respiration and glycolysis so that it is lost at some 60 μmoles/g. hr., about three times the normal rate, while lactic acid is formed at up to 100 μmoles/g. hr. The increased rates with potassium or ammonium salts are maintained for an hour or more; the increase with potassium salts requires that sodium salts also be present, which is interestingly parallel to observations with electrically-stimulated glycolysis. The effects produced by these various agents on cerebral tissues in most cases have their parallel in some muscular tissues but not in non-excitable tissues such as kidney, liver or spleen.

Among other substances which increase aerobic glycolysis in cerebral tissues are phenazine derivatives and veratrine alkaloids including protoveratrine (Dickens, 1936; McIlwain et al., 1950, 1963; Wollenberger, 1955). This latter substance has a markedly specific action in potentiating the response of cerebral tissue to electrical pulses applied at intervals of a few seconds, an effect possibly analogous to its action in delaying the re-establishment of normal resting potential in peripheral nerve after the passage of an impulse. Control of aerobic glycolysis in cerebral tissues thus shows many signs of being intricately connected with the functional activity of the tissue.

In absence of oxygen, formation of lactic acid by separated cerebral tissues increases greatly, as it does in the whole brain in vivo. Again, sustained rates of 100 μmoles/g. hr. can be reached in cerebral cortex from man or from laboratory animals. It is understandable that the accumulation of lactate is aided by absence of oxygen, as the removal of lactate or of a precursor by oxidation is not possible anaerobically; but the initial increase in lactate formation is great enough to imply also an increase in glucose consumption. Thus a normal aerobic rate of glucose utilization of some 20 µmoles/g. hr. increases anaerobically to 50 µmoles/g. hr. Looked at from another point of view, anaerobic processes of carbohydrate metabolism may thus be regarded as suppressed aerobically: this is one of several phenomena which have been called the Pasteur effect.

Anaerobic glycolysis is very differently conditioned from aerobic glycolysis in cerebral tissues. Thus electrical pulses, the presence of ammonium or of extra potassium salts, the absence of calcium salts or presence of glutamates all decrease anaerobic glycolysis; aerobically they increase it. To some extent, however, the decrease anaerobically occurs through a slow fall in glycolysis which is normal to such circumstances, being accelerated: the agents so acting can thus be regarded as accentuating this effect of anaerobiosis. Like anaerobiosis, they lower the labile phosphates of the tissue and these are required for glycolysis as well as being among its products.

Metabolic Interconnections; Inhibitors

The metabolic interchanges between glucose or other substrates detectable *in vivo* by ^{14}C-derivatives (Chapter 2) are evident also in isolated cerebral

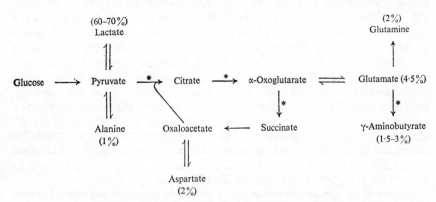

FIG. 4.7. Metabolic routes from glucose in cerebral cortical tissues (see Haslam & Krebs, 1963). Values in parentheses give the % of ^{14}C from uniformly labelled ^{14}C-glucose, found in the different compounds after incubation of about 1 hr.; rat or cat tissue in 10–20 vol. glucose saline (Beloff-Chain *et al.*, 1955; Tower, 1958, 1960). * The reactions asterisked yield CO_2, which was found to contain approx. 20% of the ^{14}C of glucose reacting. For details of the rapid and reversible reactions indicated by double arrows, see Chapters 6, 7 and 8.

tissues, and are then susceptible to further specification. Fig. 4.7 summarizes the fate of ^{14}C added as uniformly-labelled glucose to saline media containing cerebral cortical tissue. Of the ^{14}C undergoing change, 80–90% appeared as lactate and CO_2. Most of the remainder was found as amino-acids, especially as glutamate and two of its products, glutamine and γ-aminobutyric acid (see Chapter 8). These, and also aspartate and alanine which are the other amino acids appreciably labelled, can readily be understood as linked to glucose through the tricarboxylic acid cycle, described in detail in Chapter 6. Lesser amounts of ^{14}C appeared in glycogen, in phosphorylated intermediates, and in lipids and protein.

A further consequence of the equilibria of Fig. 4.7 is that $^{14}CO_2$ evolved from the tissue is of lower specific activity than the ^{14}C-glucose added to it: initially 40%, rising to 85%, in experiments of Gainer et al. (1962) with rat cerebral cortex. This follows because before addition of ^{14}C-glucose, the tissue already contains in the several compounds of Fig. 4.7 and in others linked to them metabolically, quite large reserves of materials which can yield CO_2, mainly through the tricarboxylic acid cycle. Much of the ^{14}C from glucose which enters amino-acids reappears as $^{14}CO_2$ on continued incubation; this does not however imply that these substances are obligatory intermediates in glucose oxidation. Glutamate, aspartate and alanine undergo the rapid and reversible reactions indicated (Fig. 4.7) with intermediates in the tricarboxylic cycle. In particular the aminotransferase (q.v.) acting between glutamate and α-oxoglutarate can catalyse equilibration of the two compounds, without net conversion, at the potential rate of 15,000 μmoles/g. hr. (Haslam & Krebs, 1963). As the tissue contains much more glutamate than α-oxoglutarate, transfer of much ^{14}C to glutamate occurs. Similar considerations apply to the accumulation of ^{14}C-lactate, here accentuated by the trapping effect of the incubation fluid (see above). Appearance of ^{14}C in pentose phosphate and in γ-aminobutyric acid indicates alternative, lesser, routes to $^{14}CO_2$ which are appraised in Chapters 5 and 8.

With uniformly-labelled ^{14}C-mannose as only added organic substrate for rat neocortical tissue, ^{14}C became distributed much as did ^{14}C from [U-^{14}C]-glucose (Chain et al., 1969). [U-^{14}C]fructose as only substrate at 5·5 mM, afforded notably less ^{14}C-lactate than was yielded by glucose, though this difference diminished with five-fold increase in substrate concentration. The distribution of ^{14}C from [1-^{14}C]glucosamine suggested the metabolism of the compound to resemble that of fructose. Distribution of ^{14}C from glucose and glutamate has also been examined in snail, octopus and locust ganglia (Bradford et al., 1969; Cory & Rose, 1969), giving data consistent with known pathways, though the two molluscan species appeared neither to produce γ-aminobutyric acid nor to utilize it.

2-Deoxy-D-glucose diminished glycolysis and respiration of cerebral tissues but did not cause diversion of ^{14}C from glucose to alternative oxidative routes (Tower, 1958). A number of inhibitors of carbohydrate metabolism affect the respiration or glycolysis of cerebral tissues and are referred to in subsequent chapters (see also Elliott & Wolfe, 1962): cyanides, azides, iodoacetates, arsenites, fluorides, glyceraldehyde, malonate and hydroxymalonate. Several substances without effect on the respiration or glycolysis of cerebral cortex as ordinarily studied, inhibit the increase in these processes, which is caused by electrical stimulation: barbiturates, analgesics, atropine, cocaine, and basic peptides (see McIlwain & Rodnight, 1962, and below). The data obtained emphasize in a variety of ways, the association between carbohydrate metabolism and cerebral functioning.

Metabolism of some Experimentally and Pathologically Altered Cerebral Tissues

Those seeking metabolic understanding of pathological and other changes in the functioning of the brain, have frequently investigated the major processes of carbohydrate metabolism which have just been described. This is because such metabolism is prerequisite to many other of the tissue's activities. Considering first, experimentally controlled variations (McIlwain, 1963): intact cerebral tissues kept in a moist atmosphere and between about 0–15°C retain for an hour or so most of the characteristics described in the present chapter. Respiration, glycolysis, and respiratory and glycolytic response to applied pulses are little if at all affected after 2 hr. at 0° but fall after 10 hr. Loss is accelerated by incubating at 37°, even when this is done aerobically under good metabolic conditions if glucose or a comparable substrate is absent. Loss is further accelerated by applied electrical pulses, and the first defect induced in this way is found to be in the respiratory response to applied pulses, rather than in glycolysis or in the glycolytic response. This can be seen when glucose is restored to the treated tissues; respiration is then little affected by pulses which are normally effective, and which still increase the formation of lactic acid. The respiratory response of the treated tissue can be partly restored by the further addition of fumaric or malic acids. This is probably the *in vitro* situation which corresponds most closely to that of the tissues of the brain in severe hypoglycaemia, when permanent damage to them can occur within an hour and later result in demyelination even after blood glucose has returned to its normal level. Cognate metabolic abnormalities in cerebral samples from hypoglycaemic sheep were noted above (Setchell, 1959). In cerebral tissues which have been incubated anaerobically and later are returned to aerobic conditions, response to pulses again suffers loss: a situation possibly paralleling anoxic damage to the brain.

Cerebral Tumours

Many intracranial tumours arise from non-neural cells and are not described here, though they may affect the metabolism of the brain by disturbing its blood flow (Chapter 2). Neoplasms arising from neural tissues may also have this effect and the centre of such tumours may contain many non-living cells and be of low respiratory rate. Oxygen uptake corresponding to 3–24 µmoles O_2/g. hr., in contrast to normal values of 40–55, have been found in astrocytoma, glioma, and fibroblastoma specimens (Victor & Wolf, 1937; McIlwain, 1954; Brierley & McIlwain, 1956). In these and also in others whose respiration was more normal, aerobic glycolysis was high and much closer to the anaerobic value than is usual in cerebral tissues. The metabolism of cerebral tumours thus approaches a pattern described in other neoplastic tissues by Warburg (1930). This has been examined in experimentally-induced glioblastoma and concluded to reflect a disturbance at the level of mitochondrial control mechanisms (q.v.), and to be altered towards normal by particular therapeutic treatments (Kirsch *et al.*, 1969).

Metabolic response to electrical pulses has been found low or absent in tissues from cerebral tumours. This is perhaps understandable with respect to glycolysis, which is already higher than usual (Table 4.2), but extends also to respiration in, for example, a glioma of which respiration in absence of pulses was normal, and also to an astrocytoma of low respiratory rate. These characteristics of the tumorous tissues are found to some extent in tissues of the brain of normal mammals at an early stage in their development (Chapter 13) and in areas in which glial cells have newly proliferated following injury to the brain by freezing. In all these cases respiratory rate and respiratory and glycolytic responses to pulses are low. Lack of response to electrical pulses is presumably the counterpart *in vitro* of the absence of recordable potential changes in neoplastic tissues *in vivo*, though surrounding neurons may discharge abnormally. It has been suggested that the abnormal potential changes which often come from areas around cerebral tumours and which help in the electro-encephalographic localization of the tumours, are chemically conditioned: they may be due to substances diffusing from the tumour itself.

Several types of cerebral tumours contain increased glycogen (Tiraspolskaya & Toropova, 1963) which has been found also after mechanical damage to the brain (Shimizu & Hamaro, 1958). In addition, histochemical and isoenzyme studies have been carried out with human brain tumours, and with cell-lines cultured from them (Gerhardt *et al.*, 1963; Kreutzberg *et al.*, 1966).

Epileptic and Other Conditions

The abnormal electrical phenomena induced by tumours or by other modified tissues in the brain arising from injury, may be associated with epilepsy, the changed tissue or its surroundings constituting an epileptogenic area. Such areas characterized electroencephalographically or by clinical signs have been reported to occur in parts of the brain which are apparently normal histologically, and in these cases the tissue has proved to be normal in its respiratory and glycolytic rates when examined *in vitro*. It has however been stated to be abnormal in certain aspects of its acetylcholine metabolism (Chapter 14).

Cerebral tissues obtained at neurosurgery from subjects addicted to methamphetamine have proved normal in respiratory rate when examined *in vitro*, but to utilize glucose at rates markedly lower than normal (Utena *et al.*, 1955, 1959). The change was also induced in the guinea pig by chronic administration of methamphetamine. This drug (see Chapter 15) may produce an illness closely resembling schizophrenia and cerebral tissues from schizophrenic subjects have been reported to show the same peculiarity in glucose utilization.

Metabolic Maintenance of Tissue Constituents

It has thus been shown that isolated cerebral tissues react to added substrates and to O_2 in fashions closely paralleling events in the intact brain. Much of the tissues' metabolic machinery and its control thus remain, despite the major changes caused by excision of the brain. Basis for this was first found in examining the tissues' content of labile phosphates (McIlwain *et al.*, 1951).

Phosphate Derivatives

Phosphocreatine and adenosine triphosphate are among the most labile of cerebral constituents. Their concentrations were noted in Chapter 3 to fall greatly during the minute or so occupied by exsanguinating a small experimental

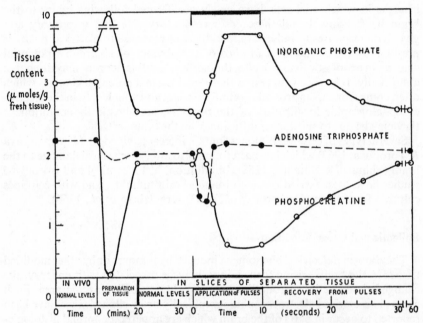

Fig. 4.8. Changes in phosphates during preparation and electrical stimulation of cerebral tissues. The tissues from guinea pigs were incubated in oxygenated glucose-salines between wire grids (**C**, Fig. 4.2) to which electrical pulses were applied for the period of 10 sec. which is indicated. Specimens removed before, during, and after stimulation by the application of electrical pulses were rapidly fixed and their phosphates determined (McIlwain *et al.*, 1951; Heald & McIlwain, 1956; Heald, 1954).

animal and removing its brain. However, it is important to the study of the separated tissue that conditions are readily obtainable for resynthesis of these substances *in vitro*. Some 75 % of the initial content of adenosine triphosphate is restored by 10 min. respiration with glucose as substrate in saline mixtures, as also is 60–70 % of the phosphocreatine (Fig. 4.8). These levels can be maintained for at least 2 hr. For the resynthesis both oxygen and glucose are necessary; glucose may be replaced by pyruvic, lactic, oxaloacetic or oxo-glutaric acids (Woodman & McIlwain, 1961), but several other substrates are less effective in the rat and guinea pig tissues which have been examined. The separated tissue thus reproduces this most important link between carbohydrate metabolism and the formation of the energy-rich phosphates. Inorganic phosphate, post-mortem, greatly increases but during respiration its level also returns to values a little below those normal *in vivo*.

After resynthesis of the labile phosphates, the levels maintained depend greatly on the composition of the surrounding fluid and on the state of the tissue. Added creatine and adenosine augment the resynthesis (Thomas, 1957; Pappius *et al.*, 1959). Agents including fluorides, malonates, and iodoacetates which interfere with carbohydrate metabolism depress the level of creatine phosphate, thus acting comparably with omission of glucose. Especially interesting, however, are the effects of a group of agents which although diverse in nature all increase cerebral respiration: these are high (30–50 mM) concentrations of potassium salts, the omission of calcium salts, the addition of 2:4-dinitrophenol or the application of electrical pulses. All these agents have also a common effect on the composition of the tissue: its level of phosphocreatine falls while that of inorganic phosphate increases.

The course of change in tissue composition after such treatment can be followed particularly closely in tissues subjected to electrical pulses (Fig. 4.8). Here, within one second of the application of pulses, breakdown of adenosine triphosphate has commenced: linkage between electrical and metabolic events is thus extremely prompt in the separated tissue as in the intact brain. The fall in adenosine triphosphate does not however involve more than about a third of its total content: the substance is resynthesized even during the continued application of pulses, apparently at the expense of the phosphocreatine. This, after an initial lag of 1–2 sec., commences to fall as the adenosine triphosphate rises: it falls continuously for some 4 sec. at the very high rate of 0·4–0·5 μmoles/g. sec. or some 1500 μmoles/g. hr. Phosphocreatine thus reaches a new lower level from which further change is not rapid; inorganic phosphate rises concomitantly with the fall in phosphocreatine. Moreover, the change in inorganic phosphate and in the other products from the labile phosphates offers one mechanism for the increase in respiration and glycolysis which results from the passage of electrical pulses (Chapter 6). Experiments with $^{32}PO_4^{3-}$ have shown that the inorganic phosphate formed on applying pulses under these circumstances is not derived directly from the phosphocreatine or adenosine triphosphate. The phosphate from these sources is, rather, transferred through compounds which probably include phosphoproteins (q.v.).

It is instructive in studying the mediation of cerebral events to compare the course of change in phosphates following electrical pulses *in vivo* (Fig. 3.7) and *in vitro*. The rate of fall *in vivo*, because the time of fixation of the intact brain even with liquid air is longer and less uniform, cannot be stated with the certainty of the rate *in vitro* but is of the same order of magnitude; probable values in the rat are 1,200–2,000 μmoles/g. hr. The electrical pulses required *in vivo* and *in vitro* are similar in frequency and in voltage-gradient, and comparable also in these respects to those employed in electroshock therapy or in inducing motor and other responses from the exposed cerebral cortex in man and in experimental animals (Fig. 4.4, McIlwain, 1956; McIlwain & Joanny, 1963). Moreover, the changes *in vitro* as *in vivo* are reversible (Fig. 4.8). Recovery of phosphocreatine *in vitro* begins within a second or so of the cessation of pulses. Its course is much slower than that of the breakdown: some 20 sec. are required for recovery and the maximal rate is about 150 μmoles phospho-creatine/g. tissue hr. Recovery *in vivo* is at a comparable rate: in Fig. 3.7 also at about 150 μmoles/g. hr.

The following approximate comparison may be made between the recovery of the energy-rich phosphocreatine and the additional energy-yielding reactions taking place during electrical excitation of the tissue. Respiration is increased in guinea pig tissues by some 60 μmoles or 120 μg.-atoms/g. hr., and lactic acid formation also by about 60 μmoles/g. hr. Observations with cell-free systems show (Chapter 6) that these could yield some 3×120, +60, or 420 μmoles/g. hr. of labile phosphate. The actual rate of accumulation during recovery is one-third of this. However, it is probable that the recovery and the fall in phosphocreatine in the separated tissue represent different balances in processes of synthesis and degradation both of which are continuous; and it is also clear that energy-consuming processes other than the formation of phosphocreatine are in progress and of these the cation movements to be described in a following section, are of major importance.

Other Constituents

Constituents which are present in the normal brain and which have been sought in incubated cerebral tissues have usually been found present, though specific conditions may be needed for their quantity *in vitro* to approximate that *in vivo*. Examples are given in several subsequent chapters, especially with respect to amino-acids, coenzymes, carbohydrate intermediates and lipids; practical aspects are detailed by McIlwain & Rodnight (1962). In general, provision of oxygen, glucose and obvious precursors is advantageous, and the separated tissue proves capable of making good many of the abnormalities induced during its preparation, as has already been exemplified in the case of phosphocreatine.

Thus lactates in the separated tissue increase during its removal from experimental animals, largely at the expense of cerebral glycogen. At the commencement of experiments with separated cerebral tissues as ordinarily prepared, glycogen has fallen from its normal level of about 1 mg./g. (equiva-lent to about 5 μmoles hexose/g.) to levels less than a tenth of this. However, the normal quantity of glycogen can be largely resynthesized by the separated tissue when it is incubated in a glucose-containing saline. In such resynthesis glucose is required not only as precursor of glycogen but also as source of energy for the reactions which yield it. Thus the synthesis in adequate media is prevented by 2:4-dinitrophenol and by electrical pulses which deplete the tissue's energy-rich phosphates (Le Baron, 1955; see also Khaikina, 1963). The glycogen synthesized *in vitro* was found to be shorter in chain-length, and with a greater degree of branching, than that native to the brain; it was more resistant to change on electrical stimulation (McIlwain & Tresize, 1956; Goncharova, 1963). The action of applied pulses in causing a very rapid formation of lactic acid in the separated tissue was noted in Table 4.2; the source of this acid is largely glucose.

Outstanding among the constituents of the brain which are maintained in isolated cerebral tissues, are the electrolytes next to be described.

Membrane Potentials, Impulse Transmission and Synaptic Phenomena in Tissues from the Brain

The many metabolic changes which can be brought about in cerebral tissues by electrical excitation lead to querying the electrical status of the tissue itself: to what degree does it maintain electrical phenomena seen in the brain *in situ*, and how does such maintenance depend on chemical factors?

Membrane Potentials

Spontaneous voltage changes corresponding to the electrocorticogram are lost when small portions of the mammalian cerebral cortex are cut from neural connections, even when blood supply remains intact. The portions will however respond to stimulation, and when they are as tissue slices thin enough for oxygenation, they show many relevant phenomena on complete removal from the brain (Fig. 4.9). On penetrating the tissue with micropipette electrodes of tip diameter 1 μ or less, negative potentials are observed in regions about the size of cellular structures. These regions occupy about one-third of the distance of travel of the electrode. The average potential in such regions is 60 mv below that of surrounding fluids, and the entry of the electrode may cause spike discharges illustrated by Li & McIlwain (1957), with potential rising to a positive overshoot of 10 to 15 mv. For such observations tissues may be maintained at the surface of fluid media with an atmosphere of moist oxygen in the chamber A of Fig. 4.9. It is then found that most constituents of typical glucose saline incubating media are necessary for optimal development of tissue potentials. Oxygen and glucose are needed; the glucose can again be replaced by a few substances including pyruvate, oxaloacetate or α-oxoglutarate but not by succinate or glutamate. When satisfactorily maintained, tissue potentials are susceptible to electrical stimulation: pulses of the characteristics needed to increase respiration or to deplete phosphocreatine, cause loss of tissue potentials; on stopping stimulation, potentials slowly recover. This sequence of depolarization and repolarization is sensitive to small quantities of a number of added substances (C, Fig. 4.9; Chapter 15).

The sodium and potassium salts of bathing media prove critical in the development of tissue potentials. Replacement of most of the sodium by choline or by tris salts which do not greatly affect respiration, prevents membrane potentials from reappearing. With normal Na, the most negative potentials are found when K is supplied at about 5 mM; below 3 mM-K potentials are smaller and less stable, and above 15 mM are progressively lost. Fig. 4.9 shows the effect of a small localized addition of KCl, which caused a transitory depolarization and subsequent recovery. In most neural systems, transitory depolarization by these means or by electrical stimulation can lead to impulse generation and comparable properties, now to be described, have been observed also in tissues from the brain.

Impulse Transmission and Synaptic Phenomena

These phenomena have now been demonstrated to occur in many preparations from the mammalian brain, appropriately maintained *in vitro*. Success came first (Yamamoto & McIlwain, 1966) with samples from the piriform cortex and corpus callosum from the guinea pig using apparatus similar to that of A, Fig. 4.9. This apparatus had been fitted with silver stimulating electrodes

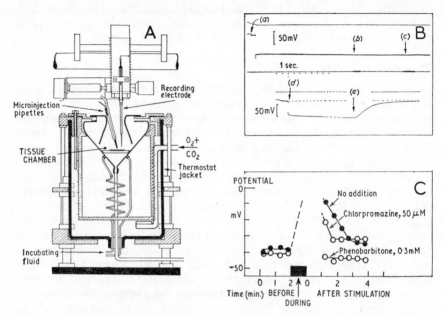

FIG. 4.9.

A. Chamber for maintaining cerebral specimens for electrical observations (Gibson & McIlwain, 1965; see McIlwain & Rodnight, 1962). During an initial period the tissue specimen is immersed in bicarbonate-buffered medium which after 20 min. is partly withdrawn to leave the specimen on a fibre grid, its upper surface in moist O_2 and its lower surface bathed by the medium. The micropipette electrode is lowered vertically into the tissue, which also may receive electrical stimulation from the wires below or added solutions from the microinjection pipettes above.

B. Potentials recorded by the micropipette electrode, in guinea pig cerebral cortex. On advancing the electrode, as measured by the upper trace, a region of negative potential, -68 mv, was encountered at (a). The potential was stable for some minutes, and unaffected by additions of $0 \cdot 2$ M-NaCl to the surface of the tissue at (b) and (c). Below: a similar penetration at (d) gives a region of -65 to -70 mv and addition of $0 \cdot 2$ M-KCl at (e) causes depolarization.

C. Displacement of membrane potential, observed as in **B**, by electrical stimulation; and subsequent recovery. The displacement is diminished in the presence of chlorpromazine, and is not seen after addition of phenobarbitone (Hillman, Campbell & McIlwain, 1963).

in place of the micro-injection pipette, and used for recording either a micropipette or a metal electrode, at defined positions on the tissue surface. By such means a rich profusion of responses was observed (Table 4.3) and indeed most unit activities seen electrically in the brain *in vivo* may be expected to have their counterparts observable in appropriate isolated systems. Particularly well-suited are those which, as the superior colliculus or piriform cortex, can easily be obtained from the brain together with a tract which provides a major neural input.

Conducted responses were readily observed in such tracts, for example in the optic and lateral olfactory tracts (Fig. 4.10) as well as in the corpus callosum. In the attached grey matter regions, electrical responses were slower and more varied. Thus in the piriform cortex of the guinea pig or rat, a surface-negative wave some 15–30 msec. in duration was of maximum amplitude a few mm. away from the tract (Fig. 4.10). On this wave were superposed several positive

Table 4.3

Electrical behaviour and chemical susceptibility of isolated systems from the mammalian brain

Part of the brain	Electrical observations	Chemical susceptibility
Neocortex[3, 4]	Direct cortical response; repetitive firing	Increased amplitude and duration on lowering [Cl⁻]
Corpus callosum[1]	Conducted response	—
Lateral olfactory tract[1, 2]	Transmission at 1 m./sec.	Little affected by 1 mм-phenobarbitone or ether
Piriform cortex [1, 2, 6, 7]	Postsynaptic responses; spike potentials; post-tetanic potentiation	Differential diminution by depressant drugs and by hypoxia
Hippocampus[4] (gyrus dentatus)	Spike responses and propagated after-discharge	Augmented after-discharge in [Cl⁻]-low media
Optic tract[5]	Conducted response	—
Superior colliculus[5]	Positive deflection and negative wave (post-synaptic)	Depressant action of serotonin, antagonized by lysergic acid diethylamide. γ-Aminobutyrate depressed

[1] Yamamoto & McIlwain, 1966. [2] Campbell, McIlwain, Richards & Somerville, 1967. [3] Richards, & McIlwain, 1967. [4] Yamamoto & Kawai, 1967, 1968. [5] Kawai & Yamamoto, 1968. [6] Richards & Sercombe, 1968. [7] Yamamoto & Kurokawa, 1968.

notches. The surface-negative wave was concluded to represent the post-synaptic potential of neurons in the cortical sample below the recording electrode. It was diminished in amplitude by hypoxia, and using glucose-saline solutions under varying O_2-tensions, correlation was found between the amplitude of the negative wave and the adenosine triphosphate content of tissue samples.

Repetitive stimulation of the tissue samples increased the complexity of the electrical responses elicited: the negative wave increased in amplitude and positive notches appeared. The positive-going potentials were correlated in time-sequence and in position in the tissue sample, with the occurrence of cell-discharge. The discharge occurred from units some 250–350 μ below the surface of the tissue. Both the cell-discharges and the post-synaptic potentials, were more susceptible to a number of applied agents than were the conducted responses which initiated them. Ether, phenobarbitone (Fig. 4.10) and chlorpromazine each showed this preferential action.

Neocortical and hippocampal preparations in simple media *in vitro*, also yielded surface-negative responses to stimulation, corresponding in some respects to direct cortical responses elicited by stimulation *in vivo*. When the

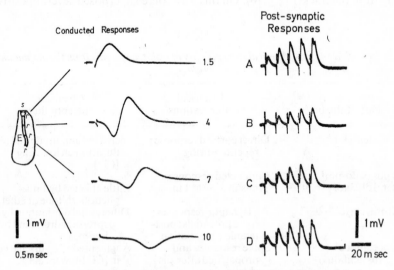

FIG. 4.10. Impulse conduction and transmission in piriform cortical samples from the guinea pig, maintained *in vitro* (Yamamoto & McIlwain, 1966; McIlwain, 1968).

Conducted responses were initiated by stimuli applied at points *s* at the anterior portion of the lateral olfactory tract, and observed at recording electrodes which were 1·5–10 mm. distant from *s* (see numbers by the oscilloscope traces); the sample of piriform lobe, outlined, is about 15 × 7 × 0·35 mm.

Post-synaptic responses were observed in similarly stimulated preparations from recording electrodes in positions E, some mm. from the lateral olfactory tract. The recordings A–D which are shown are each the result of 5 stimuli of identical characteristics given at 12 msec. intervals.

A. Tissue examined in normal medium after 40 min. incubation. The medium was then brought to 1 mM with phenobarbitone and recording B made. This medium was then replaced by normal medium lacking the drug, and recording C was made 7 min. later; D was made 7 min. after a second wash with normal medium.

Cl⁻ of the *in vitro* media was replaced by less diffusible ions, as propionate or methylsulphate, the excitability of the preparations was increased. A single stimulus then led in the hippocampal sample to a train of large spike potentials. Responses by the preparations were also modified by acetylcholine, γ-amino-butyrate and serotonin (q.v., and Table 4.3).

A major approach to understanding the complex electrical behaviour of the mammalian brain, is thus its dissection to simpler units. The variety of electrical responses shown by such derived preparations prompts the description, now to be given, of ionic phenomena which the tissues exhibit during their maintenance in simple solutions *in vitro*.

Fluid and Electrolytes of Incubated Cerebral Tissues

It is now possible to obtain incubated sections of mammalian cerebral tissues with ion content differing from that *in situ* to only a small though significant extent (Keesey, Wallgren & McIlwain, 1965). This requires specific conditions;

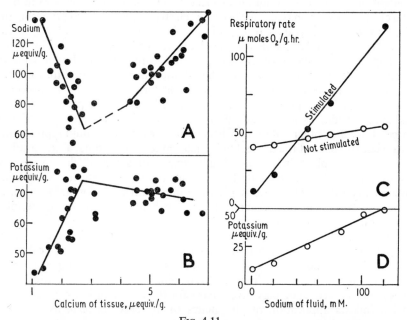

FIG. 4.11.

A, B. Sodium and potassium content of specimens of guinea pig cerebral cortex rapidly prepared and incubated for 30 min. in bicarbonate-buffered glucose salines between 0 and 5 mM in calcium salts. After incubation, tissues were rinsed rapidly in 0·3 M-sucrose at 0°, extracted with trichloroacetic acid, and their Na, K and Ca determined (Lolley & McIlwain, 1964 and see Keesey, Wallgren & McIlwain, 1965).

C, D. Showing the requirement for sodium in incubation fluids, for maintenance of their potassium content (the values quoted are those immediately after electrical stimulation) and respiratory response to electrical stimulation (Bachelard, Campbell & McIlwain, 1962).

otherwise, the large concentration gradients between tissue and surrounding fluids (Table 3.2) leads to rapid loss of K from the tissue, with gain of Na, Cl and water. Thus (i) rapid preparation of the tissue is required and immediate transfer to oxygenated glucose salines at 37°. (ii) The incubation media should be 0·75 mM in calcium salts (A, B, Fig. 4.11). Blood plasma and incubation media normally contain 2·5–3 mM-Ca, but some 30% only of that in plasma is free (unassociated with protein); cerebrospinal fluid contains about 1 mM free Ca. The media lower in Ca afford incubated tissues with 2·5 μmoles Ca/g., close to the normal *in vivo* value (Lolley, 1963). Moreover, 0·75 mM is the minimal Ca for K maintenance, and is optimal in avoiding additional uptake of Na. (iii) Potassium salts are nevertheless required at 5–6 mM, their concentration in blood plasma; media which, like cerebrospinal fluid contain 3 mM-K yield tissue not only poorer in K, but also with a lower $[K]_i/[K]_e$ ratio. (iv) An ordinary range of Na concentrations is required, but Na has specific relationships to the excitability of the tissue and to its K content, as shown in **C, D,** Fig. 4.11.

Departure from the optimal conditions described affects not only the tissue content of Na, K and Cl but also causes it to swell. Certain changes in fluid and electrolytes are unavoidable because cell structures are cut in preparing the tissue; they are equivalent to exposing to external media, about 7% of the formerly intracellular tissue volume (Keesey, Wallgren & McIlwain, 1965; see Pappius *et al.*, 1962). Much greater changes are produced by omission of glucose, oxygen or Na salts, or by the addition of metabolic inhibitors: the tissue then may nearly double in weight by absorption of fluid. Inclusion of inulin or of labelled proteins in incubation media and subsequent analysis of tissue and media, shows the additional fluid to be in part accessible to these large molecules; other data is consistent with the accessible fluid representing extracellular space of the tissue. On incubation for some hours, a very gradual increase takes place in the non-inulin space, of some 6%/hr. (Varon & McIlwain, 1961). Pyruvates or lactates can replace glucose in maintaining tissue K. Additions of solutions a few mM in neutral salts of glutamic acid, to neocortical tissues incubated in normal glucose-containing media had complex effects on tissue cations (Krebs *et al.*, 1951; Pappius *et al.*, 1962; Harvey & McIlwain, 1968). Tissue $[Na^+]$ increased; $[K^+]$ at first diminished but subsequently was recovered as Na^+ was extruded, a process which (see below) utilized tissue adenosine triphosphate and phosphocreatine. Resting membrane potential diminished (Woodman & McIlwain, 1961; Hillman & McIlwain, 1961) and this sequence may give a basis for the increased cortical cell-firing which follows application of glutamates to the brain *in vivo*, as noted in Chapters 8 and 14.

When satisfactorily prepared, isolated mammalian cerebral cortex readily maintains a gradient in potassium ions, $[K]_i/[K]_e$, greater than that corresponding to the observed membrane potential of −60 mv. Tissue heterogeneity which limits the conclusions which can be drawn from such data is considered in more detail below, but it is likely that, as *in vivo*, the opposing gradient in sodium ions is also operative. Substitution in Equation (*i*), Chapter 3, gives a value *b* for the relative tissue permeability to Na and K of 0·04–0·05 again supposing these two to be the only ions involved. Tissue chloride is distributed in the sense indicated by its electrochemical equilibrium; as an anion, the ratio corresponding to −60 mv is $[Cl]_e/[Cl]_i = 9·3$. Observed values, accepting the inulin space as the extracellular space, are 9 to 14 (Gibson & McIlwain, 1965; Keesey *et al.*, 1965).

Electrical Stimulation and Ion Movements

Stimulation promptly alters the tissue content of Na and K (Fig. 4.12). Under resting conditions, ion content can remain with little change for some hours, but electrical pulses of maximal effect double the tissue Na in 5 min.; K falls by a nearly equivalent amount and a new stable state is reached after about 10 min. When stimuli are stopped, the ion movements are reversed and in about 10 min. the original composition is nearly regained. Speeds of change, on stimulation and recovery, are impressively large, of 200–1000 μequiv./g. hr. (Fig. 4.12): clearly, major activities of the tissue are being evoked.

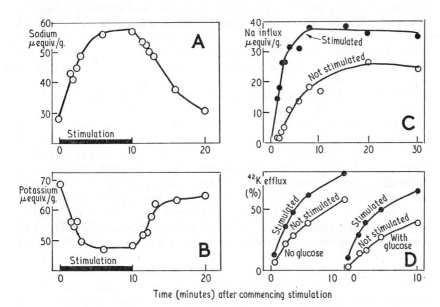

Time (minutes) after commencing stimulation

Fig. 4.12. Movements of the sodium and potassium of cerebral tissues on electrical stimulation (Cummins & McIlwain, 1961; Keesey & Wallgren, 1965; Keesey, Wallgren & McIlwain, 1965; see Krebs *et al.*, 1951).

A, B. Changes in tissue content: guinea pig cerebral cortex was incubated for 30 min. in bicarbonate glucose salines with inulin and the first samples (zero time in the figure) taken. Pulses of exponential time–voltage relationship, 0·4 msec. time constant, were applied at 100/sec. for the periods indicated, tissues promptly transferred for determination of Na, K and inulin. Other tissues were stimulated for 10 min. and allowed 1·5–10 min. subsequent recovery before sampling.

C, D. Influx or efflux of Na and K. For influx tissues were preincubated as in A, B, ^{24}NaCl added, and tissue specimens removed for analysis and measurement of radioactivity. For efflux, tissues were preincubated in media containing ^{42}KCl, transferred to fresh media and the ^{42}K appearing in the fluid determined. Pulses, when applied, were as described in A, B; glucose was omitted from the medium in the cases indicated.

The changes on stimulation diminish Na and K gradients between tissue and fluid; the potential difference at the membrane, also, diminishes (C, Figs. 4.9 and 4.12). Both changes are dependent on electrical characteristics of the pulses applied, and when these are relatively sparse, of less than 10/sec. but otherwise of maximal effect, the initial rate of loss of K$^+$ is approx. 6 nequiv./g. tissue/pulse applied (McIlwain & Joanny, 1963). With such stimuli, a new stable state is reached in a few minutes and the tissue then contains more Na,

4

less K, and has increased in respiratory rate (see above). Maximal stimulation still leaves appreciable Na and K gradients though these are not easily observable as a membrane potential. Presumably the relative tissue permeability to Na and K (and possibly to Cl) has altered, as is indeed well established in other excitable systems. The composition of the stimulated tissue is now such that Na permeability is found by Equation (i), Chapter 3, to be 0·8 that of K.

Cognate information on tissue permeability has been obtained by adding ^{24}Na and ^{42}K salts to incubation media and following their rate of exit on subsequently transferring the tissue to fresh media (C, D, Fig. 4.12). In normal unstimulated tissue the influx or efflux of each ion can proceed at rates of 200–300 μequiv./g. hr. while the tissue content of 28 μequiv. Na and 70 μequiv. K/g., remains unchanged. This contrasts with much slower rates of exchange which obtain between blood and brain in vivo (see McIlwain, 1963) emphasizing the barrier phenomenon noted in Chapter 3.

Electrical stimulation greatly increases the ion fluxes so measured, not only during the period while net changes in ion content are taking place, but also subsequently when the tissue has reached a new, stable composition. Thus ^{24}NaCl, added after 10 min. stimulation to media containing tissues whose stimulation was continued, entered at rates corresponding to an influx of 1180 μequiv. Na/g. hr.: or 5 times the rate before stimulation, despite a smaller concentration gradient in Na between tissue and fluid (Keesey & Wallgren, 1965). Potassium exchange also increased with stimulation, by a factor of about 2·5 (Cummins & McIlwain, 1961). The relative change in Na and K permeability derived from this data will be noted as in the same sense as that implied from the change in the factor b introduced into the Nernst equation in Chapter 3, but numerically smaller. In absence of glucose, the tissue content of K was smaller but underwent exchange with ^{42}K of media at approximately the same rate (the percentage change in D, Fig. 4.12 is thus larger); and, again, stimulation increases the exchange. Thus the permeability alteration caused by electrical stimulation is largely independent of the major energy-metabolism of the tissue.

The behaviour of tissue calcium contrasts markedly with that of Na and K. The normal influx and efflux of 1·2 μmoles Ca/g. tissue/hr. were increased by some 0·07 μmoles/g. on stimulation, and net content did not change (Lolley, 1963). Influx of Ca^{2+} to nerve terminal preparations was however increased when external Na^+ was replaced by Li^+, which in addition diminished Ca^{2+} efflux (Blaustein & Wiesmann, 1970). Active extrusion of Ca^{2+} was concluded to involve a mechanism by which Ca^{2+} was exchanged for Na^+, and which derived energy from the Na^+ gradient.

Tissue Compartments and the Kinetics of Ion Exchange

By following in detail the fluxes of Na, K and Cl between cerebral tissues and surrounding fluids, valuable data have been obtained which characterize different compartments within the tissue. Tissues examined as in the experiments C, D of Fig. 4.12 but with frequent sampling or in flow-systems, afford data exemplified by Fig. 4.13. Here efflux of ^{24}Na and ^{42}K is expressed semilogarithmically and subjected to analysis by methods whose application to neural systems generally is appraised by Brindley (1963). Very rapid initial outflow of these isotopes and also of Cl^- was shown; by its Na and K content, its Na/K ratio, volume and speed of exchange this initial outflow was concluded to derive from the tissue's extracellular space.

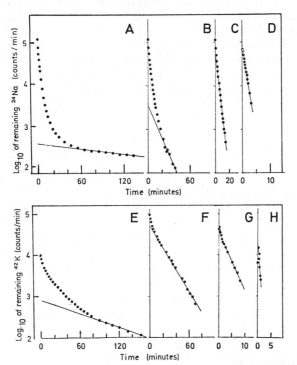

FIG. 4.13. ^{24}Na and ^{42}K remaining in neocortical tissues after their transfer from media containing the isotopes, to non-labelled media. (See Brindley, 1963; Keesey & Wallgren, 1965; Frank, 1970.)

A. Observed curve for ^{24}Na loss, with line characterizing the slowest component [(3) of Table 4.4]. The ordinate is logarithmic; the slope of the line gives the time for half-loss, $^{0.5}t$, of the component, and the extrapolation to zero time gives the quantity, q, of ^{24}Na originally present in this component.

B. Data obtained from the shorter-time results of A, by subtracting the radioactivity calculated as due at each time of observation, to the slower component; line characterizes component (2) of Table 4.4.

C. Similarly derived from B, and D from C.

E. Observed curve for ^{24}K-loss, with line characterizing the slowest component.

F, G, H, are derived successively from E by the method applied in calculating Na movements.

Among the less-rapidly exchanging components at least two, and with considerable likelihood three, fractions can be distinguished in tissues from the guinea pig, rat and frog (Keesey & Wallgren, 1965; Bradbury et al., 1968; Frank, 1970). Response to electrical excitation proved valuable in characterizing the components. Thus with the first of these cellular components, (1) of

Table 4.4, efflux of Na and K was little, if at all, affected by electrical stimulation of the tissue samples. This region (1) contained much more Na than K and was concluded to correspond to glial cells. Some 70–80 % of the tissue K was held by a component, (2) of Table 4.3, from which its efflux was relatively slow but was accelerated three- or four-fold by electrical excitation. Component (2) was low in Na but its Na was readily augmented on excitation. Thus (2) represented the major excitable component of the tissue; the quantity of K concerned showed it to represent the majority of neurons, probably including cell bodies and many cell-processes without differentiation among neuronal types. The component (3) was also richer in K than in Na, and responsive to excitation. It was however much smaller than component (2), exhibiting slower changes in Na and K, and was tentatively characterized as corresponding to the myelinated

Table 4.4

Tissue compartments characterized by cation movements

Values for rat neocortex at 37°, derived as described in Fig. 4.12. For the ascription of components (1) and (3), see text. For a corresponding analysis of Na^+ and Cl^- in the frog brain at a lower temperature, see Bradbury *et al.* (1968).

Measure	Tissue components			
	Extracellular	(1) Glial (?)	(2) Neuronal	(3) Myelineated (?)
Sodium:				
Quantity, μequiv./g.	61	32	8	2
Time for half-loss, min.	0·75	2·7	8·9	121
Potassium:				
Quantity, μequiv./g.	3	9	46	6
Time for half-loss, min.	0·5	5·5	15·2	46
Response of cation movements to electrical stimulation	None	Small	Large, Na and K	Large in K

portions of cerebral fibres. Supporting evidence for this came from its localization in the brain and the time at which it appeared during cerebral development (q.v.).

It will be recalled that microelectrode studies *in vivo* differentiated between neuronal and glial cells in terms of their relationships to electrolytes (Chapter 3): the glial cells assimilating K^+ released by neurons on stimulation. Correspondingly, it is found *in vitro* that the glia, comprising cellular compartment (1) of Table 4.4, undergo major changes when concentrations of K^+ in incubating fluids are increased (Frank, 1970; Hertz, 1968). This compartment can indeed increase four-fold in K^+ content in tissue from high-K^+ media. Such increase is necessarily accompanied by uptake of fluid, as are other circumstances in which tissues increase in electrolyte content: e.g. after addition of glutamate (Harvey & McIlwain, 1968). Here 7.2 ml. of water was absorbed for each mequiv. of cation, implying isoosmolar addition (see Table 3.2). By electron microscopic observations, uptake of fluid by cerebral tissues under several circumstances both *in vivo* and *in vitro* has been concluded to occur in astroglia; moreover, it is glia rather than neurons which respond to media of increased K^+, by increase in respiration (De Robertis & Carrea, 1965; Gerschenfeld *et al.*, 1959; Hertz, 1966).

It can thus be concluded that glial cells carry out processes of active cation transport which contribute to maintaining the extracellular fluids of the brain at their normal, relatively low K^+ content; they probably also contribute to regulating other solutes. Incubating isolated tissues in media of increased K^+ brings into operation this process of active transport, with utilization of ATP and increase in tissue respiration and glycolysis, attributable to the glial components of the tissue. On electrical stimulation in media of normal $[K^+]$, active transport is increased both in neuronal components (through Na entry) and in glia. Both categories of movement are blocked by agents which act at the neuronal components and inhibit the co-ordinated cation movements of the nerve impulse. It is presumably these factors which render the respiration, glycolysis or $\sim$P changes in electrically stimulated tissues susceptible to a wide range of blocking agents which have little effect on the same processes when these are stimulated by increased $[K^+]$.

Chemical Characterization of Systems which Control Cation Movements

Such characterization remains a fundamental need in neurochemical research in general, and is considered further in describing membrane structure in Chapter 12. The extensive cation movements induced on stimulating cell-containing cerebral tissues make such preparations valuable experimental systems, especially as the resulting Na^+ and K^+ movements have proved susceptible to minute quantities of specific inhibitors. The most active of such compounds is tetrodotoxin (Fig. 4.14), a naturally-occurring neurotoxic agent whose central actions *in vivo* received comment in Chapter 3.

Tetrodotoxin acted specifically on changes induced by excitation. It was without action on the Na^+ and K^+ content of isolated neocortical tissue maintained optimally in glucose salines, but electrical stimulation which normally doubled the tissue's Na^+ content had little or no effect in the presence of 20–50 nM-tetrodotoxin. Other responses of the tissue to stimulation were also inhibited by the toxin: loss of K^+, and increase in glycolysis and in respiration. Again, the toxin was without action on the same properties of unstimulated tissues. Tetrodotoxin was some 10^4 times more active than other acidic guanidines which were examined, and its structure must thus be judged to have a special relation to tissue processes concerned with excitation, and of these Na entry may be judged especially important (see Hille, 1968). Indeed the structural feature emphasized in Fig. 4.14 has its counterpart in phosphatidyl-serine (q.v.) and in glutamic acid which is a cerebral excitant of action partly antagonized by tetrodotoxin. Calculation showed tetrodotoxin to be active in an amount corresponding to some 100 molecules or fewer/μ^2 of neuronal surface, and each tetrodotoxin molecule supplied was concluded to block a site at which 10 or more Na^+ entered per stimulating pulse (McIlwain, 1967; McIlwain *et al.*, 1969). Actions of tetrodotoxin on the Na, K and water of cerebral tissues supported a role for glial cells similar to that outlined above (Okamoto & Quastel, 1970).

Other attempts to characterize cerebral membrane components with which entering cations might complex have been made using basic polypeptides and alkylating agents (Evans & McIlwain, 1967). Also relevant are actions of protoveratrine and of DDT or 1,1,1-trichloro-2,2-*bis*(*p*-chlorophenyl)ethane, which are believed to act by extending the period of Na entry which follows excitation (see Wollenberger, 1955; Hille, 1968; and Symposium, 1968).

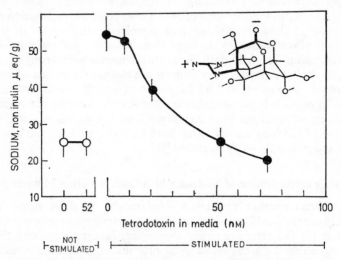

FIG. 4.14. Tetrodotoxin inhibition of electrically-induced Na⁺-entry to cerebral tissues.

In the tetrodotoxin structure shown in inset, bonds drawn heavily connect two ionic centres and are discussed further in the text. The tissue samples used were incubated in inulin-containing glucose salines, some with the tetrodotoxin concentrations stated, for 40 min. The tissues indicated were then electrically stimulated for 10 min., and at 50 min. all were rapidly transferred for analysis. Each point gives mean values from 4 samples, and vertical lines indicate the S.D. of the means (McIlwain, 1967; McIlwain, Harvey & Rodriguez, 1969).

Recovery After Stimulation

Energy-requiring processes are outstandingly involved in the changes which normally occur in the tissue when stimulation ceases. In the first 2 min. after the stimulation of Fig. 4.9 and 4.12, K is seen to re-enter the tissue, Na is extruded and membrane potential reappears. Glucose utilization is at first rapid, but then diminishes (McIlwain & Tresize, 1956). Phosphocreatine is resynthesized relatively slowly when ion recovery first commences, although it can be resynthesized in 30 sec. after a brief stimulus (Fig. 4.8) which involves little displacement of Na. In the period following the recovery of Na, phosphocreatine is resynthesized and glucose utilization returns to its lower, pre-stimulation value. Thus further experimental demonstration is given of the linkages outlined in Fig. 3.3.

Moreover, it is possible in the isolated tissue to approach the quantitative relationships between ion movements and the change in tissue phosphates or respiration. It was noted above that sparsely-applied stimuli of maximum effect caused an initial loss in K and gain in Na, of 6 nequiv./g. tissue/pulse. Subsequently Na and K concentrations were stable but respiration was increased by 1·56 nmoles/g. pulse (Fig. 4.4). Supposing that the new steady state resulted from a loss of K and gain in Na which also proceeded at 6 nequiv./g., then each mole of O_2 utilized was associated with movement of about 4 equiv. of Na and K. A different comparison may be made on the basis of events when stimuli are stopped. Fig. 4.8 shows that phosphocreatine can be resynthesized at 150 μmoles/g. tissue/hr. and A, Fig. 4.12, shows Na extrusion at 200 μequiv./g. hr. Supposing these to represent alternative ways of utilizing metabolically derived energy supplied at constant rate, 1 μmole of the phosphate is associated with extrusion of 1·3 μmoles Na. The continued investigation of this subject in preparations of cerebral membrane-structures is described in Chapter 12 (see also Symposium, 1968); the ratio quoted is minimal as it is based on net movement and not on total Na efflux.

An impressive range of electrical and metabolic characteristics of the brain *in vivo*, are thus reproduced by isolated fragments of cerebral tissue incubated in simple, chemically defined solutions. Nevertheless there are still lacking, chemically understandable linkages between the different characteristics measured and certain of these linkages are the subject of the following chapter.

REFERENCES

AHMED, K. & SCHOLEFIELD, P. G. (1961). *Biochem. J.* **81**, 45.
ASHFORD, C. A. & DIXON, K. C. (1935). *Biochem. J.* **29**, 157.
AYRES, P. J. W. & McILWAIN, H. (1953). *Biochem. J.* **55**, 607.
BACHELARD, H. S., CAMPBELL, W. J. & McILWAIN, H. (1962). *Biochem. J.* **84**, 225.
BELOFF-CHAIN, A., CATANZARO, R., CHAIN, E. B., MASI, I. & POCCHIARI, F. (1955). *Proc. Roy. Soc.* B. **144**, 22.
BLAUSTEIN, M. P. & WIESMANN, W. P. (1970). *Proc. nat. Acad. Sci., U.S.* **66**, 664.
BOURKE, R. S. & TOWER, D. B. (1966). *J. Neurochem.* **13**, 1071, 1099.
BRADBURY, M. W. B., VILLAMIL, M. & KLEEMAN, C. R. (1968). *Amer. J. Physiol.* **214**, 643.
BRADFORD, H. F., CHAIN, E. B., CORY, H. & ROSE, S. P. R. (1969). *J. Neurochem.* **16**, 969.
BRIERLEY, J. B. & McILWAIN, H. (1956). *J. Neurochem.* **1**, 109.
BRINDLEY, F. J. (1963). *Internat. Rev. Neurobiol.* **5**, 200.
CAMPBELL, W. J., McILWAIN, H., RICHARDS, C. D. & SOMERVILLE, A. R. (1967). *J. Neurochem.* **14**, 937.
CHAIN, E. B., ROSE, S. P. R., MASI, I. & POCCHIARI, F. (1969). *J. Neurochem.* **16**, 93.
CORY, H. & ROSE, S. P. R. (1969). *J. Neurochem.* **16**, 979.
CUMMINS, J. T. & McILWAIN, H. (1961). *Biochem. J.* **79**, 330.
DÉLÈZE, J. (1970). *J. Physiol.* **208**, 547.
DE ROBERTIS, E. & CARREA, R. (1965). (Ed.). *Progr. Brain Res.* **15**.
DICKENS, F. (1936). *Biochem. J.* **30**, 1233.
DICKENS, F. & GREVILLE, G. D. (1935). *Biochem. J.* **29**, 1468.
DIPIETRO, D. & WEINHOUSE, S. (1959). *Arch. Bioch. Biophys.* **80**, 268.
ELLIOTT, H. W. & SUTHERLAND, V. C. (1952). *J. cell. comp. Physiol.* **40**, 221.
ELLIOTT, K. A. C. & WOLFE, L. S. (1962). Neurochemistry, p. 177. Ed. Elliott *et al.* Springfield: Thomas.
EVANS, W. H. & McILWAIN, H. (1967). *J. Neurochem.* **14**, 35.

FIELD, J. (1948). *Meth. in Med. Res.* 1, 289.
FRANK, G. (1970). Sur la composition ionique des tranches de cerveau de rat. Liège: Université.
FRANK, G., CORNETTE, M. & SCHOFFENIELS, E. (1968). *J. Neurochem.* 15, 843.
GAINER, H., ALLWEIS, C. L. & CHAIKOFF, I. L. (1962). *J. Neurochem.* 9, 433.
GERHARDT, W., CLAUSEN, J., CHRISTENSEN, E. & RUSHEDE, J. (1963). *Acta Neurol. Scand.* 39, 85.
GERSCHENFELD, H. M., WALD, F., ZADUNAISKY, J. A. & DE ROBERTIS, E. (1959). *Neurology*, 9, 412.
GIBSON, I. M. & MCILWAIN, H. (1965). *J. Physiol.* 176, 261.
GONCHAROVA, E. E. (1963). Proc. 3rd All-Union Neurochem. Conf., Erevan, p. 455. Ed. Palladin & Buniatian. Acad. Sci. Armenian SSR.
GRAYMORE, C. N. (1969). In The Eye, p. 601. Ed. H. Davson. London: Academic Press.
HARVEY, J. A. & MCILWAIN, H. (1968). *Biochem. J.* 108, 269.
HASLAM, R. J. & KREBS, H. A. (1963). *Biochem. J.* 88, 566
HEALD, P. J. (1954). *Biochem. J.* 57, 673.
HEALD, P, J. & MCILWAIN, H. (1956). *Biochem. J.* 63, 231.
HEILBRUNN, L. V. (1952). Outline of General Physiology. London: Saunders.
HERTZ, L. (1966). *J. Neurochem.* 13, 1373.
HERTZ, L. (1968). *J. Neurochem.* 15, 1.
HILL, A. V. (1932). Chemical Wave Transmission in Nerve. Cambridge: University Press.
HILLE, B. (1968). *J. Gen. Physiol.* 51, 199.
HILLMAN, H, H., CAMPBELL, W. J. & MCILWAIN, H. (1963). *J. Neurochem.* 10, 325.
HILLMAN, H. H. & MCILWAIN, H. (1961). *J. Physiol.* 157, 263.
HIMWICH, H. E. (1951). Brain Metabolism and Cerebral Disorders. Baltimore: Williams & Wilkins.
HOROWICZ, P. & LARRABEE, M. G. (1962). *J. Neurochem.* 9, 1.
KAWAI, N. & YAMAMOTO, C. (1968). *Brain Res.* 7, 325.
KEESEY, J. C. & WALLGREN, H. (1965). *Biochem. J.* 95, 301.
KEESEY, J. C., WALLGREN, H. & MCILWAIN, H. (1965). *Biochem. J.* 95, 289.
KETY, S. S., WOODFORD, R. B., HARMEL, M. H., FREYHAN, F. A., APPEL, K. E. & SCHMIDT, C. F. (1948). *Amer. J. Pyschiat.* 104, 765.
KHAIKINA, B. I. (1963). Proc. 3rd All-Union Neurochem. Conf., Erevan, p. 447. Ed. Palladin & Buniatian. Acad. Sci. Armenian SSR.
KIRSCH, W. M., LEITNER, J. W., SCHULZ, D. & BUSKIRK, J. W. (1969). *Second Internat. Neurochem. Meeting*, p. 242. Milan: Tamburini.
KLEIN, J. R. & OLSEN, N. S. (1947). *J. biol. Chem.* 167, 747.
KOREY, S. R. & ORCHEN, M. (1959). *J. Neurochem.* 3, 277.
KRATZING, C. C. (1953). *Biochem. J.* 54, 312.
KREBS, H. A. (1950). *Biochim. Biophys. Acta*, 4, 249.
KREBS, H. A. (1961). *Biochem. J.* 80, 225.
KREBS, H. A., EGGLESTON, L. V. & TERNER, C. (1951). *Biochem. J.* 48, 530.
KREUTZBERG, G. W., MINAUF, M. & GULLOTA, F. (1966). *Histochemie*, 6, 8.
LARRABEE, M. (1958). *J. Neurochem.* 2, 81.
LARRABEE, M. G. & BRONK, D. W. (1952). *Cold Spring Harbor Symp.* 17, 245.
LEBARON, F. N. (1955). *Biochem. J.* 61, 80.
LIBET, B. & GERARD, R. W. (1939). *J. Neurophysiol.* 2, 153.
LI, C-L. & MCILWAIN, H. (1957). *J. Physiol.* 139, 178.
LOLLEY, R. N. (1963). *J. Neurochem.* 10, 665.
LOLLEY, R. N. & MCILWAIN, H. (1964). *Biochem. J.* 93, 12P.
MCILWAIN, H. (1951). *Biochem. J.* 49, 382.
MCILWAIN, H. (1953). *Biochem. J.* 55, 618; *J. Neurol. Neurosurg. Psychiat.* 16, 257.
MCILWAIN, H. (1954). *EEG Clin. Neurophysiol.* 6, 93; *Arch. Neurol. Psychiat.* 71, 488.
MCILWAIN, H. (1956). *Physiol. Rev.* 36, 355.
MCILWAIN, H. (1960). *J. Neurochem.* 6, 244.
MCILWAIN, H. (1963). Chemical Exploration of the Brain. A study of cerebral excitability and ion movement. Amsterdam: Elsevier.

McIlwain, H. (1967). *Biochem. Pharmacol.* **16**, 1389.
McIlwain, H. (1968). *Progr. Brain Res.*, **29**, 273; *Brit. med. Bull.* **24**, 174.
McIlwain, H. (1969). In Basic Mechanisms of the Epilepsies, p. 83. Ed. Jasper, Ward & Pope. New York: Little, Brown.
McIlwain, H. (1970). In Wates Symposium on the Blood Brain Barrier. Ed. R. V. Coxon. Oxford: Physiological Laboratory.
McIlwain, H., Buchel, L. & Cheshire, J. D. (1951). *Biochem. J.* **48**, 12.
McIlwain, H. & Grinyer, I. (1950). *Biochem. J.* **46**, 620.
McIlwain, H., Harvey, J. A. & Rodriguez, G. (1969). *J. Neurochem.* **16**, 363.
McIlwain, H. & Joanny, P. (1963). *J. Neurochem.* **10**, 313.
McIlwain, H. & Rodnight, R. (1962). Practical Neurochemistry. London: Churchill.
McIlwain, H. & Snyder, S. (1970). *J. Neurochem.* **17**, 521.
McIlwain, H. & Tresize, M. A. (1956). *Biochem. J.* **63**, 250.
Noell, W. K. (1951). *J. cell. comp. Physiol.* **37**, 283.
Okamoto, K. & Quastel, J. H. (1970). *Biochem. J.* **120**, 25, 37.
Pappius, H. M., Johnson, D. M. & Elliott, K. A. C. (1959). *Canad. J. Biochem. Physiol.* **37**, 999.
Pappius, H. M., Klatze, I. & Elliott, K. A. C. (1962). *Canad. J. Biochem. Physiol.* **40**, 885.
Phillips, G. B. (1964). *Proc. Soc. exp. Biol. Med.* **115**, 918.
Pirie, A. & van Heyningen, R. (1956). Biochemistry of the Eye. Oxford: Blackwell.
Richards, C. D. & McIlwain, H. (1967). *Nature*, **215**, 704.
Richards, C. D. & Sercombe, R. (1968). *J. Physiol.* **197**, 667.
Ridge, J. W. (1967). *Biochem. J.* **105**, 831.
Rodnight, R. & McIlwain, H. (1954). *Biochem. J.* **57**, 649.
Setchell, B. P. (1959). *Biochem. J.* **72**, 265, 275.
Shimizu, N. & Hamuro, Y. (1958). *Nature, Lond.* **181**, 781.
Sutherland, V. C., Burbridge, T. N. & Elliott, H. W. (1956). *Amer. J. Physiol.* **180**, 195.
Symposium (1938). *Res. Publ. Ass. nerv. ment. Dis.* **18**.
Symposium (1968). Cell Membrane Biophysics. *J. Gen. Physiol.* **51**.
Tiraspolskaya, M. M. & Toropova, M. N. (1963). *Arkh. Patol.* **25**, 34.
Thomas, J. (1957). *Biochem. J.* **66**, 655.
Tower, D. B. (1958). *J. Neurochem.* **4**, 185.
Tower, D. B. (1960). Neurochemistry of Epilepsy. Springfield: Thomas.
Utena, H., Ezoe, T. & Kato, N. (1955). *Psychiat. et Neurol. jap.* **57**, 124.
Utena, H., Ezoe, T., Kato, N. & Hada, H. (1959). *J. Neurochem.* **4**, 161.
Varon, S. & McIlwain, H. (1961). *J. Neurochem.* **8**, 262.
Victor, J. & Wolf, A. (1937). *Proc. Ass. Res. nerv. ment. Dis.* **16**, 44.
Warburg, O. (1930). The Metabolism of Tumours. Tr. F. Dickens. London: Constable.
Winterstein, H. (1929). Bethe's Handbuch, **9**. Berlin: Springer.
Wollenberger, A. (1955). *Biochem. J.* **61**, 77.
Woodman, R. J. & McIlwain, H. (1961). *Biochem. J.* **81**, 83.
Yamamoto, C. & Kawai, N. (1967). *Experientia*, **23**, 821; *Exper. Neurol.* **19**, 176.
Yamamoto, C. & Kawai, N. (1968). *Jap. J. Physiol.* **18**, 620.
Yamamoto, C. & Kurokawa, M. (1968). *Proc. Jap. Acad.* **44**, 1684.
Yamamoto, C. & McIlwain, H. (1966). *J. Neurochem.* **13**, 1333.

5 Cell-Free Cerebral Systems: Glycolysis and the Pentose Phosphate Pathway

Major metabolic problems have been left unsolved after the study of cerebral preparations with cell-structure largely intact. Thus, although interconnections have been discerned between respiration or glycolysis and phosphocreatine, inorganic phosphate or adenosine triphosphate, investigation of their nature requires other techniques. When the phosphates are added to sliced cerebral tissues, they have little or no effect on respiration or glycolysis. It is the very autonomy of the cell-containing tissues, which makes them so valuable in understanding reactions *in vivo*, which also makes it necessary to modify or destroy cell structure in order to appreciate reactions in the component systems which the cells contain. In cell-free cerebral preparations added phosphates are displayed as major reactants, necessary for carbohydrate metabolism and interconverted during its progress.

These interconversions are similar in principle in cerebral and in most other tissues of the animal body. The pathways through which carbohydrate is metabolized in the brain form intricately-linked sets of reactions of which almost all the known steps have been studied specifically in cerebral tissues. It is the specifically cerebral studies which are the primary concern of the present chapter, and other studies are mentioned only briefly and in order that those with systems from the brain should be understandable. Presenting the subject in this fashion enables gaps to be perceived in knowledge of cerebral metabolism, but carries the danger of implying more than findings in cerebral tissues themselves would warrant. This danger must not be minimized, but at the same time it can be indicated that several of the studies which first contributed to general schemes of carbohydrate metabolism were in fact initially made with cerebral tissues and later found more generally applicable. For the general schemes and their development, see Dickens (1951), Ochoa (1954), Krebs & Kornberg (1957), Symposia (1953, 1959), Boyer, Lardy & Myrback (1959–63) and Dickens, Randle & Whelan (1968).

Transition from Cell-containing to Cell-free Systems

A variety of processes may be used for breaking the cell-structure of cerebral tissues for metabolic studies: repeated freezing and thawing, rapid vibration, or treatment with organic solvents; but the simplest method, commonly used and effective, is mechanical disruption. For most metabolic studies this is best performed rapidly and just above 0°C, by rubbing the tissue between two surfaces in a mortar and pestle or with a glass or plastic pestle in a test tube "homogenizer". A fluid, which may simply be water or may carry buffers and substrates, is usually added during the rubbing so that a suspension of the tissue results, of which uniform samples can be taken. A large-scale mechanical homogenizer has been devised and appraised specifically for the production of cell-free dispersions of cerebral tissues (Rodnight *et al.*, 1969).

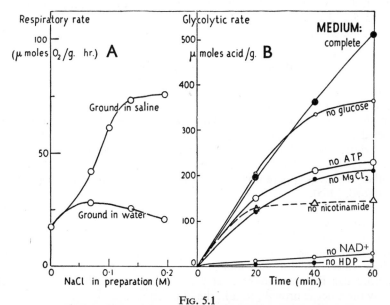

FIG. 5.1

A. Respiration of suspensions of rat cerebral cortex dispersed in fluids under different conditions. Above: in NaCl of the molarities given as abscissae. Below: ground in water and NaCl added later to the levels given as abscissae. Respiration was determined manometrically in a medium containing glucose and inorganic salts and buffered with phosphate. Data from Elliott & Libet (1942).

B. Showing the necessity for six substances in anaerobic glycolysis of dispersions from cerebral tissues of rat or mouse. The complete medium contained (mM) $NaHCO_3$, 45; Na and K phosphates, pH 7·3, 10; $MgCl_2$, 8; glucose, 28; hexose diphosphate (HDP), 2·5; adenosine triphosphate (ATP), 0·7; nicotinamide adenine dinucleotide (NAD^+), 0·5; and nicotinamide, 40 (Utter *et al.*, 1945).

At first, especially if the rubbing is carried out with an isotonic suspending medium, many cell-bodies in cerebral tissues remain intact, some with stumps of their axons but shorn of most of the axon and of dendrites. Subsequently, the cell bodies are broken; in hypotonic solutions the changes occur more quickly. Concomitantly, the metabolic properties of the preparations change. A, Fig. 5.1 shows how respiration has been found smaller and less stable with breakdown of cell structure in the more hypotonic media. Different biochemical activities of a given cell are often very clearly localized in its component parts (Chapter 12). When, in the ground tissue, all components are present many interactions occur between them and feature in the present account. Grinding a tissue of several cell types, as cerebral cortex, necessarily gives a mixture of their various components. Preliminary microdissection or other separation can avoid this but has not been carried out in the majority of cases described below.

Study of carbohydrate metabolism in cell-free systems depends on the knowledge that in spite of loss of cell structure, such metabolism can continue at rates akin to those *in vivo*. Evidence for this is presented first in the account which follows in this and the subsequent chapter. Individual metabolic stages (Tables 5.2, 5.3, and 6.2) are then described and their role in the central nervous system assessed.

Routes of Carbohydrate Metabolism

The routes of carbohydrate metabolism in the brain are similar to those which operate generally in mammalian cells, except that gluconeogenesis has not been shown to occur cerebrally. Although glucose-6-phosphatase has been detected histochemically (Tewari & Bourne, 1963) and its presence inferred also from arteriovenous differences in ^{14}C-labelled glucose-6-phosphate (Sacks & Sacks, 1968), the fructose diphosphatase necessary for gluconeogenesis in other tissues is apparently absent from the mammalian brain (Krebs & Woodford, 1965).

A further characteristic of carbohydrate metabolism in the brain is the relatively low carbohydrate store of the organ. The glycogen levels are quite small for a tissue so dependent on its sources of energy; there is also little or no intracellular glucose (see Bachelard & McIlwain, 1969). The levels of intermediates of carbohydrate metabolism are also quite low (Table 5.2). The brain therefore has little fuel reserve as carbohydrate and relies on using very rapidly the glucose brought to it in the bloodstream.

Pathway-evaluation studies have produced much evidence in support of the view that, in adult mammalian brain, carbohydrate metabolism commences almost entirely by glycolysis and that the contribution of the direct oxidative pathway, the pentose phosphate pathway, is quite small. This shunt pathway makes a greater contribution in the immature brain, when more NADPH is needed, e.g. for fat synthesis (Chapter 11) and also in the adult brain it is of greater importance in heavily myelinated tracts. For these reasons the glycolytic sequence is described first in the present chapter, and followed by a brief description of the pentose phosphate pathway.

Glycolysis

Utilization of glucose by the brain *in vivo* proceeds normally at some 18 μmoles/g. hr., and of this some 3 μmoles/g. are converted to 6 μmoles of lactic acid in each hour (Table 5.1). The formation of lactic acid can however greatly increase when oxygen is limited or when cerebral activity increases, and rates of some 400–1,000 μmoles/g. hr. are then reached during brief periods (King *et al.*, 1967; see also Chapter 3). Rates sustained anaerobically or on stimulation in sliced cerebral cortex are usually lower: of some 100 μmoles/g. hr. It is therefore especially valuable to find that under suitable conditions the high *in vivo* rates can be reproduced and maintained in the cell-free tissue.

Lactic Acid Production

For maintenance of high rates of glycolysis by cerebral dispersions it is necessary to add to the suspension many more components than glucose, as is shown by the experiment illustrated in **B**, Fig. 5.1. Here the formation of acid, shown chemically to be lactic acid, is indicated by the displacement of CO_2 from bicarbonate. It is seen that a more immediate source of lactic acid than glucose, is hexose diphosphate, for without the diphosphate little acid is formed. Glucose is however required for continued glycolysis, and as will be seen below its breakdown proceeds through the diphosphate. It is thus understandable that a phosphorylating agent such as adenosine triphosphate should be required; addition is necessary because that native to the cell has been diluted or degraded. For long-continued glycolysis, repeated addition of adenosine triphosphate has been found necessary (Meyerhof & Geliazkova, 1947). Degradation by adenosine triphosphatases (q.v.) occurs to varying degrees in differently prepared extracts of cerebral tissues and contributes to their varying behaviour towards phosphate derivatives. Thus, initially, glycolysis in the brain was erroneously described as radically different from that in other tissues in not involving phosphorylation, but fuller investigations showed the intimate connections with phosphates now to be described, which are of outstanding importance to the course of glycolysis and to its control.

The nicotinamide adenine dinucleotide (NAD$^+$; formerly DPN) and nicotinamide itself are also among the requirements for cerebral glycolysis (**B**, Fig. 5.1). Again, it is necessary to add NAD$^+$ because that native to the tissue is diluted in preparing the glycolysing suspension. The effect of the added coenzyme is however short-lived; it also is rapidly degraded by ground cerebral tissues. This degradation is inhibited by nicotinamide which is one of its products (Chapter 10), and in the presence of both the coenzyme and nicotinamide, lactic acid formation can be maintained at some 500 μmoles/g. hr. for some hours. If these two components are omitted a clear indication of point of action of the coenzyme is obtained: ground cerebral tissues with glucose, magnesium salts, and adenosine triphosphate yielded hexose diphosphate and triose phosphates, but not lactic acid (Weil-Malherbe & Bone, 1951). The NAD$^+$ as in other tissues, is required for the further metabolism of the triose phosphates.

Glycolysis and Phosphorylation in Cerebral Extracts

When cerebral tissues are ground in aqueous fluids and the resulting suspensions centrifuged, the soluble extracts so obtained, free from structural elements of the tissue, are capable of high rates of glycolysis. Again, additional substances, such as those just described, are necessary for the reaction; when these are supplied the rate per unit weight of original tissue is only a little lower than in the whole suspension (Table 5.1). Such extraction may be performed under conditions in which the subcellular particles remain intact in the precipitate removed on centrifuging; thus the enzymes yielding lactate from glucose are largely in solution in the cytoplasm of the cells (see also Chapter 12).

The glycolytic enzymes in aqueous extracts survive dialysis, so allowing the effect of many diffusible components of the reaction to be studied quantitatively (Fig. 5.1). It then becomes evident that inorganic orthophosphate plays a special role: Fig. 5.2 shows how, in absence of added inorganic phosphate, no lactate at all is produced; when inorganic phosphate is provided then, concomitantly with glycolysis, the phosphate is esterified. The necessary additions

Table 5.1.

Rate of formation of lactic acid by cerebral tissues

Conditions	Species or part	Rate (μmoles/g. hr.)
In situ, normal	Man	6
In situ, convulsing[1]	Cat or dog	400
Sliced cerebral cortex, normal	Man[2]	25
Sliced cerebral cortex, maximal sustained electrical excitation	Man[2]	75
	Rat	100
Sliced cerebral cortex, anaerobically	Rat[3]	100
	Man[5]	85
Sliced cerebral cortex, 20 sec. electrical excitation	Rat	400
Ground rat tissues, anaerobically[4]	Cerebrum	560
	Cerebellum	520
	Medulla	525
	Cord	395
Ground, centrifuged, and dialysed rat tissues[6]		300

[1] Olsen & Klein (1946). [2] McIlwain (1953). [3] Warburg (1930). [4] Utter *et al.* (1945), with some assumptions regarding the dry weight of the tissues. [5] Elliott & Penfield (1948). [6] Geiger (1940).

include also small quantities of hexose diphosphate, magnesium adenosine triphosphate and NAD^+.

As products of the esterification, adenosine di- and triphosphates, phosphopyruvates, and hexose phosphates were characterized. It is especially important to see the formation under anaerobic conditions of the important energy-rich phosphates. Their anaerobic formation has also been shown in a cerebral extract provided with hexose diphosphate and pyruvate (Ochoa, 1941); in such a mixture the addition of creatine both increased the formation of lactic acid, and allowed creatine phosphate to accumulate. The extracts presumably contained a creatine phosphokinase (q.v.) as has been indicated also by the ability of phosphocreatine to act in place of adenosine triphosphate in initiating glycolysis from glucose.

Intracellular glycogen is an important source of lactic acid in the brain *in vivo*; but because it is not diffusible it cannot effectively be made available as a substrate by adding it to the sliced tissue. It is therefore especially valuable to find that it is acted upon by cerebral extracts, yielding up to 150 µmoles lactate/hr. with an extract from 1 g. tissue (Geiger, 1940). Glycogen added to cerebral extracts already provided with glucose and other components for optimal lactate production, did not further increase the lactate, emphasizing that common steps are involved in its formation from the two components.

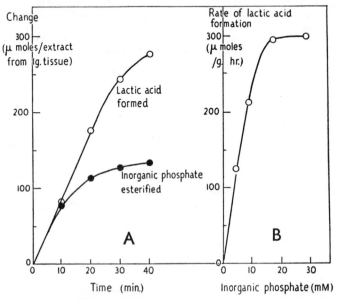

Fig. 5.2. Relation of glycolysis in cerebral extracts to inorganic phosphate (Geiger, 1940; see also Ochoa, 1941). Extracts were prepared by dispersing rat brain in 4 volumes of water; the reaction mixtures contained also $NaHCO_3$, hexose diphosphate, adenosine triphosphate, nicotinamide adenine dinucleotide, inorganic phosphate and magnesium salts, and were incubated at 37° in N_2–5% CO_2.
  A. Course of change in lactate and phosphate.
  B. Dependence of lactate formation on concentration of inorganic phosphate; the extract was dialysed.

Of substances which are unlikely to be normal sources of cerebral lactate, fructose and mannose can yield lactate as rapidly as does glucose (Geiger, 1940; Meyerhof *et al.*, 1947, 1948) but higher concentrations are required of these two sugars than of glucose. Galactose, sorbose, arabinose and xylose yielded little if any lactate.

Individual Stages in Glycolysis

The fashion in which conversion of glucose to lactic acid yields esterified phosphate can be appreciated by examining the individual enzymes concerned in the transformation. So far as is known these are similar in cerebral and in other tissues and are listed in Table 5.2. All have now been examined specific-ally in cerebral tissues, and some have been obtained from this source in a high degree of purity. Extensive surveys have been made of their activities in different parts of the brain.

Table 5.2

Glycolysis: concentrations of intermediates and rates of individual stages

Values for concentrations were obtained from rat or mouse brain rapidly frozen *in situ* (Lowry *et al.*, 1964; Passonneau *et al.*, 1969; Leloir, 1953; Merrick, 1961). The ranges of values in different species and parts of the brain are quoted in several instances in the text; see also Lowry *et al.*, 1954; Strominger & Lowry, 1955; Robins *et al.*, 1957; Buell *et al.*, 1958.

Concentrations of intermediates of glycogen metabolism were (μmoles/g.): glycogen, as glucose, 2·2–5·1; UDP-glucose, 0·1; glucose-1,6-diphosphate, 0·03–0·08.

Substance	Cerebral concentration (μmoles/g.)	Enzyme (K_m,mM)	Rate (μmoles/g. fresh wt. hr.) A[†]	B[‡]
Glucose*	1·25–1·55			
↓		Hexokinase, 0·05	600[1], 1,275[2]	660
Glucose-6-phosphate*	0·065–0·08			
↓		Glucose phosphate isomerase, 0·03	3,000[3]	3,300
Fructose-6-phosphate	0·016			
↓		Phosphofructokinase, 0·025	1,600	540
Fructose-1:6-diphosphate*	0·12			
↓		Aldolase, 0·01–0·04	345[4]	310
Glyceraldehyde-3-phosphate and dihydroxyacetone phosphate*	0·3			
↓		Triosephosphate isomerase	–	–
Glyceraldehyde-3-phosphate	–			
↓		Glyceraldehyde phosphate dehydrogenase, 0·044	1,200[1]	3,360
1:3-Diphosphoglycerate	–			
↓		Phosphoglycerate kinase, 0·01	1,600[5]	10,000
3-Phosphoglycerate* ⎫				
↓ ⎬	0·1–0·5	Phosphoglyceromutase, 0·24	2,000[5]	2,340
2-Phosphoglycerate* ⎭				
↓		D-2-Phosphoglycerate hydro-lyase (enolase), 0·033	800[6]	1,800
Phospho-enolpyruvate*	0·8			
↓		ATP-pyruvate phosphotransferase, 0·058	4,500[5]	7,080
Pyruvate*	0·1–0·2			
↓		Lactate dehydrogenase, 0·03	3,400[5]	3,540
Lactate*	2			

* Concentrations of the substances asterisked in young, anaesthetized mice are given in Fig. 7.2.
† *A.* Various species; see references above, and: [1] Laatsch, 1962, [2] Bachelard, 1967; [3] Robinson & Phillips, 1964; [4] Nicholas & Bachelard, 1969, 1971; [5] Fellenberg *et al.*, 1962; [6] Wood, 1964.
‡ *B.* Adult mice: Lowry & Passonneau, 1964.

In the present account of such enzymes, emphasis will be placed on the rates at which the individual reactions proceed, in order that their adequacy as basis for carbohydrate metabolism in the intact brain may be judged. In such assessment it is especially necessary to note whenever possible how the speed of reaction depends on the concentrations of reactants and of any activating substances, and to compare their concentrations with those found to occur in the tissue *in vivo* (see for example Bachelard & Goldfarb, 1969). To determine the maximum speed of reaction of which a given weight of tissue is capable, it must be examined with this object in view, and often in a fashion different from that which would be chosen for purifying the enzyme concerned. Assay of cerebral systems for maximum activity has been carried out with all the enzymes quoted in Table 5.2. In the following discussion, most attention will be paid to rates in preparations from the brain as a whole without separation to its parts, as such rates offer the most direct comparison with metabolic data available for the brain *in vivo*. It will be noted from data below that individual areas of grey matter often show rates up to 3 times as great as those of the mixed tissue.

Hexokinase

The most rapid cerebral reaction found to involve glucose itself is its phosphorylation by adenosine triphosphate to glucose-6-phosphate, catalysed by a hexokinase. Hexokinase (EC 2.7.1.1) has been carefully studied in cerebral preparations and its properties indicate that it can constitute a limiting or controlling factor in the metabolism of glucose by the brain *in vivo*.

Cerebral tissues show high hexokinase activity, in keeping with their dependence on carbohydrate metabolism. Long (1952) and Bennett *et al.* (1962), studying conditions for optimal activity of hexokinase, found higher levels in rat brain than in the fourteen other tissues examined; the reaction proceeded at 390 μmoles glucose/g. whole brain/hr. and reached 1400 μmoles/g. hr. in certain areas. The enzyme thus proceeds at a rate fully consistent with its participation in the formation of lactic acid at the highest rates which have been observed in the brain (Table 5.1). Its activity is not however greatly in excess of these rates, and hexokinase may thus represent a limiting factor in glycolysis in the brain *in vivo* when glycolysis is maximally stimulated, for example electrically.

The hexokinase prepared from cerebral tissues proceeds at maximal rate with glucose at 0·15 mM or higher, and with adenosine triphosphate at or above 1·5 mM (Fig. 5.3). Analysis of whole brain shows that its glucose content is about 1 mM and its adenosine triphosphate about 3 μmoles/g. Electrical stimulation of the brain permits reactions involving glucose and adenosine triphosphate at rates commensurate with these values, but in the normal tissue this does not take place. Inhibition of the enzyme by its products, glucose-6-phosphate and adenosine diphosphate, contributes to the lower values and is shown by the cerebral enzyme but not by that from yeast; it increases with increasing adenosine triphosphate and above 2mM triphosphate, 1·8 mM glucose-6-phosphate inhibited by 72% (Crane & Sols, 1953). Glucose-6-phosphate inhibition is thus very active, although the effect *in vivo* is unlikely to be as great as this in view of the low concentrations of the product which occur intracellularly in the intact tissue (Table 5.2). The inhibition exhibits noncompetitive kinetics (A, Fig. 5.4) with one of the substrates, glucose (K_i, 0·4 mM). It may also be non-competitive with regard to ATP; this was shown in the presence of excess ATP (Newsholme *et al.*, 1968) but when studied with constant excess of Mg, the inhibition appeared to be competitive with ATP (Fromm & Zewe, 1962). The importance of the Mg/ATP ratio has also been emphasized in studies on the mechanism of ADP inhibition (Bachelard & Goldfarb, 1969). Inhibition by ADP (K_i, 0·4 mM), although less potent *in vitro* than that by glucose-6-phosphate, is relevant also if the higher cerebral concentrations of ADP are considered. The inhibition is of the mixed type, both V_{max} and K_m being affected by change in ATP concentration (**B**, Fig. 5.4). Free ATP (K_i, 0·4 mM) is also inhibitory (**C**, Fig. 5.4) and the effective substrate is likely to be MgATP.

In vivo, inhibition by free ATP may condition reaction rate, as the concentrations of available Mg are likely to be less than those of ATP (Fromm & Zewe, 1962; Newsholme *et al.*, 1968; Bachelard & Goldfarb, 1969; Ning *et al.*,

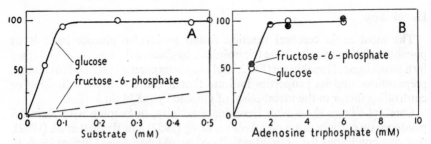

FIG. 5.3. Phosphorylation of glucose and of fructose 6 phosphate by cerebral preparations.

A. Dependence of hexokinase and phosphofructokinase on the concentration of their respective substrates glucose and fructose 6 phosphate. Reaction mixtures contained also a few mg. of aqueous extract of rat brain, 3 or 6 mM adenosine triphosphate, NaHCO₃, MgCl₂ and NaF.

B. Dependence of the two enzymes on concentration of adenosine triphosphate. Glucose was used as substrate at 1·85 mM and hexosephosphate (Robison mixture of the glucose- and fructose-6-phosphates) at 3·5 mM (Weil-Malherbe & Bone, 1951).

1969.) This pattern of inhibition by glucose-6-phosphate with mixed inhibition by ADP and by free ATP, indicates the possibility of four sites on the hexokinase enzyme: for glucose, glucose-6-phosphate, MgATP and ADP.

Systems removing glucose-6-phosphate, as phosphofructokinase, can thus appear to activate hexokinase (Long & Thomson, 1955), and the activity will depend, *inter alia*, on ATP/ADP ratios present in the tissue. The presence of other activators and inhibitors of the enzyme in body fluids in different pathological and hormonal conditions has been investigated (see Stern, 1954).

In contrast to other cerebral glycolytic enzymes, which are essentially cytoplasmic in occurrence, much of the hexokinase is attached to particulate matter and separates from tissue homogenates with mitochondria (Crane & Sols, 1953). The percentage of total hexokinase in mitochondrial fractions varies from 30 to over 75 in different preparations from various species; the remainder occurs mainly in the soluble cytoplasmic fraction. Whereas the activity in the intact mitochondria differed slightly from that of the cytoplasm

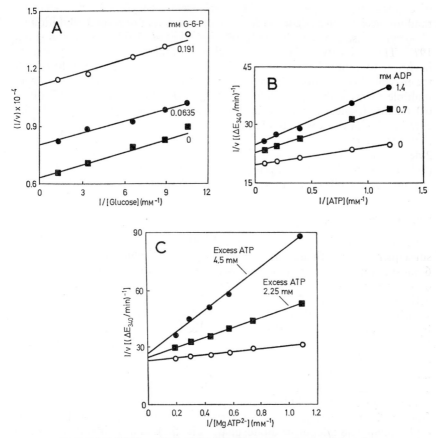

FIG. 5.4 Inhibition of cerebral hexokinase by glucose-6-phosphate, adenosine diphosphate and free adenosine triphosphate.

A. Glucose-6-phosphate (G6P) inhibition of a purified hexokinase from calf brain. Initial velocities were measured at 28° over 9½ min. in the presence of 2·24 mM–$MgCl_2$ and 1·12mM–ATP in buffered reaction mixtures at pH 7·6. The double reciprocal plots demonstrate that the inhibition is non-competitive for glucose (Fromm & Zewe, 1962).

B. Adenosine diphosphate (ADP) inhibition of purified ox brain hexokinase. Reaction mixtures were buffered at pH 7·6. and initial velocities were measured at 37° with 2mM-glucose. The Mg/ATP ratio was maintained at 2:1 (Bachelard & Goldfarb, 1969).

C. Inhibition by free adenosine triphosphate (ATP) of the cerebral hexokinase of B. Excess ATP was calculated from the amounts of Mg and ATP added to reaction mixtures.

in substrate affinity and in extent of inhibition by glucose-phosphate (Bachelard, 1967; Rose & Warms, 1967; Newsholme et al., 1968), the purified enzymes from the two subcellular sites showed little difference in kinetic properties or chromatographic behaviour (Thompson & Bachelard, 1970). The mitochondrial activity has been extracted in soluble form by the use of detergents or by osmotic shock in the presence of glucose-6-phosphate or adenosine triphosphate. It remained soluble after extensive purification which included removal of extractants. The particulate and cytoplasmic enzymes both react by a random mechanism as deduced from kinetic studies of dead-end inhibition by N-acetylglucosamine and by AMP (Bachelard *et al.*, 1971; Thompson *et al.*, 1971). The similarity between the hexokinases of mitochondria and cytoplasm in chromatographic behaviour and kinetic properties is relevant to the role of the enzymes in regulation (Chapter 7). The enzyme from both sources occurs in multiple forms with K_m values for glucose of 0·04–0·10 mM and for ATP of 0·3–0·5 mM. In sheep brain a lower K_m (0·02 mM) for glucose was suggested to be correlated with the lower circulating blood glucose level of 50 mg./100 ml. in that species (Raggi & Kronfeld, 1966). Other sugars, including fructose, 2-deoxyglucose and glucosamine are phosphorylated by cerebral hexokinase (Sols & Crane, 1954); deoxyglucose interacts with the glucose site on the enzyme and inhibits competitively with K_i, 0·25 mM (Bachelard *et al.*, 1971).

Fructose Phosphates

Glucose phosphate isomerase (EC 5.3.1.9) catalyses the step immediately subsequent to hexokinase, interconverting glucose-6-phosphate and fructose-6-phosphate; the equilibrium value is some 63–70 % in favour of the glucose derivative. All parts of the brain show very high glucose phosphate isomerase activity (Buell *et al.*, 1958). These high rates appear likely to be significant in securing the isomerization and subsequent glycolysis of the glucose phosphate in competition with two other processes (see below, Fig. 5.5): glycogen synthesis, and the alternative oxidative route. A specific study of such factors (Kahana *et al.*, 1960) in a system which actively removed the product, gave half maximal velocities with very low concentrations of substrate, 10 μM in the case of fructose-6-phosphate and 30 μM glucose-6-phosphate.

Phosphofructokinase (EC 2.7.1.11) catalyses the succeeding reaction between fructose-6-phosphate and adenosine triphosphate which forms fructose-1:6-diphosphate and adenosine diphosphate (Fig. 5.3): consuming, therefore, an equivalent of energy-rich phosphate. Under optimum conditions, including added aldolase (q.v.) to remove the diphosphate formed, rates of up to 1,600 μmoles/g. hr. have been obtained (Buell *et al.*, 1958). For these high rates, fructose-6-phosphate was required in concentrations appreciably greater than are needed of glucose for its phosphorylation by hexokinase. The enzyme mechanism is particularly complex and is relevant to its role as a major control point of glycolysis (Chapter 7). The activity is subject to inhibition, as is hexokinase, by excess of one of its substrates, namely ATP. The Michaelis constants for the two substrates, fructose-6-phosphate (0·04 mM) and ATP (0·1 mM) were found to be each independent of the concentration of the other, at non-inhibitory levels of ATP. Also like hexokinase, the inhibition by ATP depended on the Mg to ATP ratio; free ATP was considerably more inhibitory than MgATP. However the relations between activity, Mg and ATP seem more complex for phosphofructokinase than for hexokinase (Lowry & Passonneau, 1964). Citrate is also inhibitory and acts synergistically with ATP; the inhibition by both is partially relieved by fructose-6-phosphate. ATP inhibition is also decreased by orthophosphate, K^+, NH_4^+, 5'-AMP and 3',5'-cyclic AMP, some of which also appear to act synergistically. These properties confer upon the enzyme a subtlety of complex interactions suitable to its role in metabolic control (q.v.) and have led to the suggestion (Lowry, 1965; Lowry & Passonneau, 1966) that the enzyme might possess as many as 12 separate sites for substrates, inhibitors and modifiers (de-inhibitors or activators). The sites may be allosterically arranged so that occupation of one inhibitor site renders other inhibitor sites more accessible and the activator sites less accessible. Occupation of one of the activator sites could have the opposite effect.

Aldolase (Ketose-1-phosphate aldehyde-lyase)

Aldolase (EC 4.1.2.7., 4.1.2.13), which catalyses the splitting of fructose diphosphate to the two triose phosphates, is found in cerebral extracts from many species as a soluble enzyme of high activity (Palladin & Polyakova, 1949; Lowry et al., 1954; Buell et al., 1958) with a high affinity for its substrate. The enzyme was found relatively uniformly distributed in the different layers of Ammon's horn. The cerebellum and the cerebral cortex of the rabbit and the monkey showed aldolase rates ranging from 260 to 1,100 μmoles/g. hr. The enzyme of mammalian cerebral cortex occurs in at least 5 forms which differ in electrophoretic mobility from the aldolases of other tissues. All of the forms, after purification by ammonium sulphate fractionation and separation on DEAE-cellulose columns, had similar pH optima of 7·5 to 8·0 but differed in stability on storage at pH 4·4. The K_m values for fructose diphosphate depended on the enzyme concentrations and were between 3 and 20 μM at pH 8·05. Lysine and histidine residues were suggested as involved in the active centre. The distribution of the multiple forms differed in various regions of monkey brain and has been studied also in human cerebral cortex (Penhoet et al., 1966; Christen et al., 1966; Nicholas & Bachelard, 1969, 1971). The relatively low Michaelis constants observed correlate with the low concentration of substrate native to the tissue (Table 5.2). Presumably in cerebral as in other tissues, dihydroxyacetone phosphate is one product of aldolase action and is converted to the other, glyceraldehyde-3-phosphate, by a triosephosphate isomerase (EC 5.3.1.1).

Glyceraldehyde 3-phosphate: Oxidation and Phosphorylation

At this stage is formed an energy-rich phosphate capable of yielding adenosine triphosphate from the diphosphate. The oxidation does not proceed in absence of nicotinamide adenine dinucleotide (NAD^+) as coenzyme, which makes understandable the accumulation of triose phosphates observed in cerebral suspensions provided with glucose but lacking the coenzyme. The coupled phosphorylation reaction which forms 1,3-diphosphoglycerate from the triose-phosphate and orthophosphate is catalysed in cerebral extracts by an NAD^+-requiring dehydrogenase with properties similar to the glyceraldehyde-3-phosphate dehydrogenase (EC 1.2.1.12) of other tissues. A thiol enzyme, it contains in its molecule both NAD^+ and glutathione. The NAD^+ is too firmly bound to be removed on dialysis but exchanges with added isotopically-labelled coenzyme and can be removed on adsorbents. Fluorometric measurement of rates of NADH formation in cerebral extracts in the presence of 5 mM-orthophosphate and 5 mM-mercaptoethanol showed half maximal velocity to be given with 44 μM-glyceraldehyde-3-phosphate and 22 μM-NAD$^+$; orthophosphate was required at 0·4–2·2 mM, depending on the concentrations of other reactants (Lowry & Passonneau, 1964). The reaction involving glyceraldehyde-3-phosphate (R.CHO) by the dehydrogenase (Enz.SH) is considered to include the following sequence to form 1,3-diphosphoglycerate (Koeppe *et al.*, 1956):

$$\begin{array}{ccccc}
\text{R.CHO} & \text{NAD}^+ & \text{R.CO} & \text{H}_3\text{PO}_4 & \text{R.CO.OPO}_3\text{H}_2 \\
+ & \rightleftharpoons & | & \rightleftharpoons & + \\
\text{Enz.SH} & \text{NADH} & \text{Enz.S} & & \text{Enz.SH}
\end{array}$$

Measured fluorometrically in the presence of 2·5 mM-cysteine and 5 mM-arsenate, rates of the order of 12,000 μmoles/g. protein/hr. were reported for rat whole brain (Laatsch, 1962). It is of interest that adult mammalian brain contains considerably less glycerol-phosphate dehydrogenase, an enzyme which would compete with glyceraldehyde-3-phosphate dehydrogenase for triose phosphate. Cerebral glyceraldehyde phosphate dehydrogenase is inhibited by iodoacetates and indeed appears to represent one of the most sensitive sites in the body to these substances when they are administered to whole animals, especially to young animals (Himwich, 1951; Samson & Dahl, 1957), for their toxic effects indicate action at the central nervous system. That low concentrations of iodoacetates act relatively specifically at phosphoglyceraldehyde dehydrogenase explains earlier observations of their selective effect in inhibiting respiration of cerebral tissues with glucose, but not with lactate, glutamate, or succinate as substrates (Krebs, 1931). The dehydrogenase in cerebral extracts is inhibited also by glyceraldehyde (Needham *et el.*, 1951) and neurotropic viruses have been credited with action on cerebral metabolism at this point (Racker, 1954).

Production of adenosine triphosphate from the diphosphate and 1:3-diphosphoglyceric acid now depends on a *phosphoglycerate kinase* (EC 2.7.2.3) which is very active in cerebral tissues, proceeding at some 10,000 μmoles/g. fresh mouse brain/hr. (Lowry & Passonneau, 1964). It also operates at quite low substrate concentrations. When determined in presence of 5 mM-mercaptoethanol, half maximum velocity was given with only 9 μM-diphosphoglyceric acid and 2 μM-adenosine diphosphate.

Conversion to Pyruvate

The 3-phosphoglycerate produced by phosphoglycerate kinase is converted by cerebral tissues and extracts (Banga, Ochoa & Peters, 1939; Kun, 1950) to phospho-*enol*pyruvate, a reaction involving two stages. In cerebral as in other tissues, 3-phosphoglycerate is first converted by a phosphomutase to 2-phosphoglycerate. Adult mouse brain contained *phosphoglycerate mutase* (EC 2.7.5.3) activities of 200–250 μmoles/g. hr. (Lowry & Passonneau, 1964) measured in the presence of μM-2,3-diphosphoglycerate. The coenzyme requirement for the enzyme was well within the amount normally available in the brain; the Michaelis constant for 3-phosphoglycerate was 0·24 mM.

Evidence for the second stage, D-2-phosphoglycerate hydrolase or *enolase*

(EC 4.2.1.11), which catalyses dehydration to phospho-*enol*pyruvate, came first from the action of fluorides which inhibit glycolysis in cerebral preparations; in other tissues their main action is known to be at enolase. The enzyme has since been assayed in reaction mixtures containing cerebral preparations with Mg^{2+} and 2 mM-phosphoglycerate, measuring spectrophotometrically the phosphoenolpyruvate produced. Enolase was concluded to comprise 2·7% of the soluble protein in ox brain, and by solvent, salt and column fractionations was obtained essentially pure (Wood, 1964). The purified enzyme exhibited a requirement for Mg^{2+} up to a maximum activation at 1 mM. Increased Mg^{2+} caused inhibition in a fashion similar to that reported for yeast enolase (Wold & Ballou, 1957). Half maximal velocity for mouse brain was obtained with 33 μM-phosphoglycerate (Lowry & Passonneau, 1964).

The outstanding characteristic of enolase is its formation, in phospho-*enol*pyruvate, of a molecule with an energy-rich phosphate bond capable of yielding adenosine triphosphate. This is brought about by an ATP-pyruvate phosphotransferase or *pyruvate kinase* (EC 2.7.1.40) which is extremely active in cerebral tissues. It required 50 μM-phosphoenolpyruvate or 180 μM adenosine diphosphate for half-maximal velocity (Lowry & Passonneau, 1964). The overall reaction, dehydrating phosphoglyceric acid with formation of adenosine polyphosphate from adenylic acid, was demonstrated by Banga, Ochoa & Peters (1939). Later, starting with phospho*enol*pyruvate, a suspension of a few mg. of rat brain with 4 mM phosphopyruvate, 1 mM adenosine diphosphate, 4 mM magnesium chloride, and fluorides, anaerobically, transfer of phosphate was found to proceed at up to 5,600 μmoles/g. tissue/hr. (Utter, 1950, 1959; Muntz & Hurwitz, 1951), yielding adenosine triphosphate and pyruvic acid: two most important cerebral metabolites. For details of mechanism, see Rose (1960).

Ions interact interestingly in this transfer as it is exhibited by suspensions from entire or acetone-extracted cerebral tissues. Potassium and ammonium salts markedly accelerate the reaction; with 5 mM ammonium chloride rates up to 6,000 μmoles/g. were reported. Sodium chloride (70 mM) inhibited by 50%. These effects may or may not be directly on the phosphokinase; they contribute to explaining effects of NH_4^+, K^+, and Na^+, on lactic acid formation from glucose by cerebral suspensions, which are similarly affected by these ions.

The major normal fate of pyruvate is its further oxidation (Chapter 6). Before describing this, the account of glycolytic reactions and of changes in glucose phosphates will be completed in the following sections.

Lactate Dehydrogenase

This enzyme catalyses the reduction of pyruvate to lactate by reduced NAD^+: the last stage in the formation of lactate from glucose. The dehydrogenase was demonstrated in cerebral tissues many years ago and now has been purified from this source (see Peters & Sinclair, 1933; Strominger & Lowry, 1955; Winer, 1960). Under optimal conditions in cerebral cortical tissue from the monkey it reaches 4,500 μmoles/g. hr., a value many times those of the initial stages of glycolysis.

Lactate dehydrogenase (EC 1.1.1.27) from ox brain has been enriched 100-fold by adsorption and salt precipitation; an agar-gel process yields three isoenzymes (Bonavita & Guarneri, 1962). Using the purified major component, kinetic studies were made by fluorometric methods (Winer, 1960) and showed the enzyme E to react with lactate and dinucleotide in a fashion which can be represented:

$$E + NADH \hspace{8cm} E + NAD^+$$

$$\underset{1}{\Big\Updownarrow} \hspace{9cm} \Big\Updownarrow$$

$$\begin{array}{c} E.NADH \\ + \text{ pyruvate} \end{array} \underset{3}{\rightleftharpoons} \begin{bmatrix} E.NADH \\ \text{pyruvate} \end{bmatrix} \rightleftharpoons \begin{bmatrix} E.NAD^+ \\ \text{lactate} \end{bmatrix} \underset{8}{\rightleftharpoons} \begin{array}{c} E.NAD^+ \\ + \text{ lactate} \end{array}$$

Fluorescence changes showed the enzyme to form by reaction *1* a complex with the reduced coenzyme, with which pyruvate then reacted. Half-maximal velocity at stage *3* was obtained with only 30 μM-pyruvate and 3 μM-NADH; at this stage, oxamate, which was an inhibitor of the overall reaction, competed with pyruvate. On the other hand, for half-maximal velocity of the reverse reaction *8* with NAD$^+$ at 0·1 μM, lactate was required at 5 μM. The properties of the isolated enzyme thus interestingly reflect the cerebral concentrations of the reactants, of which lactate preponderates. Several aspects of the activity of lactate dehydrogenase can be inferred from effects of hydroxymalonic acid, which inhibits in cerebral tissues to about equal degrees the anaerobic formation of lactic acid from glucose, the anaerobic dismutation of pyruvic acid, and respiration with lactate (but not pyruvate) as substrate (Jowett & Quastel, 1937). Lactic dehydrogenase is evidently involved in each of these processes.

Normally, *in vitro* as *in vivo*, little pyruvate accumulates under conditions permitting formation of lactate, even anaerobically. The prompt and considerable increase in lactate during convulsive activity *in vivo* is found to be associated with relatively little increase in pyruvate beyond the normal 0·1–0·2 μmoles/g. and thus emphasizes the considerable capacity of cerebral lactic dehydrogenase (Bain & Pollock, 1949). Some of the circumstances under which pyruvate has been observed to accumulate in cerebral reaction mixtures: in presence of iodoacetates (Peters & Thompson, 1934) and of nicotine (Himwich & Fazekas, 1935), are probably due to action of the added substances at associated reactions rather than at lactic dehydrogenase itself.

Several molecular species of lactic dehydrogenase are present also in human brain; five have been characterized and two purified. These were identical in several physical and immunological characteristics with the corresponding enzymes from human heart (Nisselbaum *et al.*, 1964).

During sustained glycolysis (e.g. anaerobically) lactic acid formation is enabled to continue because the NAD$^+$ oxidized by pyruvate is reduced by glyceraldehyde 3-phosphate (q.v.). The coupling is shown in cerebral homogenates (Utter, 1950). When pyruvate is added as such anaerobically, reduction of the coenzyme can occur during oxidative decarboxylation of pyruvate to acetate and carbon dioxide (Chapter 6). Several other coenzyme-linked reactions of this type are possible with cerebral metabolites arising oxidatively.

Two reaction sequences alternative to glycolysis will now be discussed: those concerning glycogen and pentose phosphates (Fig. 5.5).

Glycogen

The breakdown of glycogen on cerebral excitation or in anoxia, and its subsequent resynthesis (Chapter 2) emphasize how change in the functional condition of the brain can evoke changes in its glycogen metabolism. There are indeed many instances of such phenomena. Glycogen levels in the brain have been reported to be decreased after administration of adrenaline or methamphetamine and to be increased by insulin, methionine sulphoximine or phenobarbitone (Chapter 15). The glycogen was doubled in fasted rats administered insulin and glucose (Prasannan & Subrahmanyam, 1965, 1968) and increased by 50% after intracisternal injections of insulin at levels which produced no change in the glycogen of other tissues, nor in the glucose of the blood (Mellerup & Rafaelson, 1969; Strang & Bachelard, 1971). Hydrocortisone caused increased rates of glycogen synthesis *in vivo* (C, Fig. 5.6) and intraperitoneal injections of phenobarbitone into mice caused the brain glycogen to treble in content (Nelson *et al.*, 1968; see also Chapter 3). Enzyme study has indeed revealed several points of control and adjustment in glycogen metabolism. This proves to involve intermediary steps recognized also in other organs, and which, in the brain, have received the specific studies now to be described.

Glycogen Synthesis

The pathway of glycogen synthesis from glucose (Fig. 5.5) in cerebral tissues has been demonstrated *in vivo* (Coxon *et al.*, 1965; Krivanek, 1958) and *in vitro* (LeBaron, 1955; McIlwain & Tresize, 1956; Kleinzeller & Rybova, 1957), although the glycogen synthesized *in vitro* was found to be shorter in chain-length, with a greater degree of branching, than the native glycogen of the brain. It was also found to be more resistant to change in tissues subjected to electrical stimulation (see Chapters 3 and 4). Rates of synthesis obtained *in vivo* and *in vitro* were similar, at 1–2 μmoles/g. hr. and are generally lower than those found in liver or muscle (Shapiro & Wertheimer, 1943; Breckenridge & Crawford, 1961). Four of the separate enzymic stages involved in producing cerebral glycogen from glucose have been investigated. The first of these, *hexokinase*, is common to three different routes of glucose metabolism, as has already been described.

The route specific to glycogen commences with the conversion of glucose-6-phosphate to glucose-1-phosphate by *phosphoglucomutase* (EC 2.7.5.1), a reversible reaction readily detectable in cerebral tissues and extracts (Shapiro & Wertheimer, 1943; Breckenridge & Crawford, 1961). From a variety of sources it requires for its activity magnesium or related ions, and glucose-1:6-diphosphate. The levels of the diphosphate in the brain (0·03–0·08 μmoles/g., Table 5.2) although low, are as high as in other tissues examined (Leloir, 1953) and are over 100 times greater than the K_m of the cerebral enzyme (Passonneau *et al.*, 1969). The speed of the reaction in cerebral tissues is evidently sufficiently great for phosphoglucomutase not to limit metabolism. It yields an equilibrium

mixture of the two hexose phosphates in which glucose-6-phosphate preponderates (95%). In other tissues its action has been found not to involve
liberation of inorganic phosphate for none is exchanged with added isotopic
phosphate. In a variety of areas of the rabbit brain, and also in other species,
phosphoglucomutase proves to have the highest activity of the four enzymes

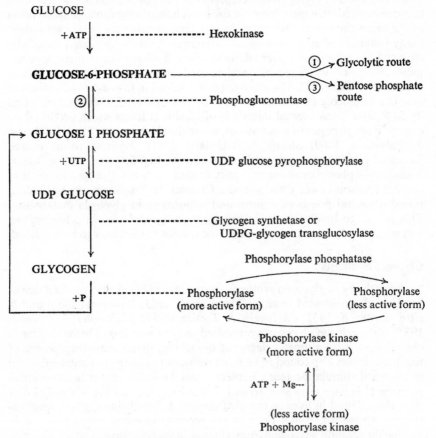

FIG. 5.5. Synthesis and breakdown of glycogen, and factors modifying
the activity of phosphorylase (see text and Krebs & Fischer, 1962;
the present figure contains only the components demonstrated in
cerebral preparations). Note the three routes from glucose-6-
phosphate, of which (1) has been described above and (3) is described subsequently. Rates of the reactions concerned are given in
Tables 5.2 and 5.3.

now being considered, being capable of interconverting 840–1900 μmoles of
substrate/g. tissue/hr. (Breckenridge & Crawford, 1961; Lowry & Passonneau,
1969): a magnitude presumably related to the need for effective competition
with the other enzymes acting on glucose-6-phosphate.

    The following stage makes specific use of uridine triphosphate (UTP)
which was noted (Chapter 3) as present in the brain in appreciable quantities,

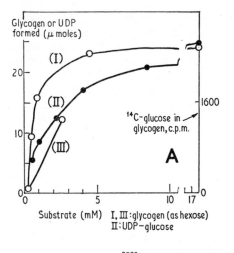

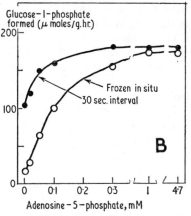

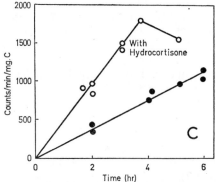

FIG. 5.6. Glycogen synthesis and breakdown.

A. The synthesis from uridine diphosphate glucose. A rabbit brain preparation in buffered cysteine mixtures was incubated with (I), 2·4 mM UDP glucose and the concentrations of glycogen primer given in abscissae; (II), with UDP glucose as quoted; (III), with UDP ^{14}C-glucose; points give the ^{14}C incorporated to glycogen with and without glycogen primer (Breckenridge & Crawford, 1960; Basu & Bachhawat, 1961a).

B. Breakdown of glycogen measured by the glucose-1-phosphate formed in reaction mixtures containing Mg and phosphate salts and glycogen with the different concentrations of adenylic acid indicated, and tissue suspensions from mouse brain. In one case the brain was frozen in situ; in the other case the head was separated 30 sec. before freezing and extraction (Breckenridge & Norman, 1962).

C. Incorporation of ^{14}C from [U-^{14}C]glucose into rabbit brain glycogen in vivo. Hydrocortisone when present was injected intramuscularly in 15 mg. doses on each of the two days preceding intravenous injection of labelled glucose (Coxon et al., 1965).

as also is glucose-1-phosphate. *Uridine diphosphate glucose pyrophosphorylase* (EC 2.7.7.9) catalyses the interconversion of these two substances with organic pyrophosphate and uridine diphosphate glucose, at rates between 150 and 450 μmoles/g. rabbit or human brain/hr. (Breckenridge et al., 1961;

Basu and Bachhawat, 1961). Conditions chosen for assay employ a few μg. of tissue in buffered media with $MgCl_2$ (concluded to act as a complex with UTP) in addition to the main reactants; half-maximal activity was obtained with 2·5 mM-UTP and 0·6 mM-glucose-1-phosphate. This assay measures the reaction in the direction which probably preponderates *in vivo*, but the tissue will also catalyse the breakdown of UDP-glucose to glucose-1-phosphate. Half-maximal velocity was then reached with uridine diphosphate glucose at 0·5 mM; reaction in this sense has been used in guiding a 30-fold purification of the enzyme from sheep brain.

Glycogen synthetase (uridine diphosphate glucose–glycogen transglucosylase, EC 2.4.1.11) now forms glycogen by adding a glucose unit from UDP-glucose to preformed glycogen, which is needed as a primer of the reaction. The synthetase proved sensitive to the range of concentrations at which the two compounds occur in the brain (Table 5.2; A, Fig. 5.6). In many of its characteristics the enzyme from the brain is similar to that from muscle or liver, which show greater synthetase potency. In the brain, the synthetase is the slowest of the four reactions involved in converting glucose to glycogen; nevertheless, when maximally exhibited, the enzyme from 1 g. cerebral tissue can incorporate 25 μmoles of glucose/hr. As this rate greatly exceeds the maximal rate of glycogen synthesis *in vivo* or in the intact tissue *in vitro* (Chapters 2 and 3), the availability of substrates and cognate factors must also play a role in conditioning the synthesis. From sheep brain, the synthetase has been purified 50-fold; it was then activated by magnesium salts and by cysteine (Basu & Bachhawat, 1961a). Two forms of the synthetase have recently been detected which differ in sensitivity to glucose-6-phosphate activation. Interconversion of the two forms, "D" (dependent on glucose-6-phosphate) and "I" (independent) occurs enzymically, which may be relevant to considerations of mechanisms which control cerebral glycogen levels (Goldberg & O'Toole, 1969; see also Chapter 7).

The pathway of synthesis of cerebral glycogen is thus similar to that operating in liver or muscle; the enzyme responsible in the brain for forming α-1,6 branches is assumed to operate in a fashion similar to the amylo-1,4 → 1,6-transglucosylase of other tissues.

Glycogen Breakdown: Phosphorylase

Glycogen breakdown in the brain proceeds by phosphorolysis. Following their demonstration that the first change undergone by glycogen in animal tissues yielded glucose-1-phosphate from glycogen and inorganic phosphates Cori *et al.* (1938) showed the enzyme system responsible, *phosphorylase* (EC 2.4.1.1), to be of widespread occurrence and at high level in cerebral tissues, provided that activating substances were present. The simplest activating substance was adenosine-5′-phosphate, required at 0·3 mM or more: levels above those of the normal brain, but reached e.g. during anoxia when breakdown of glycogen occurs. Maximally activated, the enzyme catalysed the breakdown of glycogen, and also its synthesis from glucose-1-phosphate when glycogen was present as a primer, at rates from 500 to 1200 μmoles/g. tissue/hr. (Cori *et al.*, 1938; Minard *et al.*, 1965). Glucose inhibition of the cerebral activity has been shown to be competitive for glucose-1-phosphate (Breckenridge & Norman, 1962).

Cerebral tissues also proved capable of modifying the activity of phosphorylase by other means. The brain frozen *in situ* and extracted in the cold (conditions which preserve its native glycogen: Chapter 3) shows much less phosphorylase activity when examined with a range of concentrations of adenosine-5-phosphate (**B**, Fig. 5.6). However, a few seconds at 20–37° suffice to activate the phosphorylase; in the subsequent few minutes it is again inactivated. The change at 37° was inhibited by fluorides and concluded to be due to the action of a phosphatase on the phosphorylase (Breckenridge & Norman, 1962). After its inactivation, the phosphorylase could be reactivated by adenosine triphosphate and a specific enzyme system, *phosphorylase kinase* (EC 2.7.1.38); these interactions are shown in Fig. 5.5. The activation, studied in detail in other tissues, proved to be a phosphorylation (Sutherland & Rall, 1960; Krebs & Fischer, 1962). The kinetic properties of the active and less active forms of rabbit brain phosphorylase have been compared with those of the phorphorylases a and b of muscle (Lowry *et al.*, 1967); the brain enzymes exhibited higher K_m values than the muscle enzymes and this supports the view that brain glycogen acts as an emergency store rather than as a normal reserve for energy-yielding processes.

The activity of glycogen phosphorylase in a number of tissues including those from the brain can be modified also by catecholamines (Chapter 14) and by heated tissue extracts (Rall & Sutherland, 1958). Fractionation of the extracts showed their effects to be due to their content of cyclic 3′,5′-adenosine monophosphate which acts as one factor modifying the activity of phosphorylase kinase in many tissues, although activation of the cerebral kinase by cyclic AMP has not been clearly established. The 3′,5′-adenosine monophosphate is not only present in the brain itself but undergoes rapid changes in quantity; indeed the brain is one of the richest sources of enzymes concerned with its metabolism. The cyclic AMP has major roles in the brain apart from a possible function in relation to glycogen (Butcher & Sutherland, 1962; Sutherland *et al.*, 1962; Cheung, 1967); it is described in Chapter 9 and further reference to catecholamines made in Chapter 14.

Glycogen synthesis and breakdown presumably involve the transferase branching and debranching enzymes. Since glucose phosphates are produced from glycogen breakdown in the brain, an enzyme similar to the amylo-1,6-glucosidase of muscle and liver is involved. The breakdown in the intact brain normally proceeds rapidly to lactic acid by routes already discussed: the glucose-1-phosphate yielded by phosphorylase being converted to glucose-6-phosphate by phosphoglucomutase. The glucose-6-phosphate from glycogen, as from glucose itself, then follows the sequence of Table 5.2. There is, however, a further route from glucose-6-phosphate: (3) of Fig. 5.5, which affords an alternative pathway of carbohydrate breakdown and which will be appraised in the following main section.

Glycogen Storage Disease

Two of the seven known defects of glycogen metabolism in man are associated with mental retardation: type II (α-glucosidase deficiency) and type

VII (glycogen synthetase deficiency). α-Glucosidase catalyses the last stage in breakdown of glycogen in liver and muscle, when glucose forms from oligosaccharides. The cerebral enzyme does not appear to have been studied but deposition of glycogen occurs in the brain as well as in muscle and liver in Pompe's disease (type II). In type VII disease glycogen synthetase is known to be deficient in liver and muscle but, even though the disease causes mental retardation, little is known of effects on the brain synthetase. The subject has been reviewed by Field (1966) and by Crome and Stern (1967).

Pentose Phosphate Route

Glucose-6-phosphate is acted on by ground cerebral tissues not only by the isomerization and further phosphorylation which have been described, but also by dehydrogenation. The system responsible passes to solution when the tissue is ground, and the solution retains enzyme activity after dialysis. Addition is then required of glucose-6-phosphate, nicotinamide adenine dinucleotide phosphate ($NADP^+$) and magnesium chloride, when reduction of the nucleotide takes place with oxidation of the phosphate at some 20 μmoles/g. hr. (Dickens & Glock, 1951; Glock & McLean, 1954; Dickens *et al.*, *Symposium*, 1959; Dickens *et al.*, 1968). This proved to be the initial step of a distinct sequence of reactions which could result in complete oxidation of glucose, and which was termed the pentose phosphate pathway or shunt; the sequence includes:

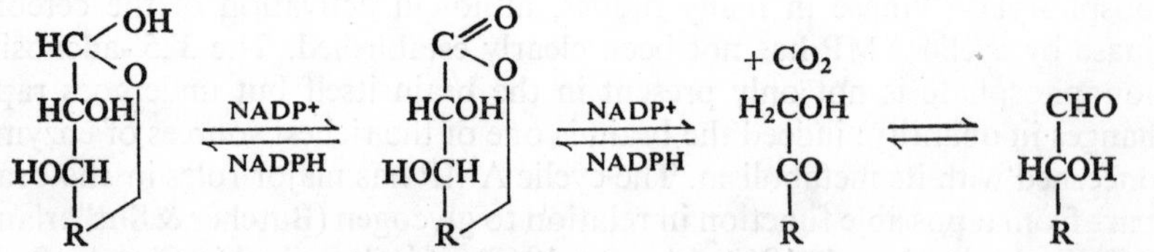

D-Glucose-6 phosphate — 6 Phospho-D-gluconolactone — D-Ribulose-5-phosphate — Ribose 5-phosphate

Glucose-6-Phosphate Oxidation

In the adult brain, the participation of the shunt pathway is small in comparison to that of glycolysis. Studies comparing the formation of $^{14}CO_2$ from 1-^{14}C-glucose and 6-^{14}C-glucose have consistently yielded values of close to 1 for the ratio of the $^{14}CO_2$ produced in normal cerebral tissues and in potassium-stimulated slices of cerebral cortex (Bloom, 1955; Sacks, 1957; Hoskin, 1960). Pathway evaluations based on the ratios of $^{14}CO_2$ formation from 1-^{14}C- or 6-^{14}C-labelled glucose are subject to limitations (Wood *et al.*, 1963) and evaluations based on ratios of ^{14}C labelling of triose phosphates are considered to be more reliable. *In vivo* studies based on the randomization of the ^{14}C from 2-^{14}C-glucose in its conversion into glycogen, also indicated only a minor contribution of the shunt (Hostetler & Landau, 1967). The small contribution of the pentose phosphate pathway to the metabolic degradation of glucose in adult cerebral tissues is suggested also by the rates of the relevant enzymes. Table 5.3 shows that glucose-6-phosphate dehydrogenase and 6-phosphogluconate dehydrogenase operate at much lower rates than the glycolytic enzymes. Also, NADP+, which is required for the shunt, occurs in much smaller concentrations in the brain than NAD+ which is required for glycolysis (Glock & McLean, 1955; Lowry et al., 1961). By themselves, comparisons of coenzyme or enzyme levels are not conclusive as the activities of glycolytic enzymes are far in

Table 5.3

Enzymes and nicotinamide nucleotide coenzymes of glycolysis or the hexose monophosphate shunt in mammalian cerebral tissue

Glycolysis			Hexose monophosphate shunt		
Enzyme	Species	Rate (μmoles/g. fresh wt./hr.)	Enzyme	Species	Rate (μmoles/g. fresh wt./hr.)
Hexokinase	Mouse	660[1]	Glucose-6-phosphate dehydrogenase	Rat	20[4]
	Guinea pig	1,275[2]		Guinea pig	35[5]
Glucose phosphate isomerase	Mouse	3,300[1]	6-Phosphogluconate dehydrogenase	Rat	13[4]
Phosphofructo- kinase	Mouse	540[1]		Guinea pig	55[5]
Glyceraldehyde phosphate de- hydrogenase	Mouse	3,360[1]			
	Rat	880[3]			

Coenzyme	Species	Content (μmole/kg. fresh wt.)	Coenzyme	Species	Content (μmole/kg. fresh wt.)
NAD+	Rat	260[6,7]	NADP+	Rat	5[6,7]
	Guinea pig	234[6]		Guinea pig	11[6]
NADH	Rat	115[6,7]	NADPH	Rat	17[6,7]
	Guinea pig	101[6]		Guinea pig	22[6]
NAD+ + NADH	Rat	375[6,7]	NADP+ + NADPH	Rat	22[6,7]
	Guinea pig	335[6]		Guinea pig	33[6]

Data from [1] Lowry & Passonneau, 1964; [2] Bachelard, 1967; [3] Laatsch, 1962; [4] Glock & McLean, 1954; [5] Yanada & Shimazono, 1962; [6] Glock & McLean, 1955; [7] Lowry et al., 1961.

excess of the normal overall rates of glucose oxidation in the brain. However, taken in conjunction with the results of the pathway-evaluation studies, it seems reasonable to conclude that only a very small proportion of the glucose oxidized is metabolized *via* the pentose–phosphate pathway in adult mammalian brain. The elevation of cerebral respiration and of rates of glucose consumption which result from electrical stimulation has been concluded (O'Neil et al., 1965) to be due to increased glycolysis rather than to increased participation of the alternative route. The participation of the shunt is of relatively greater importance in the immature brain (Guerra et al., 1967) and also in heavily-myelinated tracts (Buell et al., 1958), conditions where there is emphasis on fat synthesis for which the NADPH produced by the shunt is required.

Glucose-6-phosphate dehydrogenase (EC 1.1.1.49), which catalyses the initial reaction, proceeded in the presence of Mg^{2+} and the required coenzyme, $NADP^+$, at rates of 20–35 μmoles/g. hr. when suspensions of guinea pig or dog brain were used as source of enzyme (Khachatrian, 1961; Yanada & Shimazono, 1962). Measurements based on the use of histochemical methods gave rates of up to 150 μmoles/g. hr. in rabbit brain, with higher activities in several regions of white matter than in grey. Half-maximal velocity with the enzyme from rabbit brain was obtained with 0·24 mM glucose-6-phosphate and 3 μM-$NADP^+$ (Kuhlman & Lowry, 1957; Buell *et al.*, 1958; Roberts *et al.*, 1958).

The immediate product of the dehydrogenation, 6-phosphogluconolactone, undergoes hydrolysis to 6-phosphogluconate which is further oxidized by *6-phosphogluconate dehydrogenase* (EC 1.1.1.44); this is also an $NADP^+$ requiring step. Rates observed in suspensions of fresh rat or guinea pig brain were 13–55 μmoles/g. hr. (Glock & McLean, 1954; Yanada & Shimazono, 1962). The activity measured using histochemical techniques in rabbit brain was again higher at some 150 μmoles/g. hr. and required <0·13 mM-phosphogluconate and 2 μM-$NADP^+$ for half-maximal velocity. This second dehydrogenation forms CO_2 and a pentose phosphate (Horecker & Smyrniotis, 1951; Roberts *et al.*, 1958). Regulation of the pentose phosphate pathway is thought to occur at these two $NADP^+$-requiring dehydrogenase reactions (Kaufmann *et al.*, 1969).

Pentose Phosphate Oxidation

Ribose-5-phosphate also undergoes further reaction if added as such with magnesium salts to similar cerebral extracts, the ribose chain being lost at some 45 μmoles/g. hr. In other tissues the reactions involved are the interaction of ribose- and xylulose-5-phosphates to form a triose- and a heptulose-phosphate; these two may further yield a tetrose- and fructose-phosphate and ultimately triose-phosphate with regeneration of hexose-phosphate (see Horecker, 1953; Racker, 1954). The reaction sequence as a whole is independent of added inorganic phosphate and requires specifically $NADP^+$ and not NAD^+ as coenzyme. It requires also thiamine pyrophosphate, for the stage at which ribose-5-phosphate is converted to sedoheptulose-7-phosphate. This reaction, which is one of those catalysed by transketolase, can yield 9–35 μmoles of sedoheptulose phosphate/g. tissue/hr. from different parts of the brain of the rat and man (Bruchhausen 1964; Dreyfus, 1965).

Because cerebral tissues contain a potent NADPH-glutathione reductase (q.v.) the progress of the pentose phosphate route can depend on the availability of glutathione (GSSG; Hotta, 1962). In cerebral dispersions, 60-fold increase in the glucose so oxidized was caused by addition of GSSG, which was reduced to the thiol form, GSH, during the reaction. Provision of GSH may indeed constitute a function of the route through pentose phosphates. A further role lies in the provision of metabolically important carbohydrate derivatives: including for example the pentose phosphates themselves, which are involved in nucleotide synthesis.

Comment

The pyruvate produced from carbohydrate metabolism in the brain is oxidized further in the tricarboxylic acid cycle and by the process of oxidative phosphorylation, processes which are described in the Chapter which follows. Metabolic defects involving carbohydrates are discussed in later chapters in this book. Thus galactosaemia, which is associated with disturbance of amino acids, is described in Chapter 8; defects of polysaccharide metabolism which involve substances containing gangliosides, hexuronic acids and hexosamines are described in Chapter 11.

REFERENCES

BACHELARD, H. S. (1967). *Biochem. J.* **104**, 286.
BACHELARD, H. S., CLARK, A. G. & THOMPSON, M. F. (1971). *Biochem. J.* In press.
BACHELARD, H. S. & GOLDFARB, P. S. G. (1969). *Biochem. J.* **112**, 579.
BACHELARD, H. S. & MCILWAIN, H. (1969). In Comprehensive Biochemistry, Vol. **17**, p. 191. Ed. M. Florkin & E. H. Stotz. Amsterdam: Elsevier.
BAIN, J. A. & POLLOCK, G. H. (1949). *Proc. Soc. exp. Biol. N.Y.* **71**, 495.
BANGA, I., OCHOA, S. & PETERS, R. A. (1939). *Biochem. J.* **33**, 1980.
BASU, D. K. & BACHHAWAT, B. K. (1961). *J. Neurochem.* **7**, 174.
BASU, D. K. & BACHHAWAT, B. K. (1961a). *Biochim. Biophys. Acta* **50**, 123.
BENNETT, E. L., DRORI, J. B., KRETCH, D., ROSENZWEIG, M. R. & ABRAHAM, S. (1962). *J. biol. Chem.* **237**, 1758.
BLOOM, B. (1955). *Proc. Soc. Exptl. biol. Med.* **88**, 317.
BONAVITA, V. & GUARNERI, R. (1962). *Biochim. Biophys. Acta* **59**, 634.
BOYER, P. D., LARDY, H. & MYRBACK, K. (1959–63). *The Enzymes.* New York: Academic Press.
BRECKENRIDGE, B. M. & CRAWFORD, E. J. (1960). *J. biol. Chem.* **235**, 3054.
BRECKENRIDGE, B. M. & CRAWFORD, E. J. (1961). *J. Neurochem.* **7**, 234.
BRECKENRIDGE, B. M. & NORMAN, J. H. (1962). *J. Neurochem.* **9**, 383.
BRECKENRIDGE, B. M., SCOTT, S., STROMINGER, J. L. & CRAWFORD, E. J. (1961). *J. Neurochem.* **7**, 228.
BRUCHHAUSEN, F. v. (1964). *Arch. exper. Pathol. Pharmacol.* **264**, 330.
BUELL, M. V., LOWRY, O. H., ROBERTS, N. R., CHANG, M-L. W. & KAPPHAHN, J. I. (1958). *J. biol. Chem.* **232**, 979.
BUTCHER, R. W. & SUTHERLAND, E. W. (1962). *J. biol. Chem.*, **237**, 1244.
CHEUNG, W. Y. (1967). *Biochemistry*, **6**, 1079.
CHRISTEN, P., RENSING, U., SCHMID, A. & LEUTHARDT, F. (1966). *Helv. chim. Acta.* **49**, 1872.
CORI, G. T., COLOWICK, S. P. & CORI, C. F. (1938). *J. biol. Chem.* **123**, 375.
COXON, R. V., GORDON-SMITH, E. C. & HENDERSON, J. R. (1965). *Biochem. J.* **97**, 776.
CRANE, R. K. & SOLS, A. (1953). *J. biol. Chem.* **203**, 273.
CRANE, R. K. & SOLS, A. (1954). *J. biol. Chem.*, **210**, 597.
CROME, L. C. & STERN, J. (1967). Pathology of Mental Retardation, p. 297. London: Churchill.
DICKENS, F. (1951). The Enzymes **2**, 624. Ed. Sumner & Mybäck. New York: Academic Press.
DICKENS, F. & GLOCK, G. E. (1951). *Biochem. J.* **50**, 81.
DICKENS, F., RANDLE, P. J. & WHELAN, W. J. (1968). Carbohydrate Metabolism and its Disorders, Vol. 1. New York: Academic Press.
DREYFUS, P. M. (1965). *J. Neuropath. exp. Neurol.* **24**, 119.
ELLIOTT, K. A. C. & LIBET, B. (1942). *J. biol. Chem.* **143**, 227.
ELLIOTT, K. A. C. & PENFIELD, W. (1948). *J. Neurophysiol.* **11**, 485.

FELLENBERG, R. VON, EPPENBERGER, H., TICHTERICH, R. & AEBI, H. (1962). *Biochem. Z.*, **336**, 334.

FIELD, R. A. (1966). The Metabolic Basis of Inherited Disease, 2nd ed., p. 141. Ed. J. B. Stanbury, J. B. Wyngaarden & D. S. Fredrickson. New York: McGraw-Hill.

FROMM, H. J. & ZEWE, V. (1962). *J. biol. Chem.* **237**, 1661.

GEIGER, A. (1940). *Biochem. J.* **34**, 465.

GLOCK, G. E. & MCLEAN, P. (1954). *Biochem. J.* **56**, 171.

GLOCK, G. E. & MCLEAN, P. (1955). *Biochem. J.* **61**, 388.

GOLDBERG, N. D. & O'TOOLE, A. G. (1969). *J. biol. Chem.* **244**, 3053.

GUERRA, R. M., MELGAR, E. & VILLAVINCENCIO, M. (1967). *Biochim. Biophys. Acta* **148**, 356.

HIMWICH, H. E. (1951). Brain Metabolism and Cerebral Disorders. Baltimore: Williams & Wilkins.

HIMWICH, H. E. & FAZEKAS, J. F. (1935). *Amer. J. Physiol.* **113**, 63.

HORECKER, B. L. (1953). *J. cell. comp. Physiol.* **41**, suppl. 1.

HORECKER, B. L. & SMYRNIOTIS, P. Z. (1951). *J. biol. Chem.* **193**, 371.

HOSKIN, F. C. G. (1960). *Biochim. Biophys. Acta.* **40**, 509.

HOSTETLER, K. Y. & LANDAU, B. R. (1967). *Biochemistry*, **6**, 2961.

HOTTA, S. S. (1962). *J. Neurochem.* **9**, 43.

JOWETT, M. & QUASTEL, J. H. (1937). *Biochem. J.* **31**, 275, 565.

KAHANA, S. E., LOWRY, O. H., SCHULZ, D. W., PASSONNEAU, J. V. & CRAWFORD, E. J. (1960). *J. biol. Chem.* **235**, 2178.

KAUFMANN, F. C., BRON, J. G., PASSONNEAU, J. V. & LOWRY, O. H. (1969). *J. biol. Chem.* **244**, 3647.

KERLY, M. & LEABACK, D. H. (1957). *Biochem. J.* **67**, 250.

KHACHATRIAN, G. S. (1961). *Proc. 2nd. All-Union Neurochem. Conf.*, p. 83. Ed. Buniatian, H. Ch. Erevan: Acad. Sci. Armenian S.S.R.

KING, L. J., LOWRY, O. H., PASSONNEAU, J. V. & VENSON, V. (1967). *J. Neurochem.* **14**, 599.

KLEINZELLER, A. & RYBOVA, R. (1957). *J. Neurochem.* **2**, 45.

KOEPPE, O. J., BOYER, P. D. & STULBERG, M. P. (1956). *J. biol. Chem.* **219**, 569.

KREBS, E. G. & FISCHER, E. H. (1962). *Advances in Enzymol.* **24**, 263.

KREBS, H. A. (1931). *Biochem. Z.* **234**, 278.

KREBS, H. A. & KORNBERG, H. L. (1957). Energy Transformations in Living Matter. Berlin: Springer.

KREBS, H. A. & WOODFORD, M. (1965). *Biochem. J.* **94**, 436.

KRIVANEK, J. (1958). *J. Neurochem.* **2**, 337.

KUHLMAN, R. E. & LOWRY, O. H. (1957). *J. Neurochem.* **1**, 173.

KUN, E. (1950). *Proc. Soc. exp. Biol.* **75**, 68.

LAATSCH, R. H. (1962). *J. Neurochem.* **9**, 487.

LEBARON, F. N. (1955). *Biochem. J.* **61**, 80.

LELOIR, L. F. (1953). *Advances in Enzymology*, **14**, 205.

LONG, C. (1952). *Biochem. J.* **50**, 407.

LONG, C. & THOMSON, R. (1955). *Biochem. J.* **61**, 465.

LOWRY, O. H. (1965). In Control of Energy Metabolism, p. 63. Ed. B. Chance, R. W. Estabrook & J. R. Williamson. New York: Academic Press.

LOWRY, O. H. & PASSONNEAU, J. V. (1964). *J. biol. Chem.* **239**, 31.

LOWRY, O. H. & PASSONNEAU, J. V. (1966). *J. biol. Chem.* **241**, 2268.

LOWRY, O. H. & PASSONNEAU, J. V. (1969). *J. biol. Chem.* **244**, 910.

LOWRY, O. H., PASSONNEAU, J. V., HASSELBERGER, F. X. & SCHULZ, D. W. (1964) *J. biol. Chem.* **239**, 18.

LOWRY, O. H., PASSONNEAU, J. V., SCHULZ, D. W. & ROCK, M. K. (1961). *J. biol. Chem.* **236**, 2746.

LOWRY, O. H., ROBERTS, N. R., LEINER, K. Y., WU, M.-L., FARR, A. L. & ALBERS, R. W. (1954). *J. biol. Chem.* **207**, 39.

LOWRY, O. H., SCHULZ, D. W. & PASSONNEAU, J. V. (1967). *J. biol. Chem.* **242**, 271.

MCILWAIN, H. (1953). *J. Neurol. Neurosurg. & Psychiat.* **16**, 257.

MCILWAIN, H. & TRESIZE, M. A. (1956). *Biochem. J.* **63**, 250.

MELLERUP, E. T. & RAFAELSON, O. J. (1969). *J. Neurochem.* **16**, 777.

MERRICK, A. W. (1961). *J. Physiol.* **158**, 476.

MEYERHOF, O. & GELIAZKOVA, N. (1947). *Arch. Biochem.* **12**, 405.

MEYERHOF, O. & WILSON, J. R. (1948). *Arch. Biochem.* **17**, 153.

MINARD, F. N., KANG, C. H. & MUSHAHWAR, I. K. (1965). *J. Neurochem.* **12**, 279.

MUNTZ, J. A. & HURWITZ, J. (1951). *Arch. Biochem.* **32**, 124, 137.

NEEDHAM, D. M., SIMINOVITCH, L. & RAPKINE, S. M. (1951). *Biochem. J.* **49**, 113.

NELSON, S. R., SCHULZ, D. W., PASSONNEAU, J. V. & LOWRY, O. H. (1968). *J. Neurochem.* **15**, 1271.

NEWSHOLME, E. A., ROLLESTON, F. S. & TAYLOR, K. (1968). *Biochem. J.* **106**, 193.

NICHOLAS, P. C. & BACHELARD, H. S. (1969). *Biochem. J.* **112**, 587.

NICHOLAS, P. C. & BACHELARD, H. S. (1971). In preparation.

NING, J., PURICH, D. L. & FROMM, H. J. (1969). *J. biol. Chem.* **244**, 3840.

NISSELBAUM, J. S., PACKER, D. E. & BODANSKY, O. (1964). *J. biol. Chem.* **239**, 2830.

OCHOA, S. (1941). *J. biol. Chem.* **141**, 245.

OCHOA, S. (1954). *Advances in Enzymology*, **15**, 183.

OLSEN, N. S. & KLEIN, J. R. (1946). *Res. Publ. Ass. nerv. ment. Dis.* **26**, 118.

O'NEILL, J. J., SIMON, S. H. & SHREEVE, W. W. (1965). *J. Neurochem.* **12**, 797.

PALLADIN, A. V. & POLYAKOVA, N. M. (1949). *Ukrain. Biokhim. Zhur.* **21**, 341.

PASSONNEAU, J. V., LOWRY, O. H., SCHULZ, D. W. & BROWN, J. G. (1969). *J. biol. Chem.* **244**, 902.

PENHOET, E., RAJKUMAR, T. & RUTTER, W. J. (1966). *Proc. nat. Acad. Sci. Wash.* **56**, 1275.

PETERS, R. A. & SINCLAIR, H. M. (1933). *Biochem. J.* **27**, 1910.

PETERS, R. A. & THOMPSON, R. H. S. (1934). *Biochem. J.* **28**, 916.

PRASANNAN, K. G. & SUBRAHMANYAM, K. (1965). *Indian J. Med. Res.* **53**, 1003.

PRASANNAN, K. G. & SUBRAHMANYAM, K. (1968). *Endocrinology*, **82**, 1.

RACKER, E. (1954). *Advances in Enzymology*, **15**, 141.

RAGGI, F. & KRONFELD, D. S. (1966). *Nature*, **209**, 1353.

RALL, T. W. & SUTHERLAND, E. W. (1958). *J. biol. Chem.* **232**, 1065, 1077.

ROBERTS, N. R., COELHO, R. R., LOWRY, O. H. & CRAWFORD, E. J. (1958). *J. Neurochem.* **3**, 109.

ROBINS, E., SMITH, D. E. & JEN, M. K. (1957). *Progr. Neurobiol.* **2**, 205.

ROBINSON, N. & PHILLIPS, B. M. (1964). *Biochem. J.* **92**, 254.

RODNIGHT, R., WYNTER, C. V. A., COOK, C. N. & REEVES, R. (1969). *J. Neurochem.* **16**, 1581.

ROSE, I. A. (1960). *J. biol. Chem.* **235**, 1170.

ROSE, I. A. & WARMS, J. V. B. (1967). *J. biol. Chem.* **242**, 1635.

SACKS, W. (1957). *J. appl. Physiol.* **10**, 37.

SACKS, W. & SACKS, S. (1968). *J. appl. Physiol.* **24**, 817.

SAMSON, F. E. & DAHL, N. A. (1957). *Amer. J. Physiol.* **188**, 277.

SHAPIRO, B. & WERTHEIMER, E. (1943). *Biochem. J.* **37**, 397.

SOLS, A. & CRANE, R. K. (1954). *J. biol. Chem.* **210**, 581.

STERN, J. (1954). *Biochem. J.* **58**, 536.

STRANG, R. H. C. & BACHELARD, H. S. (1971). *J. Neurochem.* **18**.

STROMINGER, J. L. & LOWRY, O. H. (1955). *J. biol. Chem.* **213**, 635.

SUTHERLAND, E. W. & RALL, T. W. (1960). *Pharmacol. Rev.* **12**, 265.

SUTHERLAND, E. W., RALL, T. W. & MENON, T. (1962). *J. biol. Chem.* **237**, 1220.

Symposium (1953). *Brit. Med. Bull.* **9**, 85.

Symposium (1959). *Ciba Foundation Symposium on the Regulation of Cell Metabolism.* Ed. Wolstenholme & O'Connor. London: Churchill.

TEWARI, H. B. & BOURNE, G. H. (1963). *J. Histochem. Cytochem.* **11**, 121.

THOMPSON, M. F. & BACHELARD, H. S. (1970). *Biochem. J.* **118**, 25.

THOMPSON, M. F., CLARK, A. G. & BACHELARD, H. S. (1971). *Biochem. J.* In press.

UTTER, M. F. (1950). *J. biol. Chem.* **185**, 499.

UTTER, M. F. (1959). *Ann. N.Y. Acad. Sci.* **72**, 387.

UTTER, M. F., WOOD, H. G. & REINER, J. M. (1945). *J. biol. Chem.* **161**, 197.

WARBURG, O. (1930). The Metabolism of Tumours. Trans. F. Dickens. London: Constable.

WEIL-MALHERBE, H. & BONE, A. D. (1951). *Biochem. J.* **49**, 339; *J. ment. Sci.* **97**, 635.

WINER, A. D. (1960). *Biochem. J.* **76**, 5P.

WOLD, F. & BALLOU, C. E. (1957). *J. biol. Chem.* **227**, 313.

WOOD, T. (1964). *Biochem. J.* **91**, 453.

WOOD, H. G., KATZ, J. & LANDAU, B. R. (1963). *Biochem. Z.*, **338**, 809.

YANADA, K. & SHIMAZONO, N. (1962). *J. Biochem. (Tokyo).* **51**, 242.

6   Pyruvate Metabolism and Oxidative Phosphorylation

Oxidation of pyruvate was first shown to occupy a prominent position in cerebral metabolism through investigation of the action of thiamine (see Peters, 1963). In studies which constituted an important stage in understanding the actions of vitamins generally, lactate and pyruvate were shown to accumulate in the cerebral tissues of thiamine-deficient pigeons and rats *in vivo*. This occurred also during the metabolism of the tissues *in vitro* (Kinnersley & Peters, 1929; Peters & Thompson, 1934; O'Brien & Peters, 1935). Accumulation in part paralleled the severity of the impairment of the central nervous system. Both the accumulation and the central symptoms were relieved by administered thiamine. Added *in vitro*, thiamine not only increased the removal of pyruvate but also increased the uptake of oxygen by the tissue when lactate

Table 6.1

Products from pyruvic and α-oxoglutaric acids

Substance	Molar ratios of substances lost (−) and formed (+)		
	Anaerobically		Aerobically
	Sliced tissue	Ground tissue	Ground tissue
Pyruvate (added)	−2·9	−2·0	−2
Carbon dioxide	+0·97	+0·95	+4·0
Lactate	+1·0	+0·92	+0·16
Acetate	+0·78	+0·10	+0·48
Succinate	+0·18	+0·60	−
Oxoglutarate (added)	−2·0	−2·0	−
Carbon dioxide	+0·93	+1·0	−
Hydroxyglutarate	+1·20	+1·0	−
Succinate	+0·98	+0·95	−

Anaerobic experiments used about 1 g. of tissue, largely cerebral cortex from rats, in 10 ml. bicarbonate saline with 100 μmoles of substrate for 2 hr. The rate of loss of pyruvate was about 24 μmoles/g. hr. and of α-oxoglutarate, about 10 μmoles/g. hr. The aerobic experiment was in phosphate-buffered saline with pigeon cerebral tissue. (Weil-Malherbe, 1937; Krebs & Johnson, 1937; Long, 1938.)

or pyruvate was given as substrate, but not when these were replaced by succinate. Thus the continued oxidation of pyruvate appeared necessary for the functioning of the brain.

Moreover, certain but smaller quantities of pyruvate were found in mixtures in which normal cerebral tissues were respiring with glucose or lactate as substrates, and the amounts of pyruvate greatly increased when iodoacetates were added. Presumably with normal tissue, pyruvate was being both formed and oxidized at considerable rates; when added as the only oxidizable substrate, pyruvate disappeared at about 30 μmoles/g. hr. from mixtures respiring at about 60 μmoles/g. ground tissue/hr. (Table 6.1). The complete oxidation of pyruvate:

$$CH_3.CO.COOH + 2.5 O_2 \rightarrow 3CO_2 + 2H_2O$$

requires 2·5 moles O_2/mole, and thus the substance was being nearly completely oxidized at respiratory rates approaching those normal to the brain *in*

Table 6.2

Individual stages in pyruvate oxidation

Substance	Cerebral concentration[1] (μmoles/ g.)	Reaction	Free energy change[2] (ΔG, Kcal.)	Rate[1] (μmoles/ g. hr.)
Pyruvate	0·091			
↓		Pyruvate dehydrogenase†	−55	48[4]
→Acetylcoenzyme *A*	–			
↓		Condensing enzyme	− 8	30[4]
Citrate	0·327			
↓				
cis-Aconitate*	<0·01	} Aconitate hydratase	+ 1·5	90[5]
↓				
*Iso*citrate	0·016			
↓				
Oxalosuccinate*		} *Iso*citrate dehydrogenase†	−62	240[3]
↓				
α-Oxoglutarate	0·127	α-Oxoglutarate dehydrogenase,†		100[6]
↓		Succinyl CoA synthetase	−70	—
Succinate	0·686			
↓		Succinic dehydrogenase	−36	580[8]
Fumarate	0·073			
↓		Fumarate hydratase	− 1	2000[7]
Malate	0·438			
↓		Malate dehydrogenase†	−45	5300[9]
—Oxaloacetate	0·004			

[1] Concentrations were determined in the brains of mice rapidly-frozen *in situ*; rat brain gave almost identical results (Goldberg *et al.*, 1966). Rates were observed in mammalian cerebral tissues. [2] Krebs (1953). [3] Salganicoff & Koeppe, 1968. [4] Coxon & Peters (1950); Ochoa (1954). [5] Johnson (1939). [6] Holowach *et al.* (1968). [7] Lowry *et al.* (1954). [8] Aldridge & Johnson, 1959. [9] Strominger & Lowry (1955).
* Probably as enzyme-bound intermediates.
† Stages involving the formation of NADH.

vivo. The enzyme preparations responsible for the oxidation were termed the pyruvate oxidase system. Since the formulation of the tricarboxylic acid cycle or Krebs cycle it has gradually been shown, as will be evident from the account which follows, that this cycle (Table 6.2) to a large extent represents the route of pyruvic acid oxidation in the brain and that pyruvate oxidase preparations contain most if not all the components of the cycle. These components are to a large extent physically associated at the mitochondria of the tissue (Chapter 12).

Dismutation of Pyruvate

In the experiments just described, the pyruvate which was not oxidized completely was found to appear as lactate and acetate, together with smaller amounts of succinate and citrate (Tables 6.1 and 6.3). To study the formation of such substances more fully, the reactions possible were restricted by carrying out experiments anaerobically. Added pyruvate was then found to be metabolized by cerebral tissues almost as rapidly and completely anaerobically as aerobically. In this property, tissues from the brain differed from those from most other animal organs examined. Thus rat cerebral preparations consumed pyruvate aerobically at about 20 and anaerobically at 16 μmoles/g. hr. The products of the reaction (Table 6.1) were then found to appear in relatively simple ratios which suggested the reaction:

$$2 \text{ pyruvate } \rightarrow 1 \text{ lactate} + 1 \text{ } CO_2 + 1 \text{ } C_2\text{-residue}$$

the two-carbon residue appearing either as acetate itself or as succinate, and the balance between these two products depending on the integrity of the tissue.

The first alteration in the carbon skeleton of pyruvate thus appeared to be an oxidative decarboxylation; anaerobically yielding lactate through one molecule of pyruvate acting as hydrogen acceptor, while aerobically this took place to a smaller extent and further reactions occurred in the C_2-residue. Oxidative decarboxylation of α-oxobutyrate and α-oxovalerate, the homologues of pyruvate, was also catalysed by cerebral tissues (Long & Peters, 1939), as also was loss of acetopyruvic acid (Krebs & Johnson, 1937). α-Oxobutyrate reacted at almost exactly the same rate as pyruvate when judged by disappearance of substrate, though only 0·5 moles O_2 were consumed per mole of oxobutyrate; with each substrate the initial reaction was presumed to be:

$$R.CO.COOH + 0·5O_2 \longrightarrow R.COOH + CO_2$$

yielding from oxobutyrate, propionate, not further metabolized. The reaction with α-oxovalerate was much slower.

Factors Affecting the Oxidation of Pyruvate

Thiamine Pyrophosphate; Carboxylic Acids

Oxidation of pyruvate and of the two homologues, α-oxobutyrate and α-oxovalerate, was depressed in tissues from thiamine-deficient animals but was restored by addition of small amounts of thiamine pyrophosphate. This substance was already established as a coenzyme (cocarboxylase) in the decarboxylation of pyruvate by yeast; the present experiments localized its major metabolic effect in animal tissues (Table 6.3; see also Chapter 10). The complexity of the further metabolism of pyruvate in cerebral tissues was shown by the number of factors which influenced it. Thus its oxidation was catalysed by fumarate and inhibited by malonate (Banga, Ochoa & Peters, 1939). When pyruvate was formed from oxaloacetate, it was associated also with α-oxoglutarate and citrate (Krebs *et al.*, 1940). These findings are all understandable in terms of the tricarboxylic acid cycle.

Table 6.3

*Some aerobic products from pyruvate with cerebral tissues from
normal and thiamine-deficient pigeons*

Product	Formation (μmoles/g. hr.) with:			
	Tissue from normal pigeons		Tissue from deficient pigeons	
	No fumarate	3·3 mM-fumarate	No thiamine pyrophosphate	Thiamine pyrophosphate
Citrate	4	21	6*	13*
α-Oxoglutarate	10	28	5*	15*
Acetate	133	44	33	70

Pigeon brain was ground and washed by centrifuging, or dialysed, and used at about 70 mg./ml. with 10 mM-pyruvate, adenosine triphosphate, magnesium chloride and phosphate at pH 7·3. Constituents were determined after 30–40 min. at 38°C (Coxon, Liébecq & Peters, 1949; Coxon & Peters, 1950).
* 3·3 mM-Fumarate was also present.

Phosphates and Nucleotides

Further analysis of pyruvate oxidation was made possible by using finely-ground suspensions of rabbit or pigeon cerebral tissue from which components of low molecular weight were removed by dialysis. These revealed the important connection between oxidation of pyruvate and the presence of inorganic phosphate and adenine nucleotides. Maximal oxidation in this system, as Fig. 6.1 shows, was at the high rate of 120 μmoles O_2/g. tissue/hr.; to reach this, 50 mM-inorganic phosphate was required. The reaction was especially sensitive to inorganic phosphate between 1 and 10 mM. Of the adenine nucleotides, 1·4 mM-adenylic acid or 0·35 mM-adenosine triphosphate gave maximal activation. Again, succinate, fumarate, or malate was needed and these at 5 mM gave similar, maximal, effects.

The basis for the phosphate requirements was made evident when changes in the adenylic acid itself were investigated. In incubating the dialysed preparation as indicated in A, Fig. 6.1, material of the lability of adenosine triphosphate was transitorily produced. Knowing that enzymes hydrolysing adenosine triphosphate were present in cerebral tissues, fluorides were added to minimize the breakdown; and creatine, glucose, or hexose monophosphate was added to "trap" the phosphate of the newly-formed adenine polyphosphate so that it was not hydrolysed to the inorganic form. Sustained phosphorylation then took place (**C**, Fig. 6.1). The transfers of phosphate to glucose or surrogates

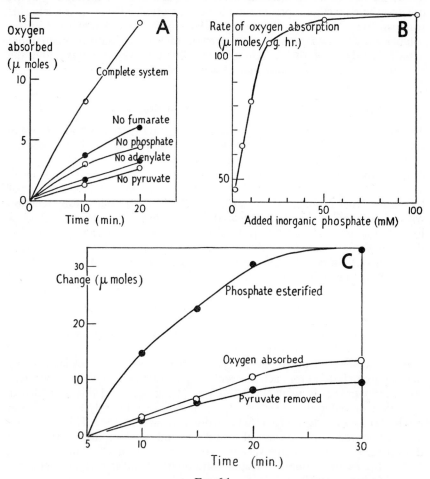

FIG. 6.1.
A, B. Necessity for inorganic phosphate, adenylic acid (9·1 mM) and fumarate (5 mM) for oxidation of pyruvate (9·1 mM) by dialysed preparations of pigeon brain. The complete system contained the components named with phosphate at 50 mM and magnesium chloride at 2 mM, in air at 38°C (Banga, Ochoa & Peters, 1939).
C. Phosphorylation coupled with oxidation of pyruvate. Reaction mixture similar to that above but containing also 20 mM-sodium fluoride and 25 mM-glucose (Ochoa, 1941).

depended on the cerebral tissue supplying the necessary phosphokinases (Chapter 5); doubtless it also supplied an adenylate kinase (q.v.).

The important link between respiration and the formation of energy-rich phosphoric esters had thus been demonstrated. These pioneering experiments with cerebral tissues were followed by many others in which oxidative phos-phorylation was studied in a variety of biological systems. Two main develop-ments have furthered such work. The systems concerned with phosphorylation as well as oxidation have been shown to be present in the mitochondria of the cell and these by careful preparation have been obtained with their adenosine triphosphate-degrading enzymes in a relatively inactive, latent form. Also, soluble extracts and pure enzyme preparations have enabled much more detailed analysis of the individual steps linking oxygen uptake and the phosphorylation. These individual steps will now be recounted.

Oxidative Decarboxylation; Pyruvate Dehydrogenase (EC 1.2.4.1)

This stage in the metabolism of pyruvate in cerebral tissues was noted above to require thiamine pyrophosphate and to yield carbon dioxide and a two-carbon fragment. In addition (see below) it is sensitive to reagents combining with dithiols. Individual stages, as in other tissues (see Ochoa, 1954; Massey & Veeger, 1963) involve interaction first of the pyruvate with catalytic amounts of thiamine pyrophosphate (TPP+; structure, Chapter 10), followed by reaction with α-lipoic acid to form the acetylated-lipoate intermediate, 6-S-acetylhydro-lipoate (Fig. 6.2). The acetyl group of the high energy thioester produced is then transferred to coenzyme A (for structure, see chapter 10) which seems to act in catalytic amounts. The reduced lipoate is regenerated by an NAD+-linked oxidation catalysed by α-lipoamide dehydrogenase, shown to be active in cerebral extracts (Giuditta & Strecker, 1963; see also p. 142). All reactions save (i), Fig. 6.2, are thought to be reversible. The thioester group in acetyl-coenzyme A contains an energy-rich bond, labile and reactive. The compound is a most important reactant, not only in the pyruvate oxidation described in the next section but also in many synthetic processes.

It is however to be noted that acetyl-coenzyme A itself is equivalent to only one energy-rich bond for each molecule of pyruvate decarboxylated, whereas much more energy is available at this step (Table 6.2), and this is yielded in oxidation of reduced NAD+. Acetylcoenzyme A is hydrolysed by ground cerebral tissues if reagents for other reactions are not provided. This is presum-ably the source of the acetate of Table 6.1, and condensation of the acetyl derivative, the source of the succinate formed anaerobically from pyruvate, and of the small amount of acetoacetate detected under certain conditions (Weil-Malherbe, 1937).

Toxic Agents

Participation of dithiols in pyruvate oxidation was first recognized through examining effects of toxic agents on the oxidation in cerebral tissues (Peters et al., 1945, 1949; Stocken & Thompson, 1946; Peters, 1963). The pyruvate oxidase system proved very sensitive to arsenites and to the chemical-warfare agent Lewisite. Like thiamine deficiency, Lewisite led to accumulation of pyruvate, and it inhibited the oxidation of pyruvate more than it did that of succinate. The cerebral pyruvate oxidase system does not necessarily represent the point of attack of arsenicals as toxic agents in vivo. It however provided an excellent test system for the development of possible antidotes to their action, which culminated in the use of 2 : 3-dimercaptopropanol (British anti-Lewisite, BAL). Thus the 50 or 70% inhibition of pyruvate oxidation brought about by

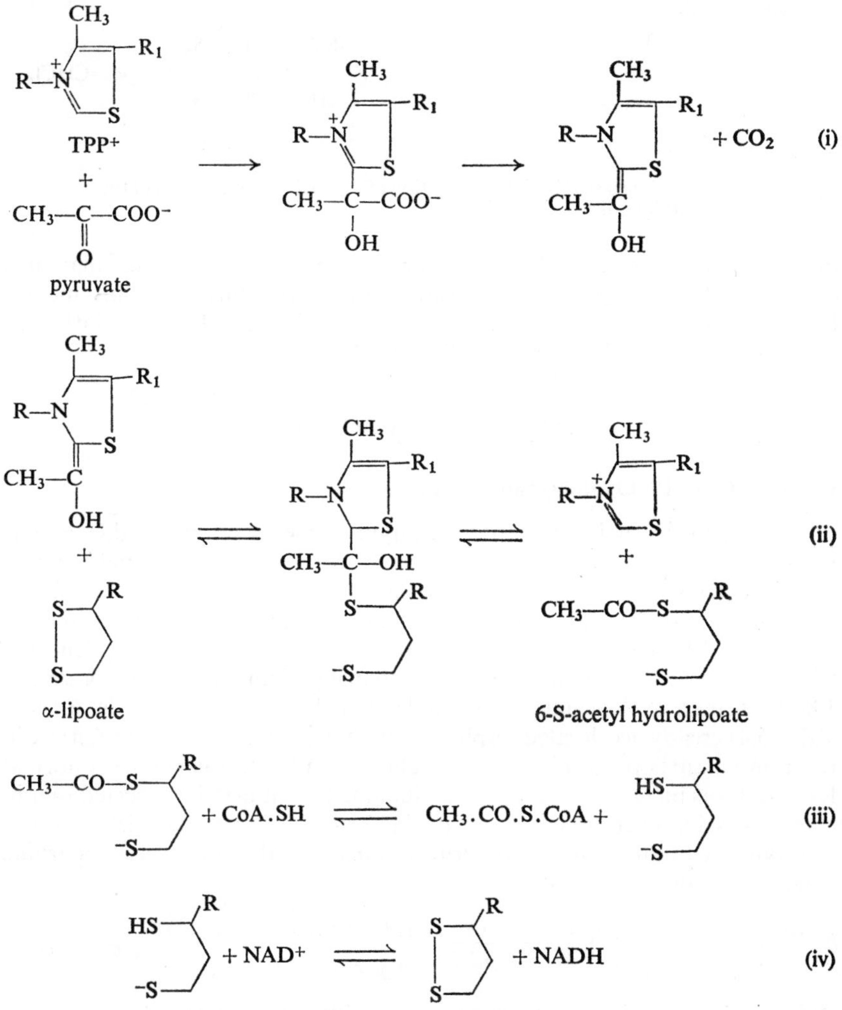

FIG. 6.2. Pyruvate dehydrogenase and formation of acetyl coenzyme A.

17 μM-Lewisite was reversed or prevented by a few equivalents of dimercapto-propanol. The changes can be represented as shown in Fig. 6.3. Monothiols were without such effect; BAL proved of great practical value (Carleton, Peters & Thompson, 1948).

The system oxidizing pyruvate in cerebral tissues is among those sensitive to oxygen at pressure of 1 to 5 atmospheres (Dickens, 1962) which in man and

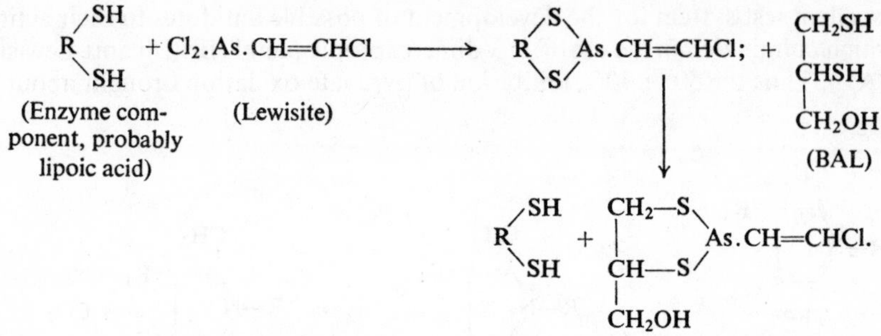

$$R\begin{array}{c}\diagup SH\\[2pt]\diagdown SH\end{array} + Cl_2.As.CH{=}CHCl \longrightarrow R\begin{array}{c}\diagup S\\[2pt]\diagdown S\end{array}As.CH{=}CHCl; \; + \begin{array}{c}CH_2SH\\[2pt]CHSH\\[2pt]CH_2OH\end{array}$$

(Enzyme com-   (Lewisite)   (BAL)
ponent, probably
lipoic acid)

$$R\begin{array}{c}\diagup SH\\[2pt]\diagdown SH\end{array} + \begin{array}{c}CH_2{-}S\\[2pt]CH{-}S\\[2pt]CH_2OH\end{array}As.CH{=}CHCl.$$

FIG. 6.3. Suggested basis for the action of the toxic arsenicals and of the antidote, BAL.

other animals cause convulsions; changes in cerebral amino acids may also be involved (see Chapter 8 and Haugaard, *Symposium*, 1964). Vesicants including mustard gas have also been studied as inhibitors of the oxidation of pyruvate by cerebral preparations (Peters, 1963).

The Tricarboxylic Acid Cycle

Condensation with Oxaloacetate to Citrate

That pyruvate in its oxidative metabolism yields citrate (Table 6.3) is indicated by several findings already recounted. Citrate is a normal cerebral constituent. It can be formed by cerebral suspensions at rates over 30 μmoles/g. hr., and for such formation required a mixture containing, with some 60 mg. tissue/ml., 10 mM-pyruvate, 6·7 mM-oxaloacetate and 0·3 mM-adenosine triphosphate with inorganic phosphate and magnesium salts (Coxon & Peters, 1950). Further, oxaloacetate (replaceable by malate or fumarate: Fig. 6.1 and Table 6.4) greatly accelerated respiration with pyruvate as substrate. Citrate in reaction mixtures from thiamine-deficient pigeon brain was below its normal level, but was increased by the added vitamin. Thus it may be expected that in cerebral as in other tissues pyruvate in forming citrate first yields acetyl-coenzyme A by the sequence described above and that the acetyl coenzyme condenses with oxaloacetate:

$$\begin{array}{c}HOOC.CO\\[2pt]HOOC.CH_2\end{array} + \begin{array}{c}CH_3.CO\\[2pt]CoA.S\end{array} \underset{\text{synthase}}{\overset{\text{citrate}}{\rightleftharpoons}} \begin{array}{c}HOOC.C(OH).CH_2COOH\\[2pt]HOOC.CH_2\end{array} + CoA.SH$$

This reaction moreover is reversible: citrate with suitable cerebral preparations can yield acetylcoenzyme A (either by this system or by an independent citrate-cleavage enzyme: Srere, 1959) and so act as an acetylating agent. This is its role during the formation of acetylcholine from citrate, choline, choline acetylase and the synthase; a catalytic amount of coenzyme A in this system yielded acetylcholine (Korkes *et al.*, 1952). Of tissues assayed for citrate synthase, cerebral are among the most active (Ochoa, 1954). Many of these features of pyruvate utilization have been reproduced in preparations of mitochondria from the brain (Deitrich & Hellerman, 1964; Tuček, 1967).

Aconitate Hydratase and *Iso*citrate Dehydrogenase

Citrate does not greatly accumulate in the normal brain nor in cell-containing preparations from it; the most rapid reaction which it is known to undergo is its conversion by aconitate hydratase (EC 4.2.1.3) to *cis*aconitate and *iso*citrate. Of the reactions involved, citrate has been observed to be formed from *cis*aconitate by extracts of rat brain, at some 90 μmoles/g. tissue/hr. *Iso*citrate yielded citrate at a slightly lower rate, and the reverse reaction has also been demonstrated (Johnson, 1939; Coxon, 1953). Studies in other tissues have shown the three acids to reach an equilibrium mixture containing about 90 % as citric acid itself.

Equilibria at aconitate hydratase have attracted attention as representing a point of action in poisoning by fluoroacetate (Buffa *et al.*, 1951; Peters, 1957, 1963). Fluoroacetate is used in rat poisons; 5 mg./kg. are toxic to several animal species including the rat. It has also been identified as the toxic principle of a South African poisonous plant, *Dichapetalum cymosum*. During poisoning with fluoroacetate, citrate was observed to accumulate in several organs of the body, and in the brain of rats to reach 1–2 μmoles/g. in place of the normal value of about 0·15 μmole/g. Acetate, pyruvate and α-oxoglutarate did not accumulate comparably. Action was thus at a point close to citrate and the suggestion was made, and since demonstrated as true, that fluoroacetate was converted *in vivo* to a fluorocitrate, by the processes normally converting acetate to citrate, and that the resulting fluorocitrate inhibited enzymes normally metabolizing citrate itself. Production of fluorocitrate could occur at the liver and kidney, and when isolated from kidney preparations fluoro-citric acid was shown to inhibit the interconversion of citric and *iso*citric acids by purified aconitate hydratase.

Symptoms of fluoroacetate poisoning in several species include electro-encephalographic disturbances culminating in convulsions, and these can be reproduced by the intracranial injection of fluorocitrate. The fluorocitrate in this situation causes accumulation of citrate in the brain, and thus as *in vitro* is presumably inhibiting the major energy-yielding reactions of the brain. Several routes of chemical mediation between this inhibition and the convulsions, have been explored. The convulsions do not appear due to accumulation of citrate as such; also at the time when they begin, changes in phosphocreatine and adenosine triphosphate are not pronounced. There is some evidence for a causal connection through cerebral ammonia, which increases in the intoxication and is further discussed in Chapter 8, but the subject is still under investigation (Pscheidt *et al.*, 1954; Peters, 1963; Lahiri & Quastel, 1963). Enzyme systems which have been separated from the brain and described in Chapter 14 can lead to the formation of acetylcoenzyme A from acetate, and also to fluoroacetylcoenzyme A from fluoroacetate. The latter reaction has been reported to occur in cerebral preparations, with subsequent formation of fluoroacetylcholine (Wollemann & Feuer, 1957).

Accumulation of citrate in cerebral tissues when aconitate hydratase is inhibited indicates that *cis*aconitate or *iso*citrate normally undergoes further change. The reaction which has been found to occur at adequate speed is the dehydrogenation of *iso*citrate followed by decarboxylation of the resulting oxalosuccinate. The dehydrogenation can be shown by reduction of methylene blue by aqueous extracts of cerebral tissues when *iso*citrate is given as substrate (Adler *et al.*, 1939). Such reduction also occurs with citrate as substrate and presumably then involves aconitate hydratase and *iso*citrate dehydrogenase (Ochoa, 1948). Two types of *iso*citrate dehydrogenase which occur in cerebral tissues have been shown to differ in coenzyme requirement and in subcellular localization. The major activity, NAD^+-linked, is exclusively mitochondrial in occurrence and is about four times more active in mitochondria than the $NADP^+$-linked enzyme which is found partly mitochondrial and partly soluble (Goebell & Klingenberg, 1964; Salganicoff & Koeppe, 1968).

NAD$^+$-isocitrate dehydrogenase (EC 1.1.1.41) requires Mn^{2+} or Mg^{2+} and 0·8 mM-*iso*citrate for full activity, which in mitochondria from rat cerebral cortex, has been estimated to be some 240 μmoles/g. hr. at 25°. The total *iso*citrate dehydrogenase activity in the brain, about 350 μmoles/g. hr. at 25°, is considerably less than that of the liver but the levels of mitochondrial NAD^+-specific activity (i.e. the enzyme directly involved in oxidation in the tricarboxylic acid cycle) are similar in the two tissues. The cerebral enzyme is activated by ADP which suggests that, like the NAD^+-linked enzyme in muscle, it may perform a regulatory role in the tricarboxylic acid cycle (Goebell & Klingenberg, 1964; Goldberg *et al.*, 1966; see Chapter 7).

The decarboxylation to oxoglutarate occurs to some extent spontaneously but is also catalysed by *iso*citrate dehydrogenase, then reaching in cerebral preparations at 15°C and pH 5·6, about 400 μmoles/g. hr. In other tissues these reactions have been found independent of phosphate and phosphate acceptors. The direction in which the reactions proceed however depends greatly on the relative proportions of oxidized and reduced coenzyme in the reaction mixture.

α-Oxoglutarate

There are many indications that α-oxoglutarate, the product of decarboxylation of oxalosuccinic acid, is an intermediate in pyruvate oxidation in the brain. It accumulates to a small extent in suspensions of cerebral tissues oxidizing pyruvate. The accumulation is increased by addition of fumarate. It is decreased when tissues from thiamine-deficient animals are used and under these circumstances its quantity is increased towards that of the normal tissue by added thiamine pyrophosphate (Table 6.3).

Alone, anaerobically, with cell-free or cell-containing preparations of rat brain, α-oxoglutarate undergoes a dismutation similar to that of pyruvate (Table 6.1). This yields three products in equimolar amounts: carbon dioxide and succinate by oxidizing one equivalent of oxoglutarate and α-hydroxyglutarate by reducing another. Production of the hydroxy acid depends on the presence of an α-hydroxyglutaric dehydrogenase which is moderately potent in cerebral tissues. Succinate is also formed aerobically from α-oxoglutarate by minced brain but a large proportion is oxidized further unless malonate is present to inhibit this (Weil-Malherbe, 1937; Coxon, Liébecq & Peters, 1949); α-hydroxyglutarate apparently is not then formed.

Investigation with cerebral systems has shown the oxidative decarboxylation to be catalysed by an *α-oxoglutarate dehydrogenase* (EC. 1.2.4.2), in a sequence akin to that concerned with pyruvate. From α-oxoglutarate is formed succinyl-coenzyme A, converted to succinate with phosphorylation of adenosine diphosphate (Holowach *et al.*, 1968; Pausescu *et al.*, 1967).

$$
\begin{array}{l}
\text{COOH} \\
| \\
\text{CO} \\
| \\
\text{CH}_2 \\
| \\
\text{CH}_2 \\
| \\
\text{COOH}
\end{array}
\quad \xrightarrow[+\text{NAD}^+]{+\text{CoA.SH}} \quad
\begin{array}{l}
\text{CO}_2 + \text{NADH} + \text{H}^+ \\
\\
\text{CO.SCoA} \\
| \\
\text{CH}_2 \\
| \\
\text{CH}_2 \\
| \\
\text{COOH}
\end{array}
\quad ; \quad \xrightarrow[+\text{P}]{+\text{ADP}} \quad
\begin{array}{l}
\text{COOH} + \text{CoA.SH} \\
| \\
\text{CH}_2 \\
| \\
\text{CH}_2 + \text{ATP} \\
| \\
\text{COOH}
\end{array}
$$

(succinyl coenzyme A)

Reversal of the latter reaction, *succinylcoenzyme A synthetase* (EC 6.2.1.4), has been shown in cerebral extracts by measuring the formation of succinyl-CoA from succinic acid and coenzyme A with either adenosine triphosphate or guanosine triphosphate, the latter being the more effective (Wollemann, 1959). Again, a large part of the free-energy change (Table 6.2) becomes available on reoxidation of the reduced nicotinamide nucleotide.

Ketoacids and Amino-acids

Interrelations of ketoacids and amino-acids are prominent in the reactions of oxoglutarate and succeeding components of the tricarboxylic acid cycle (Haslam & Krebs, 1963). The systems involved are described more fully in the following chapter, but the processes must be noted also at this point, briefly, for two reasons; see also p. 18.

(1) Transamination in cerebral systems between α-oxoglutarate and glutamate is very rapid (about 5600 μmoles/g. cerebral cortex/hr.), as is also that between oxaloacetate and aspartate. Moreover, the amino acids exist in the brain in markedly greater quantities than the ketoacids. Therefore, when ^{14}C-labelled substrates are used in investigating metabolic routes, accumulation of ^{14}C occurs in amino acids rather than in ketoacids although similar specific radioactivities have been observed in the two categories of compounds (Lindsay & Bachelard, 1966). From glucose, glutamate or α-oxoglutarate, ^{14}C can be quickly distributed among many metabolites as well as appearing in [14]CO_2. Equilibration between glutamate and α-oxoglutarate can proceed at some 15,000 μmoles/g. hr.

(2) Conversion of α-oxoglutarate to succinate can be achieved in neural systems by a characteristic series of reactions through γ-aminobutyric acid (q.v.; *Symposium*, 1960). This gives an alternative to the route through succinyl-coenzyme A which is formulated above. The mammalian brain, in distinction to other major organs, can bring about the sequence: α-oxoglutarate $\rightarrow$ glutamate $\rightarrow$ γ-aminobutyric acid $\rightarrow$ succinic semialdehyde $\rightarrow$ succinate. This has been termed the γ-aminobutyrate shunt and also leads to the appearance of ^{14}C supplied as carbohydrate intermediates, in the amino-acids named. Estimates of the rates of formation and oxidation of γ-aminobutyrate in different cerebral preparations suggest the route through γ-aminobutyrate to

account for some 10% of cerebral oxidative metabolism (*Symposium*, 1960; Haslam & Krebs, 1963).

Succinate to Oxaloacetate

Several circumstances involving succinate in pyruvate metabolism in the brain have been recounted. Succinate, again, is a normal cerebral constituent and is itself rapidly oxidized by cerebral tissues. The first stage in this oxidation, catalysed by *succinate dehydrogenase* (EC 1.3.99.1) and yielding fumarate, takes place rapidly anaerobically when a few milligrams of cerebral tissues including those from man are suspended with succinate and a hydrogen acceptor such as methylene blue or phenazine methosulphate. Any necessary carriers are present in the suspension with the dehydrogenase; aerobically flavoprotein components of the cytochrome system act as hydrogen acceptors in cerebral as in other tissues. Study of the metabolic role of succinate in the brain as elsewhere has been greatly aided by inhibition of the dehydrogenase by malonates, the lower homologues of succinates. Malonate has been used for this purpose at 20–60 mM in the presence of 5–60 mM-succinate. Inhibition at cerebral succinic dehydrogenase is probably competitive. Effects of the higher concentration must in some cases be interpreted with care, but they still have greater effects on dehydrogenation of succinate than of a wide variety of other substrates in cerebral preparations.

In anaerobic reaction mixtures of cerebral tissues with succinate and methylene blue, fumarate does not greatly accumulate as such but is found to have been converted to malate. This hydration catalysed by *fumarate hydratase* (EC 4.2.1.2) proceeds very rapidly with fumarate added as such; 20 mM-fumarate in phosphate at pH 6·8 yields malate at 2,000–3,000 μmoles/g. rat brain/hr. Rates in the grey matter of the monkey brain rise to 4,000 and in the white matter are about 1,000 μmoles malate/g. tissue/hr. (Robins *et al.*, 1956).

Aerobically, reaction mixtures of cerebral tissues and fumarate yielded not malate but a keto acid, probably oxaloacetate (Long, 1945). The conversion was accelerated by inorganic phosphate between 1 and 10 mM (Fig. 7.5) and yielded up to 10 μmoles keto acid/g. rat brain/hr. The reaction proceeds through *malate dehydrogenase* (EC 1.1.1.37), initially demonstrated by adding 0·1 M-malic acid to cerebral tissues or extracts, with nicotinamide adenine dinucleotide, methylene blue and a cyanide; oxygen is absorbed at some 200 μmoles/g. tissue/hr. and oxaloacetate is formed (Green, 1936). Subsequently, rates up to 10 mmoles malate oxidized/g. tissue/hr. have been observed and the enzyme has been obtained in a largely purified form specific to the L-acid (Robins *et al.*, 1956; Winer, 1960). Complex formation has been demonstrated between enzyme, coenzyme and substrate in a fashion analogous to that involved in lactate dehydrogenase (q.v.). About 100 μM-L-malate gave half maximal velocity.

Products from Oxaloacetate; CO_2 Incorporation

Apart from equilibration with malate, the normal fate of oxaloacetate in cerebral tissues is its condensation with acetylcoenzyme A derived from glucose

(Table 6.2), so completing the tricarboxylic acid cycle. With cerebral slices, succinate ^{14}C-labelled in the 2:3 positions formed ^{14}C-aspartate (through oxaloacetate) and $^{14}CO_2$; when in addition unlabelled glucose was supplied, the $^{14}CO_2$ increased markedly (Gonda & Quastel, 1962). The glucose was concluded to act by affording acetylcoenzyme A for condensation with oxaloacetate according to the reaction above, and in this way accelerating $^{14}CO_2$ formation by the tricarboxylic acid cycle.

Oxaloacetate added as only substrate *in vitro* can however undergo other changes. Its rapid reduction to malate has been observed in mixtures containing ground cerebral tissues (Banga, Ochoa & Peters, 1939), the reaction proceeding at about 190 μmoles/g. hr. Oxaloacetate also yields anaerobically with sheep brain, as well as the pyruvate formed at least in part non-enzymically, some 16% of α-oxoglutarate, 12% of lactate, and 3% of citrate (Krebs *et al.*, 1940). These data gave one of the first clear indications that the tricarboxylic acid cycle formed the route of pyruvate oxidation in cerebral tissues. Previously it had appeared contra-indicated (Banga, Ochoa & Peters, 1939; Krebs & Eggleston, 1940).

Products from ^{14}C-labelled pyruvate also indicate condensation with oxalo-acetate. After administering 2-^{14}C-pyruvate to rats intracerebrally, or incubating cerebral tissues with the compound, isolation of ^{14}C-products showed much accumulation of isotope in free amino-acids (see above and Smith & Moses, 1960; McMillan & Mortensen, 1963). Glutamate, aspartate, and γ-aminobutyrate showed greatest enrichment and of the different carbon atoms in the glutamate, 4-C was little labelled, the 5-C was greatly enriched, and 1, 2 and 3-C carried about one-fifth its activity. The major labelling in position 5 was concluded to result from conversion of pyruvate to acetyl CoA (q.v.), its condensation with oxalocetate and the succeeding reactions of Table 6.2. ^{14}C-Acetate was also incorporated to cerebral glutamate.

Other Reactions associated with the Tricarboxylic Acid Cycle

In the preceding section, the cycle has been described in terms of its affording a route for metabolism of pyruvate via acetylcoenzyme A. Pyruvate can enter the cycle also after conversion to oxaloacetate, and metabolites other than pyruvate can enter as acetylcoenzyme A. These processes together with a cycle-associated role for α-glycerophosphate, are now described.

Pyruvate Carboxylation

Labelling of 2-C and 3-C of glutamate by using 2-[^{14}C]-pyruvate implies also the formation of oxaloacetate by addition of CO_2. Further evidence for such carboxylation has been obtained by measuring incorporation of $^{14}CO_2$ administered to cats by intracarotid infusion (Berl *et al.*, 1962; see Chapter 2). Soon after, the highest specific activity in cerebral extracts was found in aspartic acid. The use of $^{14}CO_2$ or $H^{14}CO_3^-$ also showed the CO_2 to be rapidly incorporated into malate in lobster nerve and mammalian brain. Glutamate and especially aspartate were also rapidly labelled (Cheng & Waelsch, 1963; Berl *et al.*, 1962). Two of the enzyme systems recognized in other tissues as catalysing such incorporation, have been observed in cerebral preparations (Utter, 1959). These are carboxylation of pyruvate to form oxaloacetate and the carboxylation-reaction which forms malate, catalysed by "malic enzyme". *Pyruvate carboxylase* (EC 6.4.1.1) which requires biotin, acetyl coenzyme A and ATP, is of very low activity in the brain relative to other tissues. This is perhaps not surprising as the carboxylase is a key enzyme in gluconeogenesis (Krebs, 1964), a pathway apparently absent from the brain (see Chapter 5). Oxaloacetate formation by this route proceeds at only about 12 μmoles of pyruvate carboxylated/g. hr. in rat cerebral cortex and is confined to the mitochondria (Salganicoff & Koeppe, 1968).

It is the second CO_2-fixing system which appears to be the important one in cerebral preparations. "*Malic enzyme*", malate dehydrogenase, decarboxylating (EC 1.1.1.40), which catalyzes the NADPH-linked formation of oxaloacetate from pyruvate and CO_2, is as active in the brain as in the heart, liver or kidney. It reacts at rates from 50 to 90 μmoles/g. hr. and occurs mainly in the mitochondria (Utter, 1959; Salganicoff & Koeppe, 1968). The level of activity in the brain is sufficient to generate adequate supplies of C_4 compounds leading to the oxaloacetate required for the condensation step with acetylcoenzyme A, also produced from pyruvate by the oxidative decarboxylation reaction described earlier.

Oxidation of Ketone Bodies

Oxidation in the brain of the ketone bodies, acetoacetate and β-hydroxybutyrate, is accompanied by esterification of phosphate and in certain circumstances may be an important source of metabolic energy. *In vitro*, cerebral cortical preparations consume acetoacetate at rates which, although below those in the heart, are comparable to those observed for kidney cortex or smooth muscle (Krebs, 1961; Krebs et al., 1961). Analyses of arterial and cerebral venous blood demonstrated (Fig. 2.2) that in starvation metabolic routes in the human brain adjusted in such a way that β-hydroxybutyric acid became a major oxidizable substrate. Appreciation of the link between ketone-body oxidation and ATP generation in the brain also came indirectly from studies on rates of amino acid incorporation into mitochondrial protein when β-hydroxybutyrate was the oxidisable substrate; these were lower in adult than in immature rat brain. Deductions that the difference could be due to limited ATP generation in the mature brain as a result of lower β-hydroxybutyrate dehydrogenase activity were confirmed from a study of the mitochondrial enzymatic activities during development (Figs. 2.2 and 6.4). Studies of β-hydroxybutyrate dehydrogenase in young animals showed also that when blood concentrations of hydroxybutyrate were high as a result of fat-rich diets or of starvation, the normal fall in dehydrogenase activity which occurred on weaning, could be retarded (Fig. 6.5). This was considered likely to be due to a limited stabilization of the enzyme by its substrate (Pull & McIlwain, 1971).

Quite distinct is the mechanism by which the brain in mature animals increased its utilization of ketone bodies, for then the potency or capacity of the cerebral β-hydroxybutyrate dehydrogenase and related enzymes did not

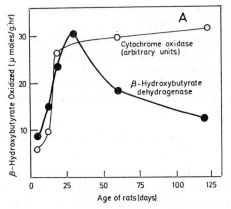
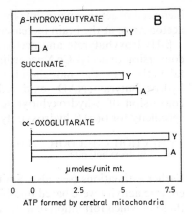

FIG. 6.4. Cerebral β-hydroxybutyrate dehydrogenase and oxidative
phosphorylation of cerebral mitochondria.
From the brain from rats of chosen ages, dispersions or mitochondrial suspensions were prepared. The mitochondria with
adenosine monophosphate, inorganic phosphate, Mg^{2+} and the
substrates indicated in **B** were incubated at 37° for 15 min. and sampled
for ATP. The dispersions (**A**) with ADP, phosphate, Mg^{2+}, NAD^+ and
β-hydroxybutyrate were used for assay of the dehydrogenase by
measurement of the acetoacetate formed (Klee & Sokoloff, 1967). In **B**,
Y refers to young and A to adult rats.

alter (Williamson, Bates, Page & Krebs, 1971; Page *et al.*, 1971; Cremer, 1971;
Pull & McIlwain, 1971) although utilization of β-hydroxybutyrate did
increase. This was due to the enzymes concerned not being saturated with
substrate at the normal, low blood levels of ketone bodies. When these were

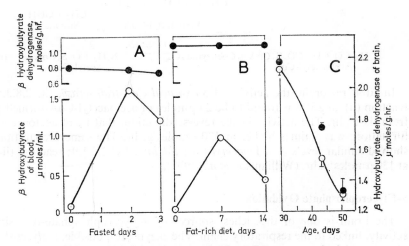

FIG. 6.5. The β-hydroxybutyrate and β-hydroxybutyrate dehydrogenase
of rats following different dietary treatments (Pull & McIlwain,
1971): A, adult rats, fasted; B, adult rats fed a fat-rich diet. C, young
rats: on normal diets, o; or fasted, ● for 2 to 3 days immediately
before sampling. Vertical lines give S.E.

increased in acute experiments by infusing acetoacetate to rats, the removal of acetoacetate at the brain increased (Hawkins, 1971).

β-Hydroxybutyrate and acetoacetate enter the tricarboxylic acid cycle by conversion to acetyl-CoA according to the following enzymic reactions which take place in the mitochondria. β-*Hydroxybutyrate dehydrogenase* (D-3-hydroxybutyrate:NAD+-oxidoreductase, EC 1.1.1.30) catalyzes the interconversion of β-hydroxybutyrate and acetoacetate (i) and shows absolute specificity for D(−) β-hydroxybutyrate.

$$CH_3.CHOH.CH_2.COOH + NAD^+ \rightleftharpoons CH_3.CO.CH_2.COOH + NADH + H^+ \qquad (i)$$
$$\text{β-hydroxybutyrate} \qquad\qquad\qquad \text{acetoacetate}$$

Earlier estimations (see also Smith, Satterthwaite & Sokoloff, 1969) of the enzyme activity were based on NADH formation and gave lower results than those in which formation of acetoacetate was followed. The latter method was concluded to be more specific in the situation and gave rates of 33 μmoles of acetoacetate formed at 25°/g. of brain/hr. in adult rat brain and 100 μmoles/g. hr. in the immature brain (Williamson *et al.*, 1971; Page *et al.*, 1971). At 37°, the rates were 70 μmoles/g. hr. in the adult and 140 μmoles/g. hr. in the immature brain (Cremer, 1971).

The acetoacetate, entering the brain or produced in the brain as a result of the above reaction, is converted to acetyl-CoA by reactions (ii) and (iii), involving intermediate formation of acetoacetyl-CoA.

$$\overset{\text{EC 2.8.3.5.}}{}$$

$$CH_3.CO.CH_2.COOH + \begin{array}{l} CH_2.CO.S.CoA \\ | \\ CH_2.COOH \end{array} \rightleftharpoons$$

Acetoacetate   Succinyl-CoA

$$CH_3.CO.CH_2.CO.S.CoA + \begin{array}{l} CH_2.COOH \\ | \\ CH_2.COOH \end{array} \qquad (ii)$$

Acetoacetyl-CoA   Succinate

$$\overset{\text{EC 2.3.1.9.}}{CH_3.CO.CH_2.CO.S.CoA + Coenzyme A \rightleftharpoons 2CH_3.CO.S.CoA} \qquad (iii)$$
$$\text{Acetoacetyl-CoA} \qquad\qquad\qquad \text{Acetyl-CoA}$$

In adult rat brain, the activity of 3-*oxo acid CoA-transferase*, EC 2.8.3.5; reaction (ii), at 25° was found to be 24 μmoles of acetoacetyl-CoA formed/g. fresh tissue/hr. The activity in the reverse direction, that is, of acetoacetate formation, was 5 times higher at 120 μmoles/g. hr. The same preparations showed similar levels of *acetoacetyl-CoA thiolase*, EC 2.3.1.9; reaction (iii), at 120 μmoles/g. hr. (Williamson *et al.*, 1971).

α-Glycerophosphate Oxidation

The brain is one of the richest sources of α-glycerophosphate-oxidising activity, linked to the respiratory chain. The enzyme responsible, L-*glycerol-3-phosphate dehydrogenase* (EC 1.1.99.5), contains tightly-bound flavin and non-haem iron and has been extracted from the mitochondria using phospholipase A, which caused 50% inactivation, or with Triton X-100. The presence of the detergent was necessary for enzyme solubility (Ringler, 1961; Dawson &

Thorne, 1968). The subcellular and regional distribution was found to be similar to that of cytochrome oxidase; the dehydrogenase was more active in the cerebellum than in frontal cortex or hypothalamus and less active in the corpus callosum (Tipton & Dawson, 1968).

Mitochondrial glycerol-3-phosphate dehydrogenase from rat brain gave rates of 850–950 μmoles of NADH oxidised/mg. of protein/hr. at 25° and, like the flavoprotein enzyme from other tissues, may be important in the oxidation of extra-mitochondrial NADH (see microsomal systems, below). Evidence that the dehydrogenase may participate in the process in rat brain has

(i)   Glyceraldehyde-3-phosphate + P_1 + NAD^+ ⟶

   1,3-diphosphoglycerate + NADH + H^+

(ii)   NADH + H^+ + dihydroxyacetone phosphate $\xrightarrow{\text{EC 1.1.1.8}}$

   NAD^+ + α-glycerophosphate

(iii) NAD^+ + α-glycerophosphate $\xrightarrow{\text{EC 1.1.99.5}}$

   NADH + H^+ + dihydroxyacetone phosphate

FIG. 6.6. The oxidation of NADH and α-glycerophosphate.

been reported (Kleitke & Wollenberger, 1969). The process (Fig. 6.6) involves the extra-mitochondrial re-oxidation by cytoplasmic glycerophosphate dehydrogenase (ii) of NADH produced in glycolysis (i). The α-glycerophosphate so formed passes into the mitochondria where the mitochondrial α-glycerophosphate dehydrogenase catalyses the reaction in reverse (iii). Dihydroxyacetone passes out from the mitochondria to complete the sequence.

The Respiratory Chain and Oxidative Phosphorylation

The tricarboxylic acid cycle and the associated reactions just described yield CO_2 and reduced flavin and nicotinamide nucleotides. Oxidation of the reduced nucleotides which regenerates their original form, is of outstanding importance because it occurs by a chain of reactions through which the energy of the oxidation is retained in utilizable form. It can be yielded as energy-rich phosphates by reaction-sequences which are common to many biological systems, and of which many components have now been demonstrated in neural tissues. The following description indicates first the sequence of carriers in the respiratory chain, and subsequently their relationship to phosphorylation.

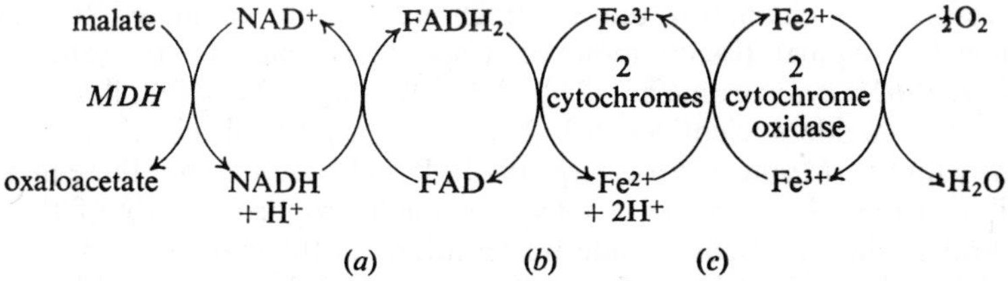

The main respiratory chain consists in cerebral as in other tissues in the oxidation of reduced nicotinamide adenine dinucleotide, NADH, through flavoproteins F and cytochromes Cyt. The scheme above, given in outline as an example, is the sequence in the oxidation of NADH produced as a result of malate dehydrogenation (*MDH*) (see Redfearn, 1961; Boyer *et al.*, 1963).

Additional features include the following.

(i) The sequence commences with NADH in the case of several substrates, in particular those indicated in Table 6.2, but certain other substrates themselves reduce flavoproteins; these include α-glycerophosphate and succinate (q.v.).

(ii) A number of cytochromes is involved, acting in a sequence which in several instances is: Cyt. b, Cyt. c_1, Cyt. c, Cyt. a, Cyt. a_3.

(iii) Components of the respiratory chain are physically associated in mitochondrial structure in fashions important to the reactions concerned; some disruption is caused by detergents and restoration by added lipids. For investigation of such factors in cerebral systems, see Giuditta & Strecker (1963). The initial stages of NADH oxidation are conditioned in this way, as is described by Singer (*Symposium*, 1964) and by di Prisco *et al.* (1965).

(iv) At three points in the chain, approximately indicated by (*a*), (*b*) and (*c*) above, the free energy change is sufficient for synthesis of an energy-rich phosphate bond.

Flavoproteins and Cytochromes

Data obtained by using mammalian cerebral tissues shows them to contain some 12 nmoles/g. of flavin adenine dinucleotide (see Chapter 10) and to exhibit light-absorption corresponding to several cytochrome components. When oxidizable substrates are added to suspensions of cerebral mitochondria, changes take place in the absorption peaks attributable to cytochromes and flavoproteins. The experiment of **A**, Fig. 6.7 shows a preparation of rat brain mitochondria to give optical changes corresponding to reduction of cyto-chrome b, while it is catalysing the oxidation of succinate. The oxidation is shown on the upper curve by the increased rate of oxygen uptake. The prepara-tion contained a quite small quantity only of cytochrome b (see below) which underwent cyclic reduction and oxidation in catalysing the uptake of oxygen. Thus on inhibition of succinate oxidation by malonate, the cytochrome became reoxidized. It was again reduced when addition was made of an alternative substrate, α-glycerophosphate, the oxidation of which is insensitive to malonate.

By measurements at wavelengths corresponding to different components of the respiratory chain, rat brain mitochondria were estimated to contain (nmoles/g. original tissue; minimal amounts calculated from Sacktor & Packer, 1962): cytochrome a, 0·7; b, 0·4; c plus c_1, 1·0; a_3, 0·8, flavoprotein, 0·7; nicotinamide nucleotides, 6·1. The levels in purified mitochondria were slightly higher (Moore & Strasberg, 1970). It will be noted that these methods exhibit in the mitochondria, a relatively small proportion only of the total cerebral flavin and nicotinamide nucleotides. As the cytochromes are iron-porphyrin derivatives, it is relevant to compare their quantity with the iron content of the brain. They contribute a few percent only. Other enzymes, e.g. α-glycerophosphate dehydrogenase (q.v.), carry iron in non-haem combination

(Ringler, 1961). The occurrence of compounds of iron in the brain, it may be noted, is not uniform and in for example the globus pallidus may be eight times that of the white matter. Only approximate correlation is to be seen between iron content and respiratory activity, and the element exists in a variety of different forms of combination (Tingey, 1938; Diezel, 1955; Hallgren & Sourander, 1958). The pathological significance of variation in cerebral iron levels has been appraised (Still *et al.*, 1969). The concentration of cytochrome c in the brain

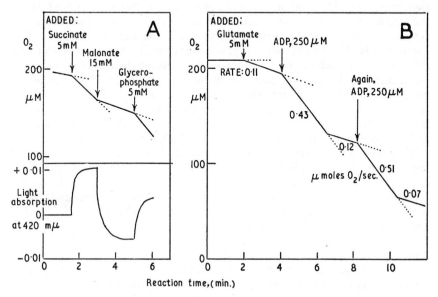

FIG. 6.7. Control of respiratory processes in cerebral mitochondria (Sacktor & Packer, 1962; see Voss *et al.*, 1961).

A. Cytochrome oxidation and reduction (lower curve) during the changes in respiration (upper curve) initiated in the mitochondrial suspensions, by the additions stated. Changes in optical density were measured at 410–430 mμ and ascribed to oxidation and reduction of cytochrome *b*.

B. Limited oxygen uptake initiated by limited additions of adenosine diphosphate, to a mitochondrial preparation from rat brain. The quantity of oxygen reacting (measured polarographically) in response to the addition of defined quantities of adenosine diphosphate, gave ADP/O ratios of 2·04, 2·04 and 2·03 in successive periods. The rates of oxygen uptake are given in μmoles O_2/sec., by numbers near the curve.

as a whole bears about the same relation to its respiratory rate as is found with content and rate in kidney or liver (Drabkin, 1950).

The oxidation of cytochromes a and a_3 has been expressed previously as a cytochrome oxidase activity and forms part of the earlier-investigated "indophenol oxidase system", by which *p*-phenylenediamine, hydroquinone or ascorbate is oxidized by cytochrome c. Oxygen uptake catalysed by cerebral tissues in such systems reached 160–190 μmoles O_2/g. tissue/hr. (Stotz, 1939), indicating that this part of the respiratory chain has a catalytic capacity more than adequate for the highest rates of cerebral respiration. Oxidation of several substrates by rat brain proceeds at rates which imply turnover of cerebral cytochrome a of 4–9 moles/mole/sec. Cytochrome oxidase activity has been found to vary greatly in different regions of the brain, being very low in the corpus callosum relative to the levels in the cerebral cortex, cerebellum or hypothalamus; this has been discussed from a phylogenetic viewpoint (Tolani & Talwar, 1963; Ridge, 1967; Tipton & Dawson, 1968).

Components of the respiratory chain can be studied spectrophotometrically in cell-containing cerebral tissues (Cummins, 1970, 1971). Electrical stimulation caused rapid reduction of the components, for increases in NADH, in reduced flavoproteins and in reduced cytochromes b, c and a–a_3 were observed. Application of acetylcholine produced similar but less marked changes. The increase in NADH and in reduced cytochrome c was inhibited by tetrodotoxin (10^{-7} M) and by ouabain (10^{-5} M). Increased K^+ caused changes in the opposite direction: NADH decreased and cytochrome c was oxidized. The action of K^+ was not affected by tetrodotoxin nor by ouabain. The studies indicated that the components of the respiratory chain in the brain respond rapidly to an increased demand for energy and that the response to electrical stimulation and to acetylcholine is different from that to high K^+.

The cerebral cytochrome system has been studied as the major site of the toxic effects of cyanides (see Chapter 3 and Himwich, 1951). Injection of even a non-lethal quantity of sodium cyanide (a few mg./kg. in dogs) reduced the cerebral arteriovenous difference in oxygen, transitorily, to one-tenth of its normal value. These quantities of cyanides did not combine appreciably with haemoglobin, which retained its normal oxygen-carrying capacity; this is in distinction to carbon monoxide which at toxic levels does so combine. When however specimens were examined from the brain of rats to which sodium cyanide at 0·1 μmole/g. had been injected, they showed an ability much less than normal in oxidizing reduced cytochrome c. Analysis of the brain showed the increase in inorganic phosphate and decrease in energy-rich phosphates which would be expected to follow inhibition of respiration. On addition of cyanide to normal cerebral tissues from untreated rats, an inhibition of cytochrome oxidase to about the extent observed in vivo (50%) was brought about by 0·02 μM cyanide. Methaemoglobin, known from clinical practice to reduce the toxic effects of cyanides, was found to reduce the effect of cyanide on the cerebral cytochrome oxidase in vitro.

Small doses of sodium cyanide (0·8 mg./kg. in cats) affect the electroencephalogram (see Fig. 3.6) and have been administered in schizophrenia with therapeutic intent, as has also malononitrile which decomposes in vivo yielding cyanides. Other nitriles induce hyperactivity and incoordination, and certain intoxications by plant products are due to cyanides (see Sourkes, 1962). Phosphorylation coupled to succinate or to cytochrome c is inhibited by chlorpromazine which also slightly inhibits cytochrome oxidase (Dawkins et al., 1959; see also Chapter 15).

Oxidative Phosphorylation

In oxidizing pyruvate, nicotinamide nucleotides are reduced at the four stages indicated in Table 6.2; in addition, oxidation of succinate involves stages similar to (b) and (c) of reactions in $FADH_2$, above. The yield of energy-rich phosphate in oxidizing 1 mole of pyruvate could thus be $4 \times 3, +2 + 1$: the latter being from the substrate-level oxidation of α-oxoglutarate. As the

Table 6.4

Oxidative phosphorylation with cerebral mitochondria and suspensions

Exp. (see below)	Additions to reaction mixtures described below	Ratios: P/O or ADP/O	Respiratory control ratio*
A	None	0	–
A	Pyruvate	0	–
A	Pyruvate + 2 mM-malate or fumarate	2·80	–
A	Pyruvate + 2 mM-malate; no hexokinase	0	–
B	Pyruvate + 1 mM-malate	3·00	7·3
A	Succinate	1·84	–
B	Succinate	1·97	3·8
B	Succinate + 1 mM-malate	2·15	3·4
A	Oxaloacetate	2·49	–
A	α-Oxoglutarate	2·38	–
B	α-Oxoglutarate	2·70	7·4
B	α-Oxoglutarate + 1 mM-malate	2·48	5·8
B	Glutamate	2·62	11·2
B	Glutamate + 1 mM-malate	2·99	10·2
A	Glutamate + 2 mM-malate	3·17	–
B	Isocitrate + 1 mM-malate	2·78	2·1
A	Alanine + 2 mM-malate	0·78	–
A	Aspartate + 2 mM-malate	0·50	–
B	Glutamine	1·94	2·7
B	Glutamine + 1 mM-malate	2·48	3·1
A**	Pyruvate + 2 mM-fumarate	2·6	–
A**	Pyruvate + 2 mM-fumarate; 50 μM-2:4-dinitrophenol	1·3	–
A**	Pyruvate + 2 mM-fumarate; 170 μM-2:4-dinitrophenol	0·1	–

Experiments A included cerebral suspensions (**) or mitochondria with glycylglycine or other buffers, adenosine phosphates, K^+, Mg^{2+} and phosphate salts and usually glucose and a hexokinase preparation. Substances added as main substrates are quoted first and were at 10–15 mM; usual reaction period, 30 min. (Case & McIlwain, 1951; Brody & Bain, 1952; Aldridge, 1957).

Experiments B were carried out using cerebral mitochondria specially prepared to produce tightly coupled oxidative phosphorylation. The oxygen uptake was measured polarographically after defined additions of adenosine diphosphate. Tris-buffered reaction mixtures contained rat brain mitochondria equivalent to 1·5–2 mg. protein/ml. with KCl and 5 mM-orthophosphate. The first named substrates were at 4 mM (Ozawa *et al.*, 1966).

* Respiratory control ratio is the ratio of the rate of respiration in the presence of ADP to the rate in its absence and is a measure of the tightness of coupling.

oxidation of 1 mole of pyruvate requires 2·5 moles O_2, the associated P/O ratio is $15/2\cdot5 \times 2$, or 3. The experiment of C, Fig. 6.1, carried out early in the subject of oxidative phosphorylation afforded a ratio of 1·5. With cerebral mitochondrial preparations and the reaction mixtures A of Table 6.4, values are reached of about 3 moles of phosphate esterified/atom of oxygen absorbed. For this result, it is seen that a dicarboxylic acid must be present with the pyruvate, and that the energy-rich products must be "trapped" by hexokinase and glucose.

Oxidation of several other metabolites of the tricarboxylic acid cycle, or related compounds, is also accompanied by esterification of phosphate. Five such substances are indicated in Table 6.4, affording results which are similar to those from other mitochondrial systems. Of substances having more specific relationship to the brain, γ-aminobutyrate causes some additional oxygen uptake, probably associated with phosphorylation (McKhann & Tower, 1961; Jobsis, 1963). Details of the production of high-energy phosphate during oxidation can at present only be suggested in outline but the phosphorylation can be dissociated from oxidation, by several added agents. 2:4-Dinitrophenol is shown to have this effect on phosphorylation catalysed by a cerebral suspension in the experiment of Table 6.4. It and the 3:5-dinitro-2-cresol owe their toxic effects *in vivo* to such actions in the mitochondria of cerebral and other tissues. After administration to the rat, the nitrocresol was shown to have its greatest effect on the labile phosphates of the brain (Parker, 1954). Cerebral cytochrome-linked *NADH dehydrogenases* (EC 1.6.2.1., 1.6.2.2) which occur with succinate dehydrogenase firmly bound to mitochondria, are inhibited by antimycin A and amylobarbitone. Flavin nucleotides and menadione (2-methyl-1,4-naphthoquinone) have been used as acceptors in following respiratory chain-linked NADH oxidation systems; inhibition by dicumarol and 2:4-dinitrophenol was also described (Levine *et al.*, 1960; Harper & Strecker, 1962; Friede & Fleming, 1962).

Adenosine diphosphate as a reactant in the oxidative phosphorylation catalysed by cerebral mitochondria has the special properties shown in **B**, Fig. 6.7. Ratios of ADP reacting per atom of oxygen absorbed are seen (Table 6.4) to be numerically similar to P/O ratios.

The highest ADP/O ratios have been observed polarographically with glutamate or α-oxoglutarate as substrate (Experiments B, Table 6.4; see also Løvtrup & Svennerholm, 1964; Millstein *et al.*, 1968). These two substrates also produced the tightest coupling (highest respiratory control ratio) between oxidation and phosphorylation; of the Krebs cycle intermediates, use of malate or succinate resulted in the lowest respiratory control ratios observed. The high degree of respiratory control when glutamate was oxidized has led to the suggestion that glutamate, produced rapidly from transamination reactions and occurring in high concentrations in the brain (Chapter 8), may be the normal endogenous energy-substrate for mitochondria *in situ* (Higgins, 1968). The data described above are consistent with mechanisms proposed for oxidative phosphorylation.

Although the components of the mitochondrial electron transport chain have been described above, the mechanisms by which ATP is synthesized from ADP and inorganic phosphate remain unclear. A number of mechanisms has been proposed (Symposium, 1970). The first of these is based on involvement of phosphorylated intermediates (Slater *et al.*, 1964; Slater, 1966). However, despite intensive study, no compound which satisfies the required criteria has so far been isolated. A distinctly different hypothesis, of chemiosomic coupling, proposes that electron transport is associated with a pH gradient across the mitochondrial membrane (Mitchell, 1967). According to this hypothesis, no common high-energy intermediates need to be postulated. This is also a feature of a proposal of Green (Penniston et al., 1968; Harris et al., 1968) that the intermediates in oxidative phosphorylation are energized complexes of the respiratory chain components which can undergo conformational changes; see also Aldridge & Rose (1969).

Microsomal systems

The brain and other tissues oxidize nicotinamide and flavin nucleotides also by components in the microsomes. Cytochromes b_5 and c have been found in the brain in concentrations lower than in mitochondria but relevant to extra-mitochondrial reoxidation of reduced nucleotides. The cytochrome b_5 of rabbit brain microsomes was concluded to occur at maximal amounts of some 40 pmoles per mg. of protein in the light microsomal fraction. The total flavoproteins of cerebral microsomes have been estimated to be also about 40 pmoles/mg. of protein. The oxidation is coupled through cytochrome c reductase; NADH oxidation was concluded to be through cytochrome b_5 to cytochrome c, while oxidation of NADPH went through flavoproteins in a naphthoquinone-requiring reaction to cytochrome c (Inouye & Shinagawa, 1965; Moore & Strasberg, 1970).

Creatine Phosphate as Energy Reserve

The amide phosphate of creatine is an important form of storage of high energy phosphate in the brain. The levels of creatine phosphate (Table 3.4) fall rapidly during ischaemia in vivo (Fig. 7.2) and also at the expense of ATP synthesis during electrical stimulation in vitro (Fig. 4.8). Examination of the data of Fig. 4.8 and Fig. 7.2 reveals that creatine phosphate is more labile than ATP and acts as an energy reserve for ATP. Energy exchange between the nucleotide and the amide is mediated by *ATP: creatine phosphotransferase* (creatine kinase, EC 2.7.3.2) which catalyses the reaction set out below.

$$
\underset{\substack{\text{creatine}}}{\overset{\displaystyle \overset{\text{NH}}{\|}}{H_2N.C.N.CH_2.COOH}} + ATP \;\rightleftharpoons\; \underset{\substack{\text{creatine phosphate}}}{\overset{\displaystyle \overset{\text{NH}}{\|}}{H_2O_3P.NH.C.N.CH_2.COOH}} + ADP
$$
$$
\underset{}{CH_3} \qquad\qquad\qquad\qquad\qquad\qquad CH_3
$$

Mg is required for maximum activity and the enzyme is activated also by thiols (e.g. thioglycollate). The enzyme is distributed equally in ox or rat cerebral cortex between the soluble cytoplasm and the mitochondria. It has been suggested that the mitochondrial activity may be in the direction of ATP utilization to form creatine phosphate and that the cytoplasmic activity may act in situ to catalyse the reverse reaction to keep constant levels of ATP at sites of ATP utilization. Only minor differences were noted in kinetic and physical properties between the particulate and soluble enzymes. Both exhibited similar pH optima: pH 8·5 for creatine phosphate synthesis and pH 6·5–7·0 for ATP synthesis (Wood, 1963; Wood & Swanson, 1964; Swanson, 1967; Sullivan *et al.*, 1968). The crystalline enzyme from calf brain has a molecular weight of 85,000 and consists of two non-covalently linked polypeptide chains of mol. wt. 40,000–45,000 (Keutel *et al.*, 1968; Yue *et al.*, 1968).

Metabolic Control

Description of cerebral metabolism in this and in preceding chapters has displayed many enzyme mechanisms of large catalytic capacity, capable of removing within seconds all substrates available to them. Reactions of this potential speed are necessarily self-limiting or are otherwise controlled, and their capacity utilized only partially or intermittently. Processes of metabolic control are indeed well developed in the brain, and are a major subject of the Chapter which follows.

REFERENCES

ADLER, E., EULER, H. V., GUNTHER, G. & PLASS, M. (1939). *Biochem. J.* **33**,1028.
ALDRIDGE, W. N. (1957). *Biochem. J.* **67**, 427.
ALDRIDGE, W. N. & JOHNSON, M. K. (1959). *Biochem. J.* **73**, 270.
ALDRIDGE, W. N. & ROSE, M. S. (1969). *FEBS Letters*, **4**, 61.
BANGA, I., OCHOA, S. & PETERS, R. A. (1939). *Biochem. J.* **33**, 1980.
BERL, S., TAKAGAKI, G., CLARKE, D. D. & WAELSCH, H. (1962). *J. biol. Chem.* **237**, 2562, 2570.
BOYER, P. D., LARDY, H. & MYRBÄCK, K. (1963). The Enzymes, 2nd ed. New York: Academic Press.
BRODY, T. M. & BAIN, J. A. (1952). *J. biol. Chem.* **195**, 685.
BUFFA, P., PETERS, R. A. & WAKELIN, R. W. (1951). *Biochem. J.* **48**, 467.
CASE, E. M. & MCILWAIN, H. (1951). *Biochem. J.* **48**, 1.
CARLETON, A. B., PETERS, R. A. & THOMPSON, R. H. S. (1948). *Quart. J. Med.* N.S. **17**, 49.
CHENG, S.-C. & WAELSCH, H. (1963). *Biochem. Z.* **338**, 643.
COXON, R. V. (1953). *Biochem. J.* **55**, 545.
COXON, R. V., LIÉBECQ, C. & PETERS, R. A. (1949). *Biochem. J.* **45**, 320.
COXON, R. V. & PETERS, R. A. (1950). *Biochem. J.* **46**, 300.
CREMER, J. E. (1971). *Biochem. J.* **122**, 135.
CUMMINS, J. T. (1970). *The Pharmacologist*, **12**, 223.
CUMMINS, J. T. (1971). Personal communication.
DAWKINS, M. J. R., JUDAH, J. D. & REES, K. R. (1959). *Biochem. J.* **72**, 204.
DAWSON, A. P. & THORNE, C. J. R. (1968). *Biochem. J.* **111**, 27.
DEITRICH, R. A. & HELLERMAN, L. (1964). *J. biol. Chem.* **239**, 2735.
DICKENS, F. (1962). In Neurochemistry. Ed. Elliott, Page & Quastel. Springfield: Thomas.
DIEZEL, P. B. (1955). *Proc. Internat. Neurochem. Sympos.* **1**, 145.
DIPLOCK, A. T., BUNYAN, J., GREEN, J. & EDWIN, E. E. (1961). *Biochem. J.* **79**, 105.
DI PRISCO, G., BANAY-SCHWARTZ, M. & STRECKER, H. J. (1965). *J. Neurochem.* **12**, 113.
DRABKIN, D. L. (1950). *J. biol. Chem.* **182**, 317.
EDWIN, E. E., DIPLOCK, A. T., BUNYAN, J. & GREEN, J. (1961). *Biochem. J.* **79**, 91.
FRIEDE, R. L. & FLEMING, L. M. (1962). *J. Neurochem.* **9**, 179.
GELBER, S., CAMPBELL, P. L., DEIBLER, G. B. & SOKOLOFF, L. (1964). *J. Neurochem.* **11**, 220.
GIUDITTA, A. & STRECKER, H. J. (1959). *J. Neurochem.* **5**, 50.
GIUDITTA, A. & STRECKER, H. J. (1963). *Biochim. Biophys. Acta*, **67**, 316.
GOEBELL, H. & KLINGENBERG, M. (1964). *Biochem. Z.* **340**, 411.

GOLDBERG, N. D., PASSONNEAU, J. V. & LOWRY, O. H. (1966). *J. Biol. Chem.* **241**, 3997.

GONDA, O. & QUASTEL, J. H. (1962). *Nature, Lond.* **193**, 138.

GREEN, D. E. (1936). *Biochem. J.* **30**, 2095.

GREENGARD, O. (1967). *Enzymologia biol. clin.* **8**, 81.

HALLGREN, B. & SOURANDER, P. (1958). *J. Neurochem.* **3**, 41.

HARPER, E. & STRECKER, H. J. (1962). *J. Neurochem.* **9**, 125.

HARRIS, R. A., PENNISTON, J. T., ASAI, J. & GREEN, D. E. (1968). *Proc. nat. Acad. Sci. U.S.* **59**, 830.

HASLAM, R. J. & KREBS, H. A. (1963). *Biochem. J.* **88**, 566.

HAWKINS, R. A. (1971). *Biochem. J.* **121**, 17P.

HIGGINS, E. S. (1968). *J. Neurochem.* **15**, 589.

HIMWICH, H. E. (1951). Brain Metabolism and Cerebral Disorders. Baltimore: Williams & Wilkins.

HOLOWACH, J., KAUFMAN, F., IKOSSI, M. G., THOMAS, C. & McDOUGALL, D. B. (1968). *J. Neurochem.* **15**, 621.

INOUYE, A. & SHINAGAWA, Y. (1965). *J. Neurochem.* **12**, 803.

JOBSIS, F. F. (1963). *Biochim. Biophys. Acta.* **7**, 60.

JOHNSON, W. A. (1939). *Biochem. J.* **33**, 1046.

KEUTEL, H. J., JACOBS, H. K., OKABE, K., YUE, R. H. & KUBY, S. A. (1968). *Biochemistry*, **7**, 4283.

KINNERSLEY, H. W. & PETERS, R. A. (1929). *Biochem. J.* **23**, 1126.

KLEE, G. B. & SOKOLOFF, L. (1964). *J. Neurochem.* **11**, 709.

KLEE, G. B. & SOKOLOFF, L. (1967). *J. biol. chem.* **242**, 3880.

KLEITKE, B. & WOLLENBERGER, A. (1969). *J. Neurochem.* **16**, 1629.

KORKES, S., DEL CAMPILLO, A., KOREY, S. R., STERN, J. R., NACHMANSOHN, D. & OCHOA, S. (1952). *J. biol. Chem.* **198**, 215.

KREBS, H. A. (1953). *Biochem. J.* **54**, 78.

KREBS, H. A. (1961). *Biochem. J.* **80**, 225.

KREBS, H. A. (1964). *Proc. Roy. Soc. B.* **159**, 545.

KREBS, H. A. & EGGLESTON, L. V. (1940). *Biochem. J.* **34**, 442.

KREBS, H. A., EGGLESTON, L. V. & D'ALESSANDRO, A. (1961). *Biochem. J.* **79**, 537.

KREBS, H. A., EGGLESTON, L. V., KLEINZELLER, A. & SMYTH, D. H. (1940). *Biochem. J.* **34**, 1234.

KREBS, H. A. & JOHNSON, W. A. (1937). *Biochem. J.* **31**, 645, 772.

LAHIRI, S. & QUASTEL, J. H. (1963). *Biochem. J.* **89**, 157.

LEVINE, W., GIUDITTA, A., ENGLARD, S. & STRECKER, H. J. (1960). *J. Neurochem.* **6**, 28.

LINDSAY, J. R. & BACHELARD, H. S. (1966). *Biochem. Pharmacol.* **15**, 1945.

LONG, C. (1938). *Biochem. J.* **32**, 1711.

LONG, C. (1945). *Biochem. J.* **39**, 143.

LONG, C. & PETERS, R. A. (1939). *Biochem. J.* **33**, 759.

LØVTRUP, S. & SVENNERHOLM, L. (1964). *Exp. cell. Res.* **29**, 298.

LOWRY, O. H., ROBERTS, N. R., WU, M-L., HIXON, W. S. & CRAWFORD, E. J. (1954). *J. biol. Chem.* **207**, 19.

McKHANN, G. M. & TOWER, D. B. (1961). *J. Neurochem.* **7**, 26.

McMILLAN, P. J. & MORTENSEN, R. A. (1963). *J. biol. Chem.* **238**, 91.

MASSEY, V. & VEEGER, C. (1963). *Ann. Rev. Biochem.* **32**, 579.

MILLSTEIN, J. M., WHITE, J. G. & SWAIMAN, K. F. (1968). *J. Neurochem.* **15**, 4111.

MITCHELL, P. (1967). *Feder. Proc.* **26**, 1370.

MOORE, C. L. & STRASBERG, P. M. (1970). *Handbook of Neurochemistry.* **3**, 53.

O'BRIEN, J. R. P. & PETERS, R. A. (1935). *J. Physiol.* **85**, 454.

OCHOA, S. (1941). *J. biol. Chem.* **141**, 245.

OCHOA, S. (1948). *J. biol. Chem.* **174**, 115, 133.

OCHOA, S. (1954). *Adv. in Enzymol.* **15**, 183.

OZAWA, K., SETA, K., TAKEDA, H., ANDO, K., HANDA, H. & ARAKI, C. (1966). *J. Biochem. Japan*, **59**, 501.

PAGE, M. A., KREBS, H. A. & WILLIAMSON, D. H. (1971). *Biochem. J.* **121**, 49.

PARKER, V. H. (1954). *Biochem. J.* **57**, 381.

PAUSESCU, E., SCHWARTZ, B., CHIRVASIE, R. & DINCA, A. (1967). *Exp. Neurol.* **19**, 455.
PENNISTON, J. T., HARRIS, R. A., ASAI, J. & GREEN, D. E. (1968). *Proc. nat. Acad. Sci. U.S.* **59**, 624.
PETERS, R. A. (1957). *Adv. Enzymol.* **18**, 113.
PETERS, R. A. (1963). Biochemical Lesions and Lethal Synthesis. Oxford: Pergamon.
PETERS, R. A., STOCKEN, L. A. & THOMPSON, R. H. S. (1945). *Nature, Lond.* **156**, 616.
PETERS, R. A. & THOMPSON, R. H. S. (1934). *Biochem. J.* **28**, 916.
PETERS, R. A. & WAKELIN, R. W. (1949). *Brit. J. Pharmacol.* **4**, 51.
PSCHEIDT, G. R., BENITEZ, D., KIRSCHNER, L. B. & STONE, W. E. (1954). *Amer. J. Physiol.* **176**, 483, 488.
PULL, I. & MCILWAIN, H. (1971). *J. Neurochem.* **18**.
REDFEARN, E. R. (1961). *Ann. Rep. Chem. Soc.* **57**, 395.
RIDGE, J. W. (1967). *Biochem. J.* **102**, 612.
RINGLER, R. L. (1961). *J. biol. Chem.* **236**, 1192.
ROBINS, E., SMITH, D. E., EYDT, K. M. & MCCAMEN, R. E. (1956). *J. Neurochem.* **1**, 68.
SACKTOR, B. & PACKER, L. (1962). *J. Neurochem.* **9**, 371.
SALGANICOFF, L. & KOEPPE, R. E. (1968). *J. biol. Chem.* **243**, 3416.
SLATER, E. C., KEMP, A. & TAGER, J. M. (1964). *Nature, Lond.* **201**, 781.
SLATER, E. C. (1966). In Comprehensive Biochemistry, Vol. 14, p. 327. Ed. M. Florkin & E. H. Stotz.
SMITH, A. L., SATTERTHWAITE, H. S. & SOKOLOFF, L. (1969). *Science*, **163**, 79.
SMITH, M. J. H. & MOSES, V. (1960). *Biochem. J.* **76**, 259.
SOURKES, T. L. (1962). Biochemistry of Mental Disease. New York: Hoeber.
SRERE, P. A. (1959). *J. biol. Chem.* **234**, 2544.
STILL, C. N., GADSEN, R. H. & HIERS, W. (1969). *Second Internat. Neurochem. Meeting*, p. 380. Milan: Tamburini.
STOCKEN, L. A. & THOMPSON, R. H. S. (1946). *Biochem. J.* **40**, 529, 535.
STOTZ, E. (1939). *J. biol. Chem.* **131**, 555.
STROMINGER, J. L. & LOWRY, O. H. (1955). *J. biol. Chem.* **213**, 635.
SULLIVAN, R. J., MILLER, O. N. & SELLINGER, O. Z. (1968). *J. Neurochem.* **15**, 115.
SWANSON, P. D. (1967). *J. Neurochem.* **14**, 343.
Symposium (1960). Inhibition in the Nervous System and Gamma-aminobutyric acid. Ed. E. Roberts. New York: Pergamon.
Symposium (1964). Oxygen in the Animal Organism. Ed. F. Dickens & E. Neil. Oxford: Pergamon.
Symposium (1970). Biological oxidation and bioenergetics, p. 137. Lucerne: 8th Intern. Congress Biochem.
TINGEY, A. H. (1938). *J. ment. Sci.* **84**, 980.
TIPTON, K. F. & DAWSON, A. P. (1968). *Biochem. J.* **108**, 95.
TOLANI, A. J. & TALWAR, G. P. (1963). *Biochem. J.* **88**, 357.
TUČEK, S. (1967). *J. Neurochem.* **14**, 531.
UTTER, M. F. (1959). *Ann. N.Y. Acad. Sci.* **72**, 454.
VOSS, D. O., CAMPELLO, A. P. & BACILA, M. (1961). *Biochem. Biophys. Res. Comm.* **4**, 48.
WEBER, G., LEA, M. A., HERD CONVERY, H. J. & STAMM, N. B. (1967). *Adv. Enzyme Reg.* **5**, 257.
WEIL-MALHERBE, H. (1937). *Biochem. J.* **31**, 299, 2080, 2202.
WILLIAMSON, D. H., BATES, M. W., PAGE, M. A. & KREBS, H. A. (1971). *Biochem. J.* **121**, 41.
WINER, A. D. (1960). *Biochem. J.* **76**, 5P.
WOLLEMANN, M. (1959). *Acta Physiol. Acad. Sci. Hung.* **16**, 153.
WOLLEMANN, M. & FEUER, G. (1957). *Acta Physiol., Hung.* **11**, 165.
WOOD, T. (1963). *Biochem. J.* **87**, 453.
WOOD, T. & SWANSON, P. D. (1964). *J. Neurochem.* **11**, 301.
YUE, R. H., JACOBS, H. K., OKABE, K., KEUTEL, H. J. & KUBY, S. A. (1968). *Biochemistry*, **7**, 4291.

7 Regulatory Processes in Intermediary Metabolism in the Brain

Neural systems exhibit a complex structural and metabolic organization; the balance and co-ordination of a large number of individual metabolic reactions is essential for neural function. Mechanisms which participate in regulation fall into two main categories: those which enable rapid change in activity of pre-existing enzymes (Table 7.1) and those causing long-term changes, in which the amount of available enzyme is regulated by modification in rates of enzyme synthesis.

The immediate regulatory responses are brought about by factors which influence the activity of pre-formed enzymes; these cause rapid, second by second, adjustments of metabolic processes to altered conditions *in situ*. Activity of pre-existing enzymes is conditioned primarily by the extent of interaction of the enzyme with components of small molecular weight, including substrates, cofactors and products. Many of the factors listed in Table 7.1 affect the amount of enzyme–substrate complex which is formed or modify the rate at which the complex is converted to product. Substrate concentration itself may limit the extent to which the enzyme–substrate complex will form; many substrates, such as glucose (q.v.), occur intracellularly at concentrations well below those required for full saturation of enzyme. This is of particular relevance in cases where more than one enzyme requires the same substrate. Examples are provided in intermediates common to more than one pathway; glucose-6-phosphate is the substrate for the isomerase of glycolysis, for the dehydrogenase in the pentose phosphate pathway and for the synthetase which forms glycogen. Acetyl coenzyme A is required for maintenance of the tricarboxylic acid cycle, for fat synthesis and for acetylcholine formation. Further involvement of metabolic intermediates is shown by direct interaction of product with the enzyme catalysing the reaction which forms that product; examples are again provided by glucose-6-phosphate in inhibition of hexokinase and acetyl coenzyme A in its inhibition of pyruvate oxidation. Regulation of metabolism in one pathway may be exerted by an intermediate of a related pathway; citrate inhibition of phosphofructokinase provides for control of glycolytic rates from the tricarboxylic acid cycle. Similar regulation of one pathway by another can be seen in the metabolism of nucleotide bases (Chapter 9). Many examples of competition between different enzymes for the same coenzyme are seen in cerebral metabolism, and the extent of metabolism of an intermediate common to competing or alternative pathways will be affected by limitations in concentration of available coenzyme in the required redox state; nicotinamide nucleotide coenzymes are especially important in this regard and are discussed in the sections which follow.

Identification of the control point of a metabolic pathway came first from detection of the "pacemaker" enzyme, i.e. that which catalysed the slowest stage in the pathway and which therefore could be regarded as rate-limiting

Table 7.1

Regulation of intermediate metabolism in the brain

The table gives examples only and these are documented more fully in the chapters indicated.

Factor influencing enzymic activity	Stage at which control is exerted	Process affected	Chapter
(1) Requirement for ions:			
Na^+ and K^+	Na^+, K^+-ATPase	Cation transport	12
K^+	Phosphofructokinase	Glycolysis	5
	Pyruvate kinase	Glycolysis, respiration	5, 6
(2) Competition for coenzymes:			
NAD^+, NADH	Various	Glycolysis, respiration, amino acid metabolism	5, 6 / 8
$NADP^+$, NADPH	Various	Pentose phosphate pathway, fat synthesis	5 / 11
(3) Interaction with metabolic intermediates:			
Glucose-6-phosphate	Hexokinase (inhibited)	Glycolysis	5
	Glycogen synthetase (activated)	Glycogen synthesis	5
Adenosine diphosphate	Hexokinase, phosphofructokinase (inhibited)	Glycolysis	5
	*Iso*citrate dehydrogenase, oxidative phosphorylation (activated)	Respiration	6
Adenosine triphosphate	Hexokinase, phosphofructokinase and pyruvate kinase	Glycolysis, respiration	5, 6
	Adenylate deaminase (activated) 5'-Nucleotidase (inhibited)	Purine nucleotide metabolism	9
Cytidine triphosphate	ATP-activated adenylate deaminase (inhibited)	Purine nucleotide metabolism	9
Acetyl coenzyme A	Pyruvate formation and oxidation (inhibited)	Glycolysis	5
	Citrate synthetase	Respiration	6
	Fatty acid synthetase	Fat synthesis	11
	Choline acetylase	Acetyl choline synthesis	14
Citrate	Phosphofructokinase (inhibited)	Glycolysis, respiration	5, 6
(4) Cytochemical:			
Enzyme localisation	Creatine kinase (mitochondrial and cytoplasmic)	ATP synthesis and utilization	6, 12

(Krebs, 1956). Kinetic studies, especially of product inhibition, have contributed valuable information on likely control points. Other approaches to the problem have included measurements of turnover rates of metabolic intermediates and estimations of equilibrium constants of individual reactions (Lowry *et al.*, 1964; Rolleston & Newsholme, 1967). Such studies of individual stages of the pathways of intermediary metabolism have provided evidence on the steps which may be assigned relevance to regulation. These steps can be seen to have importance, not only because of the chemical change which they represent, but also because they exhibit properties, suitable to involvement in regulation, which control the sequence of which they form part. These now receive attention and where possible, attempts are made to examine their interaction in regulating integrated metabolic processes (Weber, 1963; Chance et al., 1965; Rose & Rose, 1969).

Regulation of intermediary metabolism is important also in relation to the capacity of the brain to adapt promptly and efficiently to alterations in environmental conditions by rapid modification of rates of individual reactions. Thus rates of enzyme synthesis may be affected by presence of specific substrate or cofactor and also by interaction with drugs or hormones. Examples of factors which induce enzyme synthesis in the brain include the following: substrate interaction in increasing the activity of β-hydroxybutyrate dehydrogenase (Chapter 6) and of glutamate decarboxylase (Chapter 8), action of coenzyme (thiamine pyrophosphate) in pyruvate dehydrogenase synthesis (Chapter 10) and the environmental factors involved in the activity of β-hydroxyindole-O-methyltransferase (Chapter 14). The action of agents which inhibit specific stages of protein synthesis (Chapter 9) provides evidence that the factors act to affect net synthesis of enzyme protein rather than to cause modification in activity of pre-existing enzyme. Fuller documentation of these and other factors are given in subsequent Chapters.

It follows from the comments above, that the mechanisms by which control is achieved include the intracellular concentrations of metabolic intermediates and ions, which thus raises questions of how these may enter the brain. Some relevant mechanisms were discussed in Chapter 3; the entry of glucose merits the following particular attention.

Glucose Transport

Control of aspects of carbohydrate metabolism by modifying rates of glucose entry should be important in cells in which the concentrations of intracellular glucose are low and the potential activity of hexokinase is high; glucose uptake is then likely to be limiting. Such appears to be the situation in the brain. It was earlier believed that glucose entry to the brain was unimpeded, yet recent studies on factors operating to regulate rates of carbohydrate metabolism in the brain have served to indicate that the uptake may itself be a limiting factor. Glucose phosphorylation is likely to proceed at only a small proportion (3–5 %) of the rate of which brain hexokinase is potentially capable, since glucose-6-phosphate does not accumulate. Yet glucose itself also does not accumulate under normal conditions. Intracellular glucose is likely to be negligible in the brain in vivo (Bachelard, 1969); in vitro also, low concentrations have been found (Chain et al., 1960; Rolleston & Newsholme, 1967) and in some studies with incubated slices of cerebral cortex, intracellular glucose was detected only if an inhibitor of glycolysis was present (Joanny et al., 1969). It follows therefore that transport may be a control point in cerebral glycolysis. In the dog brain in vivo, over 75 % of glucose uptake was concluded to be due to facilitated transport which followed Michaelis-Menten kinetics with a K_m of 1–2 mM; the remainder was by diffusion (Gilboe & Betz, 1970).

The uptake of glucose into the brain, or cell-containing preparations derived from it, has been shown in vivo and in vitro to be a stereo-specific, saturable, carrier-mediated form of facilitated transport (Crone, 1965; Fishman, 1964; Eidelberg et al., 1967; see also Chapter 3). Evidence on the

6

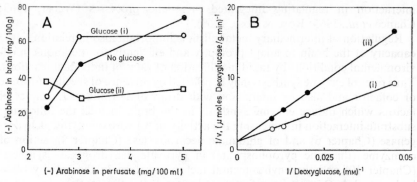

FIG. 7.1. Competition by monosaccharides for glucose uptake in the brain.

A. (−)-Arabinose uptake into perfused cat brain in the presence of glucose: (i) 31·2 mg/ml., (ii) 155 mg./ml., in the perfusing fluid (Eidelberg *et al.*, 1967).

B. 2-Deoxyglucose uptake into guinea pig cerebral cortex *in vitro* in the presence of glucose: (i) 5 mM, (ii) 15 mM, in the medium (Bachelard, 1971a).

substrate specificity of the process has come from studies on competition between sugars for entry to the brain. Thus the D-forms of the pyranose sugars, arabinose and xylose, decrease glucose uptake *in vivo* and *in vitro*, whereas furanose sugars (fructose, sorbose and ribose) do not. The relationship between arabinose and glucose in uptake by the perfused brain is illustrated in **A**, Fig. 7.1. The glucose analogues, 3-O-methylglucose and 2-deoxyglucose (**B**, Fig. 7.1), also compete but α-methylglucoside has no effect. D-mannose apparently competes for glucose uptake *in vivo* but no competition has been demonstrated *in vitro*; conversion of mannose to glucose elsewhere in the body before it reaches the brain explains the results obtained *in vivo*. Analysis of the results of specificity studies (Table 7.2) leads to the conclusion that modifica-

Table 7.2

Competition for cerebral glucose transport

Sugar	C atom modified	Method of study	Competition	Reference
α-Methylglucoside	1	*In vitro*	−	1
2-Deoxyglucose	2	*In vitro*	+	1, 2
3-O-Methylglucose	3	*In vivo*	+	3, 4
Galactose	4	*In vivo*	−	5
		In vitro	−	6
Arabinose	3, 6	*In vivo*	+	7
		In vitro	+	6
Xylose	6	*In vivo*	+	8
		In vitro	+	6

Data from [1] Bachelard, 1971a; [2] Gilbert, 1965; [3] Himsworth, 1968; [4] Bidder, 1968; [5] LeFevre & Peters, 1966; [6] Joanny *et al.*, 1969; [7] Eidelberg *et al.*, 1967; [8] Bradbury & Davson, 1964.

tion of the substituents on two of the carbon atoms of glucose affects the affinity of the substrate for the transport process. These are C atoms nos. 1 and 4, below. Substrates modified in the other positions listed in Table 7.2 compete, and the modifications may affect the rate of entry. Thus, whereas 2-deoxyglucose is taken up at rates comparable to those of glucose, the transport of xylose and arabinose is considerably slower.

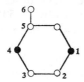

Anomeric preference for the α or β forms of D-glucose is not clearly established. *Mutarotase* (EC 5.1.3.3), which catalyses the conversion of α-D-glucose to the β-epimer, occurs in mammalian brain with activities comparable to those found in liver or kidney (Keston, 1954, 1957). Although the brain exhibits a preference for the β-epimer in its uptake from the bloodstream (Chapter 2) the importance of mutarotase as a rate-limiting step in glucose utilization has been questioned. Glucose-6-phosphate itself undergoes very rapid and spontaneous mutarotation and there is no clear evidence for anomeric preference in enzymic stages of glucose oxidation (Bailey *et al.*, 1968).

Rates of glucose uptake have been measured *in vitro*, either by disappearance of glucose from the medium or by calculations of ^{14}C incorporated into metabolites from labelled glucose, and found to be 22·5–25 μmoles/g. hr. (Gilbert, 1966; Bachelard, 1971a); this correlates well with measurements of overall rates of utilization of glucose in the intact tissue (Chapter 2). The apparent K_m for glucose in the uptake process (approximately 5 mM) is close to the concentration (80–100 mg/100 ml.) of glucose in the blood (Bachelard, 1971a). A requirement for energy to support sugar transport has not been established; although ouabain at relatively high concentration (1 mM) caused 25 % inhibition of arabinose uptake, dinitrophenol (1 mM) or phlorrhizin had no effect (Eidelberg *et al.*, 1967). Possible utilization of substrates as alternative to glucose has received comment in Chapters 2, 5 and 6; acetoacetate and β-hydroxybutyrate, which are utilized under conditions of starvation and high rates of fat mobilization in the body, have been suggested to be taken up from the bloodstream less rapidly than glucose under normal conditions (Itoh & Quastel, 1970). Intracellular glucose of the brain is increased by treatment *in vivo* with barbiturates (Mayman *et al.*, 1964); this may be due not only to decreased rates of utilization, but also to increased transport, as kinetic studies have indicated that the Michaelis constant and the maximum velocity for xylose uptake are both affected by relevant concentrations of phenobarbitone *in vitro* (Gilbert *et al.*, 1966).

Any direct effect of insulin on cerebral glucose transport is less certain (Rafaelson, 1961; Crone, 1965). Although marked decrease in cerebral glycogen content occurs as a result of insulin-induced decrease in blood sugar, the effect is probably due to the hypoglycaemia rather than to a direct effect of insulin on the brain itself. A direct involvement of insulin supplied by the blood in brain function *in vivo* is difficult to assess as the extent of penetration into the brain of the hormone, especially if it is derived from exogenous sources, appears to be very limited. *In vitro* studies on the influence of insulin on glucose uptake into isolated samples of a variety of neural tissues have yielded varying results. However, insulin, directly applied to the brain *in vivo*, has recently been shown to increase glycogen and glucose-6-phosphate. Three to four hours after intracranial injection of relatively high doses (0·1–0·2 international unit) of insulin, rat brain glycogen increased by 25–50 % and glucose-6-phosphate by 60 %, but no increase was detected in blood glucose or in muscle glycogen. Systemic injection of similar doses of insulin had no effect on brain glycogen (Mellerup & Rafaelson, 1969; Strang & Bachelard, 1971; Bachelard, 1971b). Glucose uptake into human brain *in vivo* may also be insulin-sensitive (Butterfield *et al.*, 1966).

There is increasing evidence that glucose uptake may be increased by stimulation of the brain. Increase in lactate observed as a result of electroshock *in vivo* (King *et al.*, 1967) was much greater than could be accounted for by concomitant decrease in glucose and glycogen. The evidence was thus indirect, but was taken to imply at least an eight-fold increase in the rate of glucose uptake. Direct evidence that electrical stimulation increases the rate of entry of glucose and 2-deoxyglucose has emerged from studies *in vitro* (Bachelard, 1971b).

Regulation of Energy Metabolism—General Aspects

Preceding chapters have indicated that cerebral tissues are capable of catalysing the individual stages of glycolysis, of the tricarboxylic acid cycle and of the respiratory chain at speeds much greater than those normal to the brain *in situ* or to cerebral tissues in isolation. To account for cerebral respiration with glucose as substrate and at 120 μmoles O_2/g. tissue/hr., the cycle would be required to proceed at 40 μmoles/g. tissue/hr., because one sequence of the cycle accounts for the oxidation of the acetyl group from one C_3 unit, and the overall reaction of the C_3 unit from glucose is: $C_3H_6O_3 + 3O_2 \rightarrow 3CO_2 + 3H_2O$. The majority of the individual steps of the cycle have in fact been observed to proceed at rates much greater than these (Tables 5.2 and 6.2). That they do not do so normally, but instead proceed in closer relationship to functional needs, implies specific processes of regulation. Carbohydrate metabolism as it occurs *in vivo* or in cell-containing cerebral tissues normally involves both glycolysis and oxidation of glucose. Under normal conditions the mammalian brain oxidizes 85 % of the glucose it utilizes and only about 15 % appears as lactate. Glycolysis and respiration can however constitute either alternative or parallel means of yielding energy-rich phosphates ($\sim$P) from carbohydrate, glycolysis preponderating when lack of available oxygen limits respiration. The potential yield of phosphoric esters from the two series is similar, though very different quantities of carbohydrate are consumed. Thus at its maximum rate of progress, respiration at 120 μmoles O_2/g. hr. yields about $120 \times 2 \times 3$ or some 720 μmoles $\sim$P from 20 μmoles of glucose. Glycolysis from 400 μmoles glucose/g. hr. yields 800 μmoles $\sim$P; and from glycogen, 500×3 or 1,500 μmoles $\sim$P/g. hr. The rate of glucose catabolism during maximal glycolysis in fact outruns the supply from the bloodstream.

Normally, however, the blood carries away from the brain excess glucose and oxygen, and both the glycolytic and oxidative series are self-limiting. As presented in Table 5.2 and 6.2, the two series could proceed for only a few seconds until all cerebral inorganic phosphate or adenosine esters were fully esterified. Actually, as just indicated, cerebral utilization of oxygen and glucose is continuous but limited in rate and this is reconciled with the nature of the utilizing systems through the existence of further reactions which re-form inorganic phosphate and adenosine di- or monophosphates. A major link between respiration or glycolysis, and level of functional activity, is thus made at this point: the point at which the speed of phosphorylation is limited by the speed of reactions yielding phosphate and phosphate-acceptors. Requirement of these substances by the respiratory and glycolytic enzymes secures sufficient but not excessive production of energy-rich phosphate for maintenance and for different degrees of functional activity.

This is undoubtedly a simplified picture in which other energy-rich substances which can react with adenosine diphosphate—as creatine phosphate, guanosine phosphates, or coenzyme derivatives—have their partly independent roles. Also permeability factors cannot be ignored in that glycolysis proceeds essentially extra-mitochondrially whereas the reactions of oxidation and phosphorylation take place within the organelles. Permeability factors are moreover directly related to levels of adenosine phosphates during the recovery processes consequent upon the firing of a nerve cell, in which Na^+ and K^+ are transported against concentration gradients, ATP is utilized and ADP formed through the mediation of Na^+,K^+-ATPase (q.v.) It seems possible (see Whittam, 1961, 1962; Keesey & Wallgren, 1965) that between 25% and 40% of the ATP produced from oxidative processes in the brain may be consumed in this way. The osmotic work involved in re-establishing electro-chemical gradients may therefore be comparable to the work performed in renal or gastrointestinal tissues. Direct involvement of cations with individual reactions can also be demonstrated (Chapters 5 and 6).

The net change in phosphate as computed from the individual steps of the conversion of glucose to lactate (Table 5.2) is the formation of an amount of adenosine triphosphate equimolar with the lactate, from adenosine diphosphate and inorganic phosphate. It is satisfactory to see that formation in this ratio has in fact been observed, for example, during the initial part of the experiment illustrated in Fig. 5.2. *In vivo*, little exchange of phosphate takes place between the brain and the rest of the body; the adenine nucleotides available (Chapter 3) are about 4 μmoles/g. and the inorganic phosphate about 3 μmoles/g. Thus in the absence of other changes in the nucleotides, cerebral glycolysis at 1,500 μmoles/g. hr. would rapidly be self-limiting through esterification of all available inorganic phosphate and adenosine diphosphate, leaving no reagents for phosphorylase, glyceraldehyde phosphate dehydrogenase and the phosphoglycerate and pyruvate kinases.

The glycolytic sequence as a whole *in vitro* is conditioned by level of inorganic phosphate as indicated in **B**, Fig. 5.2. Moreover, the concentrations of inorganic phosphate to which it is sensitive are in fact those observed *in vivo*. Thus participation of inorganic phosphate in control of glycolysis is certain; participation of adenosine diphosphate is extremely likely and scope remains for participation also of glucose-6-phosphate as inhibitor as well as other agents acting on hexokinase and phosphorylase (q.v.).

Of various processes which condition carbohydrate metabolism through modifying the level of inorganic phosphate, oxidative phosphorylation is of outstanding importance. This can be appreciated by examining Fig. 7.2. Here, anaerobic conditions have eliminated respiration. Fructose diphosphate, previously at a level much below that of glucose-6-phosphate, now greatly

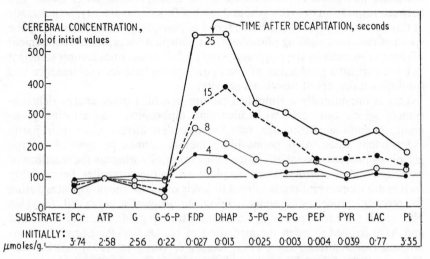

FIG. 7.2. Change in concentration of substances concerned in glycolysis, in the brain of mice kept at 38° after decapitation. Mice at 10 days of age were anaesthetized with phenobarbitone; the cerebral tissues of control animals were sampled immediately and the others at the times indicated. PCr: phosphocreatine; G: glucose; the subsequent intermediates are those asterisked in Table 5.2; P_i, inorganic orthophosphate (Lowry et al., 1964).

increases and this is accompanied by increased formation of all subsequent stages including lactate itself. The progress of this sequence under normal aerobic conditions is limited, despite the large enzyme capacity of its earlier stages as exhibited under optimal conditions (Table 5.2).

Balance Between Routes from Glucose-6-Phosphate

The factors which condition the speed of operation of the three routes from glucose-6-phosphate are interestingly varied, reflecting, presumably, their quite different metabolic roles. Thus, as examined in vitro, the glycolytic route (1, Fig. 5.5) is much the most susceptible to orthophosphate and adenosine diphosphate, and involves NAD^+. The reactions which follow (2, Fig. 5.5) and concern glycogen, involve uridine nucleotides; and although adenine nucleotides are involved in each route, adenosine-5'- and -3':5'-phosphates feature primarily in connection with glycogen breakdown. In the pentose phosphate route (3, Fig. 5.5) $NADP^+$ and its link to glutathione, are distinctive features. Ample scope is thus offered for independent control of the routes.

The enzymes which catalyse the different routes can only occasionally operate maximally *in vivo*. Thus under normal conditions about 20 μmoles glucose are utilized/g. brain/hr., and of the glucose about five-sixths is oxidized completely. This would normally be pictured as proceeding through the glycolytic pathway with subsequent oxidation of pyruvate, though the rate of enzymes of the direct oxidative pathway is adequate for metabolism at these rates. Using isotopically-labelled glucose and methods appraised by Katz & Wood (1963) and Villee & Loring (1961), estimates have been made of the proportion of CO_2 produced from glucose by the pentose phosphate route, and by the glycolytic route followed by oxidation of pyruvate. The route through pyruvate greatly preponderated in cerebral cortical tissue (DiPietro & Weinhouse, 1959; Tower, 1959). This was confirmed in studies in which tissues from the human brain, foetal and adult, were compared with other tissues of the body. In the medulla, and also in cerebral dispersions, appreciable metabolism through pentose phosphate was demonstrated (Villee & Loring, 1961; Hotta, 1962).

The various points at which regulation of these metabolic routes is likely to occur are treated in the sections which follow.

Glycogen Metabolism

During the rapid post-mortem changes that occur in the brain in the first minute or so after decapitation, glycogen remains relatively constant until most of the glucose has disappeared, after which time glycogen levels fall rapidly (Kerr & Ghantus, 1937; Lowry *et al.*, 1964). Rates of utilization of glycogen are thus controlled. It has been shown that the time taken for activation of phosphorylase (q.v.) could account partly, but not entirely, for the delay in glycogenolysis (Breckenridge & Norman, 1962), the remaining time being required for sufficient 5'-AMP to accumulate for maximum phosphorylase rates to operate (Lowry, 1966; Lowry *et al.*, 1967). So phosphorylase activity may normally be limited as the 5'-AMP usually found in the brain is below the level (0·3 mM or more) required for full enzymic activity. The pathway of glycogen synthesis (q.v.) is not the reverse of breakdown; this provides for greater flexibility of control. The activity of glycogen synthetase (Chapter 5) depends on the availability of glucose-6-phosphate as activator, so any tendency for glucose-6-phosphate to accumulate should be reflected in increased synthesis. Control may also be exerted at this stage through enzymic interconversion of the two forms of the synthetase (Goldberg & O'Toole, 1969). In the presence of saturating levels of uridinediphosphate glucose, the two forms differ in sensitivity to glucose-6-phosphate activation; increased concentrations of glucose would be expected to facilitate indirectly the synthesis of glycogen. Conditions which increase glucose would tend also to decrease rates of glycogen breakdown as glucose inhibits phosphorylase; low ATP, low glucose-6-phosphate and high 5'-AMP would be expected to diminish glycogen through lowered activation of the synthetase due to glucose-6-phosphate and the increased activation of phosphorylase by 5'-AMP.

Regulation of glycogen metabolism at the stage of phosphoglucomutase seems unlikely because the available levels of cofactor, glucose-1,6-diphosphate, though very low (Chapter 5), are not limiting; they are over 100 times greater than the K_m of the enzyme for its cofactor.

Glycolysis

The glycolytic sequence as a whole is conditioned *in vitro* by available levels of inorganic phosphate as indicated in **B**, Fig. 5.2 and in Fig. 7.5. Moreover, the concentrations of phosphate to which the sequence is sensitive are in fact those observed *in vivo*. Participation of orthophosphate occurs in individual reactions (such as glyceraldehyde-3-phosphate dehydrogenase) of the pathways and particularly in the process of oxidative phosphorylation, discussed subsequently.

The three pathways which are concerned with the consumption of glucose diverge at glucose-6-phosphate and are of different potential speed. Glycogen synthesis and the pentose phosphate pathway occur at much lesser rates than glycolysis, which proceeds normally at 20 μmoles of glucose utilized/g. tissue per hr., but capable, under maximal stimulation, of some 1,500–2,000 μmoles of lactate produced/g. hr. (thus equivalent to up to 1,000 μmoles of glucose utilized/g. hr.). During the brief period when lactate is being formed at these extremely high rates, many enzymes of the glycolytic route must be operating close to their maximal capacity. This is reached only with adequate concentrations of substrates and coenzymes, so considerable organization or adjustment for this purpose is required. Such rates can be maintained only for seconds; normally the individual glycolytic enzymes are reacting at only a few percent of their maximum capability.

Glycolytic intermediates occur in the brain at quite low concentrations as shown in Table 5.2 and Fig. 7.2; these concentrations are however commensurate with those needed for half-maximal velocity of the enzymes concerned. Kinetic studies of Lowry & Passonneau (1964) showed that tissue rate-constants for four of the glycolytic enzymes fell in a sequence appropriate to the enzymes acting efficiently in series. Examination of the levels of glycolytic intermediates during short time intervals after ischaemia (Fig. 7.2) showed that within seconds, cerebral concentrations of glucose and hexose monophosphate had decreased while intermediates subsequent to fructose-6-phosphate had increased. Such studies indicated that the likely control points between glucose and pyruvate are at the hexokinase and particularly the phosphofructokinase steps with the further possibility that pyruvate kinase may also be relevant. The possibility that control may be exerted at the three kinase reactions also emerged from aerobic incubation of cerebral cortex preparations *in vitro* (Rolleston & Newsholme, 1967).

Hexokinase

The activity of the first kinase reaction is regulated by available levels of substrates and products. Glycolytic rates are generally less than 3% of the maximum potential rate of total cerebral hexokinase activity; the inhibition available from glucose-6-phosphate, while considerable at the likely intra-cellular concentrations, is insufficient to account alone for the degree of inhibition required. Inhibitions by ADP and by free ATP also contribute but the total provided by the combination of the three phosphates is insufficient to account for a required inhibition of 97% or more. Such considerations serve to heighten interest in the distribution of hexokinase; unlike most other cerebral glycolytic enzymes, hexokinase occurs partly particulate and partly in the cytoplasm (Chapter 5). It is possible to account for adequate inhibition of the enzyme in terms of the likely intracellular levels of Mg^{2+}, ATP, ADP and glucose-6-phosphate, if it is assumed that it is the soluble cytoplasmic enzyme which is involved (Bachelard & Goldfarb, 1969). The mitochondrial enzyme exhibits similar chromatographic properties and kinetic behaviour to those of the cytoplasmic system but the possibility that changes in subcellular distribu-tion may be involved in regulation of hexokinase activity remains to be ex-plored (Thompson & Bachelard, 1970).

Phosphofructokinase

The major control point of glycolysis in the brain is considered to be at the stage of formation of fructose diphosphate. Phosphofructokinase, in the brain as in other tissues, undergoes a peculiarly complex series of interrelated modifications of its activity, involving groups of inhibitors and activators or deinhibitors, including its substrates and products, each one of which may affect the action of another (Passonneau & Lowry, 1963; Lowry & Passonneau, 1966). In this way inhibition by excess ATP, one of its substrates, is augmented by another inhibitor, citrate. The inhibition by both is decreased by the other substrate, fructose-6-phosphate. Free ATP is considerably more inhibitory than $MgATP^{2-}$; however, free Mg^{2+} itself has been shown to be slightly inhibitory. Apart from interaction with other chemicals therefore, the ratio of available Mg^{2+} and ATP is important. ATP inhibition is also decreased by inorganic orthophosphate, by the monophosphates (5'-AMP and cyclic 3',5'-AMP) and by monovalent cations (K^+ or NH_4^+) which like fructose-6-phosphate and fructose-1,6-diphosphate, can be regarded as activating or de-inhibiting agents. The extent of the inhibitory effects of citrate and ATP, which act synergistically, will depend on their availability to what is essentially a cytoplasmic enzyme (Johnson, 1960), since ATP and citrate are both gener-ated in the mitochondria. The inhibition by citrate provides a point of regulatory contact between the pathways of glycolysis and the tricarboxylic acid cycle in which accumulation of an intermediate of the cycle might decrease the rate of entry of metabolites from glycolysis to the cycle. Low ATP with increased AMP would be expected to result in increased phosphofructokinase activity as ATP inhibits and both 5'-AMP and cyclic 3',5'-AMP activate. Inhibition, enhanced by ATP, due to creatine phosphate, phosphoenolpyruvate and phosphoglycerates has also been reported (Krzanowski & Matschinsky, 1969).

Lowry (1966) has suggested that regulation of cerebral phosphofructokinase activity may normally be due to citrate inhibition without the significant involvement of other agents but under conditions likely to produce a net decrease of ATP, i.e. when the rate of ATP utilization exceeds the rate of

ATP generation, the increased levels of AMP and phosphate would become effective in increasing activity. It is possible also that the NH_4^+ released during the electrical activity of the tissue would tend to increase the activity of the enzyme. Any regulation by inhibition of phosphofructokinase would tend to produce an accumulation of glucose-6-phosphate, as the ester is in rapid equilibrium with fructose-6-phosphate, and so affect hexokinase activity in a coupled fashion.

Pyruvate Kinase

The activity of cerebral pyruvate kinase is also inhibited by free ATP; as with hexokinase and phosphofructokinase, it is the Mg:ATP ratio which is important (Rolleston & Newsholme, 1967; Wood, 1968). Pyruvate kinase activity may also depend on the intracellular cation balance; the enzyme is stimulated by K^+ and inhibited by Na^+ (Chapter 5).

The inhibitory action of free ATP on these three kinases emphasizes the relevance of available intracellular concentrations of ATP and Mg and also of ADP, to the activities of enzymes likely to participate in regulation.

The Tricarboxylic Acid Cycle

A major limitation of overall rates of metabolism through the tricarboxylic acid cycle is that imposed by restriction on the amounts of pyruvate entering the cycle *via* acetyl coenzyme A. In this respect, the inhibition by citrate of phosphofructokinase (above) is of relevance in that the control may actually be exerted through a balance between inhibition by ATP as well as citrate and deinhibition by inorganic phosphate, ADP or 5'-AMP. A general feature also will be the availability of coenzymes (nicotinamide adenine nucleotides and flavin nucleotides, Chapter 10) in the correct redox state since so many of the individual steps require the oxidised form of the coenzymes for activity.

Identification of control points in the cycle has been attempted by Goldberg *et al.* (1966) who compared the levels of cerebral tricarboxylic acid cycle intermediates during ischaemia (Fig. 7.3), anaesthesia and hyperthermia. These conditions were chosen to modify rates of metabolism without completely blocking the cycle. The level of *iso*citrate was not affected by the changes caused by any of these conditions; that of succinate rose slightly in ischaemia but not when glucose and oxygen were present (that is, in hyperthermia or anaesthesia). Likely control points were thus indicated at the *iso*citrate dehydrogenase and possibly at the succinate dehydrogenase steps.

Control of *isocitrate dehydrogenase* activity is also indicated from the involvement of ADP; as has been shown for the enzyme from insect flight muscle and rat heart, ADP is a specific activator of cerebral mitochondrial NAD^+-*iso*citrate dehydrogenase (q.v.; Goebell & Klingenberg, 1964). The low content of *iso*citrate in the brain (less than 0·02 μmoles/g.) is such as to render the activation an important feature. The stimulation of respiration by ADP is probably due, at least in part, to its direct effect on this enzyme.

Polarographic determinations of the respiratory control ratio (with glutamate as oxidisable substrate) in mitochondria prepared from rat brain

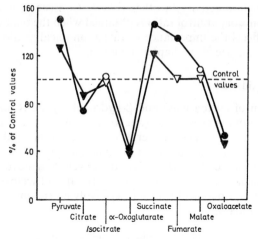

FIG. 7.3. Percentage changes of pyruvate and intermediates of the tricarboxylic acid cycle after 5 sec. (▼) and 30 sec. (●) ischaemia. The solid symbols indicate values significantly different ($P < 0.05$) from control values. The open symbols indicate non-significance (Goldberg et al., 1966).

within varying periods after decapitation showed a fall in the ratio from a normal value of about 12 (see Table 7.3) to less than half in the first minute or two. The fall was shown (Ozawa et al., 1966) to be due to the formation of endogenous inhibitors, possibly fatty acids, and thus provides an example of contribution of fat metabolism to regulation of oxidative metabolism. The inhibition is also of relevance to the known inhibitory effects of free fatty acids

Table 7.3

Respiration of cerebral mitochondria prepared at intervals after decapitation

Time after decapitation (min.)	Addition to medium	Respiration ($m\mu$atoms O_2/min. mg. of protein)	RCR
0		45·8	11·8
1		28·7	6·8
2		22·7	4·7
10		13·1	2·6
0		41·3	12·5
0	A	29·0	4·5
0	B	23·8	2·0

Respiration was measured polarographically in mitochondria from rat cerebral cortex prepared at different times after decapitation. Rates of O_2 uptake were determined at 22°C with 4 mM glutamate as substrate.

RCR: respiratory control ratio (Chapter 6).

A: endogenous inhibitor, present in mitochondria 2 min. after decapitation, prepared by ethanol extraction.

B: endogenous inhibitor, as A, 5 min. after decapitation.

Data from Ozawa et al., 1966.

on citrate synthetase activity in other tissues. Consistent observations that the highest respiratory control ratio is obtained when the oxidisable substrate is glutamate reflects the importance of this amino acid as a direct source of energy in the brain (see also Chapters 6 and 8).

Ketone-Body Oxidation

The oxidation of acetoacetate and β-hydroxybutyrate (Chapter 6) is also subject to regulatory processes relevant to entry of acetyl coenzyme A to the tricarboxylic acid cycle. The acceleration of oxidation of these substrates *in vitro* by glucose and the inhibition by malonate provide evidence that the oxidation occurs *via* acetyl coenzyme A and the cycle, and the route of metabolism has been elucidated. It proceeds through formation of acetoacetyl coenzyme A by the action of 3-oxo acid transferase, involving succinyl coenzyme A as described in Chapter 6.

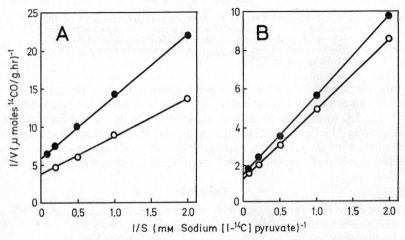

FIG. 7.4. Effect of acetoacetate on pyruvate oxidation in cerebral cortex slices from mature and immature rats. Rates were measured in O_2 at 37°C with sodium [1-^{14}C]pyruvate as added substrate, in the presence (●) or absence (○) of 5 mM-sodium acetoacetate. The results show greater inhibition of pyruvate oxidation by acetoacetate in the immature (A) than in the mature (B) rat brain (Itoh & Quastel, 1970).

Differences observed in the activity of β-hydroxybutyrate dehydrogenase between immature and adult rat brain were noted in Chapter 6; similar observations have since been made for rates of oxidation of ketone bodies in cerebral cortex slices *in vitro* (Itoh & Quastel, 1970). Metabolism of acetoacetate was more rapid in the preparations from immature brain and was less dependent on glucose for maximum rates of oxidation. In both adult and immature brain, oxidation of acetoacetate did not suppress rates of glucose utilization and was dependent upon the presence of a fully operative tricarboxylic acid cycle. In contrast to adult brain, the immature brain formed acetyl coenzyme A more readily from acetoacetate than from glucose, probably as a result of thiolase action (q.v.) on acetoacetyl coenzyme A. The accumulation of acetyl coenzyme A was concluded to cause the retardation of pyruvate oxidation (Fig. 7.4) and increase in lactate formation which were observed *in vitro* when acetoacetate was present. Pyruvate dehydrogenase (q.v.) is inhibited by acetyl coenzyme A in the heart (Garland & Randle, 1964; Davis & Quastel, 1964); presumably, cerebral pyruvate dehydrogenase is also susceptible to inhibition by acetyl coenzyme A. Any increase in lactate formation from pyruvate will tend to decrease available levels of NADH for oxidative phosphorylation, but more NAD^+ will then be available for the dehydrogenation reactions of the tricarboxylic acid cycle. Moreover the reaction in glycolysis which forms pyruvate (pyruvate kinase, q.v.) is also susceptible to inhibition by acetyl coenzyme A. Under conditions of increased ketone body oxidation resulting from increased mobilization of fat elsewhere in the body, higher rates of acetyl coenzyme A formation are therefore likely to ensue. The acetyl coenzyme A produced will influence rates of formation and of oxidation of pyruvate so providing a further point of regulatory interaction between glycolysis, fat metabolism and the tricarboxylic acid cycle.

Oxidative Phosphorylation

Respiration may be limited by the concentration of inorganic phosphate because cerebral tissues normally contain orthophosphate at concentrations below those required for maximal respiratory rates. Fig. 7.5 shows that, at the level of phosphate in the brain fixed under normal conditions (about 5 mM), oxidation of pyruvate or fumarate is probably proceeding at only half its maximal rate, but that the reactions could increase considerably were a large part of the phosphocreatine and adenosine triphosphate broken down. The data of Fig. 7.5 have been assembled from diverse sources and the correspondence between the range of inorganic phosphate in cerebral tissues, and the range of concentrations to which the different processes are most sensitive, is very evident. It is especially striking as the different investigations were not carried out with this aim in view, and their interpretation in relation to control of cerebral metabolism was made some time later (McIlwain, 1952). Requirement for adenosine derivatives, which during respiration are phosphorylated, was indicated in A and C, Fig. 6.1. More precise descriptions of their role are given by the experiments of B, Fig. 6.1. Here oxygen uptake is measured polarographically, and its rate is shown to be increased not only by oxidizable substrate, in this instance glutamate, but also by adenosine diphosphate; a limited addition of ADP was followed by increased oxygen uptake only until some 0·5 equiv. O_2 had been consumed. Respiration then reverted to its lower rate but could again be accelerated by ADP. In different experiments the rate of respiration was increased four- to seven-fold by ADP additions, indicating a "tightly coupled" system (see Chapter 6). The degree of control obtainable through adenosine diphosphate is indeed greater than ordinarily operates in the brain *in vivo* or in isolated cerebral tissues *in vitro*, when maximal stimulation may increase respiration to about double its resting rate, but not more.

Respiration may continue at maximal rate without repeated additions of

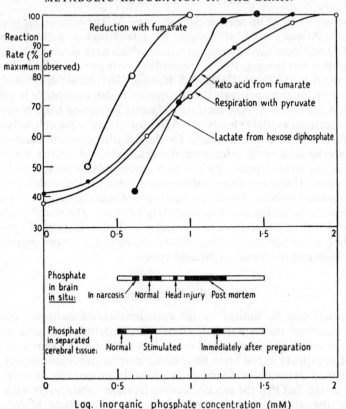

FIG. 7.5. The concentrations of inorganic phosphate to which four cerebral processes are sensitive, compared with the concentrations of phosphate found in the brain *in situ* and *in vitro*. Data from Banga, Ochoa & Peters (1939); Geiger (1940); Long (1945) and McIlwain *et al.* (1951).

orthophosphate or ADP as such, if systems are present which regenerate them. The most direct fashion in which this can occur is by hydrolysis of ATP: that is, by the presence of adenosine triphosphatases. Also, several processes in which the energy available from ATP hydrolysis is employed metabolically, have the overall effect of adenosine triphosphatases; ADP is often a product. Examples may be seen in the synthesis of glutamine or phospholipids (q.v.), in the active transport of sodium and potassium ions, or in various kinase reactions.

Suppression of Aerobic Glycolysis

Reason can thus be seen for respiration and glycolysis each paralleling cerebral activity, and the balance between the two metabolic routes may now be considered. As in many other tissues the anaerobic route, glycolysis, consumes much more substrate than the aerobic route and operates maximally only intermittently. However, a lack of glucose is not responsible for the normal inhibition of glycolysis under aerobic conditions, a phenomenon described as a "Pasteur effect".

The aerobic suppression of anaerobic processes can be interpreted as partly due to the competition between the pathways of glycolysis and oxidative phosphorylation for available ADP and orthophosphate, and to inhibition by excess ATP of kinase reactions in glycolysis. It may also result from limitations in available coenzymes required for the various reactions involved. The ratio of NAD^+ to NADH (Chapter 10) is thus of major interest; the relevance of α-glycerophosphate metabolism to continued maintenance of NAD^+/NADH ratios has been noted (Chapter 6). In cerebral tissues the anaerobic and aerobic routes compete for pyruvate, which either reacts with lactic dehydrogenase or is oxidatively decarboxylated. Anaerobically the extent of pyruvate conversion to lactate will depend on the NADH available; aerobically, continued oxidative decarboxylation of pyruvate depends on the availability of NAD^+ for regeneration of lipoic acid. Aerobically the flavoprotein and cytochromes of the respiratory chain therefore remove the NADH required by the anaerobic route and supply the NAD^+ required for the aerobic route. When both routes are progressing at moderate speed within the capacity of the cytochrome system, oxygen can thus be understood to depress glycolysis.

Differential control of glycolysis and respiration is more likely to be effected by limitations in ADP, which is present in the brain in small amounts, than in inorganic phosphate, of which appreciable amounts are found in the brains of normally respiring animals. Inorganic phosphate may conceivably be localised but the range of inorganic phosphate to which respiratory and glycolytic processes are sensitive, is similar. ADP has been implicated in various control points of the pathways: in the hexokinase and phosphofructokinase stages of glycolysis, in isocitrate dehydrogenase in the Krebs cycle and as the phosphate acceptor in oxidative phosphorylation; ATP levels are also of importance in relation to the amounts of Mg^{2+} and ADP available. Changes in the ATP/ADP ratio are minimized by creatine phosphokinase (q.v.) which acts as an energy "buffer" by regenerating ATP from ADP at the expense of creatine phosphate. On depletion of creatine phosphate, changes in the ATP/ADP ratio will affect rates of both respiration and glycolysis. A lowering of normal ATP levels will tend to promote increased flux through aerobic routes by partial release of inhibition, the increase in ADP associated with lowered ATP would increase flux through the tricarboxylic acid cycle by stimulation of isocitrate oxidation. The increased oxidative phosphorylation would regenerate further NAD^+ for aerobic glycolysis and the citric acid cycle. Anaerobic lactate formation is then restricted by limited NADH. An important general feature is the balance also between Mg^{2+} and ATP available at the precise intracellular metabolic sites as many of the relevant enzymes exhibit inhibition by excess free ATP, that is, when the available ATP exceeds the Mg^{2+} present (Rose, 1968; Bachelard & Goldfarb, 1969).

Release of Glycolysis

Under a variety of circumstances glycolysis can nevertheless continue aerobically. First among these is increased functional activity which can at its extreme supply sufficient phosphate and phosphate acceptors to permit both respiration and glycolysis to proceed at rates limited mainly by the capacity of individual enzymes. Considering control through the cytochrome system it is important that this system then proves to be capable of operating at no more than the maximal speed of phosphoglyceraldehyde dehydrogenase or lactic dehydrogenase. Its tendency to suppress aerobic glycolysis is presumably overwhelmed. The major reactions in the coenzyme then take place at the dehydrogenases which are coupled during glycolysis so that the coenzyme reduced by one is oxidized by the other.

A variety of added substances also permit aerobic glycolysis. Most direct in action is an agent such as sodium cyanide which by inhibiting cytochrome oxidase leaves reduced nucleotide and also prevents the oxidative combination of adenosine diphosphate and inorganic phosphate; all these factors increase glycolysis. 2:4-Dinitrophenol-like increased functional activity, increases both respiration and aerobic glycolysis and does so through increased supply of phosphate and phosphate acceptors, available through uncoupling phosphorylation from respiration (Table 6.4). A group of phenazine salts appears to have this effect through inhibiting reactions at the nicotinamide nucleotides (Chapter 10).

Increased functional activity can be induced in isolated cerebral tissues by the electrical stimulation which allows entry of Na^+, loss of K^+, and depolarization of the tissue cells. Evidence that this prompts the utilization of ATP in Na^+ extrusion and thus the re-establishment of membrane potentials, has been discussed previously (Chapter 4; McIlwain, 1963). Exposure of tissues to media of increased K^+ content (15–100 mM) also depolarizes tissue cells and in part simulates the effects of electrical stimulation. In the following chapters many instances will be found of processes which are important in cerebral functioning, which utilize adenosine triphosphate and which can in this way evoke additional cerebral respiration and glycolysis.

Further Aspects of Regulation

Examples will be given in subsequent parts of this book of further interactions affecting regulation of metabolic processes; thus aspects of the control of metabolism of chemical transmitters, such as their sequestration in the synaptic vesicles, are discussed in Chapter 14. The regulatory processes of genetic expression, operating through synthesis of nucleic acids and proteins (Chapter 9), are involved in growth and development of the brain (Chapter 13). These are also open to modification in the adult animal and can give the basis of metabolic adaptation. Synthesis of nucleic acids and proteins is important not only in regulating amounts of enzyme protein available for metabolism in the normal brain, but also in those cases where errors in the base sequence of nucleic acids are reflected in synthesis of abnormal enzyme protein, when disease often results. Many examples of such errors are seen in the metabolism of lipids (Chapter 11) and of amino-acids, described in the Chapter which follows.

REFERENCES

BACHELARD, H. S. (1969). Handbook of Neurochemistry, Vol. 1, p. 25. Ed. A. Lajtha. New York: Plenum Press.

BACHELARD, H. S. (1971a). *J. Neurochem.* **18**, 213.

BACHELARD, H. S. (1971b). in Brain Hypoxia (ed. Brierley, J. B.), London: Pergamon.

BACHELARD, H. S. & GOLDFARB, P. S. G. (1969). *Biochem. J.* **112**, 579.

BAILEY, J. M., FISHMAN, P. H. & PENTCHEV, P. B. (1968). *J. Biol. Chem.* **243**, 4827.

BANGA, I., OCHOA, S. & PETERS, R. A. (1939). *Biochem. J.* **33**, 1980.

BIDDER, T. G. (1968). *J. Neurochem.* **15**, 867.

BRADBURY, M. W. B. & DAVSON, H. (1964). *J. Physiol.* **170**, 195.

BRECKENRIDGE, B. M. & NORMAN, J. H. (1962). *J. Neurochem.* **9**, 383.

BUTTERFIELD, W. J. H., ABRAMS, M. E., SELLS, R. A., STERKY, G. & WHICHELOW, M. J. (1966). *Lancet*, **1**, 557.

CHAIN, E. B., LARSSON, S. & POCCHIARI, F. (1960). *Proc. Roy. Soc. B.* **152**, 283.

CHANCE, B., ESTABROOK, R. W. & WILLIAMSON, J. R. (1965). Control of Energy Metabolism. New York: Academic Press.

CRONE, C. (1965). *J. Physiol.* **181**, 103.

DAVIS, E. J. & QUASTEL, J. H. (1964). *Canad. J. Biochem.* **42**, 1605.

DiPIETRO, D. & WEINHOUSE, S. (1959). *Arch. Biochem. Biophys.* **80**, 268.

EIDELBERG, E., FISHMAN, J. & HAMS, M. L. (1967). *J. Physiol.* **191**, 47.

FISHMAN, R. A. (1964). *Amer. J. Physiol.* **206**, 836.

GARLAND, P. B. & RANDLE, P. G. (1964). *Biochem. J.* **91**, 6c.

GEIGER, A. (1940). *Biochem. J.* **34**, 465.

GILBERT, J. C. (1965). *Nature, London*, **205**, 87.

GILBERT, J. C. (1966). *J. Neurochem.* **13**, 729.

GILBERT, J. C., ORTIZ, W. R. & MILLICHAP, J. G. (1966). *J. Neurochem.* **13**, 247.

GILBOE, D. D. & BETZ, A.L. (1970). *Amer. J. Physiol.* **219**, 774.

GOEBELL, H. & KLINGENBERG, M. (1964). *Biochem. Z.* **340**, 411.

GOLDBERG, N. D., PASSONNEAU, J. V. & LOWRY, O. H. (1966). *J. biol. Chem.* **241**, 3997.

GOLDBERG, N. D. & O'TOOLE, A. G. (1969). *J. biol. Chem.* **244**, 3053.

HIMSWORTH, R. L. (1968). *J. Physiol.* **198**, 451, 467.

HOTTA, S. S. (1962). *J. Neurochem.* **9**, 43.

ITOH, T. & QUASTEL, J. H. (1970). *Biochem. J.* **116**, 641.

JOANNY, P., CORRIOL, J. & HILLMAN, H. (1969). *Biochem. J.* **112**, 367.

JOHNSON, M. K. (1960). *Biochem. J.* **77**, 610.

KATZ, J. & WOOD, H. G. (1963). *J. biol. Chem.* **238**, 517.

KEESEY, J. C. & WALLGREN, H. (1965). *Biochem. J.* **95**, 301.

KERR, S. E. & GHANTUS, M. (1937). *J. biol. Chem.* **117**, 217.

KESTON, A. S. (1954). *Science.* **120**, 355.

KESTON, A. S. (1957). *Feder. Proc.* **16**, 203.

KING, L. J., LOWRY, O. H., PASSONNEAU, J. V. & VENSON, V. (1967). *J. Neurochem.* **14**, 599.

KREBS, H. A. (1956). CIBA Foundation Symposium, "Ionizing Radiations and Cell Metabolism", p. 92. London: Churchill.

KRZANOWSKI, J. & MATSCHINSKY, F. M. (1969). *Biochem. Biophys. Res. Commun.* **34**, 816.

LeFEVRE, P. G. & PETERS, A. A. (1966). *J. Neurochem.* **13**, 35.

LONG, C. (1945). *Biochem. J.* **39**, 143.

LOWRY, O. H. (1966). Nerve as a Tissue, p. 163. Ed. K. Rodahl & B. Issekutz. New York: Harper & Row (Hoeber Medical Division).

LOWRY, O. H. & PASSONNEAU, J. V. (1964). *J. biol. Chem.* **239**, 31.

LOWRY, O. H. & PASSONNEAU, J. V. (1966). *J. biol. Chem.* **241**, 2268.

LOWRY, O. H. & PASSONNEAU, J. V. (1969). *J. biol. Chem.* **244**, 910.

LOWRY, O. H., PASSONNEAU, J. V., HASSELBERGER, F. X. & SCHULZ, D. W. (1964). *J. biol. Chem.* **239**, 18.

LOWRY, O. H., SCHULZ, D. W. & PASSONNEAU, J. V. (1967). *J. biol. Chem.* **242**, 271.

McILWAIN, H. (1952). *Biochem. J.* **52**, 289.

MCILWAIN, H. (1963). Chemical Exploration of the Brain. Amsterdam: Elsevier.
MCILWAIN, H., BUCHEL, L. & CHESHIRE, J. D. (1951). *Biochem. J.* **48**, 14.
MAYMAN, C. I., GATFIELD, P. D. & BRECKENRIDGE, B. M. (1964). *J. Neurochem.* **11**, 483.
MELLERUP, E. T. & RAFAELSON, O. J. (1969). *J. Neurochem.* **16**, 777.
OZAWA, K., SETA, K., TAKEDA, H., ANDO, K., HANDA, H. & ARAKI, C. (1966). *J. Biochem. Japan*, **59**, 501.
PASSONNEAU, J. V. & LOWRY, O. H. (1963). *Biochem. Biophys. Res. Commun.* **13**, 372.
RAFAELSON, O. J. (1961). *Metabolism*, **10**, 99.
ROLLESTON, F. S. & NEWSHOLME, E. A. (1967). *Biochem. J.* **104**, 524.
ROSE, I. A. (1968). *Proc. natn. Acad. Sci. U.S.A.* **61**, 1079.
ROSE, I. A. & ROSE, Z. B. (1969). Comprehensive Biochemistry, Vol. 17, p. 93. Ed. M. Florkin & E. H. Stotz. Amsterdam: Elsevier.
STRANG, R. H. C. & BACHELARD, H. S. (1971). *J. Neurochem.* **18**.
THOMPSON, M. F. & BACHELARD, H. S. (1970). *Biochem. J.* **118**, 25.
TOWER, D. (1959). *J. Neurochem.* **3**, 185.
VILLEE, C. A. & LORING, J. M. (1961). *Biochem. J.* **81**, 488.
WEBER, G. (1963). *Adv. Enzyme Reg.* **1**, 1.
WHITTAM, R. (1961). *Nature, London*, **191**, 603.
WHITTAM, R. (1962). *Biochem. J.* **82**, 205.
WOOD, T. (1968). *Biochem. Biophys. Res. Commun.* **31**, 779.

8 Amino Acids and Cerebral Activities

The brain at any one time contains relatively little carbohydrate, though carbohydrate metabolism is of such outstanding importance to it. Amino acids on the other hand, free or as proteins, constitute over 40% of its dry weight. This chapter is concerned more especially with the free amino acids of cerebral tissues and with mental phenomena associated with amino acid changes in the body as a whole. Cerebral proteins are rapid in their turnover, and thus, unless re-use of amino acids proceeds with complete efficiency, need for supply of amino acids to the brain continues throughout the life of an animal. Several inherited metabolic diseases which affect the brain are associated with abnormality in amino acid supply; in several instances the amino acids, supplied or synthesized intracerebrally, have their importance in relation to neurotransmission (Chapter 14). The pituitary peptides and their specialized functions are discussed in Chapter 16.

The Free Amino Acids of the Brain

Quantities Present

Cerebral amino acids or constituents for their formation derive from the bloodstream but analysis of arterial and cerebral venous blood for amino acids has not shown appreciable change at the brain; uptake from the bloodstream is less rapid than in the case of glucose or oxygen. Nevertheless, cerebral tissues like many others play a very active role with respect to the amino acids of the bloodstream, for large concentration gradients are maintained between blood plasma and the brain (Table 8.1; see also *Symposium*, 1962). The amino acids as a whole exist in rat brain at a concentration some six times higher than that of the blood plasma of the same animals. In human brain, the average value for free amino acids is about eight times that of blood plasma and concentrations have been noted to differ in different areas. Variation with cerebral location is also evident among the data for forty-two compounds in four parts of the rat brain, reported by Shaw & Heine (1965). The compounds were detected by ninhydrin after column chromatography; they were mainly amino acids and included unidentified substances.

Extraction of the mammalian brain shows the presence there of all the amino acids common to the tissues of the body. Table 8.1 lists several and

171

illustrates some unusual features in their distribution. γ-Aminobutyric acid and *N*-acetylaspartic acid are greatly enriched in the brain: sufficiently so to chemically characterize the organ. They are actively produced in the brain,

Table 8.1

Free amino acids and related compounds of the brain

Compound	Content (μmoles/100 g.)	Ratio: $\frac{[\text{brain}]}{[\text{blood plasma}]}$	References
N-Acetylaspartate	470–974	–	5, 7
Alanine	14–94	2·5	1, 4, 6, 7
β-Alanine	7	–	7
γ-Aminobutyrate	83–227	300	1, 2, 3, 5, 6, 7
Ammonia	16–26	5	5, 6
Arginine	7–16	c. 1	2, 5, 6, 7
Asparagine	11	–	7
Aspartate	153–272	300	1, 2, 4, 6, 7
Citrulline	2·5	–	6
Cystathionine[a]	4–18	–	6, 7
Cystine	4	–	9
Glutamate	781–1250	c. 150	1, 2, 3, 5, 6, 7
Glutamine	215–560	10	1, 3, 4
Glutathione	90–340	–	1, 3, 4, 5, 6, 7
Glycine	55–146	–	1, 4, 5, 6, 7
Histidine	6–9	c. 1	2, 5, 6, 7
Isoleucine	6–9	–	4, 6, 7
Leucine	7–14	0·7	2, 5, 6, 7
Lysine	11–22	0·7	2, 5, 6, 7
Methionine	8–10	–	2, 7
Ornithine	4–5	–	6, 7
Proline	6–12	–	2, 7
Phenylalanine	5–9	1·4	2, 5, 6, 7
Serine	39–177	6	1, 4, 5, 7
Taurine	125–535	40	1, 5, 7
Threonine	9–29	2	2, 5, 6, 7
Tryptophan	2·5	–	2
Tyrosine	3–11	1·4	2, 5, 6, 7
Urea	340–417	0·7	5, 7
Valine	12–18	c. 1	2, 5, 6, 7

[a] Cystathionine: 101–255 μmoles/g. human brain[7]; 575 μmoles/g. ox pineal gland.[6]

[1] Rat brain, rapidly frozen: Ansell & Richter, 1954; Richter & Dawson, 1948. [2] Rat brain, animal with Nembutal: Schurr *et al.*, 1950. [3] Rat cerebral cortex: Berl & Waelsch, 1958. [4] Guinea pig cerebral cortex: McIlwain & Tresize, 1957; Bart *et al.*, 1962. [5] Dog brain frozen *in situ*, animal with morphine: Tews *et al.*, 1963. [6] Ox cerebral cortex: LaBella *et al.*, 1968. [7] Cat, guinea pig and rat brain: Tallan *et al.*, 1954, 1956, 1958. For amino acid levels in different parts of the brain of various species, see Porcellati & Thompson (1957) and Okumura *et al.* (1959a, c).

the role of γ-aminobutyric acid (q.v.) in carbohydrate metabolism having already received comment. In general, the acidic amino acids are at high level in the brain and contribute considerably to its ion balance (Chapter 3). The occurrence there of cystathionine and homocarnosine is also notable (Tallan *et al.*, 1954, 1958; Pisano *et al.*, 1961). *N*-Acetylhistidine has been characterized as a normal constituent of the brain of fishes, amphibia and reptiles, occurring in concentrations of 0·15–6·5 μmoles/g. tissue (Erspamer *et al.*, 1965).

The cerebral content of free amino acids is labile and responsive to circumstances which affect the bodily condition of an animal. Instances are quoted in Table 8.2. In some of these instances, the total amino acid content of the brain tends to be maintained at a steady level independently of the individual amino acids which make up the total. After insulin, aspartic acid partly replaced glutamic acid. Other changes, such as fasting, chilling or physically exercising the animals, also caused appreciable changes in amino acid pattern, the levels of some of the acids rising to double or falling to half their normal values.

Table 8.2

Conditions causing change in cerebral amino acid levels

Condition	Change[a]	Reference
NH$_4$Cl infusion	Ammonia (++), alanine (++), histidine (+), aspartate (−), valine (−)	1
Anoxia	Alanine (++), γ-aminobutyrate (+), leucine (+), tyrosine (+), aspartate (−)	1
Convulsions	Alanine (+), γ-aminobutyrate (−), glutamate (−)	1, 6, 7, 8, 9
Electroshock	Glutamine (+), threonine (+)	5
Fasting	Glutamine (+), taurine (+), threonine (+), urea (−)	3, 5
Insulin	Aspartate (++), taurine (+), threonine (++), alanine (−), γ-aminobutyrate (−), glutamate (−)	2, 3, 4, 5
Post-mortem autolysis (q.v.)	Ammonia (+), alanine (+), γ-aminobutyrate (+)	1

[a] Increase: up to 50% (+); over 50% (++); decrease: (−).
[1] Tews *et al.*, 1963; [2] Knauff & Böck, 1961; [3] Cravioto *et al.*, 1951; [4] Massieu *et al.*, 1962; [5] Okumura *et al.*, 1959; [6] Roa *et al.*, 1964; [7] Wood & Watson, 1964; [8] Folbergrova *et al.*, 1969; [9] Aelony *et al.*, 1962.

A brief period of fasting can result in measurable changes in cerebral amino acids (Table 8.2). It is thus understandable that general dietary deficiencies in amino acids include among their effects, symptoms which suggest involvement of the peripheral or central nervous system as is described further in Chapter 10. Thus valine-deficient rats become abnormal in gait and posture and degenerative changes are found in their spinal cords (Ferraro & Roizin, 1947). The deficiency disease of children, termed kwashiorkor in Africa, is due predominantly to a severely inadequate intake of protein; it is accompanied by mental changes and electroencephalographic abnormalities which were found in most cases to be resolved by a high-protein diet. Of the circumstances listed in Table 8.2, anoxia and hypoglycaemia caused the greatest changes in the cerebral levels of amino acids; convulsions induced electrically or by pentamethylene tetrazole caused relatively little alteration. Thus insulin hypoglycaemia prompted changes in about fifteen amino acids and peptides of the brain of rats (Shaw & Heine, 1965). Also, during sleep or during enforced wakefulness, significant alterations were found in cerebral content of γ-aminobutyric acid and of glutamic or aspartic acids (Jasper *et al.*, 1965; Godin & Mandel, 1965).

Amino Acid Flux and Transport

Maintenance of cerebral amino acids at the levels described is the result of (i) their production and further metabolism in the brain, to be discussed below; and (ii) their influx and efflux, largely to and from the bloodstream, now to be described.

If electrochemical equilibria between cerebral cells and body fluids determined entirely the amino acid distribution at the brain, membrane potential

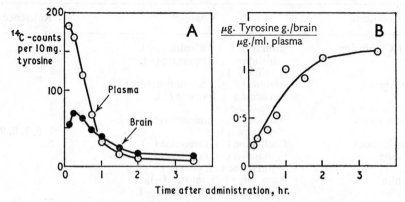

FIG. 8.1. Tyrosine of the brain and blood plasma of rats after intra-peritoneal administration. Uniformly ^{14}C-labelled tyrosine, 10 μg., was injected and samples extracted for free amino acids, determined after decarboxylation and column chromatography (Chirigos, Greengard & Udenfriend, 1960).

would bring an influx of basic amino acids, which is far from the case (Table 8.1). Special relationships between the bloodstream and the brain are thus evident in connection with amino acids as with other substances. These relationships involve appreciable flux of amino acids, as shown by the data of Table 8.3 and Fig. 8.1. For example isotopically-labelled leucine, given intra-venously to adult mice, reached its peak cerebral concentration as a free amino-acid within 10 min. The rise and fall in muscle and liver took place in about half these times. Similar time-relations are shown after a tracer dose of tyrosine in rats in Fig. 8.1 which also illustrates the approach to equilibrium between the free tyrosine of the brain and of blood plasma. The ratio at equilibrium is slightly in favour of the brain, and is similar to the ratio of the total (not only the labelled) tyrosine, quoted in Table 8.1: suggesting equilibrium with all the free cerebral tyrosine. α-Aminoisobutyric acid, a non-natural amino acid not metabolized by the brain, undergoes there a two-fold enrichment: a ratio smaller than obtains at other organs, and considered to illustrate the role of the blood-brain barrier (Kuttner *et al.*, 1961; Chapter 3).

When appreciable quantities of amino acids are injected directly to the brain (see Table 8.3, col. B), efflux again occurs, in this case at rates increasing with increasing concentration gradient. By such subarachnoid injection, about half the quantity of administered amino acid can be caused to penetrate the tissues of the brain, fairly extensively, before its later redistribution in the body (Lajtha & Toth, 1962). Direct injections of isotopically-labelled material should therefore not be assumed to result in complete penetration throughout the brain, especially in short-term experiments. However, provided the limitations are not ignored, the technique is of much value in studies of transport and metabolism of amino acids *in situ*. In some instances (leucine: Lajtha & Toth, 1961)

Table 8.3

Turnover of amino acids and proteins in brain

Amino acid	Half-life times for amino acids:		In protein
	Uncombined		
	Expt. (A) (min.)	Expt. (B) (min.)	Expt. (C) (days)
γ-Aminobutyrate	–	21	–
L-Glutamate	600	–	–
L-Leucine	34	14	4–27
D-Leucine	–	28	–
L-Lysine	20	140	3–15
D-Lysine	–	200	–
L-Methionine	–	34	14
L-Phenylalanine	–	27	–
D-Phenylalanine	–	32	–
L-Proline	–	23	–

Values are regarded as approximate only and were obtained (column A) in mice and rats by injecting intravenously the isotopically labelled amino acids; between 3 and 120 min. after administration, the issues were removed and extracted. (B): Values after subarachnoid administration. (C): in adult mice or rats. (Lajtha, 1959, 1964; Lajtha *et al.*, 1957, 1959; see also Gaitonde & Richter, 1956; Roberts *et al.*, 1958, 1959).

extrusion of an amino acid from the brain occurs against a concentration gradient and in fashions specific to the structure of a particular amino acid. Also, in experiments similar to that of **A**, Fig. 8.1, L-tyrosine was transported *in vivo* more rapidly than the D-isomer and *p*-hydroxyphenylacetic acid was not transported. *In vitro*, using isolated preparations of cerebral cortex, L- and D-tyrosine were transported at comparable rates and transport of *p*-hydroxyphenylacetic acid could also be demonstrated (Chirigos *et al.*, 1960; Guroff *et al.*, 1961). The results indicated the presence of two distinct uptake components *in vitro*: an active component, inhibited by anaerobiosis and subject to competition by other amino acids and a passive component, not so affected. Evidence has suggested (Neame & Smith, 1965; Smith, 1967) that, based on comparisons of amino acid flux and inulin uptake *in vitro*, the passive diffusional component, not subject to inhibition by dinitrophenol or by other amino acids and not stimulated by glucose, is a reflection of changes in the tissue fluid spaces (Chapter 4) which occur *in vitro* but not *in vivo*. This distinction has sometimes been ignored in studies on amino acid flux *in vitro*.

The more rapid transport of the L-isomers of amino acids, described above for alanine and tyrosine has also been demonstrated for other amino acids: leucine, lysine and phenylalanine *in vivo* (Table 8.4, Lajtha & Toth, 1961, 1962) and dihydroxyphenylalanine *in vitro* (Yoshida *et al.*, 1963). Glutamate appears to be exceptional; no stereospecificity for glutamate transport in cerebral systems has been demonstrated (Tsukada *et al.*, 1963).

Cerebral Influx and Efflux of Amino Acids

In addition to the rapid uptake of amino acids to the brain, outward transport also occurs; rates of efflux may equal those of influx. The rapid extrusion

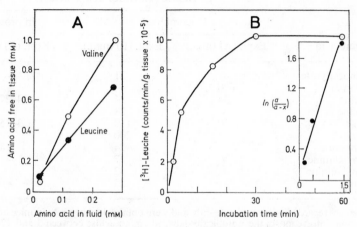

FIG. 8.2. Amino acid equilibria at isolated neocortical tissues (Jones & McIlwain, 1971).
A. The free valine and leucine of guinea pig tissue after 1 hr. incubation in fluids of the stated amino acid content. The lowest values are obtained without added amino acid and represent a fluid content of valine of 0·44 μmoles/g. and of leucine of 0·52 μmoles/g. Tissue/fluid ratios were: valine, 6·4–7·6 and leucine, 4–8.
B. Uptake of [^{3}H]leucine; after tissues had incubated for 30 min. the [^{3}H]leucine was added and incubation continued for the stated times before sampling tissues and fluid for free leucine. Inset: a logarithmic plot showing the initial uptake to approach a first-order reaction.

of amino acids against a concentration gradient has been followed *in vivo* after intracerebral injections of ^{14}C-labelled leucine, lysine or phenylalanine (Lajtha & Toth, 1961). An elevated plasma concentration of the relevant unlabelled amino acid was maintained by repeated intravenous injections. Leucine was extruded more rapidly than lysine and phenylalanine extrusion could not be detected in this study. Most of the extruded leucine or lysine went into the bloodstream; relatively little was retained in the cerebrospinal fluid or incorporated into protein. It has more recently been suggested (Schain *et al.*, 1967) from studies using ^{14}C-labelled phenylalanine and α-aminoisobutyrate *in vivo,* that equilibrium conditions in the cerebrospinal fluid do not favour isotope entry into the cerebrospinal fluid.

Influx and efflux of amino acids have been differentiated also by study of preparations from the brain, incubated *in vitro.* These preparations offer the advantage of avoiding limitations on transport imposed by the blood-brain barrier (q.v.). Care must however be exercised (i) to allow for changes in the fluid spaces of the tissue during incubation; and (ii) to determine changes in net content of amino acids which occur during the experiment. Data of Fig. 8.2 illustrate this point, and show the considerable production of free amino acid which may occur during such experiments. This will be noted to concern valine and leucine, presumably derived by proteolysis; a number of other amino acids can be synthesized in such preparations. The kinetics of entry of ^{3}H-valine to the tissue in these experiments approximated to those of a first order reaction (Jones & McIlwain, 1971).

In such studies, after a period of preincubation, stable amino acid contents can be reached when presumably net effluxes and influxes balance. Relatively short periods of subsequent incubation with an added amino acid may then be used on the assumption that efflux should be negligible, and a change should reflect true input. ^{14}C-L-Alanine was then found to accumulate more rapidly than ^{14}C-D-alanine during the first 5 min. incubation, after which the content of the D-isomer began to exceed that of the L-isomer. The results indicated that L-alanine was transported more rapidly in both directions, i.e. both into and out from the tissue. Also, after pre-incubation in the presence of ^{14}C-labelled amino-acid, the tissues were placed in media containing unlabelled amino-acid when efflux of labelled amino acid could be followed; ^{14}C-L-alanine was extruded at a faster rate than ^{14}C-D-alanine (Neame & Smith, 1965).

Competition Between Amino Acids

Evidence on the specificity of the transport process has come from studies on competition between amino acids for uptake to the brain. Thus dihydroxy-phenylalanine uptake *in vivo* was shown to be competitively inhibited by phenylalanine or tyrosine but not by alanine or glutamate. Glutamate and aspartate compete with each other for transport and therefore have been concluded to share a common route, different from that for alanine and γ-aminobutyrate (Tsukada *et al.*, 1963; Yoshida *et al.*, 1963). Also in experiments similar to those of **A**, Fig. 8.1, certain amino acids administered together with tyrosine competed with it for entry to the brain. Thus entry was delayed by tryptophan, phenylalanine or valine but not by glutamate or lysine.

It seems possible therefore that at least three carrier mechanisms are involved —for aromatic amino acids, acidic amino acids and neutral amino acids. Whether more than one mechanism is involved in the transport of neutral amino acids (Yoshida *et al.*, 1963) analogous to the two suggested for non-neural tissues (Oxender & Christensen, 1963) remains to be determined. Also, it is uncertain at present if basic amino acids are transported by a separate route.

Cations, Stimulation and Metabolic Status

Amino acid transport in cerebral preparations exhibits an absolute requirement for Na^+, which cannot be replaced by K^+, Li^+ or choline. The requirement for K^+ is less certain; Lahiri & Lajtha (1964) found no K^+ requirement for lysine, leucine or α-aminoisobutyrate uptake *in vitro* and also that the uptake was inhibited by high K^+. However ^{35}S-methionine transport was decreased at low K^+ (below 1·25 mM) or high K^+ (above 20 mM) (Folbergrova, 1961) and L-histidine uptake, which required glucose and Ca^{2+}, was inhibited by 27 mM K^+ (de Almeida *et al.*, 1965). The inhibition by high K^+ of glycine transport in the rat cerebral cortex was reversed by acetylcholine (Nakazawa & Quastel, 1968) while inhibition due to NH_4^+, ouabain, glutamate or glutamine was unaffected by acetylcholine. It was suggested that the acetylcholine might act

Table 8.4

Cerebral amino acid transport and metabolically-derived energy

Tissue	Ratio (Tissue : Medium) of L-tyrosine		
	No addition	1 mM-DNP added	10 mM-Glucose added
Cerebral cortex	1·75	1·07	2·60
Kidney cortex	1·13	1·01	1·15
Liver	0·66	0·78	0·68
Spleen	1·47	1·14	1·56
Diaphragm	0·74	0·81	–

Tissue slices of the rat were incubated for 60 min. in Krebs Ringer bicarbonate buffer which contained 1 mM tyrosine. Glucose or 2,4-dinitrophenol (DNP) was present throughout the incubation period where indicated; no addition was made to the media of the control slices (Guroff *et al.*, 1961).

by increasing permeability to Na^+. Optimal concentrations for amino acid transport would appear to be Na^+, 80 mM and K^+, 5–10 mM. With the exception of glutamate (discussed below) amino acid transport is associated with movement of Na^+ in the same direction and of K^+ in the opposite direction. Amino acid transport in cerebral preparations is inhibited by ouabain; 50% inhibition of dihydroxyphenylalanine uptake was observed with 5×10^{-6} M ouabain (Yoshida *et al.*, 1963) and 70–90% inhibition of the transport of glutamate, aspartate or γ-aminobutyrate was caused with 1×10^{-5} M ouabain (Tsukada *et al.*, 1963). Serotonin uptake in perfused brain was also inhibited (Palaic *et al.*, 1967). Similar concentrations of ouabain (Schwartz *et al.*, 1962) inhibit the cerebral Na^+,K^+-ATPase associated with active cation transport (q.v.). Cerebral amino acid transporting systems are more sensitive to ouabain than are non-neural systems. In Ehrlich ascites cells, 50% inhibition of glycine transport required $2·5 \times 10^{-4}$ M ouabain (Bittner & Heinz, 1963) and in the kidney cortex, 50% inhibition of glycine, lysine and α-aminoisobutyrate transport required 8×10^{-4} M (Fox *et al.*, 1964).

Amino acid transport in the brain occurs more rapidly than in other tissues (Neame, 1962; Guroff *et al.*, 1961; Tsukada *et al.*, 1963) and is more sensitive to interference with supply of metabolically-derived energy. This is illustrated with respect to L-tyrosine in Table 8.4. Uptake of ^{35}S-methionine also is stimulated by glucose but not by other oxidizable substrates: e.g. lactate, pyruvate or succinate (Folbergrova, 1961). Some evidence has been given for a pyridoxal phosphate requirement for cerebral amino acid transport; Tsukada *et al.* (1963) found that the compound augmented γ-aminobutyrate uptake but was without effect on glutamate transport. An energy source was needed for uptake of aspartate (but not of glycine; these two differed also in temperature-dependence), and of 5-hydroxytryptophan and γ-aminobutyrate. In addition to those already named, histidine, arginine, lysine, ornithine, proline and methionine have been found to be assimilated to isolated cerebral tissues of various species.

Table 8.5

Differential release of amino acids and related metabolites from cerebral tissues

Agent	Part of the brain	Released	Not released
Electrical stimulation	Neocortex	γ-Aminobutyrate[1, 3] Adenosine[4]	L-Leucine,[3] α-aminoisobutyrate,[3] urea[3]
	Piriform cortex	5-Hydroxytryptamine,[2] noradrenaline[2]	Glycine[2]
	Striatum	γ-Aminobutyrate,[1] glutamate,[1] lysine,[1] leucine,[1] taurine[1]	–
K[+], 25–66 mM	Striatum	Glutamate[1]	–
	Piriform cortex	Noradrenaline[2]	
Glutamate	Piriform cortex	–	Noradrenaline[2]

Tissues from guinea pigs or rats were examined in superfusion systems (see Chapter 4).
[1] Katz, Chase & Kopin (1969). [2] McIlwain & Snyder (1970). [3] Srinivasan, Neal & Mitchell (1969). [4] Chapter 9.

Amino acid/tissue relationships *in vitro* are susceptible to alteration by manipulation of the tissue as well as of the medium. In particular, electrical stimulation of the tissue causes differential release of some of its content of amino acids and related compounds (Table 8.5). The compounds released include compounds which act in or modify neural transmission and enzyme induction (McIlwain, 1970; McIlwain & Snyder, 1970). Study of their release is thus of much importance in the functioning and adaptation of cerebral systems *in vivo*, and receives further comment in Chapters 13 and 14.

Cerebral Peptides and Related Compounds

Peptides are not normally found as intermediates in the synthesis of protein, and the major free peptide of the brain, as of many other organs, is glutathione. To this the pituitary and hypothalamus constitute an exception through their content of peptide hormones, which are described in Chapter 16; the occurrence of carnosine and of homocarnosine (see below) is also noteworthy.

Glutathione

Glutathione (see McIlwain, 1959; McIlwain & Tresize, 1957) is present in the brain at 0·9–3·4 μmoles/g., so constituting up to one-third of its total non-protein, acid-extracted nitrogen and at least 95% of the thiols in this fraction. The cerebral level is similar to those of several other tissues of the body but is some ten times that of the total glutathione of blood plasma. Separated cerebral tissues in glucose salines lose one-third or one-half of their glutathione unless this is provided in the saline, when the loss is less; assimilation of glutathione as such is however not established.

Since its characterization by Gowland Hopkins as an autoxidizable component of tissues (Kosower & Kosower, 1969), much of the significance of glutathione has been pictured to lie in the oxidation and reduction of its thiol group. Reduction of the oxidized form (GSSG) occurs rapidly in cerebral tissues, catalysed by a glutathione reductase specific to the reduced nicotinamide adenine dinucleotide phosphate:

$$GSSG + NADPH + H^+ \rightarrow NADP^+ + 2GSH$$

which proceeds at some 250 μmoles/hr. g. brain. Equilibrium at the reductase is almost entirely in favour of reduced glutathione (GSH), and in the brain GSH and NADPH are at several times the concentration of their oxidized forms (a situation typical of most mammalian tissues except blood). This presumably results from a relative lack of systems oxidizing GSH and NADPH, which is a very real phenomenon in cerebral tissues. This situation can be seen as necessary if glutathione is to serve a function generally ascribed to it: that of maintaining metabolically-important thiol compounds in the reduced form on which often depends their functioning as enzymes or coenzymes. This maintenance would require the reduction of disulphides by reduced glutathione; such reduction takes place spontaneously at the pH and glutathione levels of the brain, but may also be catalysed.

A further change established as occurring at the thiol group of glutathione is its acylation. Thioesters of coenzymes were noted in the previous chapter as important intermediates in carbohydrate metabolism, and thioesters as a group are reactive compounds capable of spontaneous transacylation:

$$R^1SAc + R^2SH \rightleftharpoons R^1SH + R^2SAc.$$

A cerebral enzyme probably catalyses such changes between S-acetylglutathione and cysteine, and, further, S-acetylglutathione has been formed at some 0·1 μmoles/g. hr. from glutathione, acetate, and adenosine triphosphate by an enzyme preparation from rat brain (Feuer, 1956; Strecker et al., 1955).

Tissues of the brain can in addition bring about changes at the amide linkages of glutathione. The most active system shows an interesting specificity for the γ-peptide linkage between glutamic acid and cysteine. Breakdown of the molecule at this point:

$$HOOC.CHNH_2.CH_2.CH_2.CO\mathrel{\substack{|\\|}}NHCH(CH_2SH).CO-NH.CH_2.COOH$$

is readily shown by the Sullivan test (involving a naphthaquinone sulphonate and cyanide) which requires the free amino and thiol groupings of cysteine and is thus negative with glutathione itself. Glutathione cleavage proves not to be a simple hydrolysis, for it does not proceed unless other reactants are present. Of these the most active are amino acids and peptides (Fodor, Miller & Waelsch, 1953). The peptides presumably act as acceptors for the γ-glutamyl group; in this reaction amines are inactive, thus differentiating the present system from the glutamotransferase described below. The present system has been partly separated also from tissues of the liver and kidney where its activity is about the same as in the brain; it may operate as a stage in a γ-glutamyl cycle, with a function in the transport of amino acids (Orlowski & Meister, 1970).

Synthesis of glutathione has been demonstrated to occur in the brain by isolating and analysing the cerebral glutathione after intracisternal injection of carbon-labelled glycine; it has been similarly demonstrated in isolated cerebral tissues (Douglas & Mortensen, 1956; Takahashi & Akabane, 1961). Incorporation of the glycine took place, and the data suggested a half-life of some 70 hr. for the glutathione in experiments in which the value for liver was 4 hr. Intracisternally injected [1-^{14}C]glutamate has also been demonstrated to become incorporated in cerebral glutathione (Machiyama et al., 1970).

Blood levels of glutathione have been reported to be abnormal in certain mental diseases; large doses of glutathione have been administered intravenously without marked immediate effect on mental status (Altschule, 1957).

Other Peptides and Amides

The brain is interestingly rich in simple amino acid derivatives, some of which have not yet been detected in non-neural tissues.

The content of N-acetylaspartic acid in the brain (5–10 μmoles/g., Table 8.1) is second only to that of glutamate amongst free amino acids and related compounds. The acid is found in much lower concentration in other tissues; the characteristically high level in the brain has prompted speculation on its function. Studies on the cerebral metabolism of N-acetylaspartate using ^{14}C-labelled substrates have yielded conflicting results, due mainly to difficulty in separating N-acetylaspartate from contaminating radioactive substances in brain extracts. Thus whereas some workers detected little or no synthesis of the acid in the adult brain, others have produced evidence for synthesis involving catalysis by aspartate N-acetyl transferase (McIntosh & Cooper, 1965; Buniatian et al., 1965; Knizley, 1967). No synthesis of N-acetylaspartate has been demonstrated in non-neural tissues, although degradation with formation of CO_2 appears to be widespread in mammalian tissues, so it has been suggested that non-neural tissues may depend on supply of the acid from the brain.

Release of N-acetylaspartate from the brain has been shown to occur in vivo and in vitro; after intracerebral injection it accumulated in the kidney. In cerebral cortex slices release to the medium during incubation was increased in the presence of glucose. However, rates of turnover of the acid in adult brain are slow and its major function in the brain may be in its contribution to total anion content (Buniatian et al., 1965; McIntosh & Cooper, 1965; Berlinquet & Laliberte, 1966; Benuck & D'Adamo, 1968).

N-Acetyl-α-L-aspartyl-L-glutamate has been detected in the brains of many animals and isolated in pure form from human brain in amounts equivalent to

0·32–0·64 μmole/g. of tissue (Curatolo *et al.*, 1965; Auditore *et al.*, 1966). The dipeptide occurred in considerably greater amounts in the brains of rabbits, rats, guinea pigs and chickens (0·12–0·24 μmole/g.) than in any non-neural tissue tested (Miyamoto *et al.*, 1966). *N*-Acetyl-L-glutamyl-L-glutamate has also been detected in the brain (Kanazawa & Sano, 1967).

Homocarnosine (γ-aminobutyryl-L-histidine) has been demonstrated in the brain and spinal cord of many species (Pisano *et al.*, 1961), and 17 μmoles/kg. have been isolated in crystalline form from ox brain. Homoanserine (γ-aminobutyryl-1-methylhistidine), 4 μmoles/kg. was also isolated (Kanazawa *et al.*, 1965; Nakajima *et al.*, 1967). The authors suggested that the concentrations of these peptides isolated should be regarded as minimal levels occurring in the brain.

Amino Acid Metabolism: General Aspects

Two of the most important aspects of the metabolism of amino acids are their entry to the brain which has been described above, and their conversion to protein, which is described in the next chapter. Most of the remainder of this chapter concerns individual amino acids or peptides in their relation to the brain or to cerebral functioning, but this account is preceded by the present notes on other reactions which are common to several amino acids: their oxidation, decarboxylation, transamination and cognate reactions.

Oxidation and Decarboxylation

No amino acid adequately replaces glucose as an energy-yielding, oxidizable substrate for the mammalian brain, *in vivo* or with isolated tissues. The inability of the amino acids of the bloodstream to support normal cerebral functioning in hypoglycaemic subjects can be deduced from the observations quoted in Chapter 2; during hypoglycaemia, blood levels of amino acids fall but remain considerable. Also, the respiration of separated cerebral tissues is not increased or maintained by most added amino acids as it is with glucose. To this glutamic acid is an exception (Weil-Malherbe, 1936; Woodman & McIlwain, 1961). Eighteen amino acids, including alanine, serine or proline at 5–25 mM caused no appreciable increase in the respiration of sections of the cerebral cortex of guinea pigs and rats; some, as tyrosine, caused a slight inhibition of normal respiration. L-Glutamic acid, however, led to respiratory rates which initially were higher than in its absence, and aspartic acid showed this property to a lesser degree. The increase occurred whether or not glucose was present, but lasted for a limited period only. Examination of tissue composition showed glutamic acid to have diminished the phosphocreatine, normally resynthesized in presence of glucose, while inorganic phosphate increased in quantity. Glutamic acid thus depleted the tissue's energy-rich phosphates rather than maintaining them as does glucose or pyruvate.

Evidence for relatively slow oxidative changes in certain other amino acids has however been obtained by supplying these in high concentrations to washed cerebral tissues. In this way D- and to a lesser extent L-alanine, and also L- and D-isoleucine, phenylalanine, histidine, arginine, ornithine, lysine and tryptophan, led to increased aerobic but not anaerobic formation of ammonia (Edlbacher & Wiss, 1944). Increased respiration was evident with several of the amino acids and the system concerned appeared to be distinct from that oxidizing glutamic acid.

Formation of $^{14}CO_2$ has been observed in several instances after adding ^{14}C-labelled amino acids to cerebral tissues or dispersions (Friedberg, 1954; Roberts et al., 1962; Schepartz, 1963). This may represent decarboxylation, or more complex reactions; the corresponding ketoacids were in some cases detected in the reaction mixtures, suggesting oxidative deamination and decarboxylation. The $^{14}CO_2$ was formed from some ten amino acids including alanine, leucine, valine, serine, glycine and proline, the rates diminishing in that order and being much below those obtainable with glutamic acid. Formation of $^{14}CO_2$ was not detected from arginine, histidine or lysine; from some amino acids it was modified by a dietary change or by growth of the animals.

Cerebral preparations show D-amino acid oxidase activity, and the system responsible has been partly purified (de Marchi & Johnston, 1969; Neims et al., 1966). Activities measured in several regions showed highest values in the cerebellum, of about 2 μmoles amino acid oxidized/hr./g. tissue. Alanine, serine and glycine were the substrates most rapidly oxidized by a purified preparation from sheep cerebella.

Transmethylation and Trans-sulphuration

Two sulphur-containing amino acids, cystathionine and taurine, occur in high concentrations in the mammalian brain relative to the levels found in other tissues; interest in these amino acids has been stimulated by the characteristically high content of cystathionine in human brain (Table 8.1) and by its involvement in two neurological diseases, homocystinuria and cystathioninuria. Transmethylation and trans-sulphuration reactions are important in the metabolism of the sulphur amino acids. The pathway (Fig. 8.3) of conversion

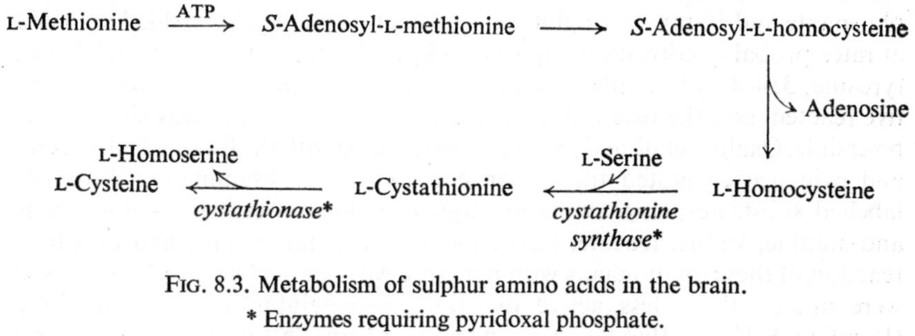

FIG. 8.3. Metabolism of sulphur amino acids in the brain.
* Enzymes requiring pyridoxal phosphate.

of methionine to cysteine has been demonstrated to occur in the brain; ^{35}S-methionine, administered intraperitoneally to rats or added to the incubation medium of in vitro preparations of the brain, is rapidly converted to form ^{35}S-labelled S-adenosyl-methionine, S-adenosyl-homocysteine and cysteine

(Gaitonde and Richter, 1957; Gaull and Gaitonde, 1967; Baldessarini and Kopin, 1966). Not all of the individual enzymes have been characterized, but those that have provided evidence in support of the presence in the brain of the pathway of Fig. 8.3.

The methionine-activating enzyme, *ATP*: L-*methionine S-adenosyltransferase* (EC 2.4.2.13) has been studied in various regions of Rhesus monkey brain. Greatest activity, 0·25–0·28 μmole/g. hr., was found in the pituitary and cerebellum whereas white matter areas showed least activity. Two of the enzymes, *cystathionine synthase* and *cystathionase*, require pyridoxal phosphate as coenzyme, a property of relevance to enzymic malfunction in the associated neurological disorders, homocystinuria and cystathioninuria, in which it is possible that the enzymic defects may be due to impaired ability to bind the vitamin. This is discussed in a subsequent section of this Chapter. Distribution of cystathionine synthase in the Rhesus monkey brain was found to be similar to that of the methionine activating enzyme; the activity was highest in the cerebellum, 1·5 μmole/g. hr., and lowest in subcortical white matter and corpus callosum (Volpe & Laster, 1970). The first intermediate in the pathway, S-adenosyl-L-methionine, is important also in other transmethylation reactions in the brain, particularly those involved in the metabolism of catecholamines (Chapter 14).

Transamination

The most potent transamination reactions in the brain as in most organs are between the ketoacids concerned in the Krebs cycle and the corresponding amino acids; the rate of 7,000 μmoles/hr./g. tissue reached in the reaction of glutamate with pyruvate has been noted above and receives further comment below.

Systems capable of transaminating many other amino acids at lesser rates have been demonstrated in the mammalian brain (Albers *et al.*, 1962; Fonnum *et al.*, 1964). In reaction mixtures containing cerebral extracts with pyridoxal phosphate and 10 mM-α-oxoglutarate, aromatic amino acids yielded ketoacids at rates probably corresponding to 0·5–5 μmoles/hr. g. tissue. Phenylalanine, tyrosine, 3:4-dihydroxyphenylalanine, tryptophan and its 5-hydroxy-derivative reacted, and the reaction with tyrosine (the most rapid) was shown to be reversible. Oxaloacetate and pyruvate also reacted with the (unpurified) extracts and evidence suggested the presence of several transaminases. With ^{14}C-labelled substrates, transamination was also shown between α-oxoglutarate and alanine, valine, leucine, isoleucine, cysteine, methionine and ornithine; reaction of these amino-acids with pyruvate was not detected. Cerebral tissues were among those less active in ornithine-oxoglutarate aminotransferase (Herzfeld & Knox, 1968), converting some 13 μmoles/hr. g. tissue in the rat. The cerebral enzyme was also little susceptible to induction by steroid hormones under the conditions examined. Transamination can yield glycine from glyoxalate in the brain; the relevant glycine-α-oxoglutarate transaminase has been observed to proceed at 12–14·5 μmoles/g. hr. and is inhibited by aminooxyacetic acid (Johnston & Vitali, 1969).

Glutamic Acid

Of individual amino acids, glutamic acid and its immediate metabolites are of oustanding importance to the brain. In most animal tissues, glutamic acid itself or as its amide glutamine, is predominant among amino acids as one occurring in high concentration and undergoing active metabolism. This is true of the mammalian brain, where the acid and amide constitute up to 60% of the free α-amino-nitrogen and undergo the varied metabolic changes summarized in Fig. 8.4.

Assimilation

To the high cerebral concentration of glutamic acid, contributions are made both by synthesis *in situ* and by assimilation from the bloodstream. The formation of ^{14}C-glutamate from ^{14}C-glucose or pyruvate in the brain makes the preponderating contribution (Chapter 6; Roberts *et al.*, 1959). Glutamate, given itself as the ^{14}C-compound, appears in the brain sufficiently rapidly to suggest entry as such at only 0·1–2 μmoles/hr. g. tissue (Lajtha *et al.*, 1959) and it is rapidly converted to glutamine (below). Little net increase in cerebral content of glutamate has been observed even when the plasma content of the acid was increased thirty-fold, but administration of glutamine could lead to higher cerebral contents of both glutamine and glutamate.

By contrast, isolated cerebral tissues actively assimilated glutamic acid when it was present aerobically in saline media (Stern *et al.*, 1949; Takagaki *et al.*, 1959; Woodman & McIlwain, 1961). Assimilation was increased by glucose and by several other oxidizable substrates and proceeded with glutamate at 2·5–20 mM, affording concentrations of glutamate up to 40 μmoles/g., in some cases fifteen times that of the medium. It occurred at rates up to 50 μmoles/hr. g. tissue, much greater than those of the assimilation *in vivo*. D-Glutamate was also assimilated, requiring glucose; uptake with either acid was markedly less in absence of sodium salts. Glutamic acid shows other important properties in relation to Na$^+$ salts in that it permits Na$^+$ entry to the intracellular compartment of cerebral tissues, and this contributes to the actions of glutamic acid as a cerebral excitant (McIlwain *et al.*, 1969; see below). Metabolic changes concomitant with glutamate uptake are discussed below in describing glutamate oxidation.

Glutamine Formation and Breakdown

These processes are important both in relation to the metabolism of glutamic acid, and also to that of cerebral ammonia. As observed in cerebral tissues (Krebs, 1935) the synthesis and breakdown appeared distinct processes, the synthesis being an energy requiring process which did not occur anaerobically. Hydrolysis, however, occurred at some 36 μmoles/hr. g. tissue without additional energy source when cerebral dispersions were mixed with glutamine and salt solutions. Using washed particulate preparations and partially purified enzymes, however, both synthesis and breakdown were found to be quite complex and to have several requirements in common (Blumson, 1957;

7

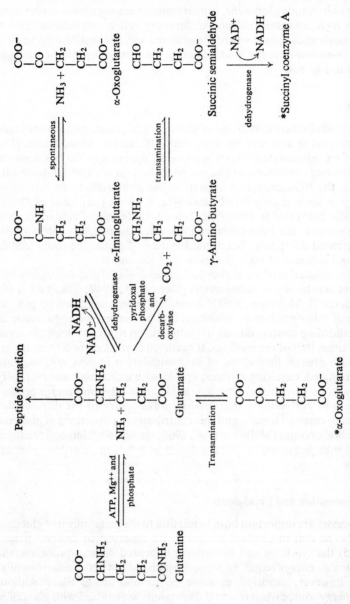

FIG. 8.4. An outline of the metabolic routes involving glutamic acid. Two transaminase reactions preponderate, with oxaloacetate and pyruvate. A lesser route leads to glutathione.

* The series of reactions from α-oxoglutarate to succinyl coenzyme A, involving γ-aminobutyrate and succinic semialdehyde, forms the "γ-aminobutyrate shunt" to part of the tricarboxylic acid cycle.

Meister *et al.*, 1962). Thus the hydrolysis required not only Mg or Mn salts, but also inorganic phosphate and adenosine di- or tri-phosphate. Also, when other bases, for example hydroxylamine, were included in this reaction mixture the amide-NH_2 could be replaced by such bases even more rapidly than by –OH in hydrolysis. Fig. 8.5 illustrates properties of this transfer reaction; with optimal activation it proceeded at 300 μmoles/hr. g. tissue. The role of the adenine nucleotides was catalytic, and when ^{14}C-labelled glutamate was added to similar reaction mixtures it was not incorporated in the γ-glutamyl hydroxamate produced.

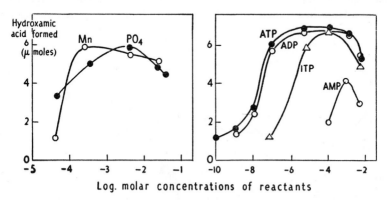

Log. molar concentrations of reactants

FIG. 8.5. Formation from glutamine of the corresponding hydroxamic acid, catalysed by an enzyme from sheep brain (Lajtha *et al.*, 1953). The complete system contained 20 mM-glutamine, 10 mM-hydroxylamine, 5 mM-phosphate, 5 mM-manganese salts, and 0·05 mM-adenosine triphosphate. Reaction was followed by the red colour yielded with ferric chloride by the glutamohydroxamic acid formed. The graphs show the effect of varying the concentrations of several of the components, and of replacing adenosine triphosphate (ATP) by the diphosphate (ADP) or monophosphate (AMP) or by inosine triphosphate (ITP).

Some explanation for the requirements of the transferase activity has been found in a coincidence of several of its properties with those of the glutamine-synthesizing system. Synthesis of glutamine was not at first observed to occur in cell-free cerebral preparations. Tissue slices required for the synthesis not only glutamic acid and ammonia but also glucose and oxygen; glutamine could then be formed at some 8 μmoles/hr. g. tissue. In this system the glucose and oxygen were found to be required as a source of energy; knowing this the synthesis of glutamine could then be brought about by cell-free systems containing adenosine triphosphate, the reaction being:

(i) $\underset{\text{acid}}{\text{Glutamic}} + \underset{\text{triphosphate}}{\text{adenosine}} + NH_3 \xrightarrow[]{\text{Enz, Mg(Mn)}} \text{glutamine} + \underset{\text{diphosphate}}{\text{adenosine}} + \underset{\text{phosphate}}{\text{inorganic}}$

The course of the reaction and some of its requirements are illustrated in Fig. 8.6, which shows their similarity with those of the transferase reaction. Moreover, a hundred-fold purification of each from sheep was achieved without separation of the two activities, which were similarly affected by a variety of reagents. The maximum rate of the synthetic reaction was 10–12 μmoles/g. hr., or about a twentieth of the transferase. The two activities were also associated in a ratio of 1:9 in pigeon liver.

The reaction outlined, (i), is likely to involve intermediates but these proved to be enzyme-bound and not at first easy to identify. Using ^{32}P derivatives, exchange between ortho-P and ATP, or ATP and ADP, could be detected only when all components were present. Further examination used at substrate level an enzyme representing a 3,000-fold purification from sheep brain, obtained as a single protein of molecular weight about 450,000 (Meister et al., 1962; Krishnaswamy et al., 1962). During purification the enzyme was found to be protected from heat inactivation by ATP and Mg; other reactants were not

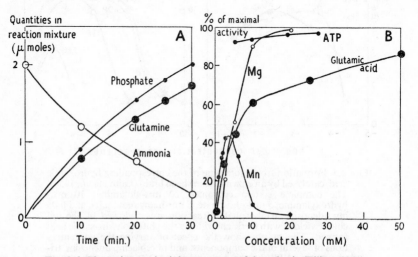

FIG. 8.6. Glutamine synthesis by an extract of sheep brain (Elliott, 1951). Reaction mixtures contained L-glutamic acid, ammonium and magnesium salts, and adenosine triphosphate (ATP). (A) The course of reaction. Values for ammonia have been decreased by 2 μmoles for convenience in drawing. (B) Dependence on the concentrations of reactants. The values with glutamic acid are expressed as percentages of that with 100 mM-glutamic acid.

comparably effective and an initial MgATP-enzyme complex was thus suggested as (a), Fig. 8.7. When to the purified enzyme, MgATP and ^{14}C-glutamate were added (but no NH$_3$) and the solution ultracentrifuged, glutamate was deposited with the enzyme. Combination did not occur when either Mg or ATP was omitted, and the glutamate passed to solution when NH$_3$ also was included; the sequence of combination a, b, d of Fig. 8.7 is thus indicated. Magnesium ions and ATP have also been shown to protect the purified enzyme against inactivation by N-ethylmaleimide; only one SH group of the 14–15 present reacted. The synthetase contains 8 identical subunits with arginine as the N-terminal amino acid (Ronzio et al., 1969).

By similar techniques, combination of enzyme and ^{14}C-glutamine was shown to require Mg or Mn and ADP indicating a sequence of steps f, e, d

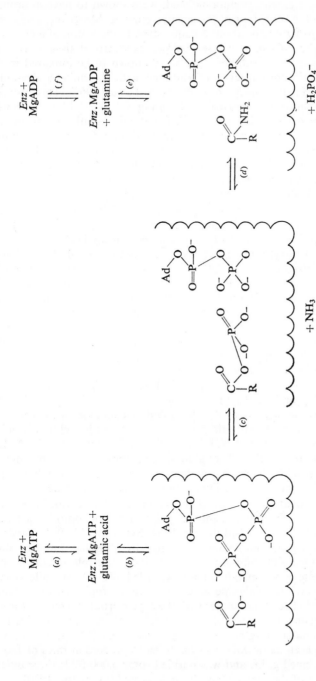

Fig. 8.7. Suggested mechanism of glutamine synthesis (Meister *et al.*, 1962; Ronzio & Meister, 1968). *Enz* and the curved line: glutamine synthetase; R–COO⁻: glutamic acid. The system *a–f* represents synthesis, while glutamine hydrolysis is suggested as proceeding by stages *f*, *e*, *d* and reaction of the product with water; for the transfer reaction of Fig. 8.4 the product from *d* reacts with hydroxylamine.

(Fig. 8.7). Several phenomena of activation and competition evident in intact cerebral tissues, e.g. with D-glutamic acid, were shown to have appropriate counterparts in the behaviour of the isolated enzyme. Moreover, study of the enzyme gave further details about a major stage in the action of a convulsive agent, *methionine sulphoximine* (see below). Neocortical tissues from cats treated with methionine sulphoximine were known to be impaired in their ability to maintain normal levels of glutamic acid, glutamine and γ-amino-butyric acid on incubation *in vitro* (Peters & Tower, 1959). This proved to involve the formation, at stages (a) and (b) of Fig. 8.7, of a stable product which inhibited the enzyme. Using the purified glutamine synthetase from sheep brain in a reaction mixture which also contained ATP, Mn^{2+} and methionine sulphoximine gave a product containing 8 moles of methionine sulphoximine phosphate and 8 of ADP per enzyme molecule (Ronzio & Meister, 1968). The inhibited enzyme was not readily re-activated; by heat or acid it was denatured with the formation of methionine sulphoximine phosphate.

The nature of reaction *c* in the scheme of Fig. 8.7 is suggested rather than rigidly proven. In a system containing the cerebral enzyme, MgATP and glutamic acid, the glutamic acid was found to be chemically labile, for it formed pyrrolidone-α-carboxylic acid much more readily than usual. Activation had apparently occurred at the γ-COOH of glutamic acid. Using ^{18}O-glutamic acid and an enzyme of vegetable origin which was similar in many respects to the cerebral enzyme, transfer of ^{18}O was observed during glutamine synthesis (Kowalsky *et al.*, 1956). Enrichment in ^{18}O occurred in the orthophosphate produced in the reaction, and not in the ADP. Reaction *c* offers an explanation of this, but other possibilities are not excluded. In the transfer reaction of Fig. 8.4, or in glutamine hydrolysis, the complex produced by reaction *d* is pictured to react with hydroxylamine or with water. As these processes involve part only of the full sequence *a–f*, scope is offered for different activation (cf. Mn), and $H_2PO_4^-$ and ADP act here as coenzymes rather than as substrates or products. Apparent K_m values for the different components in reaction (i) show the synthesis to reach half maximal velocity with L-glutamic acid at 2·5 mM, ATP at 2·3 mM, and NH_4^+ at 0·18 mM. The low value for NH_4^+ is significant in relation to the role of glutamine synthesis in removing ammonia (q.v.). Though reaction between D-glutamic acid and NH_4^+ is catalysed by the enzyme, much higher concentrations of both reactants are needed.

Study of the activation of mammalian *glutaminases* has revealed isoenzymes which differ in their requirement of polyanions for optimal activation (Katunuma *et al.*, 1967; Weil-Malherbe, 1969; Svenneby, 1969). In particular, different cerebral glutaminases were activated by phosphates and by simple organic acids. One glutaminase increased four- to five-fold in activity when *N*-acetyl aspartate or *N*-acetylglutamate was added at 10–20 mM, while *N*-acetyl-glycine or *N*-acetylphenylalanine gave seven- to ten-fold activation. Not all tissues examined gave glutaminases with these properties, which must thus be judged to be related to the notable occurrence of *N*-acetylamino acids in the brain. The glutaminase (L-glutamine aminohydrolase, EC 3.5.1.2) of pig brain, prepared as an acetone powder, was observed to proceed at rates of 130–150 μmoles NH_3 formed/g. hr. and was purified some 5,000-fold; three different molecular forms of the enzyme have been described (Svenneby, 1970).

Oxidation

Formation of glutamine accounts for only part of the changes occurring in ammonium glutamate when it is incubated aerobically with cerebral tissues. As only substrate, a large part of the glutamic acid is oxidized, through α-oxoglutarate, ultimately to CO_2 and NH_3 (Weil-Malherbe, 1936; Haslam & Krebs, 1963). Two distinct routes lead from glutamate to α-oxoglutarate: transamination, to be discussed below, and the direct oxidation which yields also NH_3. This oxidation proceeds by an initial anaerobic reaction (ii) with nicotinamide-adenine dinucleotide catalysed by glutamate dehydrogenase:

(ii) $$\text{Glutamic acid} + NAD^+ \rightleftharpoons \text{Iminoglutaric acid} + NADH + H^+$$

In the absence of secondary reactions the equilibrium of this reaction is much in favour of glutamic acid, only $1\cdot4\%$ being oxidized at pH $7\cdot4$. But equilibrium is achieved only in the presence of ammonium salts. If they are removed, the iminoglutaric acid hydrolyses spontaneously to α-oxoglutaric acid and ammonia. Thus the supply or removal of ammonia can condition the oxidation of glutamic acid. The NADH produced in the reaction is normally reoxidized through cytochromes (q.v.); the reaction is influenced also by other nucleotides (Frieden, 1965).

Glutamate dehydrogenase in dispersions of rabbit brain proceeds at rates of 400–1000 μmoles/hr. g. tissue; $0\cdot2$ mM-oxoglutarate and 15 μM-NADH gave half-maximal velocities (Copenhaver et al., 1950; Lowry et al., 1956; Lowry, 1957). The enzyme is more potent in the mammalian liver, from which source it has been purified and exhibits interesting properties (Frieden, 1963). In cerebral dispersions and mitochondrial suspensions, the greater part of glutamate oxidation is concluded to proceed through α-oxoglutarate yielded by transamination, and some 10% through glutamate dehydrogenase (Haslam & Krebs, 1963). In cell-containing preparations of cerebral cortex in saline solution, respiration with glutamic acid as substrate proceeds more rapidly than with glucose, reaching 100 μmoles/g. hr. Usually the ammonia formed by oxidation does not accumulate as such but undergoes further reactions, one of which is the formation of glutamine itself. In fact the addition of glutamic acid to cerebral tissues can result in the diminution of the ammonia content of the reaction mixture in spite of the presence of processes leading to increased formation of ammonia (Weil-Malherbe, 1936).

The formation of glutamine utilizes adenosine triphosphate and thus added glutamic acid, although supporting a high respiratory rate, diminishes the tissue's energy-rich phosphates both by this route and also because it increases the entry of Na^+ to the intracellular compartment of the tissues. The cation changes alter the membrane potential and excitability of the tissue and are discussed further in Chapter 14. Their effect on $\sim$P arises because the entering Na^+ activates the Na,K-ATPase (q.v.). Stoichiometric relationships similar to those of **A**, Fig. 8.6 have been shown to occur during the first few minutes after the addition of glutamate to cerebral tissues (Woodman & McIlwain, 1961; Harvey & McIlwain, 1968), also with breakdown of ATP. The tissues, concomitantly, swell by absorption of fluid. Such factors limit the value of glutamate as sole cerebral substrate in vivo and in vitro. The balance of the several reactions involved, however, appears to differ in different mammalian species; glutamate supported a greater respiratory response to electrical stimulation in human than in other cerebral tissues (Stern *et al.*, 1949; McIlwain 1953).

Transamination

α-Oxoglutarate has been indicated above as involved in many transaminase reactions, but two merit special emphasis here. In cerebral dispersions in absence of oxygen but with oxaloacetic acid, glutamic acid disappears and α-oxoglutaric acid and aspartic acid are formed:

$$\text{(iii)} \quad \begin{array}{cc} \text{HOOC.CH(NH}_2\text{)CH}_2\text{CH}_2\text{COOH} & \text{HOOC.CO.CH}_2\text{CH}_2.\text{COOH} \\ + & \rightleftharpoons \qquad + \\ \text{HOOC.CO.CH}_2.\text{COOH} & \text{HOOC.CH(NH}_2\text{)CH}_2\text{COOH} \end{array}$$

This transamination can proceed at the extremely high rate of 7,800 μmoles/hr. g. fresh tissue (Lowry *et al.*, 1956), which is of the order of magnitude of the most rapid reactions brought about by the brain. Among other tissues, only muscular ones are more active than the brain in this respect. The reaction proceeds at half-maximal velocity with 0·6 mM-α-oxoglutarate and 2·6 mM-aspartate and can thus operate rapidly in the normal brain. The aspartate-oxoglutarate aminotransferase concerned has been partly purified from human brain (Bonavita, 1959) and found specific to the substrates of reaction (iii). It requires pyridoxine derivatives (q.v.) as coenzymes, and probably as in other tissues includes the stages:

$$\text{(iv)} \quad \begin{array}{cc} \text{Glutamate +} & \text{α-Oxoglutarate +} \\ \text{pyridoxal phosphate-} \rightleftharpoons & \text{pyridoxamine phosphate-} \\ \text{aminotransferase} & \text{aminotransferase} \end{array}$$

and the corresponding reactions with oxaloacetate. The intermediate reaction (iv) can proceed at three times the rate of overall transamination, i.e. at over 15,000 μmoles/hr. g. tissue; this contributes to the rapid incorporation of ^{14}C from added glutamate or ketoacids among their many metabolic derivatives (Velick & Vavra, 1962; Haslam & Krebs, 1963; Simon *et al.*, 1967). Under some conditions with respiring cerebral preparations, conversion of glutamate to aspartate and CO_2 was nearly quantitative (Krebs & Bellamy, 1960) and evidence was given for its proceeding by the two ketoacids. In cerebral, but not in most other animal tissues, a route for the conversion also exists via γ-aminobutyrate and the transamination now to be described.

The second transaminase reaction to receive special emphasis is that yielding succinic semialdehyde from γ-aminobutyrate (Fig. 8.4; Bessman *et al.*, 1953). This reaction proceeds at about 40–90 μmoles/g. whole brain/hr. and appears to be the main route for removal of γ-aminobutyrate, which has notable actions on the electrical activity of several parts of the brain (Chapter 14). It is thus significant that the transaminase is most active in grey matter, especially from the lower parts of the brain which show rates up to 110 μmoles/g. hr., while white matter shows less activity (Baxter & Roberts, 1958; Salvador & Albers, 1959). After preliminary purification by acetone and ammonium sulphate, transaminase activity was enhanced by pyridoxal phosphate; half-maximal velocity was given with 3 mM-γ-aminobutyrate and 4 mM-α-oxoglutarate.

Other ketoacids examined did not react but transamination occurred with other aminobutyric acids and β-alanine. The transaminase apoenzyme has a higher affinity for pyridoxal phosphate than that of glutamate decarboxylase (Roberts *et al.*, 1958), which supports suggestions that the transaminase is less sensitive *in vivo* to convulsants of the hydrazide or semicarbazide groups (Horvath *et al.*, 1961; Killam & Bain, 1957). However hydroxylamine and aminooxyacetic acid were considered to act primarily on the transaminase, particularly *in vivo* (Baxter & Roberts, 1961). In human brain the highest activities of this transaminase (up to 200 μmoles/g. hr.) were recorded for basal ganglia, the hypothalamus, and the grey matter of both cerebral and cerebellar cortex (Sheridan *et al.*, 1967).

A similar regional distribution has been observed for *succinic semialdehyde dehydrogenase* (Miller & Pitts, 1967). This enzyme catalyses the NAD^+-linked conversion of the semialdehyde to succinyl coenzyme A and so completes the "γ-aminobutyrate shunt" (Fig. 8.4). The dehydrogenase is used as coupling enzyme in assay of the above transamination reaction (Pitts *et al.*, 1965) and has been purified 300-fold from rat brain mitochondria after extraction with detergent (Kammerat & Veldstra, 1968).

Respiration of cerebral tissues at 46 μmoles O_2/g. hr. was supported by γ-aminobutyrate in certain media, when without added substrate the rate was 21 μmoles/g. hr.: values corresponding to utilization of 6–12 μmoles γ-aminobutyrate/g. hr. Succinic semialdehyde afforded higher rates, suggesting the transamination to be a rate-limiting step; with mitochondria, both substrates gave P/O ratios of 2·7–2·9 (McKhann *et al.*, 1960). Routes involving transamination of γ-aminobutyric acid can thus make appreciable contribution to oxidative metabolism (Chapters 4 and 6).

Decarboxylation; Glutamate Decarboxylase

γ-Aminobutyrate originates from glutamic acid itself, by decarboxylation (Fig. 8.4). Table 8.1 shows cerebral tissues to contain about one-seventh of their total amino-nitrogen as γ-aminobutyric acid, and although it is much less prominent in non-neural tissues (Whelan *et al.*, 1969), among the free amino acids of the brain it is present in greater quantity than the total of eleven or more of the common amino acids such as valine, tyrosine or arginine. It was found largely uncombined and in considerable quantity in the brain of several vertebrates including man and the frog, but only in very much smaller quantities in several other organs or in blood or urine. The cerebral content of γ-aminobutyrate is associated with one of the highest [brain]/[blood] ratios among amino acids (Table 8.1). Most of the γ-aminobutyrate of the brain, while not combined in peptide form in protein, is nevertheless not in a freely-diffusible state. The form in which the acid is stored in or occluded at subcellular fractions and microsomes (Sano & Roberts, 1963) has not been established although Na^+ is known to be involved (Weinstein *et al.*, 1965; Strasberg & Elliott, 1967).

A significant proportion (over 10%) of the substrates metabolized in the Krebs tricarboxylic acid cycle may be metabolized via the "γ-aminobutyrate shunt" (Fig. 8.4)—the actual proportion may be determined by competition for NAD$^+$ (McKhann & Tower, 1961). The stoichiometric formation of γ-aminobutyrate from glutamic acid with evolution of 1 mole of carbon dioxide can be brought about by ground and acetone-dried cerebral tissues (Roberts & Fraenkel, 1950, 1951; Lowe *et al.*, 1958) yielding an average of 20–25 μmoles of γ-aminobutyrate/g. tissue/hr. Reaction rate was maximal with 25 mM glutamate, about the normal cerebral concentration, and like amino-acid decarboxylases from other sources the enzyme was sensitive to hydroxylamine and to semicarbazide. This is due to its requirement for a pyridoxal derivative, which can be demonstrated also by the lower level of decarboxylase activity found in pyridoxine-deficient rats. In cerebral preparations from deficient animals pyridoxal phosphate gave half-maximal activation at about 7×10^{-5} M at pH 6·2. The decarboxylase was at higher level in grey matter than in white, in the brain of several species including man (Müller & Langeman, 1962; Albers & Brady, 1959); highest rates were in the substantia nigra and colliculi, and of some 36 μmoles/g. hr. Under their respective assay conditions the transaminase (q.v.) which removes γ-aminobutyrate was in almost all cases of greater activity than the decarboxylase which forms it, by ratios of 1·4–50. This presumably contributes to the pattern of occurrence of γ-aminobutyrate which is discussed further in Chapter 14. Purified cerebral glutamate de-carboxylase exhibits competitive inhibition by anions, including Cl$^-$. The enzyme is enriched in the synaptosome fraction (q.v.) of rat and guinea pig cerebral cortex from which it is released by osmotic shock. Ca^{2+} is involved in its binding to synaptosomal membranes (Susz *et al.*, 1966; Fonnum, 1968).

Enzymes of the γ-aminobutyrate shunt (glutamate decarboxylase, γ-amino-butyrate transaminase and succinic semialdehyde dehydrogenase, q.v.) increase in parallel fashion in the developing brain: rat brain decarboxylase activity, 4·2 μmoles/g. hr. at birth, had increased to the adult level of 45 μmoles/g. hr. by 30 days of age (Sims & Pitts, 1970). The finding of trace amounts of γ-aminobutyrate in non-neural tissues was noted above; the decarboxylase which forms it is also present but exhibits different properties. Thus activation by pyridoxal phosphate and inhibition by Cl$^-$ and by amino-oxyacetic acid, properties which have been described for the cerebral enzyme, are not shared by the kidney enzyme. The different properties indicate that, in contrast to cerebral glutamate decarboxylase, the enzyme of non-neural tissues does not require pyridoxal phosphate (Haber *et al.*, 1970). The greater dependence of the brain enzyme on its coenzyme may be relevant to the greater sensitivity of the brain to those convulsive agents (q.v.) which act by interfering with binding of pyridoxal phosphate.

Activity of the decarboxylase has been increased by up to 70% in mouse brain *in vivo* after intraperitoneal injection of L-glutamate (1 g./kg. body weight). The enzymic activity reached its peak some 4 hr. after administration of sub-strate (Fig. 8.8). The possibility that presence of substrate had protected from inactivation was excluded and action of actinomycin D in diminishing the increase in glutamate decarboxylase activity provided evidence to support the conclusion that substrate induction of enzyme synthesis was the mechanism involved (Kraus, 1968).

Dependence of cerebral γ-aminobutyrate on glutamate decarboxylase has been concluded to be a major factor in the disturbances, featuring lethargy and terminating in convulsions, caused by exposing animals to oxygen at a few atmospheres' pressure (Wood & Watson, 1963, 1964). For the decarboxylase, but not the transaminase is sensitive to oxygen, being inhibited by 36% when measured in oxygen rather than in air. The decarboxylase was diminished in cerebral samples from mice exposed to higher oxygen pressures, and the brain of rats under these conditions contained 18–35% less γ-aminobutyrate than was found in control animals. Other amino-acids examined did not show comparable change, and the diminution in γ-aminobutyrate in a series of animals paralleled the severity of the convulsions they sustained. It is pictured

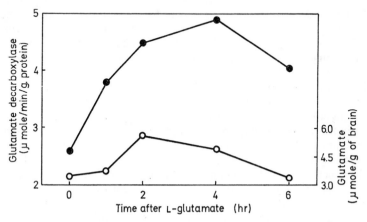

FIG. 8.8. Substrate induction of L-glutamate decarboxylase in mouse brain. L-Glutamate (o) was administered intraperitoneally. Activity of the decarboxylase (●) was measured using isotopically labelled substrate (Kraus, 1968).

that inhibition of functional activity by γ-aminobutyrate represents a protective mechanism and that when it is overwhelmed, convulsions ensue (Wood *et al.*, 1968). Other changes in γ-aminobutyrate metabolism in convulsive conditions are noted in Chapter 10.

Administration of Glutamic Acid

1. Topical. It is remarkable that glutamic acid which exists uncombined in the brain at some 10 μmoles/g., nevertheless has major effects when applied to the cortex in minute amounts. Administered iontophoretically close to cells in different parts of the cat cortex, approximately 10^{-14} mole of glutamic acid promptly accelerated the previous rate of cell discharge; the threshold concentration was calculated to be just over 0·1 mM (Curtis *et al.*, 1960; Krnjević & Phillis, 1963). Administration mechanically was comparably effective and by each route the acid was effective within 1 sec.; both the cerebral and cerebellar cortices of several mammalian species responded. With small additions of glutamate the increased firing continued for some 3–4 sec. only, stopped abruptly, and could be recommenced by a fresh addition. Sensitivity lay in the cell body or dendrites rather than axons; in the spinal cord, Renshaw cells and motoneurons could be excited. In isolated cerebral tissues, membrane potentials

measured intracellularly were promptly diminished by applied glutamate, for example from -60 to -37 mv (Gibson & McIlwain, 1965). Such depolarization gives a basis for increased excitability; in promptness and threshold to glutamate ($0\cdot2$ mM) it closely paralleled the phenomena *in situ*.

Acceleration of cell firing was caused by L- and not D-glutamate; glutamine and α-oxoglutarate were inactive but cysteic acid almost equalled glutamate in activity. The compound evidently acted as such rather than by metabolic conversion, and in spinal neurons inhibitors of a number of enzymes were without effect on the phenomenon. In particular, the reaction by which glutamic acid withdraws energy-rich phosphate, that is by glutamine synthesis, can be concluded to proceed too slowly to act as basis for the immediate depolarization, which occurs, rather, through Na^+-entry (see above; Gibson & McIlwain, 1965; Harvey & McIlwain, 1968). The excitatory actions of glutamate and congeners are in interesting contrast to inhibitory effects of γ-aminobutyrate and related compounds, and both are discussed in Chapter 14 in relation to their role in neurotransmission.

2. Intravenously or orally, glutamic acid has less direct action on the brain than might be expected, which displays well the effectiveness of the blood-brain barrier in this regard. The properties of glutamic acid make it understandable that attempts should have been made to influence mental phenomena by administering the acid. Given orally or intravenously, it or its salts have been found to increase blood pressure, pulse rate, and blood glucose: adrenergic effects probably mediated by the sympathetic nervous system (Weil-Malherbe, 1952; see Sourkes, 1962), and similar to effects of amphetamine (q.v.). These properties appear to have contributed to actions of glutamic acid in accelerating recovery from insulin hypoglycaemia, in ameliorating forms of *petit mal* epilepsy; and (with the accompanying increased alertness) in improving the performance of some mentally-retarded subjects. Glutamic acid is used on a large scale in food-manufacturing industries to improve flavour, palatability, and "acceptability" of several prepared foodstuffs (*Symposium*, 1948). In small quantities the partly neutralized acid has an attractive salty-meaty taste and in addition appears to be able to enhance the tastes of certain other foodstuffs. Its manufacture as a condiment conditioned its experimental use by making it readily available on a large scale, earlier than other amino acids. This availability has led also to glutamates occasionally being added to foods in excessive concentrations; in a minority of the population they may then induce sensory and vasomotor disturbances (Schaumburg *et al.*, 1969).

Cerebral Ammonia, Urea and Guanidines

These compounds and glutamic acid are linked metabolically and produce a number of interrelated cerebral effects.

Ammonia

Increased formation of ammonia has been known for some time to be associated with increased activity in muscle and in peripheral nerve, and has been found in the brain during convulsive activity (Richter & Dawson, 1948; Folbergrova *et al.*, 1969). Cerebral ammonia undergoes rapid changes with changed cerebral activity and is a constituent which can be determined only in tissue fixed rapidly by methods such as those described in Chapter 3. Its normal level in rat brain was found to be about 0·16 μmoles/g., which is one-sixtieth of the cerebral glutamic acid. One second after decapitation, the value had risen to 0·28 μmole/g. and it was also increased to a similar extent by one second's application of electrical impulses sufficient to lead to convulsions. Other convulsive agents had similar effects. Parallelism between levels of cerebral activity and NH_3 has been observed during sleep and the excitation and inhibition of conditioning (Vladimirova, 1964).

Ammonium salts themselves induce convulsions or coma and it has been suggested that liberation of ammonia may mediate in the actions of other convulsive agents. However, the convulsive dose of ammonium salts raises cerebral ammonia to 5 μmoles/g. Unless factors of specific localization are involved, such mediation is unlikely. For similar reasons critical mediation of ammonia in producing the symptoms of hepatic coma appears unlikely (Eiseman et al., 1959). On carotid infusion of dogs with solutions containing ammonia, the major change found in cerebral amino acids was an increase in glutamine. Also, in patients with liver disease in whom plasma NH_3 was elevated, the glutamine of the cerebrospinal fluid was markedly increased. Comparable increase in plasma glutamine did not occur, and the observations emphasize the role of glutamine synthesis (q.v.) in minimizing the accumulation of NH_3 in the brain. This interpretation is supported by experiments using cerebral and hepatic tissues from rats with CCl_4-induced damage to the liver (Barona et al., 1965). From experiments which showed that methionine sulphoximine diminished ammonia toxicity, the associated removal of adenosine triphosphate was concluded to be deleterious (Warren & Schenker, 1964).

The initial rate of formation of cerebral ammonia following application of convulsive agents is high: corresponding to some 450 μmoles/g. hr. This is, however, within the capacity of glutamic dehydrogenase (q.v.) and thus could reflect a sudden utilization of ketoacids and their reformation from glutamate; other reactions may also participate. Ammonia is formed by cerebral preparations from adenosine, guanine and guanosine at about 60 μmoles/g. hr., in reactions which in some cases require adenosine triphosphate (Muntz, 1953; Jordan et al., 1959; see also Chapter 9). Other points concerning the formation of ammonia by separated cerebral tissues in vitro are not fully understood, for the tissues can produce over 56 mg. of NH_3/100 g. (33 μmoles/g.) which is about the total amino acid nitrogen of the tissue (Table 8.1). Here proteins presumably contribute (Vrba et al., 1957). The removal of ammonia is an energy-consuming process; glutamine synthetase requires ATP and glutamate formation from α-oxoglutarate and NH_3, catalysed by glutamate dehydrogenase, utilizes NADH, thus limiting the amount of NADH available for ATP formation in oxidative phosphorylation.

Urea

The metabolism of urea cannot be invoked as a process associated with rapid cerebral change in ammonia, although urea isolated as its dixanthydryl derivative, has been found to be produced at the brain of the rat in vivo from

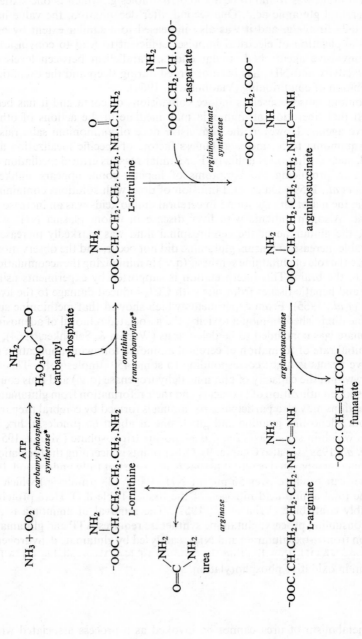

FIG. 8.9. The urea cycle. Individual stages, except those indicated by an asterisk (*), have been demonstrated to occur in the mammalian brain.

[14]C-labelled arginine (Dingman & Sporn, 1959; Sporn et al., 1959). Labelled urea is also formed in the brain in vivo when ^{14}C-labelled citrulline is the precursor (Kemp & Woodbury, 1965). There is thus good evidence that the pathway of urea synthesis from citrulline (Fig. 8.9) is present in the brain. Enzymic basis is given by the demonstration that cerebral tissues carry arginase and argininosuccinase activity (Tomlinson & Westall, 1960). The latter yields arginine and fumarate at 1–3 μmoles/g. tissue/hr., and the arginase yields urea at 7–12 μmoles/g. hr. However, the presence of the stages in Fig. 8.9 leading to citrulline has not been clearly established. Buniatian and Davtian (1966) were unable to demonstrate citrulline synthesis, but Kemp & Woodbury (1965) described conversion to arginine if highly purified 2-[^{14}C]-ornithine was used as precursor. Doubts that the complete pathway is present to any significant extent are supported by the difficulty in detecting in the brain two of the enzymes, carbamyl phosphate synthetase and ornithine trans-carbamylase, required for citrulline formation (see also Chapter 9).

The arginase of ox brain has been purified 70-fold; it was found to be of molecular weight 120,000, was activated by Mn^{2+} and inhibited by excess substrate, arginine. Half maximal velocity was obtained with 9 mM-arginine and the activity was competitively inhibited by ornithine and lysine (Gasiorowska et al., 1969).

While the presence of the complete urea cycle in the brain has not so far been confirmed, that part of the pathway known to be present, from citrulline to urea, is considered to be essential in detoxification mechanisms in the brain. The occurrence in the pathway of two genetic errors with which mental retardation is associated (argininosuccinic aciduria and citrullinaemia) lends support to this view (Kemp & Woodbury, 1965). These two conditions are discussed below.

Other Guanidines

Arginine will be noted from Table 8.1 as present in the brain at about 0·7 μmoles/g., similar to its level in blood plasma. In a systematic examination for simple mono-substituted guanidines normal to the brain (Blass, 1960) all those found were derived from amino acids, arginine preponderating. γ-Guanidobutyrate, 0·05, glycocyamine, 0·03 and taurocyamine, 0·03 μmoles/g. were also found. These concentrations are about 2–5% of those of the corresponding amino acids, which may result from the action of a transaminidase detected in cerebral dispersions (Pisano & Udenfriend, 1958).

γ-Guanidobutyrate is one of a number of related substances which, when applied at about 1 mM to the cortical surface, inhibits a particular type of electrical response to stimulation (Purpura et al., 1959). The action is given by several ω-amino acids and their guanido-derivatives, and also the guanido-derivatives of acids which do not themselves act; it is distinct from the effects produced by similar application of aspartic and glutamic acids.

Abnormal Amino Acid Metabolism and Cerebral Defect or Disorder

Abnormalities in the formation or functioning of the nervous system are prominent in inherited disorders of amino acid metabolism. Over 30 of such abnormalities have been described; Table 8.6 lists several in which cerebral abnormality is involved. Indeed a tabulation of the clinical signs and symptoms which are suggestive of inborn errors of amino acid metabolism commences with mental retardation, convulsions and ataxia and includes disorders of speech (Wolff, 1968; see also Eastham & Jancar, 1968). The causative abnormalities in amino acid metabolism usually involve alterations in enzymic activity in many organs of the body; they are thus examples of genetic or morphogenetic variation in the processes of protein synthesis and its control,

Table 8.6

Mental defect or disorder associated with abnormal metabolism of amino acids

Disease	Amino acid involved	Enzymic (or equivalent) defect	Chemicals augmented in urine
Arginino-succinic aciduria	Arginine	Argininosuccinase	Argininosuccinic acid
Citrullinaemia	Citrulline	Argininosuccinic acid synthetase[1]	Citrulline
Cystathionin-uria	Methionine	Cystathionase	Cystathionine[2]
Hartnup disease	Tryptophan	(Intestinal absorption)	Many amino acids and indoles
Histidinaemia	Histidine	Histidase	Histidine
Homocystinuria	Methionine	Cystathionine synthetase[3]	Homocystine
Hyperammon-aemia	Ornithine	Ornithine transcarbamylase	Ammonia
Maple syrup urine disease	Leucine Isoleucine Valine	Oxidative decarboxylation of corresponding branched chain α-oxo-acids	Branched chain α-oxo-acids and α-hydroxy acids
Phenylketon-uria	Phenylalanine	Phenylalanine hydroxylase	Phenylpyruvic acid; other metabolites

Other abnormalities are reviewed by Eastham & Jancar (1968) and Harris (1970).
[1] The synthetase exhibits modified kinetic properties. [2] Cystathionine accumulates in the brain also. [3] The synthetase is demonstrated to be defective in the brain.

processes which are described in more detail in Chapters 9 and 13. They may result from absence of an enzyme; alteration in kinetic properties of an enzyme (see for example, argininosuccinic aciduria); or deficient absorption of a dietary amino acid, as in Hartnup disease.

When the primary abnormality is extra-cerebral, the route by which the brain is affected usually involves the bloodstream: e.g. the 10- to 50-fold increase in the phenylalanine of the blood, which characterizes phenylketonuria. Much scope is then afforded for the chemical detection and treatment of the illnesses, which collectively form an important and not uncommon group of diseases. The evolution of treatment for many of the disorders has emphasized the critical value of accurate early diagnosis. The brain in infancy seems particularly sensitive to these conditions, which thus tend to be associated with mental retardation. A range of clinical diagnostic tests has been devised and their use for examining a high proportion of newborn infants is now routine in many communities. Legislation to make such screening compulsory has been introduced in some areas. Following early diagnosis, many of the diseases may be ameliorated by attention to dietary factors, as in phenylketonuria or galactosaemia. Here the environment is playing a part in the degree of expression of an aberrant genotype.

Argininosuccinic Aciduria

Argininosuccinic acid, an intermediate in the general metabolism of urea by the urea cycle, does not normally accumulate in appreciable amounts and its abundant excretion in the urine of subjects suffering a rare mental retardation or defect is thus noteworthy. The subjects' plasma and urinary urea were normal, and the concentration of argininosuccinic acid in their cerebrospinal fluid was greater than in their blood (Allan et al., 1958). The argininosuccinic acid excreted, 1–2 g./day, corresponds to about 1 μmole/hr. g. brain which is within the capacity of the cerebral enzymes discussed above. It is thus possible that the compound excreted originated from the brain and that urea metabolism elsewhere in the body was normal; the original patient was severely mentally retarded, showing convulsive episodes and an abnormal electroencephalogram. In studying a further family showing the defect, a defined chromosomal abnormality was found (Coryell et al., 1964). The relatives who were probably heterozygotes excreted appreciable amounts of argininosuccinic acid and feeding citrulline to a parent of a retarded child yielded the acid in greater amounts than from normal subjects. The condition of the retarded child was ameliorated by feeding a high-protein diet.

The enzymic defect is believed to be a deficiency of argininosuccinase, which catalyses the hydrolysis of argininosuccinic acid to form arginine and fumaric acid (Fig. 8.9). Although the enzymic activity has not been detected in the erythrocytes from patients it is considered unlikely that there is total absence of the enzyme because urea formation seems unimpaired. Tentative conclusions that the enzymic activity is substantially decreased rather than completely absent (Tomlinson & Westall, 1964; Moser et al., 1967) were supported by the observation that liver argininosuccinase levels, in autopsy samples from patients who died from the disease, were only 3% of normal. This abnormally low activity is sufficient to support normal rates of urea formation if the load is assumed to be evenly spread throughout the day. The load is not thus spread however, so that at times argininosuccinate presumably accumulates. Moreover, even though the argininosuccinase present might be adequate for urea formation, it may nevertheless be insufficient to provide for normal arginine production. Thus either argininosuccinic acid accumulation or arginine deficiency may cause the neural abnormality (Miller & McLean, 1967).

Citrullinaemia

Very few cases of this disease have been observed; the condition is also associated with mental retardation (McMurray *et al.*, 1962). Absence of the enzyme involved in citrulline removal, argininosuccinate synthetase, has not been demonstrated, but the enzyme in cultured fibroblasts grown from a citrullinaemic patient exhibited modified kinetic properties; the K_m was 25 times higher than in fibroblasts from controls (Tedesco & Mellman, 1967). It is of great interest that the enzyme in a genetic error of metabolism may be defective by virtue of modified kinetic properties rather than, as occurs more commonly, absence of enzymic activity—in such cases, routine enzyme determinations (normally performed at saturating concentrations of substrate) would be unlikely to detect the defect.

Phenylalanine and Phenylketonuria

It is encouraging that the chemical understanding of phenylketonuria has given simple diagnostic procedures and rational therapeutic measures described in an attractive *Symposium* (1963) and *Report* (1963). The illness is an important example of an inherited metabolic disorder, of which further instances are given in this chapter and in Chapters 10 and 11. Such conditions are discussed as part of the subject of biochemical genetics by Harris (1959), Hsia (1959) and Stanbury *et al.* (1966). The general metabolism of phenylalanine and tyrosine in relation to phenylketonuria and to other metabolic abnormalities is reviewed by Woolf (1963, 1968) and by Crome & Stern (1967).

Phenylpyruvic Acid

One approach to the study of mental disease has been to search for unusual substances in body fluids of the mentally ill. Such a search was successful in the case of about 0·5% of mental defectives. Their urine on addition of ferric chloride, gave a dark green colour found by Fölling (1934) to be due to the excretion of phenylpyruvic acid. Negligible quantities of this substance are excreted by normal individuals but the abnormal group, termed phenylketonurics or phenylpyruvic oligophrenics, excreted 0·7–2·8 g./day. Following the chemical recognition of this group of defectives, it was realized that they possessed other diagnostic characteristics including some motor disturbances, a particular stance, and light coloration of skin, hair and eyes. The condition is inherited in a fashion suggesting it to be associated with a single recessive gene with respect to which the defectives are homozygotic (Penrose, 1935); such individuals form about 1/40,000 of the population, the proportion possibly varying in different populations. Parents of the defectives, presumably with one recessive gene and constituting 1/100 of the population, showed little or no abnormality in phenylpyruvic acid.

With a substance excreted continuously in the quantities observed to be the case with phenylpyruvic acid, an origin from a dietary constituent was naturally investigated. That such is its origin is shown in the experiment of Fig. 8.10. Fasting diminished the quantity of phenylpyruvic acid excreted. Of dietary components, protein was implicated; excretion remained low on a protein-free diet but greatly increased with a high-protein diet. Of protein constituents available in the necessary quantities, phenylalanine is on structural grounds the most likely source of phenylpyruvic acid, and indeed feeding phenylalanine itself led to large excretion of the acid. Tyrosine, less likely as source of phenyl-pyruvic acid, had no comparable effect. The quantity of phenylpyruvic acid

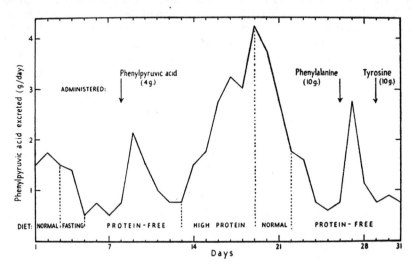

FIG. 8.10. Excretion of phenylpyruvic acid in a phenylketonuric fed various diets (data from Jervis, 1937).

normally excreted by the oligophrenics approximates to the daily intake of phenylalanine, 1·9 g., which has been found necessary to maintain nitrogen balance in normal subjects (Eckhardt *et al.*, 1948).

Phenylalanine and the Heterozygotes

Phenylalanine is indeed found at unusually high level in the blood of phenylketonurics, being between 15 and 60 mg./100 ml. plasma in place of a normal 1 mg./100 ml.; levels in cerebrospinal fluid were also much increased. With the development of methods for determining phenylalanine (see below) it has been found possible to detect a related abnormality in the parents of the defectives, presumably heterozygous for the abnormal gene. The parents differ little from normal subjects in phenylalanine level under normal conditions, but after taking a dose of phenylalanine their blood levels were for some hours about double those of normal subjects (Fig. 8.11).

In normal individuals dietary phenylalanine produces a negligible quantity of urinary phenylpyruvic acid; so also does feeding additional phenylalanine, though phenylalanine fed in large quantities to rhesus monkeys and rats can cause phenylketonuria. The phenylketonurics do not indeed possess an additional ability to convert the amino to the ketoacid. Such conversion is a normal process in the catabolism of many amino acids, although it is not normally the major route in the case of phenylalanine. A normal route (Fig. 8.12) is the introduction of a *p*-hydroxyl group by enzymes of the liver (Udenfriend & Cooper, 1952) to form a substance such as tyrosine capable of giving a Millon reaction (a red coloration with a mercuric salt and a nitrite in acid solution). The critical difference in the ketonurics is their inability to form such a *p*-hydroxy compound, as is well shown by Fig. 8.13. Tyrosine itself, fed to the oligophrenics, is dealt with in the normal manner. Their inability extends to the oxidation not only of phenylalanine but also of phenylpyruvic acid itself, which normal individuals convert to the phenol. The phenylpyruvics can, however, introduce a *p*-hydroxyl group to the more reactive aromatic nucleus of acetylsalicyclic acid, forming gentisic acid (Roseman & Dorfman, 1951). The liver is normally a major site of phenylalanine hydroxylation, the process

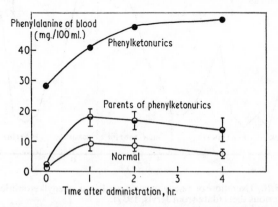

FIG. 8.11. Diminished phenylalanine tolerance in phenylketonurics and their parents (Hsia, 1959); 0·1 g. phenylalanine/kg. was fed to each group.

involving cyclic reduction and oxidation of a pteridine coenzyme and two enzyme systems. By examining biopsy specimens from the liver of phenylketonurics, they were shown to lack one of the essential enzymes, namely that which reacted with phenylalanine and the reduced pteridine (Mitoma *et al.*, 1957; Kaufman, 1963). Any residual hydroxylase activity may be decreased even further by substrate inhibition; purified rat liver phenylalanine hydroxylase may be inhibited by excess phenylalanine depending on the nature of the pteridine cofactor. The inhibition can be observed when the normal cofactor, tetrahydrobiopterin, is present but not if it is replaced by 6,7-dimethyl tetrahydropterin. Use of the dimethyl derivative in therapy has been suggested with a view to allowing maximum expression of residual hydroxylase activity (Kaufman, 1970).

Treatment and its Laboratory Control

1. Initial detection methods are still based on the simple reaction with ferric chloride, conveniently incorporated with buffers in test-papers which turn green on contact with a drop of phenylpyruvate-containing urine. Many

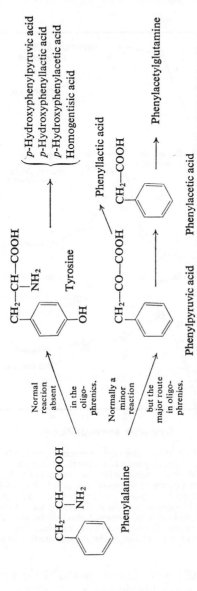

Fig. 8.12. Some metabolites from phenylalanine. For further details, see Woolf (1963), Sourkes (1962) and Chapter 14.

millions of such tests have been carried out in the course of a year or two's screening which identified about 100 cases. Phenylpyruvate can usually be first detected 2–3 weeks after birth, but occasionally only after 6 weeks. Testing at 3 weeks, 6 weeks, or both is thus recommended in order that treatment can begin promptly. Suspected phenylketonuria so detected is confirmed

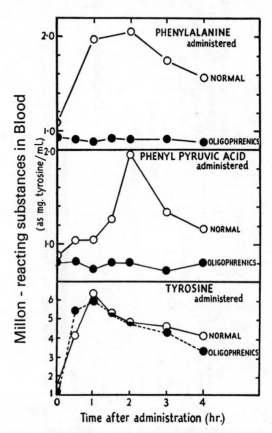

Fig. 8.13. Lack of ability on the part of phenylpyruvic oligophrenics to introduce a phenolic group to aromatic acids (data from Jervis, 1947). The oxidation is measured by the quantity of Millon-reacting substances given by the ordinates of each graph. Phenylalanine and phenylpyruvic acid in normal subjects both give rise to such substances in the bloodstream while in the oligophrenics they do not. The two groups of subjects, however, react similarly to the administration of tyrosine, the product from phenylalanine, so that they do not differ in their disposal of the substance after its formation.

by quantitative determination of phenylpyruvate. The test-papers often suffer the disadvantage of giving positive diagnosis only after the age of 3–4 weeks (see for example, Scott, 1966). Efforts to devise improved screening have been based on analysis of blood samples for phenylalanine and phenylpyruvic acid; a variety of spectrophotometric and spectrophotofluorometric methods have been developed. These have proved of value in confirmation of diagnosis but are expensive and complex for routine screening in many communities. A rapid, cheap and simple method, the "Guthrie test", is based on reversal by phenylalanine and phenylpyruvic acid of thienylalanine inhibition of bacterial growth (Guthrie & Susa, 1963). Blood is obtained by heel puncture and positive diagnosis is possible within the first week of life. The majority of States in the U.S.A. have introduced legislation which makes mass screening mandatory; many of these recommend the Guthrie test. An example is the legislation passed by the State of Ohio, which recommends that blood levels of phenylalanine above 6 mg/100 ml. from the Guthrie test be regarded as positive and that levels between 4 and 6 mg./100 ml. indicate further testing (see Legislation, 1966).

2. Treatment is dietary, by limiting the intake of phenylalanine. This itself is a dietary essential, and it is recommended that an infant first receive about 25 mg. of phenylalanine/kg. body wt./day, increasing or decreasing this quantity according to the concentration of phenylalanine found in the blood (see below); stabilization at an intake of 10–30 mg./day is usually required. Diets require planning in order to provide adequate protein or amino acids while minimizing phenylalanine, and usually need the incorporation of manufactured protein hydrolysates from which most phenylalanine has been removed by adsorption on charcoal. This removes certain other dietary essentials and accordingly the preparations contain added tryptophan, tyrosine, methionine and vitamins. Diets are designed to give as much phenylalanine as permitted from natural foods which contain little of it (listed in *Symposium*, 1963 and Report, 1963) while ensuring adequate amino acid intake from a minimum of the manufactured hydrolysate, which is the least palatable and most expensive item. Many ordinary sources of carbohydrate and fat can then give adequate calories with little phenylalanine.

3. When first establishing the diet it is recommended that blood levels of phenylalanine be determined twice weekly, and subsequently at weekly or monthly intervals. An enzymic method (LaDu & Michael, 1960; *Report*, 1963) uses an ultrafiltrate of the plasma from about 1 ml. of blood. Specimens are treated with a reagent which includes an amino acid oxidase yielding phenylpyruvic acid from phenylalanine; hydrogen peroxide formed concomitantly is decomposed by catalase. The phenylpyruvate forms in presence of arsenate and borate a complex, absorbing at 308 mμ, by which its amount is obtained. Tyrosine also reacts but absorbs differently; 0·4 μg of phenylalanine can be determined. A sensitive fluorometric method for plasma phenylalanine has developed by McCamen & Robins (1962); see also Woolf & Goodwin (1964) and Hsia *et al.* (1964).

Deficiency in phenylalanine during treatment has contributed to severe illnesses with skin disorders and failure to gain weight. Blood normally contains 0·93 ± 0·21 mg. phenylalanine/100 ml., and in phenylketonuria this may rise to 30 mg./100 ml. A level of 1–4 mg. phenylalanine/100 ml. blood is suggested as desirable in treatment.

4. Treated phenylketonurics have not yet lived a full life-span, and treatment has not always begun promptly or had satisfactory control. It is, however, concluded that almost normal development can be expected when adequate

dietary treatment is begun in the first few months of life (*Symposium*, 1963). Commenced after 6 months of age, the diet does not repair mental defects, but some development or stabilization can be expected. It is uncertain, at present, when the diet may be discontinued; but its retention up to the age of 4–10 years has been recommended. This variation in duration of treatment may be due to the occurrence of distinct groups of phenylketonurics, in view of a recent study on the frequency distribution of intelligence in children suffering from the disorder (Fuller & Shuman, 1969). The occurrence of three groups was observed which could provide an explanation for the lack of consistency experienced in assessment of the age at which dietary treatment may be discontinued.

Phenylalanine and the Brain

The therapeutic success achieved by limiting phenylalanine intake confirms phenylketonuria as an intoxication by phenylalanine. It is not a deficiency in tyrosine, a major normal product of the enzyme which is lacking in the phenylpyruvics. This enzyme is relatively specific to phenylalanine, but adequate tyrosine normally comes from dietary sources. Phenylalanine has been examined further as a toxic agent by feeding it to infant monkeys until their blood level was raised to 40–50 mg./100 ml. and they excreted up to 0·5 g. of phenylpyruvic acid/day (Waisman, *Symposium*, 1963); they then showed defects in a number of tests of discrimination and learning. It remains possible that a metabolite of phenylalanine is a more immediate toxic agent. Many metabolites including those of Fig. 8.12 have been appraised, but none has exhibited sufficiently pronounced toxic properties (Armstrong, *Symposium*, 1963). However, a metabolite formed *in vivo* from interaction of phenylalanine and pyridoxine does exhibit neurotoxic properties. Administration of ^{14}C-labelled phenylalanine with ^{3}H-labelled pyridoxine to rats resulted in the formation of doubly-labelled pyridoxylidene-β-phenylethylamine (2-methyl,3-hydroxy,5-hydroxymethyl,4-pyridylmethylene-β-phenylethylamine). The synthetic metabolite produced neurotoxic symptoms when injected into rats (Loo, 1967). Interference with pyridoxine metabolism in experimental phenylketonuria was also suggested from the effects of diets, containing large amounts of the vitamin and of phenylalanine, on the ability of rats to learn a swimming maze test (Loo & Ritman, 1967). It should be noted that doubts have been expressed as to the identity between experimentally-induced phenylketonuria in animals and the natural disorder in children (Perry *et al.*, 1965; Polidora, 1967).

Granting that phenylalanine or its metabolites act in such ways, the systems on which they act remain to be identified. Relevant at this point is the recognition of phenylpyruvic acid and its *p*-hydroxy derivative as normal cerebral constituents (Haavaldsen, 1964). Phenylpyruvic acid may specifically interfere with mitochondrial respiration in the immature brain: at 2 mM it gave 50% inhibition of oxygen consumption by the mitochondria when pyruvate was the oxidizable substrate but not when glutamate or succinate replaced pyruvate. The inhibition did not uncouple oxidative phosphorylation; P/O ratios of 2·8 were observed (Gallagher, 1969). Phenylpyruvic acid competitively inhibits human and rat brain hexokinase with $K_i = 2$–7 mM; phenylalanine itself inhibits the pyruvate kinase present with $K_i = 8$–11 mM (Weber *et al.*, 1970). Although the K_i values are of the same order of magnitude as the plasma concentrations of the metabolites in phenylketonurics, it remains to be seen if inhibition *in vivo* occurs to an extent relevant to the cerebral malfunction in the diseased state.

A defined structural defect in the brain of the phenylketonurics has not been found, though different types of lesions have been reported in different cases. Competitive relationships in which one amino acid inhibits the transport or metabolism of another, are on the other hand well established and can lead to inhibition of cell growth. Thus incomplete myelination in the central nervous system of phenylketonurics has often been described (Alvord *et al.*, 1950; Crome, Tymms & Woolf, 1962; Menkes, 1968). High circulating concentrations of phenylalanine decrease amino acid uptake to the brain and inhibit incorporation of amino acids into cerebral proteins. The effects are more marked in immature than in adult brain; in the immature brain, the greatest inhibition of amino acid incorporation was into myelin proteins (Agrawal *et al.*, 1970; see also Chapter 9). Phenylalanine has been concluded to inhibit the formation of noradrenaline and adrenaline, which were found in the blood of phenylpyruvics at about half their normal values; disturbances in 5-hydroxy-tryptamine have also been reported (*Symposium*, 1963). It is significant, in connection with adrenaline, that some phenylpyruvics suffer from *petit mal* epilepsy and are improved by amphetamine. These data are at present suggestive only, and it remains possible that further understanding of intermediation in phenylketonuria could lead to alternative treatment of the disease.

Amino Acids and Other Illnesses

The examples of inherited metabolic disease already described, arginosuccinic aciduria and phenylketonuria, offer significantly different examples of connection between amino acid abnormality and mental defect. In the first relatively rare condition, the metabolic defect appears to be in the brain itself. In phenylketonuria, a commoner condition in which the brain is affected secondarily, dietary manipulation has been successful in treatment and it is evident that this approach to therapy is more widely applicable. Thus in *maple-syrup urine disease*, again a very rare condition accompanied by mental defect, a few cases have sufficed to identify the curious urinary odour as associated with keto-acids derived from branched-chain amino acids (Mackenzie & Woolf, 1959). A dietary regimen providing minimal quantities of valine, leucine and isoleucine has taken one infant so maintained, through the stage when gross mental retardation has been exhibited in the few untreated cases examined (Westall, *Symposium*, 1964). Among the metabolites produced in the disease, α-oxoisocaproic acid shows specific inhibitory properties which may be relevant to it as a potential toxic agent. At 1 mM, the keto acid inhibited purified pyruvate decarboxylase (Dreyfus & Prensky, 1967) and at concentrations of 1–2 mM, it caused marked inhibition of myelination in myelinating tissue cultures of the cerebellum. The branched chain amino acids and other relevant keto acids had no effect (Silberberg, 1969). The concentrations of α-oxoisocaproic acid used in these studies are similar to the plasma concentration of 0·8 mM observed in patients suffering from the disorder.

Leucine features also in instances of *familial hypoglycaemia* precipitated by dietary proteins, in which electroencephalographic abnormalities and convulsive episodes are induced on eating diets rich in certain proteins. These caused the already low blood sugar of 2·2 to 3·3 mM to fall markedly, a change given also by leucine but not by some other amino acids (Cochrane *et al.*, 1956; Woolf, 1960). The effect of leucine in such patients could be simulated by isoleucine and α-oxoisocaproic acid, and was associated with an increase in the insulin-like substances of their blood plasma; normal subjects could also be sensitized to leucine by the sulphonyl ureas which induce hypoglycaemia (Grumbach & Kaplan, 1960; Fajans *et al.*, 1963).

Cystathionine, normally present in human brain in concentrations of 100 to 255 μmoles/g., is absent in *homocystinuria*. This inherited metabolic disease is of particular interest because of the clear location of the enzyme defect in the brain as well as in other tissues. The defect responsible is absence of cystathionine synthase (Fig. 8.3), resulting in increased excretion of homocystine and also of methionine; defective binding of the coenzyme, pyridoxine, may be involved (Finkelstein *et al.*, 1964; Gerritsen & Waisman, 1964; Rodnight, 1968; Cusworth & Dent, 1969). A further defect in methionine metabolism is *cystathioninuria*, in which cystathionine is excreted in the urine and has been detected in abnormally high amount in a post mortem sample of the brain of one subject. An enzymic defect has not been described in the diseased brain but deficiency of liver cystathionase supports earlier suggestions that the metabolic block occurs at the stage of cleavage of cystathionine to form cysteine and homoserine. The enzyme is also pyridoxine-requiring; the accumulation of cystathionine in the brain in vitamin B_6 deficiency, and the observation that the lowered enzymic activity in liver biopsy specimens could be partially restored by addition of the coenzyme, have served to indicate that the defect may be inability of the enzyme to bind its coenzyme (Brenton *et al.*, 1965; Berlow, 1967; Rodnight, 1968).

A different type of defective metabolism of sulphur amino acids has been indicated in an infant with increased urinary homocystine, cystathionine and methylmalonic acid. The brain content of cystathionine was also elevated but there was no change in activity of cystathionine synthase or cystathionase, in contrast to the above enzymic defects observed in homocystinuria and cystathioninuria. An abnormally low level of methionine in the diseased brain suggested the defect to be in methylation of homocysteine to form methionine. Post mortem samples of liver and kidney showed decreased activity of a specific methyl-transferase which transfers a methyl-group from methyl-tetrahydro-folate to homocysteine. The elevated urinary methylmalonate was suggested to arise from decreased *methylmalonyl-CoA-transferase* activity. Both of these transferases are vitamin B_{12}-requiring enzymes; the findings were therefore indicative of a defect in vitamin B_{12} metabolism. The investigators proposed the underlying defect to be an inability to accumulate coenzymically-active derivatives of the vitamin (Mudd *et al.*, 1969).

Histidinaemia provides another example of an inherited neurological disorder in which an enzymic defect has been demonstrated in non-neural tissues.

The disease is characterised by accumulation of histidine in the body fluids; blood levels of more than 20 mg./100 ml. have been reported. The enzyme, histidase, which normally converts histidine to urocanic acid, has been shown to be completely absent from the skin in some but not all cases; patients with normal skin histidase are suspected of having defective liver histidase (Crawhall, 1965; Crome & Stern, 1967; Woody *et al.*, 1965; Woolf, 1968).

The defects of amino acid metabolism described above involve deficiency in catabolism or anabolism of amino acid molecules. Defects may occur also in incorporation of individual amino acids into protein. One such example is possibly given by *hyperlysinaemia*, a rare disorder characterized by accumulation of lysine in the body fluids. Metabolic degradation of the essential amino acid in the patients was concluded to be normal, reabsorption of lysine was not significantly impaired; it has tentatively been suggested that the defect is a partial impairment of lysine incorporation into protein (Woody, 1964; Ghadimi *et al.*, 1965, 1966; Crawhall, 1965).

The importance of amino acids and the sensitivity of the central nervous system lead to many other instances of altered mental functioning in association with disturbances in amino acids: when, for example, their renal threshold changes. Examples of such conditions are noted briefly below; fuller accounts are available in texts on chemical pathology. Biochemical investigation of body fluids in these and other mental illness is discussed from a laboratory view-point by McIlwain & Rodnight (1962); see also Folch (1961), Sourkes (1962), Stanbury *et al.* (1966), Carson *et al.* (1963), Cumings & Kremer (1965) and Wolff (1968).

Wilson's Disease

Wilson's disease, or hepato-lenticular degeneration, is a hereditary condition showing a group of metabolic and pathological changes involving the liver, kidney and central nervous system (Wilson, 1947; *Symposium*, 1961). It usually develops in late childhood or early adult life. The disease was first characterized by hepatic changes in association with degeneration in parts of the brain especially in the lenticular bodies, with disturbances of movement and progressive intellectual deterioration. More recently two groups of metabolic characteristics have been added to the syndrome. They concern copper salts and amino acids.

Fig. 8.14 illustrates the abnormality in amino acid excretion. The cases examined included ones in which the first signs were in movement, speech, and change of expression and which were initially thought to be schizophrenic. Later there developed tremors, euphoria, salivation and difficulty in swallowing though other reflexes were normal. In other cases liver changes were more prominent and were recognized first, though clear changes were not seen on liver biopsy. The abnormalities in amino acid metabolism were in their urinary excretion, which averaged two and a half times the normal level. The level of plasma amino acids was not sufficiently raised to explain the greater excretion, which was due to a specific defect in the renal tubules. The amino acids lost were not exclusively of one type, though some were more affected than others. In one case the excretion of threonine was twelve times its normal value, while that of isoleucine was doubled. Excretion of peptides has also been found to be abnormal but glycosuria occurred in a few cases only. The abnormalities in amino acids in these instances of Wilson's disease were much more extensive than those occurring with severe liver damage, for instance in alcoholic cirrhosis of the liver.

Abnormalities of copper metabolism in Wilson's disease, reported earlier, were clearly shown to be related to the disorder by Cumings (1948, 1951). The copper content of the liver and several parts of the brain, especially the basal ganglia, was found unusually high. A normal cerebral copper content of 0·07–0·1 μmoles/g. was increased seven- or eight-fold; that of the serum was unusually low while urinary levels were high. It is probable that the basic

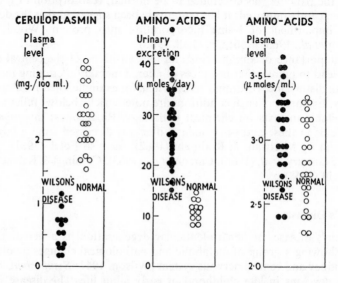

FIG. 8.14. Ceruloplasmin and amino-aciduria in Wilson's disease (Scheinberg, 1956; Cooper *et al.*, 1950; see Uzman & Hood, 1952; Cumings, 1959). Each point represents one subject.

defect in Wilson's disease is in the metabolism of copper (Scheinberg, 1956; *Symposium*, 1961). Blood plasma normally contains about 1 μg. of copper/ml., almost entirely in the form of ceruloplasmin, a specific copper-protein which has been highly purified from normal human plasma and contains eight atoms of the Cu in a protein of mol. wt. 160,000 (Kasper & Deutsch, 1963). In Wilson's disease the metabolism of ceruloplasmin is abnormal: its blood level is decreased to less than half its normal value (Fig. 8.14) and more copper occurs in a free form or combined more loosely with the major plasma proteins. This presumably allows a greater mobility of copper in the body, reflected in its then being found at unusually high levels in the urine, spinal fluid and tissues including the margin of the cornea (where pigment is visible), the brain, liver and kidney. In addition to the abnormally heavy deposition of copper observed in liver biopsy specimens, the copper in the diseased brain was found by chromatographic separation to be spread over many protein fractions. This indicated that the Cu was bound to proteins which, in the normal brain, are Cu-free (Porter, 1964). Other manifestations of the disease can be pictured to result from the deposition of copper in the tissues. Cellular changes have been reported in the brain and copper–amino acid complexes have been considered to interfere with tubular resorption of amino acids. Intraventricular injection to normal cats of 50 μg. of Cu as an albumin complex caused paralysis, and after survival of a few days marked degenerative changes were found in neural tissue adjacent to the cerebrospinal fluid (Vogel & Evans, 1961). Moreover, the bodily distribution of a small test-injection of $^{64}Cu^{2+}$ has been successfully used as an aid in diagnosis. In normal subjects at an appropriate time the liver region showed twice the radioactivity found at the thigh, while in patients suffering Wilson's disease the corresponding ratio was 0·8 (Osborn & Walshe, 1964).

Normal diets provide an excess of Cu, which is however excreted in the faeces. Ceruloplasmin may play a part in Cu transport between the organs of the body, but its administration has not proved of value in Wilson's disease. Knowing that 2:3-dimercaptopropanol (BAL: Chapter 6) was valuable in some heavy metal intoxications and could affect bodily copper (Mandelbrote et al., 1948), it was administered to subjects with the disorder. Repeated subcutaneous injection of about 200 mg. of the mercaptopropanol in some cases transitorily increased both blood and urinary copper and led to some clinical improvement. Further success has been achieved with the thiol complexing-agent D-penicillamine or ββ-dimethylcysteine, which appears to render more bodily Cu available for excretion at the kidney (Walshe, 1964; Symposium, 1961). With minimal Cu intake and administration of 0·3–1 g. D-penicillamine/day, continuously apart from interruptions for administration of mineral supplements, several patients have shown marked improvement. Their plasma Cu diminished, and urinary Cu increased. Urinary excretion data collected for over 1 year indicated that the effectiveness of penicillamine decreased gradually so that larger doses were required to maintain a negative Cu balance (Tu et al., 1965).

It may be noted that diets deficient in copper cause farm animals, notably sheep to suffer neurological disorders including ataxia, with cerebral demyelination. Examination of the brain stem and spinal cord of sheep in this condition, termed swayback, showed low copper content and lipid abnormalities (Howell et al., 1964). Ceruloplasmin catalyses the oxidation of p-phenylenediamines, and has received wider investigation in pathological conditions; claims for specific relationship to schizophrenia proved unfounded (see Kety, 1959).

Galactosemia

In infants inheriting this condition, death or severe mental retardation with other abnormalities results from feeding an ordinary milk diet (see Woolf, 1962). The illness is clearly an intoxication with galactose from the lactose of the milk, and is resolved by milk-free diets. With ordinary diets, however, galactose and amino acids appear in the urine and galactose 1-phosphate accumulates in several tissues including those of the brain, sufficiently to disturb their functioning. The metabolic defect concerns the conversion of galactose to glucose phosphates which is a normal preliminary to catabolism of galactose. In particular, the system exchanging monosaccharides between galactose 1-phosphate and uridine diphosphate glucose is lacking (UTP: α-D-galactose-1-phosphate uridyltransferase; Schwartz, Goldberg et al., 1956, 1958; Kalckar et al., 1956; Robinson, 1963). Genetic studies suggest the condition to be caused by a single autosomal gene, occurring in 0·7% of the population, for which the galactosemics (incidence: 1/70,000 births) are homozygous.

Galactitol (a polyol derived from galactose) has been detected in the brains of infants who died from galactosemia in the first month of life. The alcohol was separated by gas-liquid chromatography and was estimated to be present at a concentration of 12·9 μmoles/g. fresh tissue. No galactitol was detected in the brain of a child of the same age whose death was unrelated to galactosemia (Wells et al., 1965). Accumulation of galactitol also occurs in a rare disorder involving deficiency of galactokinase. The disease is manifested by recurrent formation of cataracts, thought to be due to the accumulation of galactitol (Gitzelmann, 1968).

In detecting galactosemia, the presence of reducing substances in urine gives initial indication, and prompt confirmation can be obtained by paper-chromatography of whether the urine contains galactose. Assay for the transferase itself can also be made by incubating washed erythrocytes, haemolysed, with uridine diphosphate glucose and galactose-1-phosphate. Determination of the residual UDPG shows none to have been consumed by the samples from galactosemics, whereas a normal utilization is 4·5–5·7 μmoles/ml. erythrocytes/hr. This assay detects also the heterozygous carriers of galactosemia, who show values of 2–2·5 μmoles/ml. hr. Dietary control should be imposed promptly and can be appraised by determining the galactose-1-phosphate content of erythrocyte samples; in untreated cases 0·5–1·5 μmoles are found/ml. erythrocytes and choice of diets which give <0·2 μmoles/ml. are recommended (Woolf, 1962; Symposium, 1964). These usually contain only a few mg. of lactose in place of the 30 g. or more of a milk diet; dietary galactolipids are tolerated and do not appear to yield galactose.

Accumulation of galactose-1-phosphate, which inhibits several enzymes concerned with glucose phosphates, appears to mediate most of the symptoms in galactosemia and also in analogous toxic conditions induced in animals by feeding excessive galactose (see Nordin & Hansen, 1963); these conditions include cataracts and epileptiform seizures.

Hartnup Disease

This hereditary condition has brought children and young adults to mental and general hospitals with psychoses and neurological disorders (Baron et al., 1956; Hersov, 1955; Rodnight & McIlwain, 1955; Jepson, 1966). The biochemical defects concern a group of amino acids in which tryptophan is prominent, and result in the appearance in the urine of neutral and aromatic amino acids (some 7 g./day) and indole metabolites: these give the disease its chemical characterization. Excretion of indole metabolites is variable; they include indole-3-acetic acid and indican, and up to 300 mg. of indican can be excreted/day. The condition may have contributed to the association, frequently reported around 1900, between indicanuria and mental disease. For one aspect of the importance of the indole metabolites is that they represent a diversion of tryptophan from a normal route of metabolism leading to nicotinic acid (Chapter 10). Sufferers from Hartnup disease are thus unusually sensitive to lack of dietary nicotinic acid, and several have presented as pellagrins, including a proportion in whom psychotic symptoms were prominent. Others have shown a cerebellar defect, changes in movement and gait not typical of pellagra and conceivably related to other aspects of the amino-aciduria.

The metabolic peculiarities of Hartnup disease were accentuated by administering a test dose of tryptophan, e.g. of 70 mg./kg. Some of this was recovered from faeces, a phenomenon not found in normal subjects. Together with the amino-aciduria, this suggested a defect in transport of amino acids, of which tryptophan is prominent (Milne *et al.*, 1960; Hersov & Rodnight, 1960). Following the test dose, certain metabolites normally produced from tryptophan diminished: kynurenine was formed in only one-quarter the normal amount. Others increased, including indican, indolylacetic acid and its glutamine derivative. These were such as could be dependent on tryptophan breakdown in the intestine by microbial action. Many of the metabolic concomitants of the disorder can thus be secondary to deranged transport; this applies also to the deficiency in nicotinamide which is derived from tryptophan through kynurenine. Thus the condition interestingly links the symptoms of amino acid deficiency referred to at the beginning of this chapter, with those of the avitaminoses which are the subject of the chapter which follows; tryptophan metabolites are further described in Chapter 14.

REFERENCES

AELONY, Y., LOGOTHETIS, J., BART, B., MORRELL, F. & BOVIS, M. (1962). *Exp. Neurol.* 5, 525.
AGRAWAL, H. C., BONE, A. H. & DAVISON, A. N. (1970). *Biochem. J.* 117, 325.
ALBERS, R. W. & BRADY, R. O. (1959). *J. biol. Chem.* 234, 926.
ALBERS, R. W., KOVAL, G. J. & JAKOBY, W. B. (1962). *Exper. Neurol.* 6, 85.
ALLAN, J. D., CUSWORTH, D. C., DENT, E. C. & WILSON, K. V. (1958). *Lancet*, i, 182.
ALTSCHULE, M. (1957). *Arch. int. Med.* 99, 22.
ALVORD, E. C., STEVENSON, L. D., VOGEL, F. S. & ENGLE, R. L. (1950). *J. Neuropath. exp. Neurol.* 9, 298.
ANSELL, G. B. & RICHTER, D. (1954). *Biochem. J.* 57, 70.
AUDITORE, J. V., OLSON, E. J. & WADE, L. (1966). *Arch. Biochem. Biophys.* 114, 452.
BALDESSARINI, R. J. & KOPIN, I. J. (1966). *J. Neurochem.* 13, 769.
BARON, D. N., DENT, C. E., HARRIS, H., HART, E. W. & JEPSON, J. B. (1956). *Lancet*, ii, 421.
BARONA, E., SALINAS, A., NAVIA, E. & ORREGO, H. (1965). *Clin. Sci.* 28, 201.
BART, B., LOGOTHETIS, J., AELONY, Y. & BOVIS, M. (1962). *Exp. Neurol.* 5, 519.
BAXTER, C. F. & ROBERTS, E. (1958). *J. biol. Chem.* 233, 1135.
BAXTER, C. F. & ROBERTS, E. (1961). *J. biol. Chem.* 236, 3287.
BENUCK, M. & D'ADAMO, A. F. (1968). *Biochim. Biophys. Acta.* 152, 611.
BERL, S., LAJTHA, A. & WAELSCH, H. (1961). *J. Neurochem.* 7, 186.
BERL, S. & PURPURA, D. P. (1963). *J. Neurochem.* 10, 237.
BERL, S. & WAELSCH, H. (1958). *J. Neurochem.* 3, 161.
BERLINQUET, L. & LALIBERTE, M. (1966). *Canad. J. Biochem.* 44, 783.
BERLOW, S. (1967). *Adv. Clin. Chem.* 9, 165.
BESSMAN, S. P., ROSSEN, J. & LAYNE, E. C. (1953). *J. biol. Chem.* 201, 385.
BITTNER, J. & HEINZ, E. (1963). *Biochim. Biophys. Acta*, 74, 392.

BLASS, J. P. (1960). *Biochem. J.* **77**, 484.
BLUMSON, N. L. (1957). *Biochem. J.* **65**, 138.
BONAVITA, V. (1959). *J. Neurochem.* **4**, 275.
BRENTON, D. P., CUSWORTH, D. C. & GAULL, G. E. (1965). *Pediatrics*, **35**, 50.
BUNIATIAN, H. Ch. & DAVTIAN, M. A. (1966). *J. Neurochem.* **13**, 743.
BUNIATIAN, H. Ch., HOVHANNISSIAN, V. S. & APRIKIAN, G. V. (1965). *J. Neurochem.* **12**, 695.
CARSON, N. A. J., CUSWORTH, D. C., DENT, C. E., FIELD, C. B. M., NEILL, D. W. & WESTALL, R. G. (1963). *Arch. dis. Childh.* **38**, 425.
CHIRIGOS, M. A., GREENGARD, P. & UDENFRIEND, S. (1960). *J. biol. Chem.*, **235**, 2075.
COCHRANE, W. A,, PAYNE, W. W., SIMPKISS, M. J. & WOOLF, L. I. (1956). *J. clin. Investig.* **35**, 411.
COOPER, A. M., ECKHARDT, R. D., FALOON, W. W. & DAVIDSON, C. S. (1950). *J. lab. clin. Invest.* **29**, 265.
COPENHAVER, J. H., MCSHAN, W. H. & MEYER, R. K. (1950). *J. biol. Chem.* **183**, 73.
CORYELL, M. E., HALL, W. K., THEVAOS, T. G., WELTER, D. A., GATZ, A. J., HORTON, B. F., SISSON, B. D., LOOPER, J. W. & FARROW, R. T. (1964). *Biochem. Biophys. Res. Comm.* **14**, 307.
CRAVIOTO, R. O., MASSIEU, G. & IZQUIRDO, J. J. (1951). *Proc. Soc. exp. Biol. N.Y.* **78**, 856.
CRAWHALL, J. C. (1965) *Ann. Rep. Chem. Soc.*, **61**, 476.
CROME, L. C. & STERN, J. (1967). Pathology of Mental Retardation, London: J. A. Churchill Ltd.
CROME, L., TYMMS, V. & WOOLF, L. I. (1962). *J. Neurol. Neurosurg. Psychiat.* **25**, 143.
CUMINGS, J. N. (1948, 1951). *Brain*, **71**, 410; **74**, 10.
CUMINGS, J. N. (1959). Heavy Metals and the Brain. Oxford: Blackwell.
CUMINGS, J. N. & KREMER, M. (1965). (Ed.). Biochemical Aspects of Neurological Disorders. Oxford: Blackwell.
CUMINGS, J. N. & KREMER, M. (1968). (Ed.). Biochemical Aspects of Neurological Disorders, 3rd Series. Oxford: Blackwell.
CURATOLO, A., D'ARCANGELO, P., LINO, A. & BRANCANTI, A. (1965). *J. Neurochem.* **12**, 339.
CURTIS, D. R., PHILLIS, J. W. & WATKINS, J. C. (1960). *J. Physiol.* **150**, 656.
CUSWORTH, D. C. & DENT, C. E. (1969). *Brit. Med. Bull.* **25**, 42.
DE ALMEIDA, D. F., CHAIN, E. B. & POCCHIARI, F. (1965). *Biochem. J.* **95**, 793.
DE MARCHI, W. J. & JOHNSTON, G. A. R. (1969). *J. Neurochem.* **16**, 355.
DINGMAN, W. & SPORN, M. B. (1959). *J. Neurochem.* **4**, 141, 148.
DOUGLAS, G. W. & MORTENSEN, R. A. (1956). *J. biol. Chem.* **222**, 581.
DREYFUS, P. M. & PRENSKY, A. L. (1967). *Nature, London*, **214**, 276.
EASTHAM, R. D. & JANCAR, J. (1968). Clinical Pathology in Mental Retardation. Bristol: Wright.
ECKHARDT, R. D., DAVIDSON, C. S. & HIRSHBERG, E. (1948). *J. clin. Invest.* **27**, 165.
EDLBACHER, S. VON & WISS, O. (1944). *Helv. Chim. Acta*, **27**, 1060, 1824.
EISEMAN, B., OSOFSKY, H., ROBERTS, E. & JELINEK, B. (1959). *J. appl. Physiol.* **14**, 251.
ELLIOTT, W. H. (1951). *Biochem. J.* **49**, 106.
ERSPAMER, V., ROSEGHINI, M. & ANASTASI, A. (1965). *J. Neurochem.* **12**, 123.
FAJANS, S. S., KNOPF, R. F., FLOYD, J. C., POWER, L. & CONN, J. W. (1963). *J. clin. Invest.* **42**, 216.
FERRARO, A. & ROIZIN, L. (1947). *J. Neuropath. exp. Neurol.* **6**, 383.
FEUER, G. (1956). *Acta Physiol. Hung.* **9**, 393.
FINKELSTEIN, J. D., MUDD, S. H., IRREVERE, F. & LASTER, L. (1964). *Science*, **146**, 785.
FODOR, P. J., MILLER, A. & WAELSCH, H. (1953). *J. biol. Chem.* **202**, 551.
FOLBERGROVA, J. (1961). *Physiol. Bohem.* **10**, 122, 130.
FOLBERGROVA, J., PASSONNEAU, J. V., LOWRY, O. H. & SCHULZ, D. W. (1969). *J. Neurochem.* **16**, 191.
FOLCH, J. (1961). Ed. *Proc. 3rd Internat. Neurochem. Symp.* Oxford: Pergamon.
FÖLLING, A. (1934). *Hoppe-Seyl. Z.* **227**, 169.
FONNUM, F. (1968). *Biochem. J.* **106**, 401.

FONNUM, F., HAAVALDSEN, R. & TANGEN, O. (1964). *J. Neurochem.* **11**, 109.
FOX, M., THIER, S., ROSENBERG, L., & SEGAL, S. (1964). *Biochim. Biophys. Acta,* **79**, 167.
FRIEDBERG, F. (1954). *Biochim. Biophys. Acta,* **11**, 308.
FRIEDEN, C. (1963). The Enzymes. 2nd. ed., Vol. 7, p. 3. Ed. P. D. Boyer, H. Lardy & K. Myrback. New York: Academic Press.
FRIEDEN, C. (1965). *J. biol. Chem.* **240**, 2028.
FULLER, R. N. & SHUMAN, J. B. (1969). *Nature,* **221**, 639.
GAITONDE, M. K. & RICHTER, D. (1956). *Proc. Roy. Soc.* B. **145**, 83.
GAITONDE, M. K. & RICHTER, D. (1957). Metabolism of the Nervous System, p. 449. Ed. D. Richter. London: Pergamon.
GALLAGHER, B. B. (1969). *J. Neurochem.* **16**, 1071.
GASIOROWSKA, I., POREMBSKA, Z. & MOCHNACKA, I. (1969). *Acta Biochim. pol.* **16**, 175.
GAULL, G. E. & GAITONDE, M. K. (1967). *Biochem. J.* **102**, 294.
GERRITSEN, T. & WAISMAN, H. A. (1964). *Science,* **145**, 588.
GHADIMI, H., BINNINGTON, V. I. & PECORA, P. (1965). *New England J. Med.* **273**, 723.
GHADIMI, H., ZISCHA, R. & BINNINGTON, V. I. (1966). *Amer. J. Dis. Child.* **113**, 146.
GIBSON, I. M. & McILWAIN, H. (1965). *J. Physiol.* **176**, 261.
GITZELMANN, R. (1968). Some Recent Advances in Inborn Errors of Metabolism, p. 129. Ed. K. S. Holt & V. P. Coffey. London: Livingstone.
GODIN, Y. & MANDEL, P. (1965). *J. Neurochem.* **12**, 455.
GRUMBACH, M. M. & KAPLAN, S. L. (1960). *J. Pediat.* **57**, 346.
GUROFF, G., KING, W. & UDENFRIEND, S. (1961). *J. biol. Chem.* **236**, 1773.
GUTHRIE, R. & SUSA, A. (1963). *Pediatrics,* **32**, 338.
HAAVALDSEN, R. (1964). *Biochem. J.* (proceedings, May).
HABER, B., KURIYAMA, K. & ROBERTS, E. (1970). *Biochem. Pharmac.* **19**, 1119.
HARRIS, H. (1959). Human Biochemical Genetics. Cambridge: University Press.
HARRIS, H. (1970). Principles of Human Biochemical Genetics. Amsterdam: North Holland.
HARVEY, J. A. & McILWAIN, H. (1968). *Biochem. J.* **108**, 269.
HASLAM, R. J. & KREBS, H. A. (1963). *Biochem. J.* **88**, 566.
HERSOV, L. A. (1955). *J. ment. Sci.* **101**, 878.
HERSOV, L. A. & RODNIGHT, R. (1960). *J. Neurol. Neurosurg. Psychiat.* **23**, 40.
HERZFELD, A. & KNOX, W. E. (1968). *J. biol. Chem.* **243**, 3327.
HORVATH, A., ORREGO, F. & McKENNIS, H. (1961) *J Pharmacol. Exp. Ther.* **134**, 222.
HOWELL, J. McC., DAVISON, A. N. & OXBERRY, J. (1964). *Res. vet. Sci.* **5**, 376.
HSIA, D. Y. (1959). Inborn Errors of Metabolism. Chicago: Year Book Publishers.
HSIA, D. Y. Y., BERMAN, J. L. & SLATIS, H. M. (1964). *J. Amer. med. Assoc.* **188**, 203.
JASPER, H. H., KHAN, R. T. & ELLIOTT, K. A. C. (1965). *Science* **147**, 1448.
JEPSON, J. B. (1966). In The Metabolic Basis of Inherited Disease, 2nd ed., p. 1283. Ed. J. B. Stanbury, J. B. Wyngaarden & D. S. Frederickson. New York: McGraw-Hill.
JERVIS, G. A. (1937). *Arch. Neurol. Psychiat.* **38**, 944.
JERVIS, G. A. (1947). *J. biol. Chem.* **169**, 651.
JOHNSTON, G. A. R. & VITALI, M. V. (1969). *Brain Res.* **15**, 201.
JONES, D. & McILWAIN, H. (1971). *J. Neurochem.* **18**, 41.
JORDAN, W. K., MARCH, R., HOUCHIN, O. B. & POPP, E. (1959). *J. Neurochem.* **4**, 170.
KALCKAR, H. L., ANDERSON, E. P. & ISSELBACKER, K. J. (1956). *Biochim. Biophys. Acta.* **20**, 262.
KAMMERAT, C. & VELDSTRA, H. (1968). *Biochim. Biophys. Acta,* **151**, 1.
KANAZAWA, A., KAKIMOTO, Y., MIYAMOTO, E. & SANO, I. (1965). *J. Neurochem.* **12**, 957.
KANAZAWA, A. & SANO, I. (1967). *J. Neurochem.* **14**, 596.
KASPER, C. B. & DEUTSCH, H. F. (1963). *J. biol. Chem.* **238**, 2325.
KATUNUMA, N., HUZINO, A. & TOMINO, I. (1967). *Advances Enz. Regul.* **5**, 55.
KATZ, R. I., CHASE, T. N. & KOPIN, I. J. (1969). *J. Neurochem.* **16**, 961.
KAUFMAN, S. (1963). The Enzymes, **8**, 373; *Proc. Nat. Acad. Sci., U.S.A.* **50**, 1085.
KAUFMAN, S. (1970). *J. biol. Chem.* **245**, 4751.

8

KEMP, J. W. & WOODBURY, D. M. (1965). *Biochim. Biophys. Acta*, **111**, 23.
KETY, S. S. (1959). *Science*, **29**, 1528.
KILLAM, K. F. & BAIN, J. A. (1957). *J. Pharmacol. Exp. Ther.* **119**, 255.
KNAUFF, H. G. & BÖCK, F. (1961). *J. Neurochem.* **6**, 171.
KNIZLEY, H. (1967). *J. biol. Chem.* **242**, 4619.
KOSOWER, E. M. & KOSOWER, N. S. (1969). *Nature, Lond.* **224**, 117.
KOWALSKY, A., WYTTENBACH, C., LANGER, L. & KOSHLAND, D. E. (1956). *J. biol. Chem.* **219**, 719.
KRAUS, P. (1968). *Hoppe-Seyler's Z. Physiol. Chem.* **349**, 1425.
KREBS, H. A. (1935). *Biochem. J.* **29**, 1951.
KREBS, H. A. & BELLAMY, D. (1960). *Biochem. J.* **75**, 523.
KRISHNASWAMY, P. R., PAMILJAMS, V. & MEISTER, A. (1962). *J. biol. Chem.* **237**, 2932.
KRNJEVIĆ, K. & PHILLIS, J. W. (1963). *J. Physiol.* **165**, 274.
KUTTNER, R., SIMS, J. A. & GORDON, M. W. (1961). *J. Neurochem.* **6**, 311.
LADU, B. N. & MICHAEL, P. J. (1960). *J. Lab. Clin. Med.* **55**, 491.
LABELLA, F., VIVIAN, S. & QUEEN, G. (1968). *Biochim. Biophys. Acta*, **158**, 286.
LAHIRI, S. & LAJTHA, A. (1964). *J. Neurochem.* **11**, 77.
LAJTHA, A. (1959). *J. Neurochem.* **3**, 358.
LAJTHA, A. (1964). *Internat. Rev. Neurobiol.* **6**, 1.
LAJTHA, A., BERL, S. & WAELSCH, H. (1959). *J. Neurochem.* **3**, 322.
LAJTHA, A., FURST, S., GERSTEIN, A. & WAELSCH, H. (1957). *J. Neurochem.* **1**, 289.
LAJTHA, A., MELA, P. & WAELSCH, H. (1953). *J. biol. Chem.* **205**, 553.
LAJTHA, A. & TOTH, J. (1961). *J. Neurochem.* **8**, 216.
LAJTHA, A. & TOTH, J. (1962). *J. Neurochem.* **9**, 199.
Legislation (1966). *Ohio State Med. J.* **62**, 822.
LOO, Y. H. (1967). *J. Neurochem.* **14**, 813.
LOO, Y. H. & RITMAN, P. (1967). *Nature*, **213**, 914.
LOWE, I. P., ROBINS, E. & EYERMAN, G. S. (1958). *J. Neurochem.* **3**, 8.
LOWRY, O. H. (1957). *Progr. Neurobiol.* **2**, 69.
LOWRY, O. H., ROBERTS, N. R. & LEWIS, C. (1956). *J. biol. Chem.* **220**, 879.
MACHIYAWA, Y., BALÁZS, R. & MÉREI, T. (1970). *J. Neurochem.* **17**, 449.
MACKENZIE, D. Y. & WOOLF, L. I. (1959). *Brit. med. J.* **i**, 90.
MANDELBROTE, B. M., STANIER, M. W., THOMPSON, R. H. S. & THRUSTON, M. N. (1948). *Brain*, **71**, 212.
MASSIEU, G. H., ORTEGA, B. G., SYRQUIN, A. & TUENA, M. (1962). *J. Neurochem.* **9**, 143.
MCCAMEN, M. W. & ROBINS, E. (1962). *J. Lab. Clin. Med.* **59**, 885.
MCILWAIN, H. (1953). *J. Neurol. Neurosurg. Psychiat.* **16**, 257.
MCILWAIN, H. (1959). *Biochem. Soc. Sympos.* **17**, 66.
MCILWAIN, H. (1970). *Nature, Lond.* **226**, 803.
MCILWAIN, H., HARVEY, J. A. & RODRIGUEZ, G. (1969). *J. Neurochem.* **16**, 363.
MCILWAIN, H. & RODNIGHT, R. (1962). Practical Neurochemistry. London: Churchill.
MCILWAIN, H. & SNYDER, S. H. (1970). *J. Neurochem.* **17**, 521.
MCILWAIN, H. & TRESIZE, M. A. (1957). *Biochem. J.* **65**, 288.
MCINTOSH, J. C. & COOPER, J. R. (1965). *J. Neurochem.* **12**, 825.
MCKEAN, C. M., BOGGS, D. E. & PETERSON, N. A. (1968). *J. Neurochem.* **15**, 23.
MCKHANN, G. M., ALBERS, R. W., SOKOLOFF, L., MICKELSEN, O. & TOWER, D. B. (1960). In Inhibition in the Nervous System and γ-Aminobutyric Acid, p. 169. Ed. E. Roberts. London: Pergamon.
MCKHANN, G. M. & TOWER, D. B. (1961). *J. Neurochem.* **7**, 26.
MCMURRAY, W. C., MOHYUDDIN, F., ROSSITER, R. J., RATHBURN, J. C., VALENTINE, G. H., KOEGLER, S. J. & ZARFAS, D. E. (1962). *Lancet*, **i**, 138.
MCMURRAY, W. C., RATHBURN, J. C., MOHYUDDIN, F. & KOEGLER, S. J. (1963). *Pediatrics*, **32**, 347.
MEISTER, A., KRISHNASWAMY, P. R. & PAMILJANS, V. (1962). *Fed. Proc.* **21**, 1013.
MENKES, J. H. (1968). *Neurology, Minneap.* **18**, 1003.
MILLER, A. L. & MCLEAN, P. (1967). *Clin. Sci.* **32**, 385.
MILLER, A. L. & PITTS, F. N. (1967). *J. Neurochem.* **14**, 579.

MILNE, M., CRAWFORD, M., GIRAO, C. & LOUGHRIDGE, L. (1960). *Quart. J. Med.* **29**, 407.

MITOMA, C., POSNER, H. S., BOGDANSKI, D. F. & UDENFRIEND, S. (1957). *J. Pharmacol.* **120**, 188.

MIYAMOTO, E., KAKIMOTO, Y. & SANO, I. (1966). *J. Neurochem.* **13**, 999.

MOSER, H. W., EFRON, M. L., BROWN, H., DIAMOND, R. & NEUMANN, C. G. (1967). *Amer. J. Med.* **42**, 9.

MUDD, S. H., LEVY, H. L. & ABELES, R. H. (1969). *Biochem. Biophys. Res. Comm.* **35**, 121.

MÜLLER, P. B. & LANGEMANN, H. (1962). *J. Neurochem.* **9**, 399.

MUNTZ, J. A. (1953). *J. biol. Chem.* **201**, 221.

NAKAJIMA, T., WOLFGRAM, F. & CLARK, W. G. (1967). *J. Neurochem.* **14**, 1107.

NAKAZAWA, S. & QUASTEL, J. H. (1968). *Canad. J. Biochem.* **46**, 363.

NEAME, K. D. (1962). *J. Neurochem.* **9**, 321; *J. Physiol.* **162**, 1.

NEAME, K. D. & SMITH, S. E. (1965). *J. Neurochem.* **12**, 87.

NEIMS, A. H., ZIEVERINK, W. D. & SMILAK, J. D. (1966). *J. Neurochem.* **13**, 163.

NORDIN, J. H. & HANSEN, R. G. (1963). *J. biol. Chem.* **238**, 489.

OKUMURA, N., OTSUKI, S. & FUKAI, N. (1959a). *Acta med. Okayama*, **13**, 27.

OKUMURA, N., OTSUKI, S. & NASU, H. (1959b). *Jap. J. Biochem.* **46**, 247.

OKUMURA, N., OTSUKI, S. & AOYAMA, T. (1959c). *Jap. J. Biochem.* **46**, 207.

ORLOWSKI, M. & MEISTER, A. (1970). *Proc. nat. Acad. Sci., U.S.A.* **67**, 1248.

OSBORN, S. B. & WALSHE, J. M. (1964). *Clin. Sci.* **27**, 319.

OXENDER, D. L. & CHRISTENSEN, H. N. (1963). *J. biol. Chem.* **238**, 3686.

PALAIC, D., PAGE, I. H. & KHAIRALLAH, F. A. (1967). *J. Neurochem.* **14**, 63.

PENROSE, L. S. (1935). *Lancet*, **ii**, 192.

PERRY, T. L., HANSEN, S., TISCHLEI, B. & HESTRIN, M. (1964). *Proc. Soc. exp. Biol. Med.* **115**, 118.

PERRY, T. L., LING, G. M., HANSEN, S. & MACDOUGALL, L. (1965). *Proc. Soc. Exp. Biol. Med.* **119**, 282.

PETERS, E. L. & TOWER, D. B. (1959). *J. Neurochem.* **5**, 80.

PISANO, J. J. & UDENFRIEND, S. (1958). *Fed. Proc.* **17**, 403.

PISANO, J. J., WILSON, J. D., COHEN, L., ABRAHAM, D. & UDENFRIEND, S. (1961). *J. biol. Chem.* **236**, 499.

PITTS, F. N., QUICK, C. & ROBINS, E. (1965). *J. Neurochem.* **12**, 93.

POLIDORA, V. J. (1967). *Proc. natn. Acad. Sci. U.S.A.* **57**, 102.

PORCELLATI, G. & THOMPSON, R. H. S. (1957). *J. Neurochem.* **1**, 340.

PORTER, H. (1964). *Arch. Neurol.* **11**, 341.

PURPURA, D. P., GIRADO, M., SMITH, T. C., CALLAN, D. A. & GRUNDFEST, H. (1959). *J. Neurochem.* **3**, 238.

Report (1963). Treatment of Phenylketonuria. Report to the Medical Research Council. London: British Medical Association.

RICHTER, D. & DAWSON, R. M. C. (1948). *J. biol. Chem.* **176**, 1199.

ROA, P. D., TEWS, J. K. & STONE, W. E. (1964). *Biochem. Pharmacol.* **13**, 477.

ROBERTS, E. & FRAENKEL, S. (1950, 1951). *J. biol. Chem.* **187**, 55; **188**, 789.

ROBERTS, E., ROTHSTEIN, M. & BAXTER, C. F. (1958). *Proc. Soc. exp. Biol. N.Y.* **97**, 796.

ROBERTS, E. & SIMONSEN, D. G. (1963). *Biochem. Pharmacol.* **12**, 113.

ROBERTS, R. B., FLEXNER, J. B. & FLEXNER, L. B. (1959). *J. Neurochem.* **4**, 78.

ROBERTS, S., SETO, K. & HANKING, B. H. (1962). *J. Neurochem.* **9**, 493.

ROBINSON, A. (1963). *J. exp. Med.* **118**, 359.

RODNIGHT, R. (1968). Applied Neurochemistry, p. 377. Ed. A. N. Davison & J. Dobbing. Oxford: Blackwell.

RODNIGHT, R. & McILWAIN, H. (1955). *J. ment. Sci.* **101**, 884.

RONZIO, R. A. & MEISTER, A. (1968). *Proc. natn. Acad. Sci. U.S.A.* **59**, 164.

RONZIO, R. A., ROWE, W. B., WILK, S. & MEISTER, A. (1969). *Biochemistry*, **8**, 2670.

ROSEMAN, S. & DORFMAN, A. (1951). *J. biol. Chem.* **192**, 105.

SALVADOR, R. A. & ALBERS, R. W. (1959). *J. biol. Chem.* **234**, 922.

SANO, K. & ROBERTS, K. (1963). *Biochem. Pharmacol.* **12**, 489.

SCHAIN, R. J., COPENHAVER, J. H. & CARVER, M. J. (1967). *J. Neurochem.* **14**, 195.

SCHAUMBURG, H. H., BYK, R., GERSTL, R. & MASHMAN, J. H. *Science, N.Y.*, **163**, 826.
SCHEINBERG, I. H. (1956). *Progr. Neurobiol.* **1**, 52.
SCHEPARTZ, B. (1963). *J. Neurochem.* **10**, 825.
SCHURR, P. E., THOMPSON, H. T., HENDERSON, L. M. & ELVEHJEM, C. A. (1950). *J. biol. Chem.* **182**, 29.
SCHWARTZ, A., BACHELARD, H. S. & MCILWAIN, H. (1962). *Biochem. J.* **84**, 626.
SCHWARZ, V., GOLDBERG, L., KOMROWER, G. M. & HOLZEL, A. (1956). *Biochem. J.* **62**, 34.
SCHWARZ, V., HOLZEL, A. & KOMROWER, G. M. (1958). *Lancet*, **i**, 24.
SCOTT, J. (1966). *Lancet*, **i**, 875.
SELLINGER, O. Z. & DE BALBIAN VERSTER, F. (1962). *J. biol. Chem.* **237**, 2836.
SELLINGER, O. Z., DE BALBIAN VERSTER, F., SULLIVAN, R. J. & LAMAR, C. (1966). *J. Neurochem.* **13**, 501.
SHAW, R. K. & HEINE, J. D. (1965). *J. Neurochem.* **12**, 151, 527.
SHERIDAN, J. J., SIMS, K. L. & PITTS, F. N. (1967). *J. Neurochem.* **14**, 571.
SHIMADA, M. & NAKAMURA, T. (1966). *J. Neurochem.* **13**, 391.
SILBERBERG, D. H. (1969). *J. Neurochem.* **16**, 1141.
SIMON, G., DRORI, J. B. & COHEN, M. M. (1967). *Biochem. J.* **102**, 153.
SIMS, K. L. & PITTS, F. N. (1970). *J. Neurochem.* **17**, 1607.
SOURKES, T. L. (1962). Biochemistry of Mental Disease. New York: Hoeber.
SMITH, S. E. (1967). *J. Neurochem.* **14**, 291.
SPORN, M. B., DINGMAN, W., DEFALGO, A. & DAVIES, R. K. (1959). *J. Neurochem.* **5**, 62.
SRINIVASAN, V., NEAL, M. J. & MITCHELL, J. F. (1969). *J. Neurochem.* **16**, 1235.
STANBURY, J. B., WYNGAARDEN, J. B. & FREDRICKSON, D. S. (1966). The Metabolic Basis of Inherited Disease, 2nd. ed. New York: McGraw-Hill.
STERN, J. R., EGGLESTON, L. V., HEMS, R. & KREBS, H. A. (1949). *Biochem. J.* **44**, 410.
STRASBERG, P. & ELLIOTT, K. A. C. (1967). *Canad. J. Biochem.* **45**, 1795.
STRECKER, H. J., MELA, P. & WAELSCH, H. (1955). *J. biol. Chem.* **212**, 223.
SUSZ, J. P., HABER, B. & ROBERTS, E. (1966). *Biochemistry*, **5**, 2870.
SVENNEBY, G. (1969). Second Int. Mtg. of Int. Soc. for Neurochem, Sept. 1–5, p. 386. Milan.
SVENNEBY, G. (1970). *J. Neurochem.* **17**, 1591.
Symposium (1948). Monosodium Glutamate. Chicago: Quartermaster Food and Container Institute for the Armed Forces.
Symposium (1961). Wilson's Disease: Some Current Concepts. Ed. J. M. Walshe & J. N. Cumings. Oxford: Blackwell.
Symposium (1962). Amino Acid Pools. Ed. J. T. Holden. Amsterdam: Elsevier.
Symposium (1963). Phenylketonuria. Ed. Lyman, F. L. Springfield, Illinois: Thomas.
Symposium (1964). Neurometabolic Disorders in Childhood. Ed. K. S. Holt & J. Milner. Edinburgh: Livingstone.
TAKAGAKI, G., HIRANO, S. & NAGATA, Y. (1959). *J. Neurochem.* **4**, 124.
TAKAHASHI, Y. & AKABANE, Y. (1961). *J. Neurochem.* **7**, 89.
TALLAN, H. H., MOORE, S. & STEIN, W. H. (1954). *J. biol. Chem.* **211**, 915, 927.
TALLAN, H. H., MOORE, S. & STEIN, W. H. (1956). *J. biol. Chem.* **219**, 257.
TALLAN, H. H., MOORE, S. & STEIN, W. H. (1958). *J. biol. Chem.* **230**, 707.
TEDESCO, T. A. & MELLMAN, W. J. (1967). *Proc. Natn. Acad. Sci. U.S.A.* **57**, 829.
TEWS, J. K., CARTER, S. H., ROA, P. D. & STONE, W. E. (1963). *J. Neurochem.* **10**, 641.
TOMLINSEN, S. & WESTALL, R. G. (1960). *Nature*, **188**, 235.
TOMLINSON, Y., NAGATA, Y., HIRANO, S. & MATSUTANI, T. (1963). *J. Neurochem.* **10**, 241.
TSUKADA, Y., NAGATA, Y., HIRANO, S. & MATSUTANI, T. (1963). *J. Neurochem.* **10**, 241.
TU, R. J. B., BLACKWELL, S. & WATTEN, R. H. (1965). *Metab., Clin. Exptl.* **14**, 653.
UDENFRIEND, S. & COOPER, J. R. (1952). *J. biol. Chem.* **194**, 503.
UZMAN, L. & HOOD, B. (1952). *Amer. J. med. Sci.* **223**, 392.
VELICK, S. F. & VAVRA, J. (1962). The Enzymes, 2nd Ed., **6**, 219. Ed. P. D. Boyer, H. Lardy & K. Myrback. New York: Academic Press.

VLADIMIROVA, Y. A. (1964). In Problems of the Biochemistry of the Nervous System, p. 135. Ed. A. V. Palladin. Trans. H. Hillman & R. Woodman. London: Pergamon.

VOGEL, F. S. & EVANS, J. W. (1961). *J. exp. Med.* **113**, 997.

VOLPE, J. J. & LASTER, L. (1970). *J. Neurochem.* **17**, 413, 425.

VRBA, R., FOLBERGROVA, J. & KANTUREK, J. (1957). *Nature*, **179**, 470.

WALSHE, J. M. (1964). *Clin. Sci.* **26**, 461.

WARREN, K. S. & SCHENKER, S. (1964). *J. lab. clin. Med.* **64**, 442.

WEBER, G., GLAZIER, R. I. & ROSS, R. A. (1970). *Adv. Enzyme Reg.* **8**, 13.

WEIL-MALHERBE, H. (1936). *Biochem. J.* **30**, 665.

WEIL-MALHERBE, H. (1952). *J. ment. Sci.* **98**, 565.

WEIL-MALHERBE, H. (1969). *J. Neurochem.* **16**, 855.

WEINSTEIN, H., VARON, S., MUHLEMAN, D. R. & ROBERTS, E. (1965). *Biochem. Pharmacol.* **14**, 273.

WELLS, W. W., PITTMAN, T. A., WELLS, H. J. & EGAN, T. J. (1965). *J. biol. Chem.* **240**, 1002.

WHELAN, D. T., SCRIVER, C. R. & MOHYUDDIN, F. (1969). *Nature, Lond.* **224**, 916.

WILSON, S. A. K. (1947). Neurology. London: Arnold.

WOLFF, O. H. (1968). In Cumings & Kremer, 1968.

WOOD, J. D. & WATSON, W. J. (1963). *Canad. J. Biochem. Physiol.* **41**, 1907.

WOOD, J D & WATSON, W J (1964). *Canad. J. Physiol. Pharmacol.* **42**, 277.

WOOD, J. D., WATSON, W. J. & DUCKER, A. J. (1968). *J. Neurochem.* **15**, 603.

WOODMAN, R. J. & MCILWAIN, H. (1961). *Biochem. J.* **81**, 83.

WOODY, N. C. (1964). *Amer. J. Dis. Child.* **108**, 543.

WOODY, N. C., SNYDER, C. H. & HARRIS, J. A. (1965). *Amer. J. Dis. Child.* **110**, 606.

WOOLF, L. I. (1960). *Clin. Chim. Acta.* **5**, 327.

WOOLF, L. I. (1962). *Advan. Clin. Chem.* **5**, 1.

WOOLF, L. I. (1963). *Advan. Clin. Chem.* **6**, 97.

WOOLF, L. I. (1968). In Cumings & Kremer, 1968.

WOOLF, L. I. & GOODWIN, B. L. (1964). *Clin. Chem.* **10**, 146.

YOSHIDA, H., KANIKE, K. & NAMBA, J. (1963). *Nature*, **198**, 191.

9   Metabolism of Nucleic Acids and Proteins

Earlier chapters have included comments on numerous cerebral proteins in terms of their enzymic reactions; their properties as substrates and products now receive attention. The adult brain is rich in cytoplasmic ribosomes which are seen under the electron microscope to occur both free and bound to the endoplasmic reticulum. The possession of large numbers of the classical morphological sites for protein synthesis correlates well with active rates of incorporation of labelled precursors into protein of both neurons and glial cells. The brain does not synthesize a high proportion of material for secretion to the bloodstream as do the liver or pancreas, yet measurements of relative rates suggest that protein synthesis may be as active in the brain as elsewhere in the body. A tissue with a generally high metabolic rate may be expected to require a rapid turnover of enzyme protein and there is evidence for renewal of protein also in cell processes including axons and dendrites. Moreover cerebral tissues have also a high rate of RNA turnover.

The greater recent interest in mechanisms of protein synthesis in the brain comes from a desire to understand the unique functional features of the organ. The underlying processes of adaptation, learning and memory may involve change in the structure of nucleic acids and proteins. Whereas a decade ago knowledge of protein synthesis in the brain lagged behind that of other tissues, studies on cerebral nucleic acid and protein metabolism are now well developed. Various aspects of DNA and RNA metabolism are gradually being investigated in neural as in other mammalian systems. Initial considerations have therefore been given to the cerebral occurrence and metabolism of nucleic acid components.

Purine and Pyrimidine Nucleotides

The brain contains adenine, cytidine, guanine and uridine nucleotides (Table 3.3) of which, as in other tissues, ATP preponderates at 3 μmoles/g. of fresh tissue; ATP and to a lesser extent, ADP are amongst the most labile constituents of the brain (see Chapter 3). Guanine nucleotides occur in quantities about one-quarter of those of the adenine nucleotides (Kerr, 1942; Tarr et al., 1962). Uridine nucleotides, which occur in total amounts of about 1 μmole/g., include not only the mono-, di- and triphosphates, but also uridine diphosphate glucose, important in glycogen metabolism (Chapter 5).

Some preformed purine bases and nucleosides can enter the brain. Adenosine acts as precursor for adenine nucleotides when it is added to incubation media with cerebral cortex preparations *in vitro*. The ATP content of the tissues was observed to increase by about 0·4 μmoles/g. fresh tissue after incubation for 100 min. in glucose-salines with added 1 mM-adenosine; adenine gave a smaller increase (Thomas, 1957). Incubation for 1 hr. with lower concentrations (5 to 13 μM) of isotopically-labelled precursors gave rapid incorporation of radioactivity into purine nucleotides and RNA; ^{14}C-adenine gave specific activities more than twice the values observed when ^{14}C-adenosine was the precursor. Over 90% of the isotope taken up in each case was incorporated into purine nucleotides (Santos *et al.*, 1968; Shimizu *et al.*, 1969). Interpretation of the extent and ease of entry of adenine and adenosine to the brain awaits further information on the intracellular pool sizes of these compounds. Evidence for the existence of more than one pool of purine nucleotides has come from a comparison of the effects of adenine and adenosine, *in vitro*, on cerebral levels of cyclic AMP. After 5 min. incubation in the presence of 50 μM adenosine, the content of the cyclic nucleotide was increased from 1 to 30 μmoles/g. of tissue. Adenine was ineffective in this respect; adenosine acted in part as precursor of cyclic AMP (q.v., and see Sattin & Rall, 1970; McIlwain, 1971).

Formation of Nucleotide Bases

The complete pathways of biosynthesis of purines and pyrimidines have not been demonstrated in the brain, but the stages that have been described serve to indicate that at least the complete purine pathway is present. Labelled adenine derivatives have been isolated from the brains of mice within 30 min. of intraperitoneal injection of ^{14}C-glycine. Incorporation of glycine into adenine nucleotides has also been demonstrated *in vitro* by incubating minced cerebral tissue with 2-[^{14}C]-glycine in the presence of glucose, fumarate and glutamine. The first stage of purine biosynthesis from ^{14}C-glycine has been specifically demonstrated by the use of L-azaserine to block further metabolism of the product, L-N-formylglycinamide ribonucleotide. The reaction in minced rat brain required Mg^{2+}, glucose and glutamine (Henderson & Le Page, 1959; Wells *et al.*, 1963; Howard *et al.*, 1970).

The brain is indeed one of the most active tissues in nucleotide and nucleic acid synthesis; this is discussed subsequently under RNA synthesis. The lack of detectable amounts of carbamylphosphate synthetase in the brain (Kemp & Woodbury, 1965; Appel & Silberberg, 1968; see also Chapter 7) throws doubt on the presence of the complete apparatus for pyrimidine biosynthesis. However, rapid formation from an intermediate precursor (orotic acid) occurs (Fig. 9.1). After intraventricular injection of 6-[^{14}C]-orotic acid (0·15 μmole) into cats, incorporation of ^{14}C into uridine nucleotides and uridine diphosphate glucose was observed within 3 hr. The incorporation was equivalent to about 0·3% of the specific activity relative to the orotic acid administered and was diminished by pretreatment of cats with 6-azauridine, also given intraventricularly (Wells *et al.*, 1963). The related azauracil attracted attention by causing cerebral disturbances during its use in treating neoplasms. In the brains of azauridine-treated cats the concentration of uridine nucleotides fell by 30–60 % and the precursor, orotidine, accumulated. Localization of the point of action of the inhibitor (orotidylic acid decarboxylation, q.v. and Fig. 9.1) was further indicated by the finding that ^{3}H-uridine conversion to uridine phosphates was not affected by azauridine.

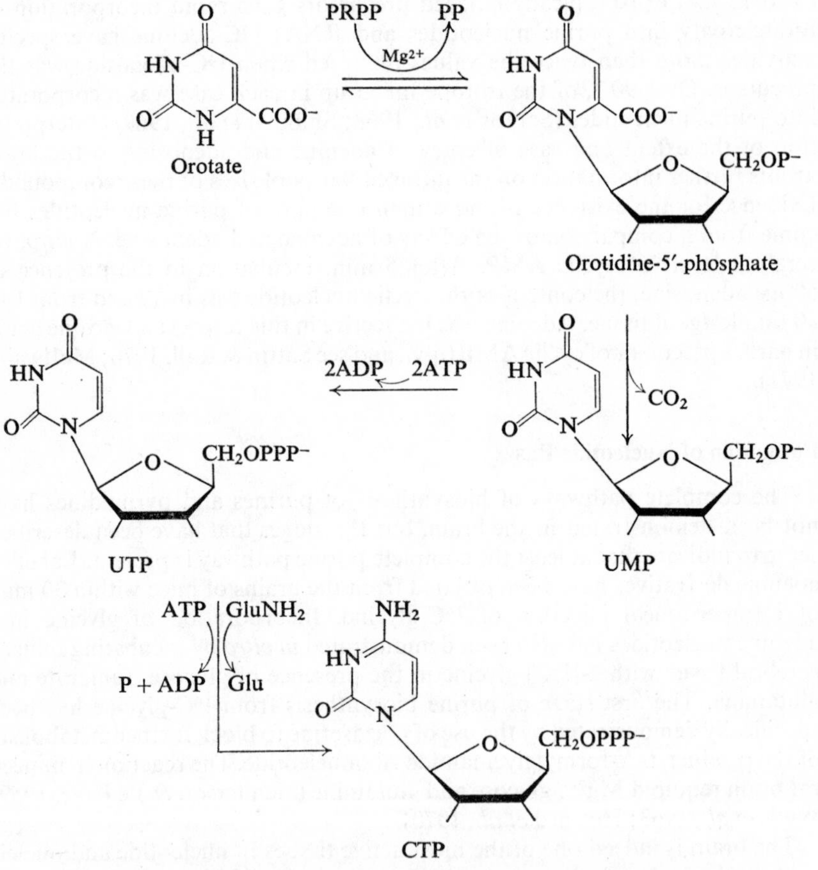

FIG. 9.1. Formation of pyrimidine nucleotides. Note that the sequence of reactions prior to orotate has not been clearly established in the brain.
UMP: uridine monophosphate; UTP: uridine triphosphate; CTP: cytidine triphosphate; PRPP: phosphoribosylpyrophosphate; P: inorganic orthophosphate; Glu: glutamate; GluNH$_2$: glutamine.

During these experiments ^{14}C from orotic acid was also incorporated into cytidine nucleotides. However no labelling of cytidine nucleotides was detected when guinea-pig cerebral cortex preparations were incubated with tritiated uracil or UMP (Cain, 1967). This is consistent with observations that cerebral systems produce RNA more readily from orotate than from uracil; further comment appears subsequently in the description of RNA synthesis.

The sole route established for cytidine nucleotide formation, in the brain and in other tissues, involves the amination of UTP; enzymic production of CTP by amination of UTP has recently been demonstrated in the brain (Dawson, 1968). Enzymes which phosphorylate thymidine to form TMP, TDP and TTP are also present (Weissman *et al.*, 1960).

Orotidine 5'-phosphate decarboxylase (EC 4.1.1.23) catalyses the irreversible decarboxylation of orotidine 5'-phosphate to form uridine 5'-phosphate (Fig. 9.1). The purified enzyme from cow brain was inhibited by nucleoside monophosphates (CMP and UMP) more strongly than by the di- or triphosphates (Appel, 1967). The cytidine nucleotides were more effective inhibitors than the uridine nucleotides; the inhibitions have been suggested to be relevant to regulation of pyrimidine levels in the brain (below).

Degradation of Nucleotide Bases

Little information is available on the pathways of degradation of pyrimidines in the brain; much more evidence is available for purine degradation (Fig. 9.2). In the brain, like most mammalian tissues, the principal end-product of purine degradation is uric acid. The NH_3 produced by deamination reactions (Table 9.1), which occur at 35–320 μmoles/g. hr. (Jordan *et al.*, 1959; Setlow & Lowenstein, 1967), is unlikely to account for the total NH_3 produced in the brain (Weil-Malherbe & Green, 1955). Enzymes for dephosphorylation of purine nucleotides and for deamination of the nucleotides and nucleosides have been characterized and are described in the following sections. The most active of these is adenylic acid deaminase (Table 9.1) which converts AMP to IMP and has been the deamination step most intensively studied.

Dephosphorylation: 5'-Nucleotidase. The first report of cerebral 5'-nucleotidase was the observation of orthophosphate formation from adenylic acid hydrolysis in human brain (Reis, 1951). Sheep brain 5'-nucleotidase (EC 3.1.3.5), as active in dephosphorylating IMP as 5'-AMP, has been purified free from phosphatase activity against 2'-AMP, 3'-AMP and nucleoside di- and tri-phosphates. The purified enzyme, which contained no adenosine deaminase or AMP deaminase activity, exhibited allosteric inhibition by ATP, UTP or CTP (Fig. 9.3). Inorganic orthophosphate, without effect alone at concentrations of up to 10 mM, reversed at 0·2 mM the inhibition due to ATP; no effect was observed on the inhibition caused by CTP or UTP (Ipata, 1967, 1968). Such interactions with nucleotide triphosphates are relevant to the regulation of nucleotide levels in the brain. This receives further comment below.

Deamination Reactions

Guanase (guanine deaminase, EC 3.5.4.3), which forms xanthine by hydrolytic deamination, occurs in the mammalian brain mainly as a soluble cytoplasmic enzyme (Jordan *et al.*, 1959), although significant activity is present also in mitochondria. The particulate activity, after extraction with Triton X-100 (*iso*octylphenoxypolyethoxyethanol), was found to differ in electrophoretic mobility and immunochemical and kinetic behaviour from the

FIG. 9.2.

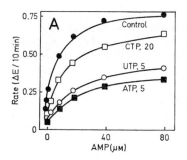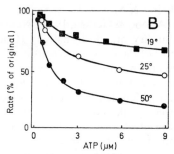

FIG. 9.3. Nucleoside triphosphates and cerebral 5'-nucleotidase.
A. Inhibition of 5'-nucleotidase activity, estimated using 5'-AMP as substrate, by ATP, UTP or CTP: concentrations, μM.
B. Temperature dependence of 5'-nucleotidase inhibition by ATP, estimated with 80 μM-AMP as substrate (Ipata, 1967, 1968).

cytoplasmic system, which resolved into two activity peaks on DEAE-cellulose columns (Kumar *et al.*, 1967). Activity, 115 μmoles/g. hr. in the cerebral hemispheres, was not detected in the cerebellum in which an endogenous inhibitor, a heat-labile protein, was found to occur. Guanase is highly active in human basal ganglia (Kelley, 1968) and in rat brain was reported (Jordan *et al.*, 1959) to be more active (61·5 μmoles of NH_3 formed/g. hr.) than *guanosine deaminase* (35·2 μmoles/g. hr.) which produces xanthosine (Jordan *et al.*, 1959; Table 9.1).

Adenosine deaminase (EC 3.5.4.4) activity in rat and rabbit brain is only about one-third of that of adenylate deaminase. It occurs mainly in the soluble fraction and catalyzes the formation of NH_3 from adenosine at rates of 57·5 μmoles/g. hr. (Jordan *et al.*, 1959). Unlike adenylate deaminase, the activity of adenosine deaminase appears to be unaffected by ATP or GTP (Setlow *et al.*, 1966). The most active of the deamination reactions is due to *adenylate deaminase* (EC 3.5.4.6). This enzyme catalyzes the hydrolytic deamination of AMP to form IMP and is found in both mitochondrial and soluble cytoplasmic fractions of cerebral tissues (Muntz, 1953; Weil-Malherbe & Green, 1955;

FIG. 9.2. Metabolism of purine nucleotides.
The stages illustrated are all thought to be present in the brain; those clearly established, as described in the text, are signified by heavy lines (——). Structures are shown as the preponderant tautomeric form at neutral pH.

(1) Adenine phosphoribosyl transferase
(2) 5'-Nucleotidase
(3) Adenylic acid deaminase
(4) Adenosine deaminase
(5) Guanase
(6) Hypoxanthine-guanine phosphoribosyl transferase (HGPRT)
(7) Xanthine oxidase.

ATP: adenosine triphosphate; AMP: adenosine monophosphate; IMP: inosine monophosphate; XMP: xanthosine monophosphate; GMP: guanosine monophosphate; GDP: guanosine diphosphate; GTP: guanosine triphosphate; Glu: glutamate; $GluNH_2$: glutamine; PRPP: phosphoribosylpyrophosphate; PP: pyrophosphate; P: orthophosphate.

Mendicino & Muntz, 1958; Setlow & Lowenstein, 1967) and in rat peripheral nerve (Abood & Gerard, 1954). Neural tissues were reported to be second only to voluntary muscle in activity (Conway & Cooke, 1939). A characteristic property of the deaminase is its activation by ATP (Fig. 9.4) shown originally for the enzyme in acetone powders of dog and ox brain (Muntz, 1953; Weil-Malherbe & Green, 1955). The requirement for ATP, which is specific but not absolute (Mendicino & Muntz, 1958; Cunningham & Lowenstein, 1965), is increased by alkali metal ions (Fig. 9.4), particularly Li^+ and, to a lesser extent, Na^+, the effects being on the affinity of the enzyme for ATP rather than on the maximum velocity of the reaction. Under conditions of maximal activation the enzyme in calf brain catalyzed the removal of NH_3 at rates equivalent to 320 μmoles/g. hr. and was more active than in the other tissues tested, which

Table 9.1

Enzymes of purine degradation in the brain

Enzyme	Reaction catalyzed	Rate (μmole/g. hr.)
Guanine deaminase	Guanine + H_2O → Xanthine + NH_3	61·5
Guanosine deaminase	Guanosine + H_2O → Xanthosine + NH_3	35·2
Adenosine deaminase	Adenosine + H_2O → Inosine + NH_3	57·5
Adenylate deaminase	AMP + H_2O → IMP + NH_3	320
5′-Nucleotidase	AMP + H_2O → Adenosine + P_i	*ca* 12

Values from rat, rabbit and calf brain: Jordan *et al.* (1959); Setlow & Lowenstein (1967); Ipata (1968).

did not include muscle. ATP activation (Fig. 9.4) of the purified enzyme was reversed by CTP competitively; both nucleotides afforded protection against heat inactivation in contrast to the nucleoside diphosphates which were ineffective (Setlow *et al.*, 1966; Setlow & Lowenstein, 1967, 1968).

Xanthine oxidase, which has been shown to be present in cerebral preparations, catalyses the formation of uric acid from hypoxanthine and xanthine and represents the final stage of purine catabolism (Villela, 1968; Fig. 9.2). Due to its structural similarity to caffeine (1,3,7-trimethylxanthine) and theobromine (3,7-dimethylxanthine), suggestions have been made that uric acid may have a stimulatory action on the central nervous system. Earlier tentative reports (Stetton & Hearon, 1959) of a possible correlation between serum uric acid levels and intelligence have not been clearly substantiated by subsequent study (Bland *et al.*, 1968; Stetton, 1968). Uric acid of cerebrospinal fluid, normally 2 μg./ml., has been reported to be elevated in progressive cerebral atrophy but no changes have been observed in schizophrenia or in non-progressive cerebral atrophy (Farstad *et al.*, 1965a, b).

A defect in purine metabolism, associated with a familial neurological and behavioural disorder, has been shown to involve excessive production of uric acid resulting from an accelerated rate of purine biosynthesis. Known as the "Lesch-Nyhan Syndrome", the defect is due to an absence of hypoxanthine-guanine phosphoribosyl transferase activity (HGPRT) (Nyhan *et al.*, 1967;

Seegmiller *et al.*, 1967; see Fig. 9.2). Normally the enzymic activity is higher in neural tissue than in any other (Rosenbloom *et al.*, 1967); using a highly sensitive radiochemical assay based on 8-[^{14}C]-guanine, no HGPRT could be detected in the erythrocytes from nine patients, nor in the brain or basal ganglia of one patient (Kelley, 1968).

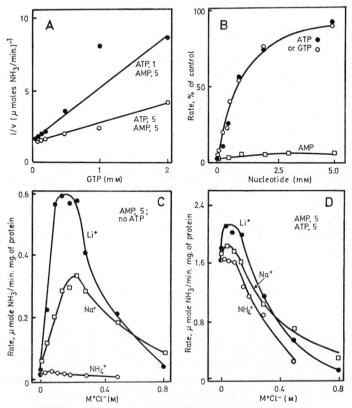

Fig. 9.4. Factors influencing brain adenylate deaminase.
    A. Dixon plots (1/v *vs.* GTP) show the kinetics of GTP inhibition of the ATP-activated enzyme.
    B. Protection against heat inactivation by ATP or GTP. The enzyme was pre-incubated at 50°C for 30 min. in the presence of ATP, GTP or 5′-AMP and then estimated for residual activity.
    C. Activation by cations, especially by Li$^+$ in the absence and in the presence (**D**) of ATP (Setlow *et al.*, 1966, 1967, 1968).
    Concentrations of nucleotides are mM.

A defect in an enzymic reaction which forms guanylic acid from guanine (and IMP from hypoxanthine) would cause a decreased formation of GMP; lack of normal levels of GMP could result in increased purine synthesis by diminished regulatory feed-back inhibition of glutamine phosphoribosyl-pyrophosphate amidotransferase, the initial step of purine synthesis. In patients suffering the defect, an associated increase in adenine phosphoribosyl-transferase (see Fig. 9.2) has also been observed. The precise cause of the neurological damage is unknown—it could be due (Sweetman, 1968) either to a decrease in an essential purine nucleotide or an increase in an unusual purine metabolite since methylated purines are known to be centrally-active.

The relationship with gout, in which overproduction of uric acid is well-characterized, is not clear. Though HGPRT activity is partly deficient in some patients suffering from gout, it is normal in others.

Cyclic AMP and Cyclic GMP

Interest in 3′,5′-adenosine monophosphate (cyclic AMP) came initially from the discovery by Sutherland and coworkers of its role in activation of liver glycogen phosphorylase. Since then the nucleotide has been shown to mediate many of the actions of a number of hormones in a variety of mammalian tissues (Robison et al., 1967, 1968, 1971; Breckenridge, 1970). Cerebral systems have been much investigated in this regard; collected sources of information for the following account include Costa & Greengard (1970), Rall & Gilman (1970), Robison et al. (1971) and McIlwain (1971).

When examined in cell-free preparations, the metabolism of cyclic AMP is superficially simple and can be expressed as:

$$\text{ATP} \xrightarrow{\textit{adenyl cyclase}} \text{cyclic 3′, 5′-AMP} \xrightarrow{\textit{3′, 5′-phosphodiesterase}} \text{5′-AMP}$$

The quantities of cyclic AMP in the brain under normal conditions are a few nmoles/g: that is, about one-thousandth of the concomitant ATP. This is in keeping with the relatively small capacity of *adenyl cyclase*, which in preparations from the brain of a number of mammals forms cyclic AMP at rates of 1–4 μmoles/g. tissue/hr. For reaction to occur at these rates, about 1 mM-ATP is required; at 0·1 mM-ATP, formation is diminished. The brain has been found to contain the highest adenyl cyclase activity of many mammalian tissues examined; the cerebral enzyme occurs almost exclusively in association with particulate matter, especially subfractions rich in nerve endings (q.v.) (Sutherland et al., 1962; de Robertis et al., 1967; Weiss & Costa, 1968).

The various neurohumoral agents which can cause major increases in the cyclic AMP content of cell-containing cerebral preparations are described below; these affect the adenyl cyclase of broken cell preparations to a smaller extent. In the cell-free systems, cyclic AMP accumulates only if methylxanthines or related compounds are added to prevent breakdown by *3′, 5′-phosphodiesterase*. Cyclic nucleotides are not affected by several other phosphatases; the specific phosphodiesterase activities are of high potency in cerebral preparations and are capable of hydrolysing 2–2·5 mmoles of cyclic AMP/g. tissue/hr. The mammalian cerebral cortex was the most potent of some 20 tissues examined and required Mg^{2+} for activity. Relatively high concentrations of cyclic AMP, approximating to 1–2 mM, were also needed to attain the high rates quoted; at normal levels of cyclic AMP rates were much lower: 10 nmoles/g.hr. when cyclic AMP was at 5·5 μM. The K_m of the enzyme, which was soluble and apparently of cytoplasmic origin, was about 0·1–0·3 mM. Its ability to inactivate cyclic AMP was limited also by its susceptibility to inhibition by ATP (half-maximal at 1 mM-ATP), by other nucleotide triphosphates and by inorganic pyrophosphate.

An endogenous activator of the phosphodiesterase was revealed in cerebral preparations during the course of enzyme purification. The purified phosphodiesterase showed marked decrease in activity after removal of the activator, which proved to be protein of molecular weight about 40,000. Re-addition of the activator to the purified enzyme increased activity in a linear fashion

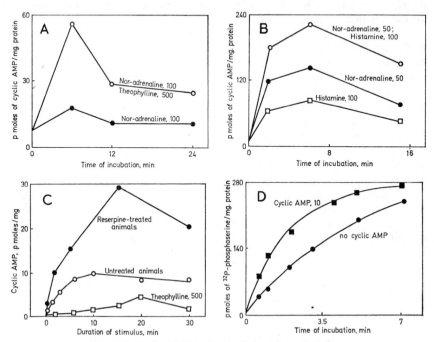

FIG. 9.5. Cyclic AMP and preparations from the brain.
A. Effect of noradrenaline and theophylline on accumulation of cyclic AMP in rabbit cerebellum. The chopped tissue was incubated in glucose-bicarbonate for 42 min. before addition of the agents shown.
B. Effect of noradrenaline and histamine, singly or together, on accumulation of cyclic AMP under the conditions of A (Kakiuchi & Rall, 1968) with theophylline.
C. Increase of cyclic AMP in slices from cerebral cortex with electrical stimulation. Electrical pulses were applied for varying periods after an incubation period of 50 min. in glucose-bicarbonate. Animals treated with reserpine were injected with 0·5 mg./kg. and 2 mg./kg., 44 hr. and 20 hr. respectively, before death (Kakiuchi et al., 1969).
D. Activation of cerebral protein kinase by cyclic AMP. A preparation of synaptosome membranes from ox cerebral cortex was incubated in Tris-HCl with 1 mM-γ-^{32}P-MgATP in the presence or absence of 10 μM cyclic AMP (Weller & Rodnight, 1970).
All concentrations of agents shown are μM.

suggesting a stoichiometric relation between them; a lowered K_m for cyclic AMP resulted. Kinetic examination of the original rat brain enzyme, using a sensitive radioassay, indicated the occurrence of second phosphodiesterase activity with a lower K_m for cyclic AMP of about 1 μM. At present only the kinetic evidence for its occurrence is available; whether it is a type of phosphodiesterase distinct from the enzyme of higher K_m or whether it reflects a different state of activation of the same enzyme requires further study (Butcher and Sutherland, 1962; de Robertis *et al.*, 1967; Weiss and Costa, 1968; Honda and Imamura, 1968; Brooker *et al.*, 1968; Cheung, 1967, 1970).

The role of cyclic AMP in cerebral tissues appears to be consistent with the "second messenger" concept of Sutherland *et al.* (1965). It is possible that many, if not all, of the actions of cyclic AMP are mediated through protein kinase reactions; the brain is one of the most active tissues in histone kinase activation by cyclic AMP (Kuo & Greengard, 1969) and a specific membrane-bound protein kinase in the brain is stimulated by the nucleotide (Weller & Rodnight, 1970; **D**, Fig. 9.5). Indeed cyclic AMP is unusual energetically: calorimetric measurement of the enthalpy of hydrolysis of its 3' bond gave a value of -14 kcal/mole, which is close to the calculated value of -12 kcal/mole (Greengard *et al.*, 1969). It has been suggested that this energy might be necessary for activation by the cyclic nucleotide of the protein kinases, although as far as is known, cyclic AMP is not consumed during its action as a catalyst in phosphorylation processes. Its importance has been noted in histones, which may condition genetic expression (below) and also in carbohydrate metabolism, which received comment in Chapter 5.

3'-5'-Guanosine monophosphate (cyclic GMP) is also present in the brain; the level found there, 0.2 μmole/kg., was higher than in any other mammalian tissue examined. Associated with cyclic GMP is the enzyme which forms it, *guanyl cyclase*. The enzyme is soluble, in contrast to adenyl cyclase which occurs in particulate fractions. Guanyl cyclase activity in the brain (0.1 μmole/g. hr.) is considerably lower than that of adenyl cyclase (1.3 μmoles/g. hr.) but is higher than most mammalian tissues; only lung contained more. The enzyme has an apparent K_m for GTP of 0.02 to 0.1 mM and for Mn^{2+}, 0.5 mM (Goldberg *et al.*, 1969; Hardman & Sutherland, 1969).

Cyclic AMP and cellular regions of the brain

In the brain *in vivo* or in isolated tissues from it, the level and the turnover of cyclic AMP are greatly affected by factors which often have little or no action on the isolated enzymes just described. These factors include (i) neural and electrical excitation; (ii) other agents which modify the Na^+ and K^+ content and membrane potential of tissue cells: e.g. ouabain, 40 mM-K^+ or veratrine; (iii) adenosine and some related compounds and (iv) neurohumoral agents especially noradrenaline, histamine and serotonin.

The cyclic AMP of isolated cerebral tissues under normal metabolic conditions was close to the value of 1–2 nmoles/g. tissue found *in situ*. Electrical excitation greatly increased this value (**C**, Fig. 9.5). This increase was not due only to liberation of the neurohumoral agents (iv), though this liberation occurred concomitantly (see Chapter 14). Excitation in the presence of added noradrenaline caused still greater increase; and, also, the increase induced electrically was diminished by the further addition of 0.5 mM-theophylline (**A** and **B**, Fig. 9.5) (Klainer *et al.*, 1962; Kakiuchi and Rall, 1968; Kakiuchi *et al.*, 1969; Krishna *et al.* 1969; Shimizu *et al.*, 1970).

Fractionation of cerebral extracts led however to characterization of an endogenous constituent which when added to incubating tissues increased their cyclic AMP by a process augmented by noradrenaline and inhibited by theophylline. This constituent was adenosine itself. With the addition of 0·125 mM-adenosine, the cyclic AMP of incubating neocortical tissues could rise to 30 nmoles/g. within a few minutes; on transferring such tissues to adenosine-free media their cyclic AMP fell and the rates and properties of the two changes suggested them to operate through adenyl cyclase and the phosphodiesterases. After using [8-^{14}C]-adenosine and isolating both ATP and cyclic AMP from the tissue, the specific activities of these nucleotides were consistent with the cyclic AMP being derived from ATP, its normal precursor. However, the conversion of ^{14}C-ATP derived from ^{14}C-adenosine (and also, in parallel experiments, from ^{14}C-adenine), into ^{14}C-cyclic AMP proved to have an unexpectedly high efficiency. Up to 20–40% of the ^{14}C-ATP could yield ^{14}C-cyclic AMP. The cyclic AMP resulting was at about 30 nmoles/g., and thus the precursor pool of ATP was about 0·1 μmoles/g., or about 5% of the tissue's total ATP. The uptake of adenosine, and to an even greater extent that of adenine, were thus to quite limited regions of the tissue.

To obtain the high yields of ^{14}C-AMP which have been quoted, cortical tissues were treated with agents in categories (ii) and (iv), above: in particular, with 40 mM-K$^+$ and noradrenaline. These agents presumably mimic the depolarization and transmitter release which accompany excitation *in vivo*, and act by modifying the membrane-sited adenyl cyclase so that it more effectively acts on ATP. Adenosine may in part have such an action though this is not proven; it certainly acts as actual precursor for cyclic AMP, and does so through forming ATP. As this formation is in a limited region it may be associated with a sufficient increase in ATP concentration there, to explain the increased tissue concentration of cyclic AMP. Electrical stimulation releases from a given neocortical sample both adenosine and related compounds (iii, above) and the neurohumoral agents (iv). This is an association reminiscent of the joint release of adrenaline and 5′-AMP from the adrenal on its excitation. With neocortical tissues, release of compounds (iii) and (iv) is presumably presynaptic and their action in augmenting cyclic AMP, postsynaptic (Shimizu and Daly, 1970; Shimizu *et al.*, 1961, 1970; Pull and McIlwain, 1971; McIlwain, 1971).

Regulation of Purine Nucleotide Levels

Adenylate deaminase activity provides IMP for subsequent synthesis of guanyl compounds and requires ATP specifically as activator. GTP inhibition of the ATP-activated reaction provides a mechanism for the metabolic regulation of guanine nucleotide levels according to the relative concentrations of ATP and GTP present. Concentrations of 5′-AMP may be regulated in two ways by ATP: by activation of 5′-AMP deamination and also by the competitive inhibition of 5′-nucleotidase discussed above, which would tend to prevent breakdown of 5′-AMP to adenosine and inorganic phosphate. The involvement of orthophosphate in reversing ATP inhibition of the nucleotidase should also be noted. These interactions are therefore of relevance to mechanisms by which the relative balance of adenine and guanine nucleotides may be maintained or adjusted in the brain (Fig. 9.6).

Regulation specifically of ATP is conditioned by a variety of interactions, including individual stages of glycolysis and respiration and also the reactions catalysed by creatine phosphokinase and Na^+,K^+-ATPase which received comment in preceding Chapters. Regulation of adenine nucleotides may also depend on the following reaction, catalysed by *adenylate kinase* (myokinase, EC 2.7.4.3).

$$ATP + 5'-AMP \rightleftharpoons 2 ADP$$

Problems arise in studying this enzyme since the activity is difficult to distinguish experimentally from Na^+,K^+-ATPase and ATP-ADP exchange reactions. Early attempts to measure activity were based on spectrophotometric assay of ATP production from ADP using excess hexokinase in a

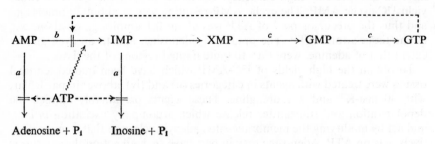

Fig. 9.6. Factors involved in regulation of purine nucleotide levels in the brain.
  a. 5'-Nucleotidase, inhibited by ATP.
  b. Adenylate deaminase, activated by ATP and inhibited by GTP.
  c. Reactions requiring ATP (see Fig. 9.2).

coupled reaction (Smillie, 1957) or by use of a combined ATPase assay, when adenylate kinase was deduced by difference (Rappoport *et al.*, 1963). Negligible activity was found in cerebral nuclei but whole brain homogenates appeared to be very active. More recently, isotopic exchange between ^{14}C-AMP and ADP has been used to measure adenylate kinase activity in cerebral microsomes where rates of 30 μmoles of nucleotide converted/mg. of protein per hr. were recorded (Swanson & Stahl, 1966).

Nucleic Acids

DNA occurs as deoxyribonucleoprotein in the cellular nuclei of the brain where it is a major component of the chromosomes. A small proportion of the cerebral DNA (some 1–2% of the total DNA) is found in mitochondria (Balazs & Cocks, 1967). Estimations of the DNA content of the brain are important in affording a chemical estimate of cell numbers and are discussed in Chapter 13. Certain of the determinations are subject to interference by phosphoinositides and gangliosides; methods which avoided this gave levels of 0·92 mg/g. of calf brain and 0·7 mg/g. for adult rat brain (Zamenhof *et al.*, 1964). From histochemical studies on the regional distribution in human brain areas, the highest concentrations of DNA were found in the calcarine cortex (4·3 μg./mg. dry weight); the lowest were in dorsal funiculi (0·92 μg./mg.)

(Landolt *et al.*, 1966). The elevated DNA levels found in rat cerebellum are of interest; it is the Purkinje neurons of human cerebellum in which tetraploid DNA has been detected (Lapham, 1968). Methods for isolation and purification of cerebral DNA have been described; the DNA was separated from various species of RNA and proved to be in a highly-polymerized state with little contamination of protein or RNA (Mori *et al.*, 1970, Oesterle *et al.*, 1970).

The regional distribution of RNA in human brain areas is similar to that of DNA. The calcarine cortex contained the highest RNA concentration (6·4 μg./mg. dry weight) and the lowest was in the dorsal funiculi (1·56 μg./mg.) (Landolt *et al.*, 1966). The RNA per cell, from the RNA/DNA ratio, was highest in the frontal cortex. Total RNA of the rat cerebral cortex has been estimated to be 0·7–0·8 mg./g. of fresh tissue (Adams, 1965). The subcellular distribution of cerebral RNA is widespread (Table 9.2), with nuclear and microsomal fractions most enriched.

Table 9.2

Subcellular distribution of RNA in rat cerebral cortex

Fraction	RNA (% of that in homogenate)			
	1	2	3	4
Nuclear	41·6	24·8	18·0⎫	24·7
Mitochondrial	17·9	17·4	16·5⎭	
Microsomal	42·2	33·9	36·3	46·6
Supernatant	5·9	24·0	21·3	16·5

Values vary according to the conditions used for subcellular fractionation: [1] Aldridge & Johnson (1959); [2] Barkowski *et al.* (1961); [3] Balazs & Cocks (1967); [4] Adams (1965).

The decreases in RNA content of the brain which occur during maturation are discussed in Chapter 13.

Ribonucleoprotein of the Ribosomes

Ribonucleoprotein particles have been separated from cerebral microsomal fractions by treatment with deoxycholate, which disperses away the associated membrane structures, or by the use of EDTA which detaches the granules from the membranes (Hanzon & Toschi, 1959; Datta & Ghosh, 1963; Yamagami *et al.*, 1963). The polydisperse particles contain 30% of their dry weight as RNA; no DNA, lipid or hexose derivatives were detected but phosphomonoesterase and ribonuclease activities were present. The phospho-monoesterase proved to be tightly-bound to the purified ribosomes and catalysed the hydrolysis of nitrophenol phosphate esters at rates of 7·5 μmoles/ g.hr. Phosphodiesterase activity, also tightly bound, was estimated to occur at 1 μmole/g.hr. The preponderant phosphodiesterase exhibited an alkaline pH optimum and was less stable to heat than the acid phosphodiesterase. Attempts to solubilize the activities were unsuccessful so no separation of the two was achieved (Datta *et al.*, 1969a). The proteins of the ribosomes not only carry the enzymic activities just described but may also be associated with ribosomal stability. Spermidine and spermine have been detected in purified ribosomes; when added to the separated particles, these bases also gave significant protection against heat and against enzymic degradation (Datta *et al.*, 1969b).

Spermine (4 nmol/mg. of protein) was found to be the preponderant poly-amine of microsomal preparations from rat cerebral cortex; spermidine was also present (1·2 nmole/mg.). At concentrations equivalent to these, spermine and spermidine each gave over 200 % stimulation of ^{14}C-valine incorporation into the protein of the microsomes, incubated *in vitro* with the pH 5 enzyme fraction (q.v.). At higher concentrations (10- to 100-fold), these bases caused inhibition of the incorporation. Spermine also increased the rate, but not the extent, of formation of amino-acyl transfer-RNA in the pH 5 enzyme fraction. Although spermine and spermidine also occur in the cytoplasmic fraction, the main site of action of the polyamines was concluded to be at the microsomes (Giorgi, 1970).

Table 9.3

Proportion of nucleotides in ribosomal RNA from the brain

Source of RNA	GMP	CMP	AMP	UMP	$\dfrac{G+C}{A+U}$
Rat brain polysomes[1]	31·6	28·6	18·0	21·8	1·51
Rat brain microsomes[2]	29·6	29·7	20·8	19·8	1·46
Mouse brain ribosomes[3]	32·4	27·2	18·7	21·8	1·48
Goat brain ribosomes[4]	32·6	30·3	22·7	14·6	1·68
Human globus pallidus ribosomes[5]	29·1	33·7	19·0	18·2	1·69

Values are expressed as percentage of each nucleotide in RNA: [1] Jacob *et al.* (1966); [2] Balazs & Cocks (1967); [3] Kimberlin (1967); [4] Datta & Ghosh (1963); [5] Hydén (1963).

Nucleotide composition of cerebral ribosomes from a variety of species was similar (Table 9.3) and of the order of GMP 31 %, CMP 30 %, AMP 20 % and UMP 19 %. The ratio $(G + C)/(A + U)$ for brain ribosomal RNA was close to 1·6, which is higher than the ratios reported for other RNA species of the brain, or the ratio $(G + C)/(A + T)$ for DNA (see below and Table 9.4).

Ribosomal protein synthesis in the brain, as in other tissues, has been shown to occur preferentially in *polyribosomes* (Murphy, 1966; Campagnoni & Mahler, 1967; Jacob *et al.*, 1967) and is discussed subsequently. Preparation of undissociated polyribosomes ideally requires techniques which avoid the use of detergents. Even with mild deoxycholate treatment only, about 20 % of the total ribosomal population of post-mitochondrial fractions is in monomer form. *In vivo* the proportion is conceivably considerably less than 20 % as the experimental conditions are thought to be more likely to cause disruption of polyribosomes rather than aggregation of monomers. The polyribosomes occur as aggregates of 80S monomer particles probably linked by RNA chains. Partial separation of rat cerebral cortex polyribosomes according to size was achieved using sucrose density–gradient centrifugation. Sizes ranged from $S_{20,w}^0$ values of 76–238 with the majority in the 100–125 region (Campagnoni & Mahler, 1967; Jacob et al., 1967). Electron microscopy showed occurrence of clusters, mainly consisting of four to five ribosomes, but much larger clusters have also been observed in separated preparations from rat brain and in neurons of rabbit Deiter's nuclei (Ekholm & Hydén, 1965; Campagnoni & Mahler, 1967).

The number of polysomes, relatively high in rat brain at birth, declines slowly during development (Murthy, 1966) in contrast to the liver in which the number, relatively small at birth, increases with development. This, as will be seen later, has been correlated with changes in rates of protein and nucleic acid turnover. The proportion of polyribosomes and monoribosomes found at any one time may depend on the functional state of the tissue. Convulsions produced by methionine sulphoximine or by electroshock were found to cause disaggregation of polyribosomes (Vesco & Giuditta, 1968; Sellinger & Azcurra, 1970). Study of the time course of electroshock showed a decrease in the number of polyribosomes during the first 15 min. and an increase over the following 15–30 min. (MacInnes et al., 1970). The number of polyribosomes in the brain stem and rates of RNA synthesis were decreased after hypophysectomy (Gispen et al., 1970). External stimuli may also affect the polyribosomes: the number in the occipital cortex, but not in the liver, decreased when rats were deprived of light for 3 days and increased after the animals had been exposed to light. In view of the known role of messenger RNA (q.v.) in polyribosome aggregation in other systems, the authors suggested that the changes in numbers of polyribosomes may reflect changes in amounts of messenger RNA; similar changes in rates of incorporation of amino acids to the polyribosomal protein were observed (Appel et al., 1967).

Identification of RNA Species

The types of RNA which have been detected in mammalian cerebral tissues are summarized in Table 9.4. A major effort in studies on cerebral RNA metabolism has been on attempts to characterize different RNA types, in particular to detect and distinguish messenger RNA from precursors of ribosomal RNA. Evidence for sub-ribosomal particles or ribosome precursors of 35S and 45S has been obtained in a number of laboratories. Difficulties in such studies arise from the changes in size of RNA likely to occur as a result of extraction of the RNA from ribonucleoprotein particles. Aggregation of low molecular weight RNA molecules as well as degradation of ribosomal RNA to smaller species is possible; changes may also occur according to the functional state of the tissue.

To date, messenger RNA has not been isolated and purified from the brain, but its existence and certain of its properties have been inferred. Total RNA has been extracted from nuclear or cytoplasmic ribonucleoprotein fractions using phenol-sodium dodecylsulphate-8-hydroxyquinoline mixtures. Kimberlin (1967) found hot extraction advantageous and used at 70–75°C a mixture of

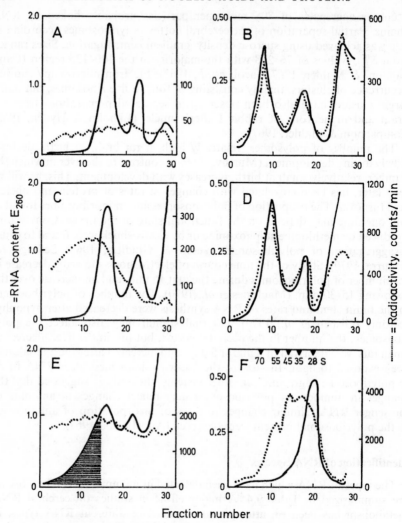

FIG. 9.7. Separation of cerebral RNA species on sucrose density
gradients.

Microsomal or nuclear RNA was isolated and purified after incorporation of labelled precursor for 30 min. or 18 hr. Species of RNA were
separated on gradients of 5–20% sucrose containing 100 mM sodium
chloride and 10 mM sodium acetate at pH 5. The curves show the RNA
(———) and radioactivity (----) in fractions obtained after centrifugation
for 13–15 hr. The heavier RNA populations are to the left, with lower
fraction numbers (Vesco & Giuditta, 1967).

A. Microsomal RNA after 30 min. incorporation of ^{14}C-orotate was
found labelled in polydisperse populations including those heavier than
28S. The heavier fractions had DNA-like base ratios: $(G + C)/
(A + U) = 0.96$, and were found to stimulate valine incorporation into
protein in cell free systems.

B. Microsomal RNA as in A, after 18 hr. incorporation. Labelling
then coincides with peaks of 28S and 18S ribosomal RNA and also of
soluble RNA.

0·5% dodecylsulphate and 0·1% 8-hydroxyquinoline in 90% phenol. Use has also been made of the LiCl technique for separating soluble RNA (Barlow *et al.*, 1963). Different RNA populations have been partially separated by sucrose density-gradient centrifugation of the extracts (Fig. 9.7) and populations of messenger RNA have been suggested on a basis of relative rapidity of isotopic labelling, polydispersity, sedimentation rates, base composition ratios and stimulation of protein synthesis (described below). Species of 18S

Table 9.4

RNA species detected in mammalian brain

Type of RNA	Size*	Base ratio $\left(\dfrac{G + C}{A + U}\right)$
(1) Ribonucleoprotein from:		
Polysomes (containing an average of 4 to 6 ribosomes)	100–170S	1·5–1·6
Monoribosomes	76–80S	1·5–1·6
Ribosomal precursors	35S, 45S	
(2) Ribonucleic acid from:		
Ribosomal RNA	18S	1·3
	28S	1·8
Messenger RNA	Polydisperse (usually >28S)	0·9

* $S_{20,w}^{0}$ values are quoted. No transfer RNA (approx. 4S in size in other mammalian tissues) has so far been fully characterized.

and 28S have been identified in ribosomal RNA extracted from sub-ribosomal particles (Table 9.4; Jacob *et al.*, 1966; Dawson, 1967; Vesco & Giuditta, 1967; Schneider & Roberts, 1968). The separated RNA species contained $(G + C)/(A + U)$ base ratios of 1·34 for the 18S and 1·82 for the 28S, in comparison to ratios of 1·5–1·6 for total unfractionated ribosomal RNA. Electrophoretic separation of cytoplasmic RNA extracted from rat brain resulted in detection of 4S RNA, in addition to 18S and 28S, which were present in equal amounts. Transfer RNA of other mammalian tissues is

FIG. 9.7.—*cont.*

C. Nuclear RNA, after 30 min. incorporation of ^{14}C-orotate, was labelled mainly in populations of size greater than 28S.

D. Nuclear RNA as in C, after 18 hr. incorporation. The distribution was similar to that of the microsomal RNA (B) in that label appeared in 28S, 18S and soluble RNA.

E. Nuclear RNA after 30 min. incorporation of ^{32}P-orthophosphate. The populations labelled were polydisperse; those of the shaded area were examined further in F.

F. Nuclear RNA populations from E were re-centrifuged in density gradients of 25–42% sucrose. Label was mainly in 45S and 35S populations, thought to be ribosomal RNA precursors (see text). Fractions above 45S in size had base ratios similar to those for DNA: $(G + C)/(A + U) = 1·05$.

considered to be about 4S but clear identification of the 4S fraction with transfer RNA in the cerebral cortex has not been described (Tencheva & Hadjiolov, 1969). Convincing evidence for the occurrence of one species of transfer RNA has been reported; a ^{14}C-valyl RNA was separated by chromatography on methylalbumin-coated kieselguhr columns after incubation of cerebral extracts with ^{14}C-valine (Dellweg et al., 1968). Many specific transfer RNA molecules have been isolated from non-neural systems and their primary structure determined. For a discussion of structure and function of these, see Philipps (1969) and Levitt (1969).

A further species of RNA in rat brain has been described. The total nucleic acids were prepared from the brain, frozen in situ, by a combination of cold and hot extraction with phenol-8-hydroxyquinoline-dodecylsulphate reagents and precipitation with 1·5 M-NaCl. Chromatography of the extracts gave five separate fractions in a highly-purified state, one of DNA and four of RNA. One of the RNA fractions exhibited properties, not previously described, which indicated that it was distinct from messenger RNA, transfer RNA or or ribosomal RNA. The new fraction was of high molecular weight, and its solubility in 1·5 M-NaCl was taken as evidence of a double-stranded, possibly helical, structure. It accounted for some 30% of the total cerebral RNA and analysis of its base composition showed a high guanine content. The base ratio $(G + C)/(A + U)$ of 1·59 was similar to the ratio found for ribosomal RNA (1·60) in the extracts (see also Table 9·5) but expressed as $(A + G)/(C + U)$, the ratio was higher in the new RNA (1·21) than in the ribosomal RNA (1·11). The origin of this RNA is uncertain but its properties suggested occurrence in the nucleus (Oesterle et al. 1970).

Axonal RNA

RNA occurs in very low concentrations in nerve axons but the total RNA of the nerve cell processes exceeds that of the perikarya. The axons of the giant Mauthner neurons in young goldfish contained concentrations some 2·5% of that in the cell bodies but the total axonal RNA was estimated to be about four times the total present in the perikarya (Edström et al., 1962). Considerably lower RNA concentrations were found in adult cat peripheral nerve: 80–225 pg./10 cm. length, which was equivalent to 0·1–0·2% of the cell body concentration (Koenig, 1965). The differences between the two studies may have been due to variations in age or in the species studied. Axonal RNA was concluded to be of ribosomal type from nucleotide analysis; due to difficulties encountered in pyrimidine analysis, the purine ratio (A/G) was used to indicate the RNA type. For sciatic nerve axonal RNA, the A/G ratio was 0·47 for axoplasmic RNA and 0·55 for myelin sheath RNA (Edström, 1964). The ratios are closer to those for ribosomal RNA (0·58) than for "messenger" RNA (0·96) or DNA (1·08). These results do not exclude the possibility that messenger RNA also is present in the axon; difficulties of isolation, separation and analysis in such studies are great but the conclusion drawn was that axonal RNA is essentially of ribosomal type. The RNA extracted from axons exhibited properties indicative of the presence of at least two populations: ribonuclease-digestible and ribonuclease-resistant; 85–96% of the total RNA labelled from

[3]H-adenine or ^{3}H-orotate was present in the ribonuclease-resistant RNA, an incorporation which was sensitive to actinomycin D (Koenig, 1967).

Such evidence for axonal ribosomal RNA poses problems since electron microscopists have failed to detect ribosomes in axons (Pick *et al.*, 1964; Palay & Palade, 1965; van Breeman *et al.*, 1958). The possibility that the axonal RNA which has been described is due to RNA of axonal mitochondria is at present difficult to assess; this is discussed below in the section on protein synthesis.

Metabolism of Nucleic Acids

Changes in the deoxyribonucleic acid content of the brain during development are described in Chapter 13. DNA synthesis is a prerequisite for cell duplication which does not occur in the differentiated neurons of the adult brain. Cell maintenance but not replication would be expected to be associated with metabolic stability of neuronal DNA, which is observed in incorporation studies using ^{3}H-thymidine: autoradiographic examination of cerebral tissues of the cat after intraventricular injection of the precursor showed it to be incorporated mainly into glial cell nuclei (Altman & Chorover, 1963). However, autoradiographic studies have shown post-natal formation of new neurons (neurogenesis) to continue in various regions of the brain, especially in the granular layer of the cerebellum (Altman, 1969).

Rapid labelling of neurons, formed by proliferation of undifferentiated cells, occurs in mouse foetuses after administration of ^{3}H-thymidine; the isotope was detected in the pyramidal cells of layers V and VI of the cortex and in Purkinje neurons of the cerebellum (Gavriovla, 1968). DNA formation in the immature central nervous system may depend on dietary factors; the DNA content of neonatal brain cells has been reported to be decreased if protein in the maternal diet was restricted to 8% throughout gestation (Zamenhof *et al.*, 1968). Levels of DNA, and of RNA, have been shown to increase rapidly in Schwann cells associated with regenerating peripheral nerve (Oderfeld & Niemierko, 1969).

Deoxyribonuclease occurs in the brain in two forms which differ in pH optima and have been separated by ammonium sulphate fractionation (Sung, 1968). One form had an optimum pH of 5·0 and acted preferentially on native DNA. The second form exhibited optimal activity between pH 7·4 and 8·9 and acted preferentially on heat-denatured DNA. The two forms of the enzyme differed also in the Mg^{2+} required for maximum activity.

Ribonucleic Acid Synthesis

The synthesis of RNA in brain cell nuclei (Fig. 9.8) is catalyzed by *DNA-dependent RNA polymerase* in similar fashion to that established for the more extensively-studied microbial systems. The enzyme, similar in properties in rat, rabbit and monkey brain, was shown to be more active in immature than in adult brain and more active in grey matter than in white. In the adult mammalian brain the polymerase exhibits activity at levels similar to those found in the liver of the same animals (Barondes, 1964; Bondy & Waelsch, 1965).

Brain nuclear RNA-polymerase has a pH optimum of 8·0, requires all four nucleotides for activity and is inhibited by actinomycin D or by pretreatment with deoxyribonuclease. Dependence on the presence of spermidine and of an ATP-generating system has been demonstrated and maximum activity requires Mg^{2+} and K^+, which were not satisfactorily replaced by Mn^{2+} and Na^+ respectively. High ionic strength of incubation media caused decrease in activity of the enzyme. Rates observed for the cerebral cortex were: for UTP incorporation, 135–242 pmoles/min. per mg. of DNA and for ATP incorporation, 156–308 pmoles/min. per mg. of DNA (Bondy & Waelsch, 1965; Dutton & Mahler, 1968).

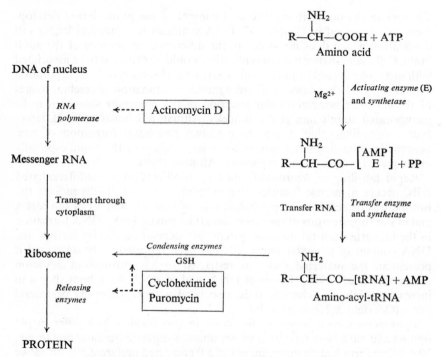

FIG. 9.8. Nucleic acids and ribosomal protein synthesis. Broken arrows indicate sites of action of inhibitors.

Increase in quantity of RNA, active in the developing brain, does not seem to occur in the adult tissue although the RNA continues to turn over rapidly. Net synthesis of cerebral RNA ceases at about the same stage as does that of DNA (18 days of age in the rat). The RNA content of the cerebral cortex is then about 0·6 mg./g. fresh weight of cortex. Thereafter the RNA content decreases to an eventual level of 0·3–0·4 mg./g.; the DNA content remains constant (Adams, 1966). The decrease in RNA is probably correlated with the decline in the number of polysomes (q.v.) seen during development (Murthy, 1966). RNA synthesis has been studied using ¹⁴C- or ³H-labelled purine or pyrimidine precursors and ³²P-labelled inorganic orthophosphate. Use of the latter has been concluded to be less specific because non-RNA constituents of isolated ribosomes may also be labelled with ^{32}P. The rate of ^{14}C-orotate incorporation into rat brain RNA was 5 times more rapid than that of ^{14}C-uracil (Adams, 1965), thus emphasizing the care that needs to be exercised in comparison of rates observed using different precursors even if other conditions seem comparable, and especially if endogenous levels of precursor are not measured.

Incorporation of UMP and dihydro-UMP into microsomal RNA *in vitro* required an ATP-generating system, was inhibited by orthophosphate, by pyrophosphate or by pretreatment with ribonuclease (Carr & Grisolia, 1964). Comparison with non-neural tissues showed the brain to be very active in RNA synthesis; about 25% of uridylic acid residues were concluded to be labelled from UMP within 5 min. and rates of UMP incorporation into RNA were estimated to be 13–45 mμmoles/min. per mg. of RNA in rat and ox brain. Soluble RNA was labelled more rapidly than microsomal RNA. Migration of labelled RNA from the nucleus to the cytoplasm was followed by autoradiography of mouse and kitten brain after administration of ^{3}H-uridine. The rates of migration were similar for different types of neuron (Shimada & Nakamura, 1966). In this study, subcutaneous injection of precursor was more satisfactory than the intracerebral route, after which very limited penetration was observed. Altman & Chorover (1963) also reported isotopic penetration to be localized when ^{3}H-adenine, ^{3}H-uracil or ^{3}H-thymidine were injected intraventricularly. Autoradiographic examination showed the labelled precursors to diffuse by ventricular as well as by subarachnoid routes; diffusion by both routes was sluggish and variable.

Categories of Cerebral RNA

Turnover times for *ribosomal RNA* estimated as a result of *in vivo* studies vary from less than 1 day (^{3}H-uridine incorporation into mouse brain ribosomes; Kimberlin, 1967) to 6 days (^{14}C-orotate incorporation into rat brain microsomes; Dawson, 1967). The RNA extracted had base ratios $(G + C)/(A + U)$ of 1·5–1·6 (Tables 9.3 and 9.5). Attempts to distinguish ribosome precursors during short time incorporation studies in rabbit brain *in vivo* were based on the sedimentation properties of the nuclear and cytoplasmic RNA populations labelled at different times (Fig. 9.8). The label appeared first in RNA of sub-ribosomal particles or ribosome precursors, possibly of 35S to 45S in size, and subsequently in polysomal RNA. Free ribosome monomers (80S) were labelled last and led to the suggestion that free monomeric ribosomes arise from degradation of polysome aggregates rather than as intermediates in polysome formation from sub-ribosomal precursors (Vesco & Giuditta, 1967; Dutton *et al.*, 1969).

Turnover times for the rapidly-labelled RNA suggested to be *messenger RNA* are of the order of $\frac{1}{2}$-2 hr. (Jacob *et al.*, 1966, 1967; Kimberlin, 1967; Singh, 1965) although some evidence for a slightly more stable population of messenger RNA with a half-life of 10–12 hr. has also been suggested (Appel, 1967). Jacob *et al.* (1967) calculated that 80% of the total RNA labelled within the first hour was messenger; at 2 hr. the proportion was slightly less, at 70%.

Synthesis of the rapidly-labelled RNA was inhibited by actinomycin D. Its identity as messenger RNA was suggested by the base ratio; $(G + C)/(A + U)$ was about 0·9 (Table 9.5) compared with 1·5 for ribosomal RNA. The ratio of 0·9 is closer to the $(G + C)/(A + T)$ ratio for DNA of 0·7 (Table 9.5) and to the ratio of 0·75 found for liver DNA (Hoyer et al., 1963). Further support for the identity of this RNA as messenger RNA came from hydridization studies of the rapidly-labelled RNA with homologous DNA (Jacob et al., 1967; Bondy & Roberts, 1967, 1968).

Table 9.5

Nucleotide base ratios of RNA species from the brain

Source of RNA	Type* of RNA	GMP	CMP	AMP	UMP	Base ratio $\left(\dfrac{G + C}{A + U}\right)$
Rat brain[1]	mRNA	22·4	24·7	24·5	28·5	0·89
	rRNA	31·6	28·6	18·0	21·8	1·51
Mouse brain[2]	mRNA	26·9	20·9	21·9	30·2	0·92
	rRNA	32·4	27·2	18·7	21·8	1·48
Rat cerebral cortex[3]	rRNA (18S)	31·4	25·8	19·8	22·9	1·34
	rRNA (28S)	36·0	28·9	16·6	19·0	1·82
Rat brain[1]	DNA	21·5	20·0	29·1	29·4	0·71

* mRNA: proposed messenger RNA (see text); rRNA: ribosomal RNA. It should be noted that DNA contains thymine (T) in place of uracil (U). [1] Jacob et al. (1966). [2] Kimberlin (1967). [3] Schneider & Roberts (1968).
Values are expressed as percentage of each nucleotide in RNA (or DNA).

Part of the labelled RNA is degraded very rapidly after administration of actinomycin D: the half-life of $\frac{1}{2}$–4 hr. was similar to the half-life of messenger RNA observed *in vivo* and was taken to indicate that a population of messenger RNA was involved (Appel, 1967; Cain, 1967). The half-life (1 hr.) of the rapidly-degraded, high-molecular-weight RNA of the cytoplasm was only slightly longer than that of the nuclear RNA (20–30 min.) (Singh, 1965). It should be noted that the RNA of ribosome precursors may also be labelled within the first hour. However, the base ratios and the polydispersity can be regarded as evidence for a population of labile messenger RNA in the brain with a turnover time of $\frac{1}{2}$–2 hr.

Careful attempts to distinguish between rapidly-labelled messenger RNA and precursors of ribosomal RNA have proved more difficult than with more rapidly-dividing or neoplastic cells such as microorganisms, Hela cells or tumour cells. The absence of comparably clear evidence of 35S or 45S precursors of ribosomal RNA in rapidly-labelled fractions of cerebral nuclear RNA (Dutton et al., 1969) led to the suggestion that 35S and 45S material may not accumulate in the nucleus due to a very rapid turnover rate of the ribosomal precursors. It was calculated that synthesis of messenger RNA might occur at three times the rate of precursor ribosomal RNA synthesis.

Since the isolation of characteristic messenger RNA has not proved possible so far, the evidence for its presence has been based on certain of the properties of the rapidly-labelled species; included in these has been observation of the stimulatory activity of cerebral nuclear RNA on cerebral ribosomal protein synthesis (q.v.). The view that protein synthesis in the brain is more active than in certain other tissues received support from the observation that the RNA fractions derived from rat brain nuclei were more active in this regard than those from the liver. By the use of various ^{14}C-labelled amino acids and analysis of the labelled peptide fractions insolated from cerebral ribosomes, the RNA-stimulated incorporation into protein was concluded to be qualitatively as well as quantitatively different from the incorporation in the absence of added nuclear RNA and was taken to provide further evidence for the presence of messenger RNA in the nuclear RNA (Bondy & Roberts, 1967, 1968). The $(G + C)/(A + U)$ ratios of the nuclear RNA, together with hybridization studies, suggested that a higher proportion of messenger RNA was present in cerebral than in liver nuclear RNA.

RNA methylase occurs in the soluble cytoplasm of rat and kitten brain in association with soluble RNA. The enzyme was separated into three types by chromatography on hydroxyapatite columns. The enzymes were purified 25-fold and differed in pH optima. RNA methylase activity was found to be eight times more active in foetal than in adult brain. Using S-adenosyl-L-^{14}C-methionine as donor, the purified enzyme from adult brain methylated RNA from bacterial methyl-deficient mutants but showed only slight activity in methylating homologous soluble RNA from rat brain. It was concluded that the RNA is fully methylated in adult brain and so cannot be methylated further (Simon *et al.*, 1967). However, there is evidence that ribosomal RNA can be methylated when labelled methionine is used as the methyl donor. RNA species were separated from the brain after combined injections of ^{3}H-methyl-L-methionine and ^{14}C-uridine. RNA of ribosomal type contained both labels; the 18S-RNA was more heavily labelled than the 28S-RNA and indicated that greater methylation of the 18S species had occurred. In contrast to the ribosomal RNA, messenger RNA was concluded to be non-methylated because ^{14}C but not ^{3}H was incorporated (Saborio & Aleman, 1970).

The role of cerebral nucleic acids receives further comment in the subsequent section in this chapter on protein synthesis.

Ribonucleotide Metabolism

The precursor nucleotides required for RNA synthesis in the nucleus may be stored in the nucleus, or alternatively be made available by transport of the nucleotides from the cytoplasm to the nucleus. At present the evidence suggests that both may operate. Double-labelled (^{14}C and ^{32}P) ATP has been used to demonstrate that nucleotides can pass through the nuclear membrane without requiring prior dephosphorylation to form the nucleoside. Also, nucleotides may be stored in the nucleus as "homopolymers"; polyadenylate, polycytidylate, polyguanylate and polyuridylate are all synthesized in the nucleus. ^{32}P-Polyadenylate added to nuclear extracts is rapidly converted to labelled ATP, ADP and AMP. Mechanisms are thus available there for storage of nucleotides as homopolymers in the nucleus and for rapid release of the mononucleotides from the storage polymer (Simler *et al.*, 1967; Mandel, 1967, 1969).

Ribonucleotides are formed from RNA in the brain by the action of *ribonuclease*; two forms of the enzyme have been detected, an acid and an alkaline ribonuclease. In goat brain, the acid ribonuclease is the more active. The optimum pH is 5·4 and interaction of cations was noted. Removal of Mg^{2+} by EDTA caused increase in activity and Ca^{2+} caused inhibition (Datta *et al.*, 1965). An endogenous inhibitor of ribonuclease is present in the soluble cytoplasmic fraction of brain preparations. An acidic protein of molecular weight 60,000, it contains SH groups and is similar in these properties to an inhibitor found in the liver (Takahashi *et al.*, 1970).

Cerebral Proteins

Their multitudinous functions as enzymes, structural elements, hormones, and probably in transporting systems result in many references to proteins throughout this book. The present concern is with their more general properties as chemical substances and metabolites: the categories of protein found in the brain, and their synthesis and breakdown. Protein categories were first investigated by examining the brain as an organ, after separations no more exacting than to grey and white matter. Increasingly it is now realized that more enlightenment can come from initial division to smaller regions, or to subcellular components. The description which follows reflects these different phases of study.

Categories of Proteins Present

Proteins constitute some 40 % of the dry weight of the whole brain. Many classes of protein found elsewhere have, when sought in the brain, been found there. Others which occur in the brain may be specific to the brain, since so far they have not been detected elsewhere. Separation and characterization was initially by differential solubility, as indicated in *A*, Table 9.6, which includes a summary of earlier investigations. Maximal extraction by such procedures (often not desirable if fractionation is to follow) was examined systematically by LeBaron & Folch (1959). In parts of the brain of several species, proteins which are soluble and not deposited on centrifuging have been separated into some fifteen fractions differing in mobility on electrophoresis or on chromatography (Bailey & Heald, 1961; Bondy & Perry, 1963). These methods have shown the brain in four mammalian species to carry soluble proteins not found in the liver of the same species; in general the cerebral extracts contained a greater proportion of acidic proteins than did those from the liver (Moore & McGregor, 1965).

Many of the fractions of Table 9.6 represent materials of considerable metabolic activity. Thus the phosphorus of cerebral phosphoproteins, characterized by lability to alkali, can undergo rapid exchange in the intact tissue (see Chapter 12). Neurokeratin, also, is very distinct from the keratins of hair or horn. Though resembling them in resistance to proteolytic enzymes, it differs in amino acid composition and has been shown, when prepared from

Table 9.6

Cerebral protein fractions

Fraction	Type of protein in fraction	% of total protein*
A. By extraction		
Soluble in barbitone, pH 8·6	Two, albumin-like[1]	15
	Three, globulin-like[1]	35
Soluble in saline	Two globulins[2], nucleoprotein[2]	–
Soluble in 4·5% KCl	Isoelectric point[3] pH 5·6	28 (g); 24 (w)
Soluble in water	Isoelectric point[3] pH 4·6	30 (g); 19(w)
Soluble in water	A phosphoprotein[4]	12
Soluble in dilute alkali	Phosphoprotein[4]	25
Insoluble in water, acid or alkali	Mixed[4]	50
Insoluble in water after treatment with pepsin and trypsin	Neurokeratin[5]	4 (g); 15 (w)
Insoluble in 0·1 N-NaOH at room temperature; soluble on autoclaving with water	Collagen[6]	3·3
Insoluble in 0·1 N-NaOH at 100°	Elastin[6]	3·5
Insoluble in water; soluble in chloroform-methanol	Proteolipids[7]	20 (g); 50 (w)
B. After dispersion in isotonic sucrose[8, 9]		
Deposited first with nuclei	Basic proteins (including histones); acidic proteins and myelin	15–20 (g)
Deposited with mitochondria (q.v.)	Wide variety of enzymes and proteins of:	35–45 (g)
	mitochondria	10–15 (g)
	nerve ending particles	15–20 (g)
	myelin	10–15 (g)
Deposited with microsomes	Partly soluble in detergents and separable to many fractions	15–20 (g)
Not deposited	Wide variety of enzymes and proteins separable by electrophoresis; acidic proteins; much globulin	25–30 (g)

* Of whole brain unless indicated: (g), of grey matter; (w), of white.
[1] Robertson (1957); this separation was by electrophoresis, and those following by solubility. [2] Halliburton (1894). [3] Palladin (1949). [4] McGregor (1916–17); Logan, Mannell & Rossiter (1952). [5] Kuhne & Chittenden (1890). [6] Lowry, Gilligan & Katersky (1941). [7] Folch & Lees (1951). [8] McIlwain & Rodnight (1962); see also Chapter 12 of the present book. [9] Bondy & Perry (1963); De Robertis *et al.* (1962, 1963).

the tissue by milder methods, to be part of more complex substances: (a) of the proteolipids described below and (b) of a complex containing inositol phosphate (LeBaron & Folch, 1956). The collagen and elastin on the other hand appear to be similar to those found in the structural elements of other organs and to be associated in the brain with blood vessels.

The brain is unusual among organs in its content of proteins which can be extracted from the fresh tissue by chloroform–methanol mixtures. Such proteins are found to be in association with lipids. Of these proteolipids, a fraction A separated from chloroform–methanol solution at $-10°$ and could be further fractionated; a fraction B was precipitated from methanol–chloroform by acetone, contained 50 % of protein and was obtained in crystals; and a proteolipid C containing 75 % of protein was soluble in chloroform itself. The protein components of each of the proteolipids could be separated by drying aqueous chloroform–methanol mixtures and the proteins were found to be resistant to proteolytic enzymes. Phosphatidopeptides have been characterized in such extracts (LeBaron, 1963): associations having phosphoinositides prominent among the lipid moiety, and separable to their components by acid, non-polar solvents. The efficiency of the extraction of lipoproteins by chloroform–methanol is increased if the tissue preparations are pretreated by thorough washing in water or by prolonged dialysis, due possibly to removal of electrolytes (Lees, 1968). Salts have also been shown to affect the chloroform–methanol solubility of purified myelin (Autilio et al., 1964; Lees, 1966). A lipoprotein with different properties has been obtained by chloroform–methanol extraction at pH 2 (Wolfgram, 1966). This material differed from the chloroform–methanol extracted lipoproteins described by Folch & Lees (1951) in solubility characteristics, trypsin digestibility and amino acid composition. It contained 13 % nitrogen and 1–1·7 % phosphorus. Water-soluble lipoproteins, which do not require chloroform–methanol for extraction, also occur; these differ from soluble serum proteins in lipid composition, density and in immunochemical properties. Certain of the cerebral nucleoproteins are also found in association with lipids (Steel & Gies, 1907–8); they contain both pentose and deoxypentose nucleotides (Folch & Uzman, 1948).

Further protein fractions, present in small amounts, are characterized by association with copper and of them a cerebrocuprein I has been highly purified (Porter & Folch, 1957); it contains two atoms of copper in a compound about 35,000 in molecular weight. There is little to record which is specific to the brain generally in the amino acid composition of its proteins, though much interest attaches to the detailed analyses of proteins of cerebral origin, and references to such data are quoted. Analyses are available for proteins of the whole or of different parts of the brain in a variety of animal species and for specimens from human subjects in several pathological conditions (see Block & Bolling, 1945; Bogoch, 1969). The isolation from rat and cat brain of a protein with properties similar to those of muscle actomyosin has also been described. It super-precipitated with Mg^{2+} and ATP and contained Mg^{2+}- and Ca^{2+}-activated ATPase (Puszkin et al., 1968).

Proteins of Cerebral Subcellular Components

Distribution of cerebral proteins among subcellular fractions is shown in B, Table 9.6. The characteristic nucleoproteins and histones of the *nuclear* fraction are described in Chapter 12. Cerebral histones are relatively stable metabolically with turnover rates ($t_{1/2}$ of 54 or 104 days) much slower than those generally found for the proteins of the nucleus or cytoplasm of the brain, and slower also than for the histones of liver nuclei. The half-lifetimes for cerebral histones are of similar order to those for populations of cerebral DNA and this provides support for suggestions that histones and DNA are replaced concurrently. The types of histone separable by electrophoresis and their amino acid composition in brain and liver are indistinguishable; organ specificity of brain histones is thus unlikely (Piha et al., 1966).

Cerebral nuclear fractions also contain acidic proteins, found in neurons and glial cells. The soluble acidic "S 100" protein (below) was not detected in these fractions (Dravid & Burdman, 1968). A brain-specific basic protein, 27,000 in molecular weight, has been extracted from pig brain (Tomasi & Kornguth, 1968). Immunohistological evidence for its localization in neuronal nuclei was presented and there was no fluorescent antibody reaction with kidney, liver, spleen or ovarian cells. It should be noted that cerebral nuclear fractions contain material other than nuclei (see Chapter 12).

A high proportion of the total protein (some 40 % of grey matter) occurs in primary *mitochondrial* fractions. In contrast to mitochondrial preparations from other tissues, less than half of the protein in the cerebral fractions is mitochondrial, the rest being due mainly to the presence of myelin and nerve ending particles (Table 9.6; see also Chapter 12). The mitochondria contain a large number of enzymes which include those concerned with such major pathways of intermediary metabolism as fat metabolism, the tricarboxylic acid cycle, electron transport and oxidative phosphorylation. Some are loosely associated and can be relatively easily extracted; others are more tightly bound. The proteins of cerebral mitochondrial membranes have been extracted using phenol-acid mixtures and resolved into over 20 bands on acrylamide gels. The pattern was quite distinct from that in extracts of nerve-ending membranes. Myelin contained a much simpler protein pattern; only four or five bands were detected (Cotman & Mahler, 1967; Mehl, 1968).

The encephalitogenic basic proteins, which when injected into animals cause allergic encephalomyelitis, are found only in *myelin* and have been demonstrated there immunochemically. The purified encephalitogenic proteins are of molecular weight 15,000–20,000 and are non-globular with a disordered non-helical structure. The protein isolated from the myelin of ox spinal cord forms a stoichiometric reversible complex with triphosphoinositide and other phospholipids (Chapter 11) with properties which indicate that the complex may be the state in which the encephalitogenic proteins occur in the myelin *in vivo* (Martenson et al, 1969a, b; Palmer & Dawson, 1969; Chao & Roboz-Einstein, 1970).

Cerebral *microsomal* preparations, heterogeneous in source and in morphology, also contain a large number of proteins difficult to extract (Got et al., 1967; Cotman & Mahler, 1967). Between 16 and 20 bands have been resolved on acrylamide gels after extraction of ox brain microsomes with pentanol, which was concluded to be more satisfactory than a range of detergents tested (Brackenridge & Bachelard, 1969). Proteins have also been extracted from brain microsomes using phenol-acid mixtures. Similar solvent systems were used for resolution on acrylamide gels (Cotman & Mahler, 1967; Mehl, 1968); a number of proteins was separated but the acidic solvents used prevent comparison of mobilities with other systems.

9

Soluble Proteins

These are defined usually by their presence in supernatant liquors after centrifugation of tissue homogenates at 100,000 *g* for 1 hr. Preparation has most typically been in media containing iso-osmotic concentrations of sucrose; proteins present in such soluble fractions do not necessarily reflect those originally present as soluble proteins in the cytoplasm. The proteins of the soluble fraction which remains after deposition of particulate matter (Table 9.6) have received most attention, since they present fewer difficulties of extraction and subsequent removal of extractant. In earlier studies proteins were classified by electrophoretic mobility equivalent to serum proteins; the convenience of terminology does not imply that similarly-named proteins from different sources are identical. From 70 to over 100 protein peaks or bands have been detected, or separated by column chromatography of aqueous extracts, from the brain (Bogoch *et al.*, 1964; Moore & McGregor, 1965); some of the peaks may have been due, however, to protein–protein or protein–buffer interactions.

Supernatant fractions have also proved to be a rich source of proteins apparently specific to neural tissues. The best characterized of these is the "S 100" protein, so called because of its solubility characteristics in saturated ammonium sulphate solutions (Moore & McGregor, 1965; Moore, 1965). The yield from beef brain was 10 mg./100 g. and the protein had an apparent molecular weight of about 30,000 (from G 100 Sephadex columns). Amino acid analysis showed a high content of glutamate and titration analysis indicated the presence of one cysteinyl-SH group per 11,000 molecular weight. Shown immunologically to be brain-specific, its presence has been detected in many parts of the nervous system and in both neurons and glial cells (Hydén & McEwan, 1966; Moore *et al.*, 1968). The acidic protein resolved into two components on acrylamide-agarose electrophoresis. The major component was about 15,000 in molecular weight (Vincendon *et al.*, 1967). Rapid labelling in rabbit brain ribosomes of S-100 protein with ^{14}C-leucine has been demonstrated by immunological reaction with S-100 antibody (Rubin & Stenzel, 1965), indicating a dynamic role in the brain. The S-100 protein has also been reported to cause inhibition of RNA synthesis (q.v.) in the chromatin of rat brain nucleoli (Bondy & Roberts, 1969). Another acidic soluble protein with slightly different properties has been detected; named "14-3-2", it is also specific to the brain and is larger, with a molecular weight of 40,000. The use of specific lesions leading to neuron degeneration provided evidence which indicated enrichment of the S-100 protein in glial cells and of the "14-3-2" protein in neurons (Cicero *et al.*, 1970).

A brain-specific *glycoprotein* is neuraminic acid-rich and migrates during electrophoresis at rates similar to α_2-globulin. It occurs at higher concentration in white than in grey matter, and in white matter, the rate of its appearance during development suggested a temporal relationship with myelination (Warecka & Bauer, 1967, 1968). Further brain-specific soluble proteins have been detected by electrophoresis. Five distinct species were separated from aqueous cerebral extracts; three of these migrated towards the anode and in this sense were also acidic proteins (Kosinski & Grabar, 1967). Immunoelectrophoresis has also shown the presence of proteins in cerebrospinal fluid which are absent from serum (Clausen, 1961; Burtin, 1964).

One of the soluble protein constituents has been isolated by virtue of its *colchicine-binding* ability (Weisenberg *et al.*, 1968). Some 5–10% of the protein of the soluble fraction of pig brain, it exists as a dimer of molecular weight 120,000 and binds, and is stabilized by, 1 mole of colchicine and 2 moles of guanosine triphosphate per dimer. On the basis of molecular weight, sediment-ation characteristics, binding properties and a relatively high content of glutamate, aspartate, glycine, leucine and proline, it has been suggested to be the protein unit of microtubules (Chapter 12).

The interaction of colchicine with axonal protein has helped to reveal aspects of axonal function; small doses (1–10 μg.) of colchicine injected to a peripheral nerve inhibited the axonal flow of protein. Two types of protein flow were involved; one at a fast rate of some 300 mm./day and the second at a slow rate of 2 mm/day (James & Austin, 1970; James *et al.*, 1970; see p. 259 and Chapter 12).

Protein Breakdown

The rates of protein breakdown *in vivo* have been studied by following the overall rates of disappearance of protein-bound ^{14}C after labelling by the inclusion of ^{14}C-lysine in the diet. The average half-life of the cerebral proteins was close to 14 days, and is comparable to the time calculated from studies of rates of amino acid incorporation into proteins in the brain. The calculations of rates of protein breakdown indicated that approximately 90% of the total protein of the tissue had a turnover time of between 10 and 20 days; small populations would be expected to be turning over faster or slower than the mean rate (Lajtha & Toth, 1966). The rates of catabolism of pre-labelled cerebral proteins were not significantly affected by electroshock (Minard & Richter, 1968).

Proteolytic enzymes are quite active in cerebral preparations: more so than in muscle though less than in kidney or liver. The cerebral enzymes can liberate amino acids from endogenous materials, from added proteins or from simple peptides. Cerebral proteinases are most active at pH 3·5–3·8; dispersions of rat brain liberated some 20–25 μmoles of amino acid/g. tissue/hr. from endogen-ous protein. On centrifugation, activity was enriched in a particular mito-chondrial subfraction in distinction to nuclear, nerve-terminal, myelin, or soluble fractions. The enriched fraction may contain lysosomes (q.v.); it was of high proteolytic activity, forming 620 μmoles amino acid/g. protein/hr. from endogenous substrates, and 4500 μmoles/hr. from added haemoglobin (Marks & Lajtha, 1963). Other added proteins were also degraded, though less rapidly. This enzyme has been enriched from the brain of the cow by extraction from an acetone powder, precipitation with ammonium sulphate, adsorption and electrophoresis, yielding material which formed 180 μmoles tyrosine/mg. protein/minute (Palladin *et al.*, 1963).

At pH 7–7·8, liberation of amino acids from endogenous substrates in cerebral dispersions proceeded at about 12 μmoles/g. tissue/hr. It was most rapid in fractions containing nuclei and myelin fragments, then reaching

160 μmoles/g. protein/hr., increased to 600 by added haemoglobin. Albumin and casein did not act as substrates but globin was particularly effective, a specificity different from that found at pH 3·5. Hydrolysis of simple peptides also occurs at pH 7; a system splitting DL-alanylglycine was more potent in certain layers of the cerebral and cerebellar cortex than in the brain stem or spinal cord, its distribution suggesting nerve cell bodies or their dendrites to have higher activity than axons. Peptidase activity was shown by mouse and human brain towards a variety of simple peptides containing an amino acid with a lipophilic sidechain, e.g. glycylleucine; evidence for the presence of more than one such enzyme was obtained by examining some thirty peptides and by inhibitors; thus a system hydrolysing tripeptides, as glycylglycylphenyl-alanine, appeared distinct from that hydrolysing dipeptides (Pope & Anfinsen, 1948; Uzman *et al.*, 1962; Lajtha, 1964). More recently, an aminopeptidase specific for leucylglycylglycine has been isolated from rat brain (Marks *et al.*, 1968); arylaminidase and carboxypeptidase B activities are also present, but so far have not been fully characterized (Marks, 1970).

Amino Acid Incorporation to Proteins

Several amino acids have been demonstrated to be incorporated to the proteins of the brain, *in vivo*, under the experimental conditions of Table 9.7. Thus after administering isotopically labelled amino acids intracerebrally and extracting other materials, the protein residue has proved to contain labelled amino acids in peptide linkage. In adult animals as well as those still growing,

Table 9.7

Turnover of labelled L-*leucine in subcellular fractions from the brain*

Fraction	Half-lifetime
Whole homogenate or tissue	4–27
Mitochondria	20
Synaptic vesicles	21
Synaptic membranes	21
Ribosomes	12
Soluble fraction	16

Values (half-lifetimes are in days) are regarded as approximate only, and were obtained after intracerebral or intraventricular administration. Data from Gaitonde & Richter (1956;) Lajtha (1959, 1964); von Hungen *et al.* (1968).

incorporation of leucine, phenylalanine, methionine, glutamic acid and lysine has been shown. Relations between the specific activities of the free cerebral amino acids and those of the protein sampled at the same time can be expressed, with many reservations, as turnover rates and a half-lifetime given for the isotope in the protein. These values, even when a single amino acid is involved, inevitably cover a wide range, not fully represented in Table 9.7, by virtue of the different protein types and cellular situations which are involved. The differing rates of incorporation in different species and parts of the brain and in different levels of cerebral activity have been examined and discussed (Lajtha, 1964; Palladin, 1964; Piha et al., 1963). The brain as a whole shows moderate activity in this respect, its rates of incorporation lying between those found with liver and muscle. Administration of ^{14}C-lysine has displayed even in the cerebral histones a slow turnover, less than that of other nuclear proteins but interestingly similar to that of cerebral deoxyribonucleic acid (Piha et al., 1965).

Examining valine, uniformly ^{14}C-labelled and given subcutaneously to young mice, ^{14}C was found in samples taken 40 min. later in the proteins from a number of cerebral areas (Flexner et al., 1962). Such incorporation specifically to the brain was inhibited up to 90% by the antibiotic puromycin administered intracerebrally. Connection between this inhibition and the performance of animals in learning and retention was sought but not found; performance was later found to be disturbed by longer exposure to puromycin. 2-^{14}C-Glycine given subcutaneously is also incorporated promptly to cerebral proteins of mice, as well as to purines and pyrimidines of the brain, as is described on p. 223, above. Amino acid incorporation to the proteins of goldfish brain in vivo was inhibited to a similar extent (80–90%) by puromycin and by cycloheximide (Brink et al., 1966).

Rates of protein synthesis in the brain in vivo are sensitive to external stimuli. Thus marked effects have been observed with animals reared in the dark and subsequently exposed to light (Brattgård, 1952; Singh & Talwar, 1967, 1969; Appel et al., 1967). In the monkey, labelling of protein in the occipital cortex was increased by exposure of the animals to flickering light but not when the stimulus was continuous light. However further clarification of the response to light stimulation is required; use of a split-brain preparation in the monkey revealed no effect of unilateral light stimulation on rates of incorporation of ^{3}H of ^{3}H$_2$O into cerebral protein (Metzger et al., 1967). Spreading cortical depression, evoked by a single topical application of 25% KCl, caused 42% inhibition of protein synthesis in the brain in vivo (Krivanek, 1970).

Cerebral tissues in vitro also incorporate amino-acids to the protein which they contain. With ^{14}C-glycine, the process was inhibited by lack of oxygen or the presence of 2:4-dinitrophenol in incubating salines, and the incorporation was concluded to require adenosine triphosphate (Mase et al., 1962). The incorporation into isolated cell-containing preparations of the cerebral cortex is inhibited by puromycin and cycloheximide and thus proceeds by the mechanisms described below. Although rates of incorporation of labelled amino acids into cerebral proteins in vivo may be increased be electroshock (Pryor et al., 1967) application of electrical pulses to cerebral cortex preparations in vitro caused decrease in the rates of ^{14}C-valine incorporation (Orrego & Lipmann, 1967; Jones & McIlwain, 1971). Study of the time-course of incorporation showed changes secondary to modified rates of amino acid entry induced by stimulation (Jones & Banks, 1970). The ATP required to support protein synthesis, some 4–5 μmoles ATP consumed/g. hr., is not large and thus not likely to mediate the diminution of incorporation caused by stimulation (Jones &

McIlwain, 1971). The inhibition may be secondary to changes in RNA (q.v.) which occur on electrical excitation.

After incubation of cerebral cortex preparations with ^{3}H-leucine *in vitro*, the tissues were disrupted by passage through a sieve and fractionated by density-gradient centrifugation in Ficoll. Fractions enriched in neuronal perikarya and in clusters of glial cells were obtained. The neuronal-enriched fractions were 6 times more active in incorporating labelled amino acid per mg. of protein than the glial fractions and were more sensitive to hypoxia, dinitro-phenol and cycloheximide. Similar studies *in vivo* of incorporation of ^{3}H-cytidine or ^{3}H-orotic acid to cerebral RNA also showed the neuronal-enriched fractions to be the more active (Blomstrand & Hamberger, 1970; Flangas & Bowman, 1970; see also Rose, 1969). Greater activity of neuronal nuclei in protein synthesis has been demonstrated; the nuclei were fractionated by density-gradient centrifugation of crude nuclear fractions prepared at various times after intraperitoneal injection of ^{3}H-leucine. Fractions enriched in neuronal nuclei showed activity comparable to that of the microsomes (q.v.) in amino acid incorporation per mg. protein and considerably higher than the activity of the fractions enriched in glial nuclei (Burdman, 1970).

The requirements of cerebral preparations for adenosine triphosphate and other components in their amino acid incorporation to proteins have been examined further in cell-free systems; the incorporation has been shown to be catalysed most rapidly by fractions rich in polyribosomes and is described in detail below.

Mechanisms of Protein Synthesis in Neural Systems

The principles which underly the general mechanisms of protein synthesis are summarized in Fig. 9.8. The sequence of nucleotide bases in the DNA of the nucleus can be described as carrying information for directing the synthe-sis of specific protein molecules. The mechanisms of protein synthesis result in accurate translation of the DNA nucleotide sequence into the amino-acid sequence of the synthesized protein. Messenger RNA, which passes from the nucleus to the cytoplasmic sites of protein synthesis, is formed as a result of DNA-directed RNA-polymerase action, described above. At the polyribo-somes, the complementary nucleotide sequence in messenger RNA conditions the order of insertion of the activated amino acids (as amino-acyl transfer RNA) into the growing polypeptide chain. Although this has been generally accepted as the normal sequence of events, it is possible that categories of DNA may themselves also act as intermediaries, passing from the nucleus to cytoplasmic sites and conditioning protein synthesis there (Bell, 1969).

The available evidence indicates that the mechanisms of protein synthesis in the brain are no different from those of other mammalian tissues. It is possible, however, that protein synthesis in the nerve axon is exceptional and this is discussed subsequently. The importance of synthesis of genetically-conditioned specific proteins in the brain is evident from the consequences which arise when its progress is modified. Many genetically-determined errors of metabolism cause severe mental abnormality or neurological disease. The genetic alterations are due to minor changes in the sequence of nucleotide bases in the DNA of the gene which, by the normal mechanisms of protein synthesis, results in formation of protein molecules with corresponding alteration in amino acid sequence. If the protein is an enzyme, the alteration is usually sufficient to cause complete absence of catalytic activity, although the possibility that modified catalytic activity might result should not be ignored (see, for example, argininosuccinic aciduria).

$$A \xrightarrow{\alpha} B \xrightarrow{\beta} C \xrightarrow{\gamma} D \qquad \text{(i)}$$

potential inhibition

$$A \xrightarrow{\alpha} B \xrightarrow{\beta} C \xrightarrow{/\!/} D \qquad \text{(ii)}$$
$$\searrow E$$

Sequence (i) represents a hypothetical pathway for synthesis of metabolite **D**. If enzyme (γ), responsible for catalysing the conversion of **C** to **D**, is defective, metabolite **D** will not be formed (unless an alternative pathway for its synthesis is available). Metabolite **C** would therefore tend to accumulate. Substance **D**, the end product of the pathway, is frequently found to exert "feed-back" inhibition of the enzyme (α) which catalyses the first stage specific to the pathway. Absence of product **D** in such cases means that this mechanism for regulating the rate of metabolism in the pathway will be absent, so that **C** will accumulate to a still greater extent. Accumulated **C** may be converted to an abnormal metabolite **E** as indicated in sequence (ii). Abnormal quantities of **C** or detection of unusual metabolites **E** are the signs which have frequently led to the identification of the defect in a genetic error of metabolism. An example of this is the detection of unusual metabolites of phenylalanine in phenylketonuria (q.v.) and several further examples are given in Chapters 8 and 11.

Ribosomal Protein Synthesis

Isolated microsome preparations from rat or guinea pig cerebral cortex incorporate labelled amino acids at rates of 0·05–0·35 nmole/mg. of protein per hr. (Sataki *et al.*, 1964; Suzuki *et al.*, 1964; Zomzely *et al.*, 1964), which are similar to those reported for microsomes from other mammalian tissues. There is good evidence that cerebral microsomal protein synthesis occurs on the polyribosomes (q.v.); *in vivo*, ^{14}C-leucine incorporation in the first 5 min. was found on subcellular fractionation to have occurred solely in the polyribosomes and only after much longer periods in proteins of microsomal membranes (Jacob *et al.*, 1967). Polyribosomal systems, as was earlier found for microsomal preparations, clearly exhibit a requirement for ATP and for the "pH 5 enzyme" fraction from the soluble cytoplasm (Table 9.8 and Fig. 9.9). A full complement of exogenous amino acids has also been shown to be necessary for maximum rates; guanosine triphosphate (GTP) seems also to be required, although some workers have found addition of GTP to be without effect on their systems. Some evidence for competition between amino-acids for incorporation to protein of brain homogenates has been reported. Thus phenylalanine inhibited incorporation of ^{14}C-tyrosine and leucine of ^{14}C-isoleucine into the proteins of particulate fractions (Peterson & McKean,

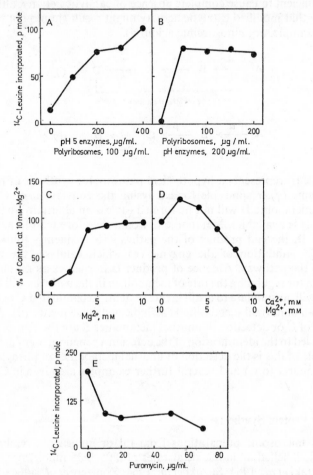

FIG. 9.9. Requirements for protein synthesis in cerebral polyribosomes.

The polyribosomes were isolated from rat cerebral cortex and incubated for 60 min. at 37°. Optimal rates of ^{14}C-leucine incorporation into polyribosomal protein (100 μg./ml.) required 10 mM-Mg^{2+}, 40 mM-NaCl, 100 mM-KCl, 6 mM-glutathione, 5 mM-ATP, 1 mM-GTP and the pH 5 enzyme fraction.

The curves illustrate the requirement for the pH 5 enzymes and polyribosomes (A and B) and for Mg^{2+} (C); D shows inhibition by Ca^{2+}. Puromycin inhibition of amino acid incorporation is shown in E (Campagnoni & Mahler, 1967).

1969). The effects of variation in rates of amino acid entry on incorporation to protein in whole-cell-containing preparations, noted above, are unlikely to contribute significantly in cell-free systems, so the inhibition described for dispersions indicates that competition between amino-acids for incorporation may occur.

Cerebral polyribosomal protein synthesis is consistent with protein synthesis generally in its inhibition by puromycin and its dependence upon the presence of Mg^{2+}. Optimum concentrations of Mg^{2+} are about 10 mM (Fig. 9.9) and the process is inhibited by Ca^{2+}. The involvement of other cations, particularly the monovalent cations, has been studied, but no clear-cut requirement has been established. Stimulation of incorporation rates by rapidly-labelled species of RNA, suggested to be messenger RNA, has been observed in many laboratories (see Vesco & Giuditta, 1967; Kimberlin, 1967). Further support for the involvement specifically of polyribosomes came indirectly from the observation that changes in rates of protein synthesis in the brain and liver correlated well with

Table 9.8

Requirements for leucine incorporation into protein of cerebral polyribosomes

Change in conditions	^{14}C-Leucine incorporated (pmole)	% of control value
No change	123	100
Omission of:		
ATP	44	36
GTP	79	64
pH 5 Fraction	10	8
Polyribosomes	0	0
Addition of:		
ATP generating system	132	107
Nineteen amino acids	—	*ca* 200

The polyribosomes were incubated *in vitro* under the conditions of Fig. 9.9 (Campagnoni & Mahler, 1967).

the number of polyribosomes present (Murthy, 1966). The occurrence of polyribosomes both free and bound to the endoplasmic reticulum was noted above; protein synthesis has been shown to occur in all polyribosomes, free or bound, to a similar extent (Sellinger & Ohlsson, 1969).

In common with other mammalian systems, protein synthesis in the brain seems more active on polyribosomes larger than tetramers, although it is not clear at present if the size of protein molecule synthesized is related to the size of polyribosome involved. Comparison of the process in cerebral cortex and liver of the rat suggested that the cerebral messenger RNA–ribosome complex may be less stable in brain than in liver. Subsequent to incorporation of labelled amino acids into heavy polyribosomes, a larger proportion of the radioactivity became associated with lighter ribosome fractions of the brain (Zomzely *et al.*, 1968).

The overall process of ribosomal protein synthesis in the brain follows therefore the sequence of events described for other systems. Certain of the steps have been inferred rather than clearly demonstrated, as no transfer RNA or messenger RNA molecules have been isolated to the extent achieved with less complex tissues, although as seen from the description above, much evidence on RNA species has accumulated. The presence also of ATP-requiring amino acid activation reactions has been shown in preparations from several cerebral areas (Lipmann, 1957; Takahashi & Abe, 1963); these reactions were more active in newborn than in adult rats (Murthy & Rappoport, 1965; Murthy, 1966). Inhibition by reduced glutathione also indicated the presence of glutathione-dependent binding of aminoacyl-transfer RNA to the messenger RNA–ribosome complex, by analogy with other, more fully characterized systems (Fig. 9.8).

In view of suggestions that methylation of histones may provide a mechanism for modification of histone structure in relation to genetic function, methylation of proteins was compared in various organs of the rat *in vitro*. Using S-adenosyl-L-[methyl-^{14}C]-methionine as methyl donor, the brain proved to be the most active in protein methylation; the methyl groups were found mainly in the arginine of the cerebral histones with lesser amounts in the lysine (Paik & Kim, 1969).

Protein Synthesis in Mitochondria and Nerve Endings

Independent mechanisms for protein synthesis are present also in cerebral mitochondria and in isolated nerve ending particles. Mitochondrial fractions, purified by sucrose density-gradient centrifugation, incorporated amino acids at rates up to 75 pmoles/mg. of protein per hr., which are similar to those obtained for the mitochondria from liver or heart and only slightly lower than those reported for cerebral microsomal systems. The cerebral mitochondria did not require exogenous ATP or the "pH 5 soluble" fraction essential for microsomal protein synthesis. Pretreatment of intact mitochondria with ribonuclease had no effect and the incorporation into mitochondrial protein was inhibited by DNP, rotenone, antimycin A and partially by chloramphenicol (Bachelard, 1966; Campbell *et al.*, 1966; Morgan & Austin, 1968). The lack of effect of certain treatments, e.g. actinomycin D or ribonuclease, could be due to lack of access of the agent, and not necessarily to lack of sensitivity of the system. Chloramphenicol, which inhibits microbial protein synthesis, is generally accepted as an inhibitor also of mitochondrial but not ribosomal protein synthesis in mammalian tissues. Partial inhibition of the process by chloramphenicol has been reported for mitochondria from the brain and adrenal medulla and for nerve endings (Bachelard, 1966; Garren & Crocco, 1967; Austin & Morgan, 1968; Autilio *et al.*, 1968), although one group of workers reported no effect of the inhibitor on cerebral systems (Gordon & Deanin, 1968).

Amino acid incorporation into the proteins of nerve ending particles is less active than with purified mitochondria *in vitro* (Fig. 9.10; Bachelard, 1966; Austin & Morgan, 1967). Ribosomes have not been demonstrated within nerve endings and it is possible that the activity observed in the particles is due to their constituent mitochondria. The evidence is at present inconclusive: Austin & Morgan (1968) reported some activity, inhibited by cycloheximide but not by actinomycin D, in non-mitochondrial elements from nerve endings, but Gordon & Deanin (1968) found all of the activity of their nerve ending preparations to be due to the mitochondria present

The relevance of protein synthesis in cerebral cytoplasmic mitochondria is uncertain. Mitochondria of other mammalian tissues contain a fully independent machinery for protein synthesis, including characteristic mitochondrial DNA, RNA polymerase and ribosomes, but the proteins synthesized within the mitochondria seem to be restricted to structural rather than enzymic proteins (Haldar *et al.*, 1966). Whether the same is true of cerebral mitochondria remains to be elucidated.

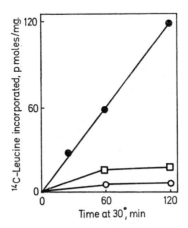

FIG. 9.10. Amino acid incorporation into proteins of cerebral mitochondrial and nerve ending preparations.
    The fractions were separated by sucrose density gradient centrifuga-
tion and incubated with ^{14}C-leucine in the presence of 7·5 mM-MgSO$_4$.
The rate of incorporation into protein over 2 hr. is shown for purified
mitochondria (●), nerve ending particles (□) and myelin (○) (Bachelard,
1966).

Such considerations are important in regard to mechanisms of protein renewal in the axon, in which mitochondria are present but ribosomes appear to be absent. This is discussed in the following section.

Protein Synthesis in the Axon; Axonal Flow

For many years it was assumed, with good reason, that all renewal of macromolecules in nerves at sites far removed from neuronal cell bodies was effected by synthesis in the cell body and subsequent transport through the axon, i.e. that the materials were synthesized at classical cytoplasmic ribosomal sites very remote from their functional sites. Much evidence has been presented in favour of axonal transport, and is discussed in Chapter 12. However, the renewal of proteins and enzymes in axons is unlikely to be entirely due to transport subsequent to synthesis in the perikaryon. After irreversible inactivation by organophosphates of acetylcholine esterase, the enzymic activity appeared at the same rate all along the nerve, and if anything slightly more rapidly in more distal segments (Koenig & Koelle, 1961; Clouet & Waelsch,

1961). Carefully applied local applications of puromycin in cat hypoglossal nerve provided evidence for local synthesis of the enzyme independent of the cell body. The rate of esterase reappearance in the Mauthner giant axon of the goldfish occurred at rates which, if due to axonal flow, would necessitate rates of the order of 1,000 mm./day, i.e. some two to three times the maximum rates of movement through the axon (Edström, 1966). Use of inhibitors of protein synthesis suggested the process to be of DNA-directed ribosomal type (Koenig, 1965, 1967; Edström, 1967; Edström & Sjöstrand, 1969), yet no ribosomes have been detected in the axon. The possibility that the observed synthesis was due to synthesis in supporting cells such as Schwann cells or oligodendroglia is considered unlikely, since the studies described were designed to exclude them.

Although mitochondria, which possess the full capability for protein synthesis described above, are present within the axoplasm, inhibition studies, particularly using chloramphenicol, have indicated that the axonal synthesis is ribosomal rather than mitochondrial (Edström & Sjöstrand, 1969; Koenig, 1969). Some evidence has emerged for the presence of extramitochondrial RNA within the axon; extramitochondrial axonal RNA was more rapidly labelled than mitochondrial RNA and the possibility that RNA had been transferred from the Schwann cell to the axon was excluded by pulse-labelling experiments (Koenig, 1969). Thus, while at present the precise mechanism of local axonal protein synthesis remains to be elucidated, there can be little doubt that such a mechanism exists and that renewal of proteins and enzymes at sites far removed from the cell body is contributed to partly by local synthesis and partly by the transport of pre-synthesized material from the cell body.

REFERENCES

ABOOD, L. G. & GERARD, R. W. (1954). *J. cell. comp. Physiol.* **43**, 379.
ADAMS, D. H. (1965). *J. Neurochem.* **12**, 783.
ADAMS, D. H. (1966). *Biochem. J.* **98**, 636.
ALDRIDGE, W. N. & JOHNSON, M. K. (1959). *Biochem. J.* **73**, 270.
ALTMAN, J. (1969). *Handbook of Neurochem.* **2**, 137.
ALTMAN, J. & CHOROVER, S. L. (1963). *J. Physiol.* **169**, 770.
APPEL, S. H. (1967). *Nature*, **213**, 1253.
APPEL, S. H., DAVIS, W. & SCOTT, S. (1967). *Science*, **157**, 836.
APPEL, S. H. & SILBERBERG, D. H. (1968). *J. Neurochem.* **15**, 1437.
AUSTIN, L. & MORGAN, I. G. (1967). *J. Neurochem.* **14**, 377.
AUTILIO, L. A., APPEL, S. H., PETTIS, P. & GAMBETTI, P. L. (1968). *Biochemistry*, **7**, 2615.
AUTILIO, L. A., NORTON, W. T. & TERRY, R. D. (1964). *J. Neurochem.* **11**, 17.
BACHELARD, H. S. (1966). *Biochem. J.* **100**, 131.
BAILEY, B. F. S. & HEALD, P. J. (1961). *J. Neurochem.* **6**, 342.
BALAZS, R. & COCKS, W. A. (1967). *J. Neurochem.* **14**, 1035.
BARKOWSKI, T., HARTH, S., MARDELL, R. & MANDEL, P. (1961). *Nature*, **192**, 456.
BARLOW, J. J., MATHIAS, A. P., WILLIAMSON, R. & GAMMACK, D. B. (1963). *Biochem. Biophys. Res. Communs.* **13**, 61.
BARONDES, S. H. (1964). *J. Neurochem.* **11**, 663.
BARONDES, S. H. & JARVICK, M. E. (1964). *J. Neurochem.* **11**, 187.
BELL, E. (1969). *Nature*, **224**, 326.
BLAND, J. H., JARRETT, F. A., PLUNKETT, G. E., RAVARIS, G. L. & SYLWESTER, D. (1968). *Feder. Proc.* **27**, 1087.

BLOCK, R. J. & BOLLING, D. (1945). The Amino Acid Composition of Proteins and Foods. Springfield, Illinois: Thomas.
BLOMSTRAND, C. & HAMBERGER, A. (1970). *J. Neurochem.* **17,** 1187.
BOGOCH, S. (1969). *Handbook of Neurochem.* **1,** 75.
BOGOCH, S., RAJAM, P. C. & BELVAL, P. G. (1964). *Nature,* **204,** 73.
BONDY, S. C. & PERRY, S. V. (1963). *J. Neurochem.* **10,** 593, 603.
BONDY, S. C. & ROBERTS, S. (1967). *Biochem. J.* **105,** 1111.
BONDY, S. C. & ROBERTS, S. (1968). *Biochem. J.* **109,** 533.
BONDY, S. C. & ROBERTS, S. (1969). *Biochem. J.* **115,** 341.
BONDY, S. C. & WAELSCH, H. (1965). *J. Neurochem.* **12,** 751.
BRACKENRIDGE, C. J. & BACHELARD, H. S. (1969). *Int. J. Protein Res.* **1,** 157.
BRANNEN, T. P. (1968). *J. theoret. Biol.* **20,** 358.
BRATTGÅRD, S. O. (1952). *Acta Radiol. (Suppl.)* **96,** 1.
BRECKENRIDGE, B. McL. (1970). *Ann. Rev. Pharmacol.* **10,** 19.
BRETSCHNER, M. S. (1969). *Nature,* **217,** 509.
BRINK, J. J., DAVIS, R. E. & AGRANOFF, B. W. (1966). *J. Neurochem.* **13,** 889.
BROOKER, G., THOMAS, L. J. & APPLEMAN, M. M. (1968). *Biochemistry,* **7,** 4177.
BURDMAN, J. A. (1970). *J. Neurochem.* **17,** 1555.
BURTIN, P. (1964). In Immuno-Electrophoretic Analysis, p. 244. Ed. P. Graber & P. Burtin. Amsterdam: Elsevier.
BUTCHER, R. W. & SUTHERLAND, E. W. (1962). *J. biol. Chem.* **237,** 1244.
CAIN, D. F. (1967). *J. Neurochem.* **14,** 1175.
CAMPAGNONI, A. T. & MAHLER, H. R. (1967). *Biochemistry,* **6,** 956.
CAMPBELL, N. K., MAHLER, H. R., MOORE, W. J. & TEWARI, S. (1966). *Biochemistry,* **5,** 1174.
CARR, D. O. & GRISOLIA, S. (1964). *J. biol. Chem.* **239,** 160.
CHAO, L.-P. & ROBOZ-EINSTEIN, E. (1970). *J. Neurochem.* **17,** 1121.
CHEUNG, W. Y. (1967). *Biochemistry,* **6,** 1079.
CHEUNG, W. Y. (1970). *Biochem. Biophys. Res. Commun.* **38,** 533.
CICERO, T. J., COWAN, W. M., MOORE, B. W. & SUNTZEFF, V. (1970). *Brain Res.* **18,** 25.
CLAUSEN, J. (1961). *Proc. Soc. Exp. Biol. & Med.* **107,** 170.
CLOUET, D. H. & WAELSCH, H. (1961). *J. Neurochem.* **8,** 201.
CONWAY, E. J. & COOKE, R. (1939). *Biochem. J.* **33,** 479.
COSTA, E. & GREENGARD, P. (1970). *Adv. Biochem. Psychopharmacol.* **3.**
COTMAN, C. W. & MAHLER, H. R. (1967). *Arch. Biochem. Biophys.* **120,** 384.
CUNNINGHAM, B. & LOWENSTEIN, J. M. (1965). *Biochim. Biophys. Acta,* **96,** 535.
DATTA, R. K., BHATTACHARYYA, D. & GHOSH, J. J. (1964). *J. Neurochem.* **11,** 87.
DATTA, R. K. & GHOSH, J. J. (1963). *J. Neurochem.* **10,** 363, 611.
DATTA, R. K., GHOSH, J. J. & BHATTACHARYYA, K. C. (1969a). *J. Neurochem.* **16,** 875.
DATTA, R. K., SEN, S. & GHOSH, J. J. (1969b). *Biochem. J.* **114,** 847.
DAWSON, D. M. (1967). *J. Neurochem.* **14,** 939.
DAWSON, D. M. (1968). *J. Neurochem.* **15,** 31.
DELLWEG, H., GERNER, R. & WACKER, A. (1968). *J. Neurochem.* **15,** 1109.
DEROBERTIS, E., ARNAIZ, G. R. DE L., ALBERICI, M., BUTCHER, R. W. & SUTHERLAND, E. W. (1967). *J. biol. Chem.* **242,** 3487.
DEROBERTIS, E., ARNAIZ, G. R. DEL., SALGANICOFF, L., DE IRALDI, A. P. & ZIEHER, L. M. (1963). *J. Neurochem.* **10,** 225.
DEROBERTIS, E., PELLEGRINO DE IRALDI, A., RODRIGUEZ DE LORES ARNAIZ, G. & SALGANICOFF, L. (1962). *J. Neurochem.* **9,** 23.
DRAVID, A. R. & BURDMAN, J. A. (1968). *J. Neurochem.* **15,** 25.
DUTTON, G. R., CAMPAGNONI, A. T., MAHLER, H. R. & MOORE, W. J. (1969). *J. Neurochem.* **16,** 989.
DUTTON, G. R. & MAHLER, H. R. (1968). *J. Neurochem.* **15,** 765.
EDSTRÖM, A. (1964). *J. Neurochem.* **11,** 309.
EDSTRÖM, A. (1966). *J. Neurochem.* **13,** 315.
EDSTRÖM, A. (1967). *J. Neurochem.* **14,** 239.
EDSTRÖM, A. & SJÖSTRAND, J. (1969). *J. Neurochem.* **16,** 67.
EDSTRÖM, J.-E., EICHNER, D. & EDSTRÖM, A. (1962). *Biochim. Biophys. Acta,* **61,** 178.

EKHOLM, R. & HYDÉN, H. (1965). *Ultrastructure Res.* **13**, 269.
FARSTAD, M., HAUG, J. O., LINDBAK, H. & SKAUG, O. E. (1956a). *Acta. Neurol. Scand.* **41**, 52.
FARSTAD, M., SKAUG, O. E. & SOLHEIM, D. M. (1965b). *Acta. Neurol. Scand.* **41**, 59.
FLANGAS, A. L. & BOWMAN, R. E. (1970). *J. Neurochem.* **17**, 1237.
FLEXNER, J. B., FLEXNER, L. B., STELLAR, E., DE LA HABA, G. & ROBERTS, R. B. (1962). *J. Neurochem.* **9**, 595.
FOLCH, J. P. & LEES, M. B. (1951). *J. biol. Chem.* **191**, 807.
FRIEDE, R. (1959). *Expl. Neurol.* **1**, 441.
GAITONDE, M. K. & RICHTER, D. (1965). *Proc. Roy. Soc. B.* **145**, 83.
GARREN, L. D. & CROCCO, R. M. (1967). *Biochem. Biophys. Res. Communs.* **26**, 722.
GAVRIOVLA, T. N. (1968). *Bull. expl. Biol. Med.* **65**, 110.
GIORGI, P. P. (1970) *Biochem. J.* **120**, 643.
GISPEN, W. H., DE WIED, D., SCHOTMAN, P. & JANSZ, H. S. (1970). *J. Neurochem.* **17**, 751.
GOLDBERG, N. D., DIETZ, S. B. & O'TOOLE, A. G. (1969). *J. Biol. Chem.* **244**, 4458.
GORDON, M. W. & DEANIN, G. G. (1968). *J. biol. Chem.* **243**, 4222.
GOT, K., POLYA, G. M., POLYA, J. B. & COCKERILL, L. M. (1967). *Biochim. Biophys. Acta*, **117**, 42.
GREENGARD, P., RUDOLPH, S. A. & STURTEVANT, J. M. (1969). *J. biol. Chem.* **244**, 4798.
HALDAR, D., FREEMAN, K. & WORK, T. S. (1966). *Nature*, **211**, 9.
HALLIBURTON, W. D. (1894). *J. Physiol.* **15**, 90.
HANZON, V. & TOSCHI, G. (1959). *Expl. cell. Res.* **16**, 256.
HARDMAN, J. G. & SUTHERLAND, E. W. (1969). *J. biol. Chem.* **244**, 6363.
HENDERSON, J. F. & LEPAGE, G. A. (1959). *J. biol. Chem.* **234**, 2364.
HONDA, F. & IMAMURA, H. (1968). *Biochim. Biophys. Acta.* **161**, 267.
HOWARD, W. J., KERSON, L. A. & APPEL, S. H. (1970). *J. Neurochem.* **17**, 121.
HOYER, B. H., MCCARTHY, B. J. & BOLTON, E. T. (1963). *Science*, **140**, 1408.
HYDÉN, H. (1963). *Brain*, **86**, 773.
HYDÉN, H. & MCEWAN, B. (1966). *Proc. Natl. Acad. Sci. U.S.A.*, **55**, 354.
IPATA, P. L. (1967). *Biochem. Biophys. Res. Communs.* **27**, 337.
IPATA, P. L. (1968). *Biochemistry*, **7**, 507.
JACOB, M., STEVENIN, J., JUND, R., JUDES, C. & MANDEL, P. (1966). *J. Neurochem.* **13**, 619.
JACOB, M., SAMEC, J., STEVENIN, J. & MANDEL, P. (1967). *J. Neurochem.* **14**, 169.
JAMES, K. A. C. & AUSTIN, L. (1970). *Biochem. J.* **117**, 773.
JAMES, K. A. C., BRAY, J. J., MORGAN, I. G. & AUSTIN, L. (1970). *Biochem. J.* **117**, 767.
JONES, C. T. & BANKS, P. (1970). *Biochem. J.* **118**, 801.
JONES, D. A. & MCILWAIN, H. (1971). *J. Neurochem.* **18**, 41.
JORDAN, W. K., MARCH, R., BOYD-HOUCHIN, O. & POPP, E. (1959). *J. Neurochem.* **4**, 170.
KAKIUCHI, S. & RALL, T. W. (1968). *Mol. Pharmacol.* **4**, 367, 379.
KAKIUCHI, S., RALL, T. W. & MCILWAIN, H. (1969). *J. Neurochem.* **16**, 485.
KELLEY, W. N. (1968). *Feder. Proc.* **27**, 1047.
KEMP, J. W. & WOODBURY, D. M. (1965). *Biochim. Biophys. Acta*, **111**, 23.
KERR, S. E. (1942). *J. biol. Chem.* **145**, 647.
KIMBERLIN, R. H. (1967). *J. Neurochem.* **14**, 123.
KLAINER, L. M., CHI, Y.-M., FREIDBERG, S. L., RALL, T. W. & SUTHERLAND, E. W. (1962). *J. biol. Chem.* **237**, 1239.
KOENIG, E. (1967). *J. Neurochem.* **14**, 429, 437.
KOENIG, E. (1969). Abstr. 2nd Int. Soc. Neurochem. Conf. (Milan), p. 12. Ed. R. Paoletti, R. Fumagalli & C. Galli.
KOENIG, E. & KOELLE, G. B. (1961). *J. Neurochem.* **8**, 169.
KOSINSKI, E. & GRABAR, P. (1967). *J. Neurochem.* **14**, 783.
KRISHNA, G., FORN, J. D. & GESSA, G. L. (1969). Abstr. 2nd Int. Soc. Neurochem. Conf. (Milan), p. 258, 259. Ed. R. Paoletti, R. Fumagalli & C. Galli.
KŘIVÁNEK, J. (1970). *J. Neurochem.* **17**, 531.

KUHNE, W. & CHITTENDEN, R. H. (1890). *Z. Biol.* **26**, 292.
KUMAR, S., JOSAN, V., SANGER, K. C. S., TEWARI, K. K. & KRISHNAN, P. S. (1967). *Biochem. J.* **102**, 691.
KUO, J. F. & GREENGARD, P. (1969). *Proc. natn. Acad. Sci. U.S.A.* **64**, 1349; *J. biol. Chem.* **244**, 3417.
LAJTHA, A. (1959). *J. Neurochem.* **3**, 358.
LAJTHA, A. (1964). *Internat. Rev. Neurobiol.* **6**, 1.
LAJTHA, A. & TOTH, J. (1966). *Biochem. Biophys. Res. Communs.* **23**, 294.
LANDOLT, R., HESS, H. H. & THALHEIMER, C. (1966). *J. Neurochem.* **13**, 1441.
LAPHAM, L. W. (1968). *Science*, **159**, 310.
LEBARON, F. N. (1963). *Biochim. Biophys. Acta*, **70**, 658.
LEBARON, F. N. & FOLCH, J. (1959). *J. Neurochem.* **4**, 1.
LEES, M. B. (1966). *Feder. Proc.* **25**, 767.
LEES, M. B. (1968). *J. Neurochem.* **15**, 153.
LEVITT, M. (1969). *Nature*, **224**, 659.
LIPMANN, F. (1957). *Proc. Internat. Neurochem. Sympos.* **2**, 329.
LOGAN, J. E., MANNELL, W. A. & ROSSITER, R. J. (1952). *Biochem. J.* **51**, 470.
LOWRY, O. H., GILLIGAN, D. R. & KATERSKY, E. M. (1941). *J. biol. Chem.* **139**, 795.
McGREGOR, H. H. (1916–17). *J. biol. Chem.* **28**, 403.
McILWAIN, H. (1971). In: Effects of Drugs on Cellular Control Mechanisms. Edit. Rabin, B. R. In Press.
McILWAIN, H. & RODNIGHT, R. (1962). Practical Neurochemistry. London: Churchill.
MACINNES, J. W., McCONKEY, E. H. & SCHLESINGER, K. (1970). *J. Neurochem.* **17**, 457.
MANDEL, P. (1967). *Bull. Soc. Chim. Biol.* **49**, 1491.
MANDEL, P. (1969). The Future of the Brain Sciences, p. 191. Ed. S. Bogoch. New York: Plenum.
MARKS, N. (1970). *Handbook of Neurochem.* **3**, 133.
MARKS, N., DATTA, R. K. & LAJTHA, A. (1968). *J. biol. Chem.* **243**, 2880.
MARKS, N. & LAJTHA, A. (1963). *Biochem. J.* **89**, 438.
MARTENSON, R. E. & GAITONDE, M. K. (1969a). *J. Neurochem.* **16**, 889.
MARTENSON, R. E., DEIBLER, G. E. & KIES, M. W. (1969b). *J. biol. Chem.* **244**, 4261, 4268.
MASE, K., TAKAHASHI, Y. & OGATA, K. (1962). *J. Neurochem.* **9**, 281.
MEHL, E. (1968). Macromolecules and the Function of the Neuron, p. 22. Ed. Z. Lodin & S. P. R. Rose. Amsterdam: Excerpta Med. Found.
MENDICINO, J. & MUNTZ, J. A. (1958). *J. biol. Chem.* **233**, 178.
METZGER, H. P., CUENOD, M., GRYNBAUM, A. & WAELSCH, H. (1969). *J. Neurochem.* **14**, 183.
MINARD, F. N. & RICHTER, D. (1968). *J. Neurochem.* **15**, 1463.
MOORE, B. W. (1965). *Biochem. Biophys. Res. Communs.* **19**, 739.
MOORE, B. W. & McGREGOR, D. (1965). *J. biol. Chem.* **240**, 1647.
MOORE, B. W., PEREZ, V. J. & GEHRING, M. (1968). *J. Neurochem.* **15**, 265.
MORGAN, I. G. & AUSTIN, L. (1968). *J. Neurochem.* **15**, 41.
MORI, K., YAMAGAMI, S., AKAHANI, Y. & KAWAKITA, Y. (1970). *J. Neurochem.* **17**, 1691.
MORRIS, N. R., AGHAJANIAN, G. K. & BLOOM, F. E. (1967). *Science*, **155**, 1125.
MUNTZ, J. A. (1953). *J. biol. Chem.* **201**, 221.
MURTHY, M. R. V. (1966). *Biochim. Biophys. Acta*, **119**, 586, 599.
MURTHY, M. R. V. & RAPPOPORT, D. A. (1965). *Biochim. Biophys. Acta*, **95**, 121.
NYHAN, W. L., PESEK, J., SWEETMAN, L., CARPENTER, D. G. & CARTER, C. H. (1967). *Pediatric Res.* **1**, 5.
ODERFELD-NOWAK, B. & NIEMIERKO, S. (1969). *J. Neurochem.* **16**, 235.
OESTERLE, W., KANIG, K., BUCHEL, W. & NICKEL, A.-K. (1970). *J. Neurochem.* **17**, 1403.
ORREGO, F. & LIPMANN, F. (1967). *J. biol. Chem.* **242**, 665.
PAIK, W. K. & KIM, S. (1969). *J. Neorochem.* **16**, 1257.
PALAY, S. L. & PALADE, G. E. (1955). *J. Biochem. Biophys. Cytol.* **1**, 69.
PALLADIN, A. V. (1949). *Chem. Zbl.* **1**, 217 (from *J. Physiol. USSR*, **33**, 727).

PALLADIN, A. V. (1964). Problems of the Biochemistry of the Nervous System. Trans. F. S. Freisinger, H. Hillman & R. Woodman. Oxford: Pergamon.
PALLADIN, A. V., POLYAKOVA, N. M. & LISHKO, V. K. (1963). *J. Neurochem.* **10**, 187.
PALMER, F. B. & DAWSON, R. M. C. (1969). *Biochem. J.* **111**, 629, 637.
PETERSON, N. A. & McKEAN, C. M. (1969). *J. Neurochem.* **16**, 1211.
PHILIPPS, G. R. (1969). *Nature,* **223**, 374.
PICK, J., DeLEMOS, C. & GERDIN, C. (1964). *J. comp. Neurol.* **122**, 19.
PIHA, R. S., BERGSTROEM, R. M., BERGSTROEM, A., UUSITALO, A. J. & OJA, S. A. (1963). *Ann. Med. Exptl. Biol. Fenniae,* **41**, 485.
PIHA, R. S., CUENOD, M. & WAELSCH, H. (1965). Proc. XIII Colloq. Prot. Biol. FLUIDS, Brugge, p. 66.
PIHA, R. S., CUENOD, M. & WAELSCH, H. (1966). *J. biol. Chem.* **241**, 2397.
POPE, A. & ANFINSEN, C. B. (1948). *J. biol. Chem.* **173**, 305.
PORTER, H. & FOLCH, J. (1957). *J. Neurochem.* **1**, 260.
PRYOR, G. T., OTIS, L. S., SCOTT, M. K. & COLWELL, J. J. (1967). *J. comp. physiol. Psychol.* **63**, 236.
PULL, I. & McILWAIN, H. (1971). Unpublished observations.
PUSZKIN, S., BERL, S., PUSZKIN, E. & CLARKE, D. (1968). *Science,* **161**, 170.
RALL, T. W. & GILMAN, A. G. (1970). *Neurosciences. Res. Prog. Bull.* **8**, 821
RAPPOPORT, D. A., FRITZ, R. R. & MORACZEWSKI, A. (1963). *Biochim. Biophys. Acta,* **74**, 42.
REIS, J. L. (1951). *Biochem. J.* **48**, 548.
ROBERTSON, D. M. (1957). *J. Neurochem.* **1**, 358.
ROBISON, G. A., BUTCHER, R. W. & SUTHERLAND, E. W. (1967). *Ann. N.Y. Acad. Sci.* **139**, 703.
ROBISON, G. A., BUTCHER, R. W. & SUTHERLAND, E. W. (1968). *Ann. Rev. Biochem.* **37**, 149.
ROBISON, G. A., BUTCHER, R. W. & SUTHERLAND, E. W. (1971). Cyclic AMP. New York: Academic Press.
ROSE, S. P. R. (1969). *Handbook of Neurochem.* **2**, 183.
ROSENBLOOM, F. M., KELLEY, W. N., MILLER, J. M., HENDERSON, J. F. & SEEGMILLER, J. E. (1967). *J. Amer. Med. Assoc.* **202**, 175.
RUBIN, A. L. & STENZEL, K. H. (1965). *Proc. natn. Acad. Sci.* **53**, 963.
SABORIO, J. L. & ALEMAN, V. (1970). *J. Neurochem.* **17**, 91.
SANTOS, J. N., HEMPSTEAD, K. W., KOPP, L. E. & MIECH, R. P. (1968). *J. Neurochem.* **15**, 367.
SATAKE, M., TAKAHASHI, Y., MASE, K. & OGATA, K. (1964). *J. Biochem. Japan,* **56**, 504.
SATTIN, A. & RALL, T. W. (1970). *Mol. Pharmacol.* **6**, 13.
SCHNEIDER, D. & ROBERTS, S. (1968). *J. Neurochem.* **15**, 1469.
SEEGMILLER, J. E., ROSENBLOOM, F. M. & KELLEY, W. N. (1967). *Science,* **155**, 1682.
SELLINGER, O. Z. & AZCURRA, J. M. (1970). Protein Metabolism of the Nervous System, p. 517. Ed. A. Lajtha. New York: Plenum.
SELLINGER, O. Z. & OHLSSON, W. G. (1969). *Life Sci.* **8**, 1083.
SETLOW, B., BURGER, R. & LOWENSTEIN, J. M. (1966). *J. biol. Chem.* **241**, 1244.
SETLOW, B. & LOWENSTEIN, J. M. (1967). *J. biol. Chem.* **242**, 607.
SETLOW, B. & LOWENSTEIN, J. M. (1968). *J. biol. Chem.* **243**, 3409.
SHIMADA, M. & NAKAMURA, T. (1966). *J. Neurochem.* **13**, 391.
SHIMIZU, H., CREVELING, C. R. & DALY, J. (1970). *Proc. nat. Acad. Sci. U.S.A.* **65**, 1033.
SHIMIZU, H., DALY, J. & CREVELING, C. R. (1969). *J. Neurochem.* **16**, 1609.
SHIMIZU, H. & DALY, J. (1970). *Biochim. Biophys. Acta.* **222**, 465.
SIMLER, S., POPOVIC, D. & MANDEL, P. (1967). *Bull. Soc. Chim. Biol.* **49**, 1509.
SIMON, L. N., GLASKY, A. J. & REJAL, T. H. (1967). *Biochim. Biophys. Acta,* **142**, 99.
SINGH, U. N. (1965). *Nature,* **206**, 1115.
SINGH, U. B. & TALWAR, G. P. (1967). *J. Neurochem.* **14**, 675.
SINGH, U. B. & TALWAR, G. P. (1969). *J. Neurochem.* **16**, 951.
SMILLIE, R. M. (1957). *Arch. Biochem. Biophys.* **67**, 213.
STEEL, M. & GIES, W. J. (1907–8). *Amer. J. Physiol.* **20**, 378.

STEIN, H. & YELLIN, T. (1967). *Science*, **157**, 96.

STETTON, D. (1968). *Feder. Proc.* **27**, 110.

STETTON, D. & HEARON, J. Z. (1959). *Science*, **129**, 1737.

SUNG, S.-C. (1968). *J. Neurochem.* **15**, 477.

SUTHERLAND, E. W., ØYE, I. & BUTCHER, R. W. (1965). *Rec. Progr. Hormone Res.* **21**, 623.

SUTHERLAND, E. W., RALL, T. W. & MENON, T. (1962). *J. biol. Chem.* **237**, 1220.

SUZUKI, K., KOREY, K. R. & TERRY, R. D. (1964). *J. Neurochem.* **11**, 403.

SWEETMAN, L. (1968). *Feder. Proc.* **27**, 1055.

SWANSON, P. D. & STAHL, W. L. (1966). *Biochem. J.* **99**, 396.

TAKAHASHI, Y. & ABE, S. (1963). *Experientia*, **19**, 186.

TAKAHASHI, Y., MASE, K. & SUZUKI, Y. (1970). *J. Neurochem.* **17**, 1433, 1521.

TARR, M., BRADA, D. & SAMSON, F. E. (1962). *Amer. J. Physiol.* **203**, 690.

TENCHEVA, Z. S. & HADJIOLOV, A. A. (1969). *J. Neurochem.* **16**, 769.

THOMAS, J. (1957). *Biochem. J.* **66**, 655.

TOMASI, L. G. & KORNGUTH, S. E. (1968). *J. biol. Chem.* **243**, 2507.

UZMAN, L. L., VAN DEN NOORT, S. & RUMLEY, M. K. (1962). *J. Neurochem.* **9**, 241.

VAN BREEMAN, V. L., ANDERSON, E. & ROGER, J. F. (1958). *Exp. cell. Res. Suppl.* **5**, 153.

VESCO, C. & GIUDITTA, A. (1967). *Biochim. Biophys. Acta*, **142**, 385.

VESCO, C. & GIUDITTA, A. (1969). *J. Neurochem.* **15**, 81.

VILLELA, G. G. (1968). *Experientia*, **24**, 1101.

VINCENDON, G., WAKSMAN, A., UYEMURA, K., TARDY, J. & GOMBOS, G. (1967). *Arch. Biochem. Biophys.* **120**, 233.

VON HUNGEN, K., MAHLER, H. R. & MOORE, W. J. (1968). *J. biol. Chem.* **243**, 1415.

WARECKA, K. & BAUER, H. (1967). *J. Neurochem.* **14**, 783.

WARECKA, K. & BAUER, H. (1968). *Dtsch. Z. Nervenheilk.* **194**, 66.

WEIL-MALHERBE, H. & GREEN, R. H. (1955). *Biochem. J.* **61**, 210, 218.

WEISENBERG, R. C., BORISY, G. G. & TAYLOR, E. W. (1968). *Biochemistry*, **7**, 4466.

WEISS, B. & COSTA, E. (1968). *Biochem. Pharmacol.* **17**, 2107.

WEISSMAN, S. M., PAUL, J., THOMSON, R. Y., SMELLIE, R. M. S. & DAVIDSON, J. N. (1960). *Biochem. J.* **76**, 1P.

WELLER, M. & RODNIGHT, R. (1970). *Nature*, **225**, 187.

WELLS, W., GAINES, D. & KOENIG, H. (1963). *J. Neurochem.* **10**, 709.

WOLFGRAM, F. (1966). *J. Neurochem.* **13**, 461.

YAMAGAMI, S., MASUI, M. & KAWAKITA, Y. (1963). *J. Neurochem.* **10**, 849.

ZAMENHOF, S., BURSZTYN, H., RICH, K. & ZAMENHOF, P. J. (1964). *J. Neurochem.* **11**, 505.

ZAMENHOF, S., MARTHENS, E. & MARGOLIS, F. (1968). *Science*, **160**, 322.

ZOMZELY, C. E., ROBERTS, R., GRUBER, C. P. & BROWN, D. M. (1968). *J. biol. Chem.* **243**, 5396.

ZOMZELY, C. E., ROBERTS, R. & RAPAPORT, D. (1964). *J. Neurochem.* **11**, 567.

10 Nutritional Factors and the Central Nervous System

The science and practice of nutrition are concerned with outstandingly important relationships between organism and environment: relationships which in higher animals involve the central nervous system in numerous ways. Aspects of this neural involvement are outlined first in the present section, after which nutritional factors are considered specifically in relation to the brain and according to their chemical nature. Many matters which are mentioned only briefly here, receive fuller attention in texts of physiological psychology (cf. Deutsch & Deutsch, 1966); eating and drinking are important to many test-systems in animal psychology. In natural populations, relationships between animal and food become part of ecological studies and the nervous system is both sensor and target; in human populations nutritional effects on learning and behaviour evoke social and administrative study (see Scrimshaw & Gordon, 1968).

Sensory Appraisal of Potential Foods

The chemical senses of taste and smell with their peripheral receptors and cerebral representation, evolved in relation to feeding and these senses remain, in present-day animals including man, of extreme importance in appraising and selecting food. Indeed, food technology gives much impetus to their current study (Amerine *et al.*, 1965; Ottoson & Shepherd, 1967).

Neural pathways involved in *taste* extend from buccal receptors through the medulla and thalamus before reaching the cerebral cortex in areas which include the insula and subtemporal regions, apparently without a single area specialized for taste. Interruption of the pathway named has been observed to raise thresholds for specific taste sensations. Chemical interaction between tissue-components and the compound giving a particular taste sensation may be illustrated by sweet-tasting substances. Structural and stereochemical similarities shown by certain sugars, amino acids and synthetic imides make it possible to specify interaction at a common site (Schallenberger *et al.*, 1969). In extracts from taste-buds of the ox tongue, difference-spectroscopy showed a component to interact with sucrose sufficiently to afford a basis for isolation. The sucrose-combining component was protein-like, was purified by ammonium sulphate precipitation and the free-energy change of the combination indicated H-bonding as probably involved in the reaction with sucrose (Dastoli & Price, 1966; Dastoli, 1968; see however Koyama & Kurihara, 1971). The binding of the protein with five sugars and saccharin was found to be directly related to their sweetness as determined in human and other mammalian species.

The tasting of sweetness is susceptible to chemical modification. A plant-derived material, gymnemic acid, when held as a 1 mM solution in the mouth (Stocklin et al., 1967; Stocklin, 1967) depressed the sweet sensation given by sucrose. A "miracle fruit" (Synsepalum dulcificum) yielded a taste-modifying protein which was itself tasteless but which, when held in the mouth for a few minutes, caused acidic substances to taste sweet (Kurihara & Beidler, 1968, 1969). The protein was required at 0·1–0·5 μM for this effect, which lasted for a few minutes or a few hours and specifically altered perception of sourness; perception of salty or of bitter tastes, or of sweetness resulting from sucrose itself, was unaffected. The taste-modifying protein contained 6·7 % of arabinose and xylose and these pentoses themselves, in about 1 M solution, taste sweet to an extent comparable to the sweetness induced by the taste-modifying protein in much more dilute solutions. Thus the pentoses are unlikely to act in free solution after release from the protein, and it is pictured that they are first brought to the neighbourhood of sweet-receptors by the protein, and subsequently are enabled to combine after the pH change by the sour, acidic substances has caused a conformational change in the receptor.

Conceivably the interaction in taste-receptors is by membrane distortion causing change in permeability and hence of polarization and cell-firing. Lack of vitamin A (cf. in relation to membrane structure, p. 300) causes abnormal taste-responses by rats to quinine and salt. Administration of the vitamin promptly restored NaCl discrimination, supporting an action at the taste-sensitive cells. Vitamin-A alcohol may also ameliorate anosmia in certain instances (Bernard et al., 1961; Duncan & Briggs, 1962). Penetration of phospholipid-protein or -cephalin monolayers by odourous substances has shown some promise as a model system (Friedman et al., Symposium, 1964). Capsaicin, a compound contributing to the pungency of red pepper, on ingestion acts not only peripherally but also at hypothalamic temperature-sensitive regions. Here it can cause long-term insensitivity of cells concerned with detection of warmth, and histological examination of preparations from the rat has shown this to be accompanied by cellular changes (Szolcsányi et al., 1971). These are remarkably specific to a category of neurons in the pre-optic nucleus, which are presumably concerned with temperature-detection.

The neural apparatus involved in smell extends from the sensory epithelium to the olfactory bulb and from the bulb to the piriform lobe of the brain, largely by the lateral olfactory tract. Damage to these structures can impair olfactory discrimination, which normally is highly developed, as has been shown by observing olfactory responses to pure compounds with a great variety of chemical structures (Symposium, 1964; Harper et al., 1968; Zotterman, 1967). Complex odours have been separated by gas chromatography to components which elicited specific electrophysiological responses on application to the olfactory mucosa (Ottoson & Shepherd, 1967). Neural organization in the olfactory bulb and cortex is complex, involving recurrent fibres and inhibitory as well as excitatory synapses which have been examined in relation to several transmitting and pharmacological agents (Baumgarten *et al.*, 1963; Legge *et al.*, 1966).

The lateral olfactory tract and piriform cortex obtainable from rodents as a slice 0·3–0·4 mm. thick, form an excellent *in vitro* system for study of neural conduction and synaptic transmission in the brain (Yamamoto & McIlwain, 1966; McIlwain, 1968). Electrical stimulation at the anterior end of the tract is shown by observing metabolic and electrical responses, to excite about one-third of the attached cortex.

Cerebral Involvement in Protein and Calorie Intake

Among the bodily adjustments in which the CNS functions throughout life, are those which condition the quantity and type of food intake. Much of this subject is recounted more fully in writing on nutrition (Davidson & Passmore, 1966; Scrimshaw & Gordon, 1967; Symposia, 1967, 1969); the neuronal and hormonal controls involved are complex and can receive only brief comment here.

Hypothalamic regions contribute to regulation of mammalian food and fluid intake; lesions in specific regions can cause animals to cease to eat, or to eat to excess. Various interactions between peripheral and central systems are proposed in interpretation: for example, that the kidneys release a humoural factor inducing thirst (Fitzsimmons, 1969). Regulation of body weight is normally remarkably accurate, but lesions in ventromedial nuclei of the hypothalamus of mice can quickly cause obesity. Means by which central sensing of general nutritional status may occur are discussed by Hervey (1969): one theory suggests the production at defined rate of a preferentially fat-soluble substance, possibly steroid, to which a hypothalamic region is sensitive. The blood level of such a substance would then be dependent on the quantity of body fat.

Nutritionally-important substances are in addition subject to individual control at the hypothalamus. On supplying glucose from microcapillaries close to individual firing units in the rat brain (Oomura *et al.*, 1969), 40 % of units examined in the ventromedial nucleus of the hypothalamus increased their rate of firing. None of the units, presumably cells, diminished in firing rate but in lateral hypothalamic regions the units which increased in activity with glucose were sparser, and some units decreased in firing-rate when glucose was applied. Cells were also encountered which responded to hypertonic solutions of both glucose and NaCl and were of possible significance as osmoreceptors. Glucose-sensitive regions appear to be affected by intracerebral gold thioglucose, which causes localized hypothalamic lesions.

The amino acid content of surrounding fluids can also affect the firing of cerebral cells; aspects of this subject are considered in describing neural transmitting agents and in referring to glutamic acid, which is particularly active in this respect. Peripheral taste receptors also show unusual sensitivity to glutamates, as is evidenced by the commercial use of glutamates in enhancing the flavour of foodstuffs.

Dietary Imbalance and Anorexia

Diets which are unsatisfactory for any one of a variety of causes may induce anorexia (Milne, 1968; *Symposium*, 1965). This behavioural change has been observed in rats when the protein content of a diet is too high or too low: that is, outside the range of 10–20 % protein which is preferred. More specifically, anorexia is also induced when any one of the eight essential amino acids is omitted: absence of valine, leucine, isoleucine, threonine, methionine, lysine, phenylalanine or tryptophan can be effective. Remarkably, food intake was diminished in rats within 24 hr. of the omission of one of the amino acids. As force-feeding a deficient diet exacerbated lesions and shortened an animal's life, the anorexia was protective.

Kwashiorkor, a protein and calorie deficiency in man, also involves anorexia. Serum-protein concentration falls; the blood level of most amino acids diminishes, the change being greatest in essential amino acids, especially in valine and leucine (Milne, 1968). Electroencephalographic changes are observed, including an increased proportion of slow α-wave frequencies and the condition is associated with mental apathy or irritability. It is rapidly relieved by administering a preparation of essential amino acids. Bodily signs similar to those of kwashiorkor have been produced experimentally in pigs fed a low-protein diet (Stewart & Platt, 1967) and were associated with cerebral oedema and diminution of brain weight. Undernourished rats and pigs display behavioural changes (see Scrimshaw & Gordon, 1967).

High-protein diets also induce anorexia. While most of the common amino acids become toxic at high doses (e.g. of L-tryptophan, 8 mmoles/kg. body weight, or L-alanine, 57 mmoles/kg. in rats), smaller doses of amino acids given singly, caused profound anorexia, often with prostration or uncoordinated movements (Milne, 1968). Blood ammonia level rose in the animals, but not to levels associated with toxicity from ammonium salts themselves. The anorexia induced in animals by a high-protein diet diminished after some days, and recovery was associated with increased formation of amino acid metabolizing enzymes. Indeed organs including the liver and kidney could change markedly in relative size during such adaptation and the readjustment of hormonal balance which was involved, included participation of the pituitary hormones (*Symposia*, 1965, 1969).

The self-imposed restriction of food intake which is characteristic of the mental illness *anorexia nervosa* can produce extreme emaciation and patients, frequently girls and young women, become little more than half normal weight. Quantitative appraisal of the food and calorie intake of such persons (Russell, 1967) showed it insufficient to maintain even the diminished body weight. Nevertheless, plasma proteins remained approximately normal; the plasma content of 18 amino acids was within normal range, in contrast to the diminution observed in kwashiorkor. Interestingly, the patients were selecting a diet severely depleted in carbohydrate but relatively high in protein and this (see preceding paragraph) may contribute to maintaining the abnormally low intake of food.

Vitamins and the Central Nervous System

When the vitamins required by man and by most experimental animals are listed, placing first those of which deficiency most prominently affects the central nervous system, the list begins with thiamine and nicotinic acid. These are followed by vitamins B_6 and B_{12}, and then by pantothenate and riboflavin. Of indirect or lesser effect are vitamins A, D, E, and ascorbic acid.

The substances are described below in the order quoted. This order is not that of their importance in cerebral metabolism; riboflavin is as important in this regard as is thiamine, but lack of riboflavin affects first other parts of the body and necessarily receives a briefer notice here. Sources of general information on the vitamins and other nutritional essentials include Follis (1963), Davidson & Passmore (1966), Dickens *et al.* (1968) and Sebrell & Harris (1968). The *Symposia* (1953, 1957), Blackwood *et al.* (1963), Brozek *et al.* (1960, 1961) and Kare & Muller (1967) are concerned specifically with nutritional factors and neural systems.

The first six substances quoted above all belong to the B group of vitamins. They have this collective name because they tend to occur together in natural products and their separate effects were not at first differentiated. Though they are now characterized and effects of the lack of each have been studied separately their collective name is a reminder that they occur together and may be lacking together, and thus deficiencies as they are seen clinically are still very likely to involve two or more of the vitamins at once.

Thiamine

Investigation of how lack of thiamine brings about changes in cerebral functioning has extended throughout the past 50 years during which most of the current knowledge of cerebral metabolism has been acquired. As can be judged from Chapter 6, studies of thiamine by R. A. Peters and his colleagues contributed much to such knowledge, for great stimulus came from finding in thiamine deficiency, defects in the main energy-yielding reactions of cerebral tissues themselves. In the following account the cerebral effects of thiamine deficiency will first be outlined, and their metabolic basis then discussed. More general and peripheral aspects of thiamine avitaminoses, including beri-beri, receive only incidental comment here; accounts of thiamine from which information has been drawn include those of Williams *et al.* (1950), Williams (1961), the *Symposia* (1961, 1969) and the Study Group (1967) and *Conference* (1962).

Effects of Deficiency

When considered from the point of view of changes caused in the functioning of the brain, thiamine deficiency has been described as leading to the two types of disorder summarized in Table 10.1. The two types differ in the circumstances of their development. They were in part differentiated in earlier observations on beri-beri and many of their symptoms have been reproduced in experimental animals. In the different forms of beri-beri, many organs of the body are affected by a deficiency of thiamine which is aggravated by other factors including protein deficiency; the neural lesions are preponderantly peripheral but damage to the central nervous system also plays a role.

(1) The neurasthenic syndrome appears in normal subjects maintained on a diet suboptimal in thiamine but otherwise fully adequate. It can be completely cleared by administered thiamine. The anorexia of this condition appears in thiamine deficiency in a variety of experimental animals and is in

Table 10.1

The central nervous system and lack of thiamine in man

Effect	Conditions of development	Symptoms
(1) *Neurasthenic syndrome*		
(Jolliffe *et al.*, 1939; Wilder, and Bowman & Wortis, in *Symposium*, 1943)	Developed in 4–5 days on less than 150 µg. thiamine/day. Developed in some weeks on diet giving 450 µg./day. Lost 3–6 days after administering 1–2 mg./day thiamine	Lassitude, irritability, anorexia. Precordial pain, dyspnoea on exertion, palpitation, electrocardiogram abnormalities, muscle cramps and tenderness, skin hyperaesthesia. Basal metabolic rate lowered 14–33%, and intolerance to cold
(2) *Wernicke's syndrome*		
(Alexander *et al.*, 1938; Alexander, 1940; Jolliffe *et al.*, 1941; *Symposia*, 1943, 1961; Williams, 1961; Study Group (1967)	Developed with a small intake of thiamine and of normal foodstuffs during alcoholism, persistent vomiting, or high fever	Ophthalmoplegia and peripheral neuropathy; ataxia (always respond to thiamine). Clouding of consciousness (may require factors in addition to thiamine). High blood pyruvate (responds to thiamine). When arrested by thiamine, may leave permanent cerebral lesions

part protective, for forced feeding of deficient animals leads to an earlier development of polyneuritis. The symptoms reported in man include also personality changes and lowered performance in memory and dexterity tests.

(2) The more severe condition described by Wernicke in 1881, but only much later shown to involve thiamine, occurs when the intake of thiamine is very low and usually when other aggravating factors are present. Thus Wernicke's original cases were of persistent vomiting and alcoholism; for more recent discussion see Victor & Adams (*Symposium*, 1961). The condition appeared also in prisoner-of-war camps (Davidson & Passmore, 1966). When the deficiency has progressed to the stage involving peripheral neuritis and changes in consciousness, irreversible damage appears to have occurred in cerebral structures. Lesions are found especially in the periventricular grey matter consisting of haemorrhage, proliferation of blood vessels and glial cells with

degeneration of neurons. These changes were described by Wernicke and have been reproduced in experimental animals kept on diets deficient specifically in thiamine. Administered thiamine at this stage is not fully curative, though it relieves several symptoms. There may remain a clinically-observed defect termed the Korsakoff syndrome: failure in memory of recent events, a tendency to confabulate, and disorientation in time and place. This syndrome is produced also by certain types of physical damage to the brain and by some toxic agents which also cause changes in cerebral structure. Its occurrence in thiamine deficiency may thus be an indication of the need for thiamine in maintaining cerebral structure as well as functioning.

A cerebro-cortical necrosis observed in calves has been found to be due to deficiency in thiamine. In its initial stages, when anorexia and ataxia were followed by coma, the condition could be alleviated by administration of thiamine alone (Pill et al., 1966). Investigation of untreated animals showed many of the biochemical signs of thiamine deficiency in man, which are described below: diminution in cerebral thiamine, an elevation of blood pyruvate and a fall in the transketolase of the blood. Characteristics of the disorder, including the cerebral lesions, were induced in a normal calf by placing it on a thiamine-deficient diet and administering pyrithiamine.

Very many factors influence thiamine requirement but only a few can be recounted here. Experimental animals may be maintained on diets with little or no added thiamine while carbohydrate intake is low; the requirement increases with increase in dietary carbohydrate, and thiamine requirement can be expressed to a considerable extent in terms of the carbohydrate intake. This reflects a major point of metabolic utilization of thiamine, as its pyrophosphate, in carbohydrate metabolism; and the considerable dependence of the brain on specifically carbohydrate metabolism is likely to be a factor which makes symptoms in the central nervous system so prominent in the deficiency.

Effects of thiamine-lack can be induced in experimental animals on diets normally adequate in thiamine, by substances which destroy or antagonize the vitamin. Thus an intoxication by diets containing raw fish involved many of the characters of Wernicke's syndrome including the specifically localized haemorrhagic lesions in the brain. The toxic agent proved to be an enzyme which degraded thiamine and could catalyse also the replacement of the thiazole part of thiamine by other bases (Fig. 10.1). "Thiaminase diseases" may be due to the presence of this enzyme in intestinal bacteria and other natural sources (Hayashi, 1957; Dreyfus & Victor, 1961). Also, certain substances including pyrithiamine (see below) which are structurally related to the vitamin can cause signs of thiamine deficiency within a day of their administration to small animals (Rindi et al., 1961). The effects of pyrithiamine are prevented by increased intake of thiamine. The two substances compete for entry to the brain, presumably at specific transport mechanisms, because of their similarity in structure but the similarity is not sufficiently close for pyrithiamine to lead to a derivative functioning as thiamine pyrophosphate: a deficiency in thiamine thus results. A comparable inhibitory analogue may be formed under some circumstances by a thiaminase of the rumen microflora, and produce cerebrocortical necrosis in sheep and cattle (see above; Edwin & Jackman, 1970).

Placing relatively strong solutions of thiamine or cocarboxylase on the cerebral cortex can result in convulsions, and large intravenous doses bring paralysis and respiratory disturbance. These curare-like effects are relatively unspecific and require quantities some thousands of times those needed to cure the avitaminosis.

Thiamine (I)

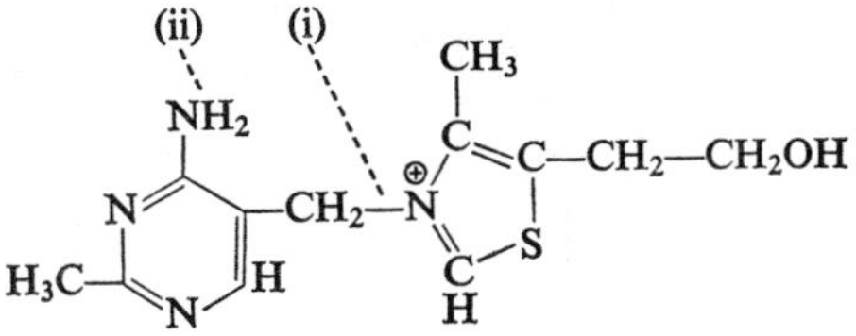

Thiamine pyrophosphate

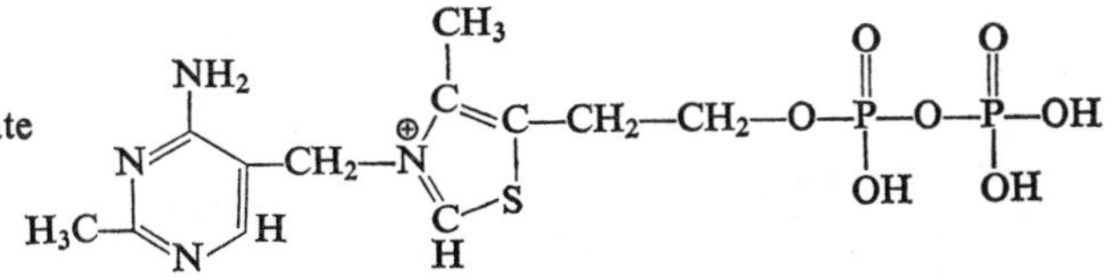

Pyrithiamine

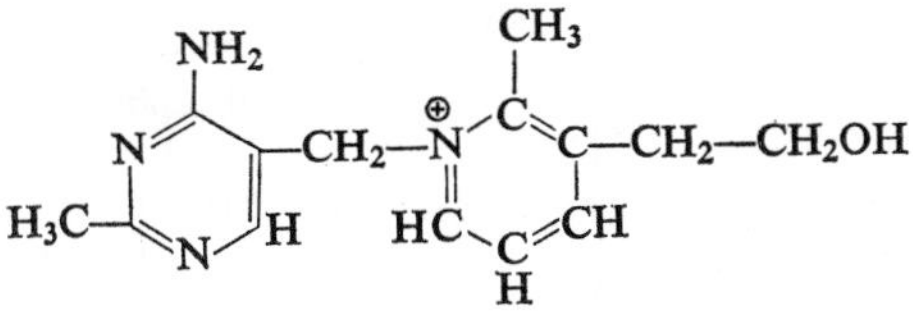

FIG. 10.1. Thiamine structure and analogues. In structure I, (i) represents the point of degradation by fish thiaminases (see Yudkin, 1949; Harris, 1951), and (ii) the amino group which is replaced by hydroxyl to give oxythiamine.

Thiamine of the Blood

In tracing dietary deficiency in thiamine to its effects in the brain, the thiamine of the bloodstream is an important intermediary. In the blood, thiamine exists at about one-tenth of its level in other tissues, and largely as its pyrophosphate, cocarboxylase (Fig. 10.1). In foodstuffs thiamine is present mainly in the free form; vegetable foods contain little cocarboxylase and thiamine itself preponderates in muscle. After recent intake of food, free thiamine can be detected in the blood, but at other times the level is undetectable or no more than about 20 nmoles/l. The pyrophosphate, on the other hand, is present at about 150–400 nmoles/l. (Sinclair, 1939; Lowry, 1952). The dietary thiamine has thus been promptly phosphorylated, and the liver plays a large part in this although cerebral and most other tissues can themselves carry out the reaction.

The thiamine pyrophosphate of the blood is largely in its formed elements. An upper limit for the thiamine derivatives in plasma appears to be about 30 nmoles/l.; erythrocytes contain some 270 and white blood cells and platelets about 2,200 nmoles/l. In cell-containing cerebral preparations, added thiamine pyrophosphate has a less immediate metabolic effect than has thiamine itself; presumably the pyrophosphate is less diffusible than thiamine. Its assimilation to cerebral tissues may therefore be aided by an enzyme which the tissues contain and which splits phosphate from the pyrophosphate (Fig. 10.2). The thiamine pyrophosphatase activity of cerebral tissues is potentially quite high. Phosphate liberation at 12 μmoles/g. rat brain/hr. has been observed but

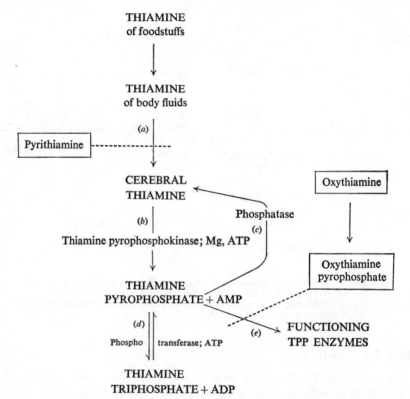

Fig. 10.2. Thiamine metabolism and functioning. The point of action shown for pyrithiamine describes its main inhibitory effect, but it has a subsidiary action by the route indicated for oxythiamine (Steyn-Parvé; Gubler & Johnson in *Study Group*, 1967; Johnson & Gubler, 1968; Itokawa & Cooper, 1968).

required 0·5 mM substrate; at lower levels approaching those possible *in vivo*, liberation was very much slower (Westenbrink *et al.*, 1943; Pratt, 1953). More than one enzyme appears to be involved in liberation of phosphate from thiamine pyrophosphate, and the systems concerned may have functions apart from assimilation of thiamine. They are not uniformly distributed in the brain, but occur especially in cell bodies, in granules in the cytoplasm rather than in the nucleus.

When dietary thiamine is withheld, the thiamine of the blood falls fairly promptly. This occurs in most species which have been examined and the blood or erythrocyte content in thiamine derivatives has been used in assessing the nutritional status of animals in relation to thiamine. The fall in the level of thiamine in the blood is accompanied or followed fairly closely by a fall in most organs of the body. In this respect the thiamine of the brain is exceptional and will now be considered in more detail.

Cerebral Thiamine

The brain compared with other organs of the animal body is moderately rich in thiamine (Table 10.2), in man containing about 5 and in the mouse about 12 nmoles/g. of tissue. It occurs in four forms: as thiamine and as its mono-, di- and tri-phosphoric esters. The greater part of the cerebral

Table 10.2

Thiamine content of human tissues

Condition of subject	Thiamine (μg./g.) in:				
Investigation A	Cerebral cortex	Heart	Skeletal muscle	Liver	Kidney cortex
Normal	1·0	2·2	0·4	1·1	1·5
Receiving additional thiamine	1·2	3·3	–	2·4	–
Poor nutrition: High fever and vomiting	0·5	0·6	–	0·3	0·4
Poor nutrition: Alcoholism	0·6	0·5	0·1	0·5	0·5

Investigation B	Cortical grey matter	Cortical white matter	Basal ganglia	Cerebellum
Normal*	$1·3 \pm 0·14$	$0·77 \pm 0·15$	$1·48 \pm 0·23$	$1·54 \pm 0·11$

Investigation C	Form of thiamine (%)				
	Total thiamine (μg./g.)	Free	Mono-phosphate	Pyro-phosphate	Tri-phosphate
Normal (frontal lobe)	1·6	11	10	68	9
Subacute necrotizing encephalomyelopathy	0·4	8	14	78	<0·1

Investigations (A) and *(B)*: data from Ferrebee *et al.* (*Symposium*, 1943), by analysis of tissues obtained post-mortem from subjects between 30 and 50 years of age, except those asterisked (*) who ranged between 6 and 74 years. Thiamine distribution in the tissues of other species has been recorded by, among others, Villela *et al.* (1949), Martin & Lissak (1950) and Dreyfus (1959, 1961).

Investigation (C): data from Cooper *et al.* (1969), by fluorometric methods after electro-phoretic separation of thiamine and its derivatives.

thiamine occurs as the di- or pyrophosphoric ester and has the coenzyme properties of cocarboxylase (Chapter 6), which have been used as one method for its determination. Although, normally, only small quantities of free thiamine are found in the brain (Table 10.2), much more can be measured shortly after administering the free vitamin (Ochoa & Peters, 1938). Some 10% of cerebral thiamine has been found as the triphosphate (Kiessling, 1961; Cooper et al., 1969) and receives more detailed discussion below.

The thiamine and its derivatives in cerebral tissues are relatively stable after removal of the brain from experimental animals, and rapid freezing appears not to be necessary for their determination (Ochoa & Peters, 1938; Dreyfus, 1961). Certain species of fish contain in several organs, thiaminases which

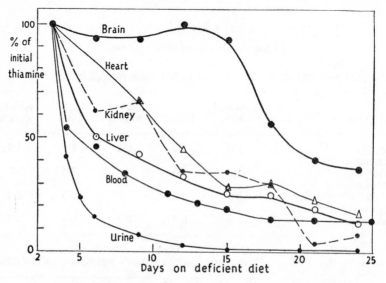

Fig. 10.3. Course of depletion of the rat in thiamine (Lowry, 1952). Initial levels were (in µg./g. or ml.): brain, 2·7; heart, 5·3; kidney, 3·7; liver, 4·2; blood, 0·21; urine, 3·3.

degrade the vitamin, and in these species the cerebral tissues also possess some, but relatively little, of the degrading enzyme (Harris, 1951). The cerebral content of thiamine derivatives may vary over a two- or three-fold range in different parts of the brain (Table 10.2), in general being greater in the parts of greater respiratory rate.

The level of thiamine derivatives in a given part of the brain, normally varying only moderately, falls markedly in severe thiamine deficiency. This has been found in several studies with experimental animals and as the data of Table 10.2 show, occurs also in man. The cerebral thiamine is seen in this study to be more stable than is that of other organs, increasing less when excess thiamine is administered and falling less in deficiency. The same phenomenon is seen in Fig. 10.3 which gives the time-course of thiamine depletion in the rat. Cerebral thiamine remained constant during 15 days on a thiamine-free diet, whereas in the first few days that of other organs had, like urinary excretion, fallen considerably. The fall in cerebral thiamine appears to correspond to the time when signs of disturbance in the nervous system begin, and also the time when urinary thiamine falls to a very low, constant level which is suggested as a chemical measure of the progress of the deficiency.

In pigeons the normal level of thiamine derivatives in the brain could be reduced to one-half without considerable change in behaviour; such changes were produced by further deficiency and with severe symptoms cerebral thiamine was found at one-tenth of its normal level. Similar relationships were shown in thiamine-deprived rats (Dreyfus, 1961) and in addition the losses of thiamine in ten different parts of the brain were found to be similar, despite the localized nature of the resulting pathological changes. Pyrithiamine (Fig. 10.1) in the course of producing in rats and pigeons effects similar to those of thiamine-deficiency, also caused the cerebral content of thiamine pyrophosphate to fall to about one-fifth of its normal value (Koedam, 1958; Rindi et al., 1961).

Details of how neural tissues recover from thiamine deficiency have received recent examintion. The diminished activity of pyruvate dehydrogenase is recovered in a few hours, and involves protein synthesis (Reinauer & Hollman, 1969). Thiamine-deficient rats, fed [^{14}C]leucine and [^{14}C]thiamine yielded mitochondria from which the two labelled compounds were recovered at maximum specific activity. A sub-mitochondrial fraction showed enrichment of the two compounds and also of pyruvate dehydrogenase; increase in this enzyme on administering thiamine was inhibited by actinomycin D or by cycloheximide. Thus coenzyme-mediated enzyme induction is involved.

Interconversion of Thiamine and its Phosphates

Five or more distinct processes are involved in the uptake and interconversion of thiamine and its phosphate derivatives in the brain (a–e, Fig. 10.2). They have been revealed by enzyme investigations, by the use of structurally related inhibitors, and by pathological studies.

(a) Effects of pyrithiamine, especially, have emphasized the uptake of thiamine as a distinct process (Rindi et al., 1961; Steyne-Parvé, Study Group 1967). Thiamine derivatives in the brain as in other organs could be diminished to 30–40% of their normal value by including pyrithiamine in normally adequate diets, and polyneuritic symptoms resulted. The cerebral thiamine was restored to normal in the presence of pyrithiamine by addition of further thiamine; polyneuritic symptoms were then prevented and the elevated levels of ketoacids which had been caused by pyrithiamine, were also restored to normal (Holowach et al., 1968).

(b) A specific thiamine pyrophosphokinase (ATP: thiamine pyrophosphotransferase, EC 2.7.6.2) catalyses the subsequent conversion of cerebral thiamine to the major form in which it functions in intermediary metabolism, namely thiamine pyrophosphate, the diphosphate. The kinase reaction in a cerebral dispersion proceeded at about 0·6 μmoles converted/g. tissue/hr. and the enzyme concerned was partly purified from a rat brain acetone powder (Johnson & Gubler, 1968). Half-maximum velocity was given by about 0·1 μM thiamine; or, with excess thiamine, by 20 mM adenosine triphosphate. Mg^{2+} was also required; assay depended on the transketolase reaction (q.v.).

Certain thiamine analogues are also pyrophosphorylated by the phosphokinase. Oxythiamine (Fig. 10.2) was indeed concluded to have its main action as a thiamine antagonist in organs other than the brain, after conversion to oxythiamine pyrophosphate while pyrithiamine acted partly in the form of its pyrophosphate. The two analogues differ interestingly in the physiological and pathological changes which they induced, oxythiamine having little cerebral effect and each analogue eliciting part of the consequences which result from withholding dietary thiamine (*Study Group*, 1967).

(*c, d*) Of enzymes acting on thiamine pyrophosphate, the *phosphatase* (*c*, Fig. 10.2) received comment above and is distinct from thiamine phosphokinase which catalyses the reverse reaction. The further phosphorylation of thiamine pyrophosphate to yield the triphosphate has been investigated in cerebral dispersions (*d*, Fig. 10.2; Itokawa & Cooper, 1968), and here as in other organisms the reaction proved to be reversible. The *phosphotransferase* concerned catalysed both the conversion of thiamine pyrophosphate and adenosine triphosphate to thiamine triphosphate and ADP, as well as the phosphorylation of ADP by thiamine triphosphate. Most of the thiamine pyrophosphate phosphotransferase activity of the dispersion was found in its mitochondrial subfraction.

Study of body fluids from a patient with subacute necrotizing encephalomyelopathy (q.v., below) showed both blood and urine to inhibit a preparation of the phosphotransferase from rat brain (Cooper *et al.*, 1969). These fluids from normal subjects did not inhibit the enzmye; the inhibitory factor was glycoprotein in character. Such inhibition is consistent with the lowered quantity of thiamine triphosphate found cerebrally in the encephalomyelopathy.

(*e*) Attachment of thiamine pyrophosphate as coenzyme to the apoenzymes with which it functions, has been demonstrated as a distinct and reversible step by the effects of oxythiamine pyrophosphate. Thiamine pyrophosphate was displaced by this analogue, from carboxylase and transketolase (q.v.; *Study Group*, 1967).

Cerebral Metabolism in Thiamine Deficiency

Diminution in the cerebral concentration of thiamine phosphates in thiamine-deficient animals is associated with major disturbances in cerebral metabolism. The first of these to be demonstrated was an accumulation of lactic acid in thiamine deficient pigeons (Kinnersley & Peters, 1929; Peters, 1963; *Study Group*, 1967); subsequently, transketolase was shown to lose activity. Lactate accumulated because its oxidation was defective, the respiration of separated cerebral tissues of deficient animals, provided *in vitro* with lactic acid as substrate, was below normal. Oxidation of lactate proceeds through pyruvate, and this substance also accumulated *in vivo* and when added *in vitro* was oxidized at an abnormally slow rate. As reactions involving ketoacids are the main source of energy for cerebral activities, failure of cerebral function in the deficient animals is understandable.

(1) The relationship between lack of thiamine and lowered oxidation of pyruvate is a very direct one. Thiamine itself or its pyrophosphate, added *in vitro* to cell-containing tissue preparations from deficient animals, increases their oxidation of pyruvate (**B**, Fig. 10.4). In a preparation which is probably cytolysed (**A**, Fig. 10.4), thiamine has less effect but thiamine pyrophosphate remains fully active, which indicates it to be, or to be closer to, the form in which the vitamin functions; the nature of this functioning has been recounted (Chapters 5 and 6). Moreover, in experiments similar to those of Fig. 10.4 in which thiamine itself increased respiration, subsequent extraction of the

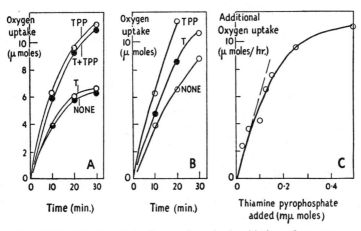

Fig. 10.4. Thiamine derivatives and cerebral oxidation of pyruvate (Banga, Ochoa & Peters, 1939). A and **B**, the time-course of oxygen uptake by dispersion of cerebral tissues from thiamine-deficient pigeons, in salines with about 20 mM-pyruvate and 4 mM-fumarate and either with no further addition; or with: T, 30 μM-thiamine; TPP, 0·5–2 μM-thiamine pyrophosphate. The dispersion used in **B** was made in isotonic solution but that in A involved treating the tissue with water. C, the acceleration in respiration in similar mixtures brought about by graded additions of thiamine pyrophosphate; the mixtures contained 0·3 g. tissue.

reaction mixture to which thiamine had been added showed thiamine pyrophosphate to have been synthesized. The synthesis was at the rate of at least 1 nmole/g. tissue/hr. Several other metabolic sequelae of thiamine deficiency can be attributed to its role in pyruvate oxidation. Thus during *in vitro* metabolism of cerebral tissues from deficient animals, the formation of acetate, citrate, and α-oxoglutarate is decreased (Table 6.3). Also, rats maintained on diets containing pyrithiamine (as well as on diets lacking thiamine) afforded cerebral dispersions with diminished ability in oxidizing pyruvate (Gubler, 1961). This and other defects were made good by thiamine pyrophosphate. Acetylcoenzyme A, which is the precursor of each of the acids specified above and also of acetylcholine, is an immediate product of the thiamine-catalysed pyruvate oxidation. This makes understandable the depression in acetylcholine synthesis observed in extracts from the brain of thiamine-deficient rats (Bhagat & Lockett, 1962), a depression made good by added acetylcoenzyme A.

(2) Other cerebral processes involving thiamine pyrophosphate also concern α-keto acids or diketones. Thus it functions in oxidation of α-oxoglutarate, in the production of acetoin and in transketolase. The activity of this latter system (Chapters 5 and 7) may be rate-limiting in the cerebral metabolism of hexose phosphates by the pentose phosphate pathway. The activity of transketolase in the white matter of the brain is rather greater than in grey matter, and both are diminished in thiamine deficiency (Dreyfus, 1962 and in *Study Group*, 1967). A survey of transketolase activity in several parts of the rat nervous system showed greatest proportional decrease in the pons, and this correlated with the site of visible lesions. The time-course of development of ataxia in thiamine-deficient rats was also correlated with fall in cerebral transketolase activity.

An estimate of the proportion of cerebral thiamine which is involved in pyruvate oxidation may be made as follows. Fig. 10.4 shows that the first addition of 0·2 nmole thiamine pyrophosphate to cerebral tissues results in a respiratory increase of some 11 μmoles O_2/hr. This corresponds to 55,000 moles O_2/hr./mole thiamine. Human cerebral tissues contain some 4 nmoles of thiamine/g. (Table 10.2), and their maximal respiratory rate is about 100 μmoles/g./hr. This corresponds to 25,000 moles O_2/hr./mole thiamine. Granted that the *in vitro* conditions allow thiamine pyrophosphate to exhibit an effect similar to that *in vivo*, these values would indicate about half the cerebral thiamine to be brought into play in pyruvate oxidation. As it is involved also in other metabolic processes in the brain, there is clearly little if any excess of thiamine and disturbance of function with moderate depletion is understandable.

Related Effects of Deficiency

In thiamine deficiency pyruvate metabolism is restricted not only in the brain but also in other organs of the body, notably in the muscles which collectively contain the greatest quantity of thiamine. Consequently the level of keto acids in the body as a whole tends to increase and this is reflected in their level in the bloodstream. In a resting condition the blood keto acids of deficient animals may not be greatly abnormal, but when their turnover is increased by administering glucose the metabolic defect is emphasized. Instances in which this was observed in subjects showing Wernicke's syndrome are illustrated in Fig. 10.5. Here blood keto acids in several subjects were high even before glucose ingestion. The glucose caused only a small and transitory rise in keto acids in the normal subjects but a greater and more prolonged rise in the deficient subjects, so that at 2 hr. their mean keto acid level was 3·5 times its normal value. These abnormalities were completely removed by administered thiamine.

Considering the wider subject of high levels of blood keto acids in neurological disorders, response to thiamine occurs only in certain subjects who are presumably deficient in it (Thompson & Cumings, 1964); the keto acids of the blood include as well as pyruvate which preponderates, α-oxoglutarate and acetoacetate. The diminished thiamine pyrophosphate of the blood in thiamine deficient rats (Fig. 10.3), is manifested in a considerable lowering of erythrocyte transketolase activity (Brin *et al.*, 1958). This leads to a three-fold increase in pentose derivatives in the cells; administration of thiamine to the animals, or its addition to the erythrocyte suspensions, diminished this abnormality and thus contributed to its characterization. Several transketolase assays are available and their value in diagnosis has been appraised (*Study Group*, 1967).

The many metabolic and other disturbances of thiamine deficiency make it understandable that hormonal changes should also occur, either through

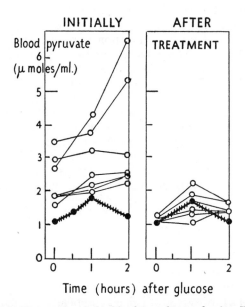

Fig. 10.5. *Keto acids of the blood in subjects showing Wernicke's syndrome* (Bowman & Wortis: Symposium, 1943 and *Study Group*, 1967). The keto acids, expressed as pyruvate, were determined at different times quoted, after the ingestion of 10 mmoles glucose per kg. body weight. Treatment consisted of the administration of 0·3 mmole thiamine with in some cases other B vitamins. The barred line gives the mean data for twenty-seven normal subjects; each of the other lines refers to one subject showing Wernicke's syndrome.

the endocrine organs reacting to these disturbances or becoming themselves deficient in thiamine. Both the islets of Langerhans and the adrenal medulla hypertrophy in beri-beri; hyperglycaemia and reduced glucose tolerance have been found. Combined observation of changes in blood lactate, pyruvate and glucose may give an early indication of mild thiamine deficiency and has been applied to mentally disturbed subjects (Horwitt, 1948).

The widespread metabolic changes of the deficiency also make it possible that cerebral functioning is disturbed in part indirectly, for example by high blood pyruvate or methylglyoxal or by changed hormone levels. The deleterious effect of carbohydrate-containing diets in thiamine deficiency may in part arise in this way, for the cerebral cocarboxylase of animals dying from

10

thiamine deficiency was less depleted when their diet contained more carbo-hydrate. Further, deficiency signs in surviving animals were much more severe on carbohydrate-containing than on carbohydrate-free diets, although both groups had similar levels of thiamine in the brain and in other organs (Yudkin, 1949, 1951; Gruber, 1953; Salem, 1954). For alternative suggestions, see *Conference* (1962), *Study Group* (1967) and Itokawa & Cooper (1969).

Subacute Necrotizing Encephalomyelopathy

In first describing this condition, Leigh (1951) drew attention to the re-semblance between its histological lesions and those of Wernicke's disease. Mental retardation and motor disfunction were also involved. Leigh's en-cephalomyelopathy typically commences at 1 or 2 years of age, though the 40 or 50 cases now recorded include an adolescent (Hardman *et al.*, 1968) and they demonstrate the disease to be familial, possibly being inherited through a single autosomal recessive gene (Ebels *et al.*, 1965; Clayton *et al.*, 1967; Montpetit *et al.*, 1971). It develops while subjects are receiving normal thiamine intake, but nevertheless they show metabolic abnormalities cognate to those of thiamine-lack: persistent acidosis and increased blood lactate and keto acids (Worsley *et al.*, 1965; Procopis *et al.*, 1967; Clayton *et al.*, 1967). Three thiamine pyrophosphate-requiring enzymes were at normal levels in blood samples from a girl suffering the encephalomyelopathy: pyruvate dehydrogenase, α-oxoglutarate dehydrogenase and transketolase (Cooper *et al.*, 1969). In expectation that a cofactor metabolically-linked with thiamine in keto acid metabolism might have therapeutic value, lipoate (q.v.) was administered to a case 2 years of age. This markedly ameliorated the condition, with associated fall in keto acids of the blood (Clayton *et al.*, 1967); the patient lived a further 4 years and although she died of the condition results may be judged encouraging.

Examination of a further case of Leigh's encephalomyelopathy has revealed a cerebral abnormality closer to thiamine itself (Table 10.2; Cooper *et al.*, 1969, 1970 and see page 278). Parts of the brain of a child who died of the condition were found to contain quantities of thiamine below the normal range. The different forms of thiamine were present in their usual propor-tions, except that the triphosphate could not be detected. Knowing the route of formation of the triphosphate (Fig. 10.2), the TPP-ATP phospho-transferase of a cerebral preparation was measured in the presence and absence of body fluids from the patient. Both blood and urine were found inhibitory to the transferase while these fluids from normal subjects were not. The inhibitory properties appeared to be associated with glycoprotein frac-tions. A cerebral enzymic role for thiamine triphosphate has not been specified; the abnormalities previously reported in Leigh's disease included an 85% diminution of muscle phosphofructokinase (Clayton *et al.*, 1967).

Nicotinic Acid

Although several observers had concluded by the middle of the nineteenth century that pellagra was closely connected with poor diets, bacteriological theories of its origin nevertheless developed; important in refuting these theories and in providing a basis for present knowledge were Goldberger's observations of 1914 in asylums in the south of the U.S.A. These showed pellagra to be rife among patients but not among medical staff and to be closely correlated with diet (for a re-publication and appraisal of this work which includes much social study, see Terris, 1964). Pellagra has remained an appreciable cause of secondary illness among patients in mental hospitals and in senile conditions (Hardwick, 1943; Leigh, 1952; Gregory, 1955; Hersov, 1955). Probably contributing to this are the faulty feeding habits found among such patients and also the greater difficulty of recognizing in them, the mental changes which are prominent among the signs of pellagra.

Effects of Deficiency

Lack of nicotinic acid is the main cause of pellagra, though deficiencies in other B-vitamins are frequent concomitants of the disorder. Human requirements for dietary nicotinic acid are about 10–30 mg./day. In treatment of deficiency, some 300 mg. are given per day; 12–16 mg. usually suffice to maintain a normal blood level of some 50 μmoles/l. A considerable proportion of the daily requirement of nicotinic acid need not be provided preformed but can be derived from tryptophan (see below).

Signs of disturbed cerebral functioning are among the earliest symptoms of pellagra or of nicotinamide deficiency induced experimentally. The symptoms include depression, sometimes with morbid fears, dizziness and insomnia. More severe or prolonged deficiency brings with the apprehension, hallucinations, disorientation or delirium. At several stages and in many subjects nicotinic acid deficiency has proved difficult to differentiate from other psychoses, and indeed nicotinic acid can be regarded as a therapeutic agent for a disease which in its initial stages is often largely a mental disorder.

The symptoms described often precede the dermatitis and other effects of nicotinic acid deficiency, especially as the dermatitis requires for its development exposure to sunlight or to a comparable stimulus. The disorder responds to nicotinamide unless it is too far advanced. Moreover, in an experiment in which nicotinamide was administered to a group of deficient subjects under close observation, not only did the mental disturbances cease promptly with administration but also they reappeared when the nicotinamide was stopped (Spies et al., 1938; Gregory, 1955). The therapeutic effect of nicotinamide was specific to the pellagrins and did not take place in subjects with somewhat similar symptoms due to alcoholism or schizophrenia.

If the disturbances described are not terminated by making available nicotinic acid or a surrogate, permanent structural changes take place in the brain. The morphological lesions seen in chronic pellagra include central chromatolysis, degeneration especially in the large neurons of the motor cortex, the brain stem and the anterior horn of the spinal cord; it has been termed retrograde degeneration as it involves changes in the Nissl bodies of the cells similar to those seen after section of the axon (Leigh, 1952; Meyer *in* Blackwood *et al.*, 1963). Histologically-similar lesions have been found in dogs suffering the condition of black-tongue caused by nicotinic acid deficiency.

Metabolic Causes of Nicotinamide Deficiency

Many years after nicotinic acid was characterized as a dietary essential, various animals including man were found capable of deriving half or more of their minimal requirements from sources other than the nicotinic acid derivatives preformed in their food. Thus when the total bodily nicotinic acid of groups of growing rats was determined before and after 28 days' growth on a diet low in nicotinic acid, their collective nicotinic acid increased from 2·3 to 7·4 mg., to which the diet contributed only 0·13 mg. (Dann, 1941; Henderson in *Symposium*, 1956a). The synthesis has been shown to proceed from tryptophan (Fig. 10.6) and to occur in man, either in the tissues or in intestinal micro-organisms. Administration of tryptophan leads to increased excretion of nicotinic acid or amide, and its metabolites N-methylnicotinic acid and N-methyl-2-pyridone-5-carboxyamide (Sarett & Goldsmith, 1950; Brown & Price, 1956).

The classical pellagra of maize (corn) diets was the result of deficiency both in nicotinic acid derivatives and in tryptophan; some 60 mg. of tryptophan, by metabolic routes noted in Fig. 10.6 are normally the dietary equivalent of 1 mg. of nicotinic acid. Some situations in which tryptophan intake is normal but in which the compound is metabolically diverted or is inaccessible can also induce pellagra-like syndromes (see Milne, 1968; Sebrell & Harris, 1968, and below). The conditions include a carcinoid state, when proliferation of the abnormal cell-type results in 60% of dietary tryptophan being converted to serotonin and its metabolites in place of a normal 1% conversion. Also poor intestinal absorption of dietary tryptophan in Hartnup disease (q.v.) can result in sufferers from this condition showing the signs of nicotinic acid deficiency. Indeed, before Hartnup disease was recognized as a distinct entity, some probable cases were described as pellagrins.

The altered amino acid levels of phenylketonuria and maple-syrup urine disease (q.v.) are also concluded to cause diminished efficiency in the use of dietary tryptophan for producing nicotinamide. Many factors, indeed, may affect such efficiency: adrenocortical steroids were found to prevent or give remission to a nicotinamide deficiency disease in rats and dogs (Greengard *et al.*, 1968). Prolonged isoniazid therapy, also, can diminish the conversion of tryptophan to nicotinic acid through producing a deficiency in pyridoxine coenzymes which are necessary for the conversion.

Nicotinic Acid Derivatives in the Brain

Compared with other organs, the brain is moderately rich in nicotinic acid derivatives. This is shown to be the case in rat tissues in Table 10.3, and has been observed also in man. The cerebral nicotinamide exists very largely in the form of the catalytically-active nicotinamide adenine dinucleotides, NAD^+ and $NADP^+$ (Fig. 10.6). These through their participation in the main energy-yielding reactions of the tissue make understandable the importance of nicotinic acid to cerebral functioning (Chapters 5 to 7).

The cerebral content in nicotinic acid derivatives has been observed to fall considerably during deficiency. This is shown in the experiment of *A*, Table 10.3; the fall of 37% was avoided in animals fed the same diet supplemented with 0·1 mg. of nicotinic acid per rat, daily. In other studies, a comparable fall in cerebral nicotinic acid derivatives has not always been found; the experiment of Table 10.3 employed a diet containing maize which is associated in man with incidence of pellagra, as has been noted above. Respiration of

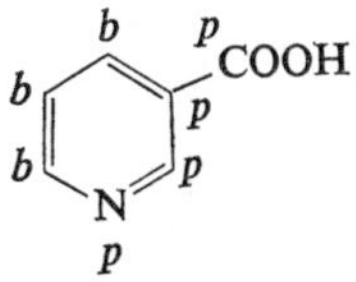

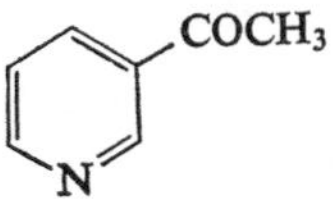

FIG. 10.6. I, Nicotinic acid indicating the parts of the molecule derived from the pyrrole (*p*) and benzene (*b*) rings of tryptophan.
II, 3-Acetylpyridine, a nicotinic acid antagonist (Woolley, 1952; see Beher & Anthony, 1953).
III, R = H: Nicotinamide adenine dinucleotide (NAD$^+$); R = PO$_3$H$_2$, nicotinamide adenine dinucleotide phosphate (NADP$^+$). The line (i) shows the point of action of NAD(P)$^+$ deoxyribosyltransferase, which catalyses also the hydrolysis of the two nucleotides with loss of coenzyme activity (Mann & Quastel, 1941; McIlwain & Grinyer, 1950); (ii) specifies the —NH$_2$ which is replaced by —OH in desamido-NAD$^+$.
IV, The reduced forms NADH and NADPH, of the coenzymes.

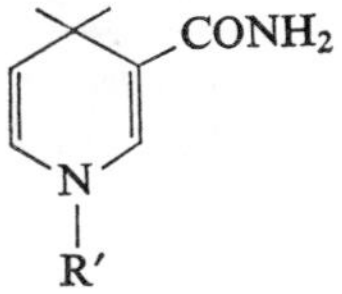

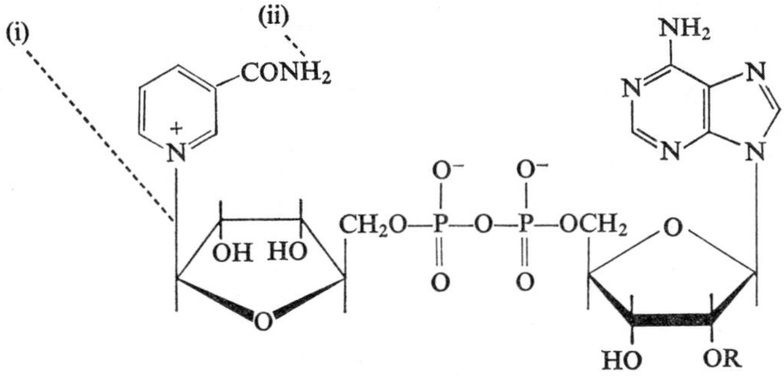

separated cerebral tissues from dogs deficient in nicotinic acid has been measured but not found to be depressed (Kohn *et al.*, 1939). In these experiments the cerebral tissues did not appear to be deficient in nicotinamide nucleotides, though other tissues were depleted and showed respiratory changes. Both loss of nicotinamide nucleotides and changed enzyme levels have however been observed in the cerebral tissues of young rats which were kept 8 weeks on a deficient diet, and which showed severe deficiency signs (Garcia-Bunuel *et al.*, 1962). The nicotinamide-adenine dinucleotide of the brain had again fallen by 30–40%, thus giving a basis for the altered cerebral

Table 10.3

Nicotinic acid and coenzyme content of animal tissues

Organ	On full diet	On deficient diet	
		alone	with 0·1 mg. nicotinic acid/ rat/day
A			
Rat brain (Wistar strain)	380	240	380
Rat heart	930	850	870
Rat skeletal muscle	630	370	620
Rat blood	110	98	95

Nicotinic acid content (nmoles/g.) — column heading spanning On full diet and On deficient diet.

Organ	Nicotinic acid (nmoles/g.)	Nicotinamide-adenine nucleotides (nmoles/g.)			
		NAD+	NADH	NADP+	NADPH
B					
Mouse brain	590	510		–	–
Rat brain	–	298	95*	11†	24†
Rat liver	–	668	41	374	386
Rat blood	–	110*	87*	14*	12*
Guinea pig brain	275	257		–	–
Rabbit cerebral hemisphere	200	150		–	–
Human brain	160	–		–	–

A: Singal *et al.* (1948). Other data: Axelrod *et al.* (1941).

B: Gore, Ibbott & McIlwain (1950); Taylor *et al.* (1942) and Burch *et al.* (1963); values given for oxidized and reduced forms by Garcia-Bunuel *et al.* (1962) are probably in some cases affected by conditions of fixation, but the values * are quoted from their results; see also Minard & Hahn (1963).

† For additional data, and discussion of problems of measurement, see Burch *et al.*, 1967.

functioning. Certain apoenzymes may also change: preparations from the deficient brains, examined in the presence of added coenzymes, showed a level of α-glycerophosphate dehydrogenase 60% above normal. This was ascribed to delayed maturation; glutamate and *iso*citrate dehydrogenases were un-changed in level.

Cerebral Synthesis of Nicotinamide Nucleotides

Administration of large doses of nicotinamide or of NAD+ to mice can cause moderate increase of the nucleotide in the brain (Kaplan *et al.*, 1956). Cerebral tissues themselves can to some extent incorporate labelled inorganic phosphate to the NAD+ which they contain (Heald, 1956), though they do not increase their content of the nucleotide when incubated with additional nicotinic acid or its amide, as do for example human erythrocytes.

Synthetic routes (Fig. 10.7) have been established by administering iso-topically-labelled precursors *in vivo*, mainly to rats and mice. On systemic administration of [14C]nicotinic acid and its derivatives, only a small propor-tion of the 14C which was incorporated into tissues was found in the brain. Nicotinic acid itself gave promptest incorporation, followed by NAD+ and nicotinamide (Deguchi *et al.*, 1968). Administering [14C] nicotinic acid intra-cisternally gave much greater cerebral incorporation and enabled the sequence of synthesis to be specified (Fig. 10.8); it is similar to that occurring in the liver. The small amount of nicotinate injected was almost completely utilized in 15 min., and 14C increased most rapidly in nicotinic ribonucleotide, followed by desamido-NAD+ and by NAD+ itself, which at the end of the experiment retained 10% of the 14C administered.

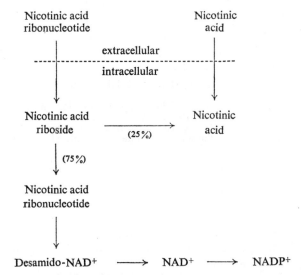

FIG. 10.7. Processes leading to nicotinamide nucleotides in the brain, based on the data of Fig. 10.8 and cognate studies.

This sequence was confirmed by giving intracisternally to other rats, the supposed intermediates, some doubly labelled with [14C]nicotinamide and 32P. Thus the 32P in nicotinate ribonucleotide was lost more rapidly than the 14C, while the ribonucleoside was utilized to a large extent directly in producing NAD+. [7-14C]-Nicotinamide given intracisternally (Fig. 10.8) was incor-porated very rapidly to NAD+, but was not stable in this combination. The labelled NAD+ is seen from **B**, Fig. 10 to diminish by 50% in an hour, whereas that labelled by nicotinic acid remained stable for 20 hr. (**A**, Fig. 10). Incorporation of the nicotinamide was concluded to be due to the deoxy-ribosyl transferase involved in degrading NAD+ (see below) and not to net synthesis.

Nicotinamide adenine dinucleotide phosphate (NADP+) has been demon-strated to be produced by cerebral extracts from NAD+ and ATP, at some 4 nmoles/mg. protein/hr.

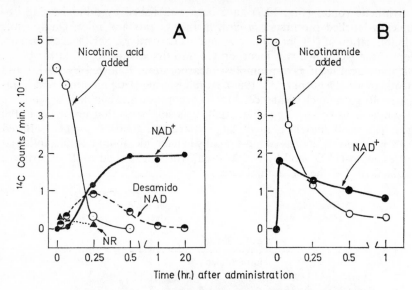

Fɪɢ. 10.8. Biosynthesis of nicotinamide ribonucleotides in the brain of the rat and mouse (Deguchi *et al.*, 1968).

A. [7-^{14}C]Nicotinate was given intracisternally to groups of rats, and the brain sampled at the subsequent times indicated. NR: nicotinate ribonucleotide.

B. [7-^{14}C]Nicotinamide was similarly administered, and cerebral samples extracted; no ^{14}C was detected in NR or in desamido NAD$^+$.

Nicotinamide Nucleotide Degradation

Loss of the nicotinamide nucleotides from cerebral preparations is very readily observed; it proves to be an enzymic process in which the molecules are hydrolysed with formation of nicotinamide (Fig. 10.6). An unexpected feature of the reaction is its high speed. With NAD$^+$ at 0·4 mM, a concentration comparable to that occurring in the brain itself, ground cerebral tissues can inactivate the coenzyme at 200 μmoles/g. hr. This would halve the tissue's coenzyme content in 2 to 5 seconds. Glycolysis in cerebral tissues requires the coenzyme and in the ground cell-free tissue, glycolysis proceeds maximally only in the presence of nicotinamide or a comparable inhibitor of the hydrolysis of NAD$^+$ (Chapter 5).

The nucleotides are however relatively stable in cerebral preparations in which cell structure is largely intact. Possibly enzyme and substrate are separated; but the degrading enzyme probably has other functions *in situ*, for it has been found capable of catalysing the exchange of the nicotinamide of diphosphopyridine nucleotide with other bases as well as with the hydroxyl ion (Fig. 10.6), i.e. it shows the properties of a deoxyribosyltransferase. Thus cerebral preparations can form from the nucleotides their acetylpyridine analogues. To such formation is attributed the central actions of *N*-acetylpyridine, which include in rats and mice hypothalamic lesions and abnormal gait (Kaplan, 1960; Woolley, 1952). In particular, the rates of reactions requiring $NADP^+$, including glucose-6-phosphate dehydrogenase and glutathione reductase (q.v.) were markedly lower when the 3-acetylpyridine analogue replaced the coenzyme, and this analogue was found in appreciable quantities in the brain of affected animals (Coper *et al.*, 1963). The cerebral deoxyribosyltransferase forms also the isonicotinic acid hydrazide analogue of NAD^+, and may play a role in the central actions of the hydrazide (see also pyridoxine).

The transferase appears at a particular stage in cerebral development and has been extensively purified (Nemeth & Dickerman, 1960; Windmueller & Kaplan, 1962). It is firmly attached to particulate matter in cerebral suspensions but extractable from acetone-powders, especially after a limited treatment with trypsin (McIlwain, 1950; Swislocki & Kaplan, 1967). After chromatography using modified celluloses, a preparation hydrolysing 7·6 μmoles $NAD^+/\mu g$. protein/hr. was obtained (1 mg./10 lb. pig brain). This was shown immunochemically to be a single component of some 95% purity; the molecular weight, 26,000, and amino acid composition were determined. That the enzyme plays a role in the intact tissue is suggested by the action of substances which inhibit it. These inhibitors, such as 50 mM-nicotinamide or 10 μM-phenosafranine, release aerobic glycolysis when added to the cell-containing tissue respiring in glucose salines. The mechanism of this, and the function of the enzyme, are not fully understood; but it is relevant that the degradation is specific to the oxidized form of the coenzymes and thus alters the E_0 in systems containing both the oxidized and reduced forms. The potential rate of the breakdown is about equal to that at which the pyridine nucleotides undergo oxidation and reduction during their functioning as respiratory carriers; a function in metabolic regulation appears likely.

Other Effects of Nicotinic Acid

Nicotinic acid in oral or intravenous doses only a little greater than the daily requirement as a vitamin, is a potent vasodilator: 20–60 mg. in man may cause flushing. Nicotinamide is without this action but equally potent as a vitamin and is therefore the preferred form for administration as an essential nutrient; most nicotinic acid of foodstuffs is present as the amide or as its higher derivatives. Nicotinic acid has been deliberately used as a vasodilator in the expectation that this action extended to the cerebral blood vessels, and beneficial effect reported in depressive states. Improvement has also been reported in numerous instances of mental disorder when the subjects were not regarded as pellagrous but may nevertheless have been deficient in nicotinic acid (Lehmann, 1952).

With knowledge of nicotinamide as a vitamin, pellagra is now relatively uncommon but instances are reported of subjects with mental symptoms akin to those of pellagra often responding to nicotinic acid though an apparently normal diet is being consumed. As indicated above, abnormality in tryptophan metabolism has been demonstrated in several such people. Early observations emphasized the association of pellagra with diets rich in maize and it is suspected that this is due not only to the lack in such diets of nicotinic acid and of tryptophan, but also to the presence of a toxic agent whose effects are antagonized by nicotinic acid: thus these diets increase the requirement for the vitamin.

The Vitamin B_6 Group: Pyridoxine

Among the many effects on the nervous system which are produced by deficient diets, those now known to be due to lack of vitamin B_6 were characterized in 1934 (*Symposium*, 1956). Major differentiating characteristics were the convulsive and ataxic states caused by avitaminosis-B_6, which have now been demonstrated in at least twelve mammalian species including man. The course of the convulsive seizures in pigs and rats was impressively similar to that of grand mal epilepsy in man, and when the diet was supplemented with vitamin B_6, no more attacks occurred (Chick *et al.*, 1938, 1940). Also, before other neurological signs of pyridoxine deficiency are evident, rats and dogs show disturbances in learning and conditioning (Brožek *et al.*, 1960, 1961). Vitamin B_6 is needed preformed by all species of animals examined, and general effects of its deficiency are extensively documented (see Sebrell & Harris, 1968).

Pyridoxine Requirement

The vitamin B_6 group includes the three compounds of Fig. 10.9 which until recently were also called pyridoxine (IUPAC–IUB Commission, 1970), together with their phosphates; pyridoxal phosphate and pyridoxamine phos-

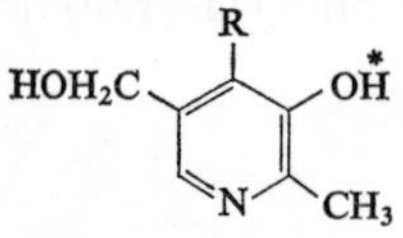
R
HOH₂C
OH*
N
CH₃

Vitamin B_6 group:
pyridoxol, R = —CH_2OH
pyridoxal, R = —CHO
pyridoxamine, R = —CH_2NH_2
Pyridoxal phosphate:
esterfied at OH*
Deoxypyridoxine: R = —CH_3

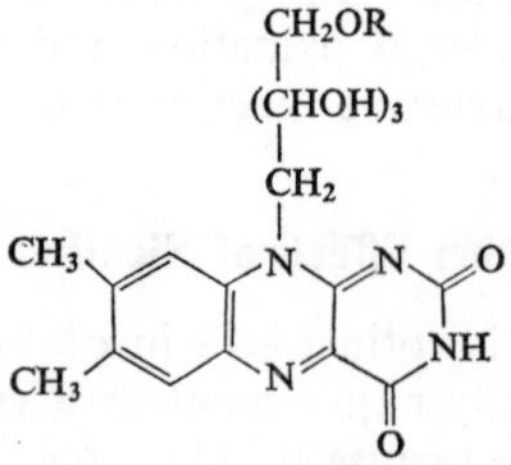
CH₂OR
(CHOH)₃
CH₂
CH₃
CH₃
N
N
O
NH
N
N
O

Riboflavin: R = —H.
Flavin-adenine dinucleotide:
R— = $PO_3H.PO_3H.C_{10}H_{12}O_3N_5$

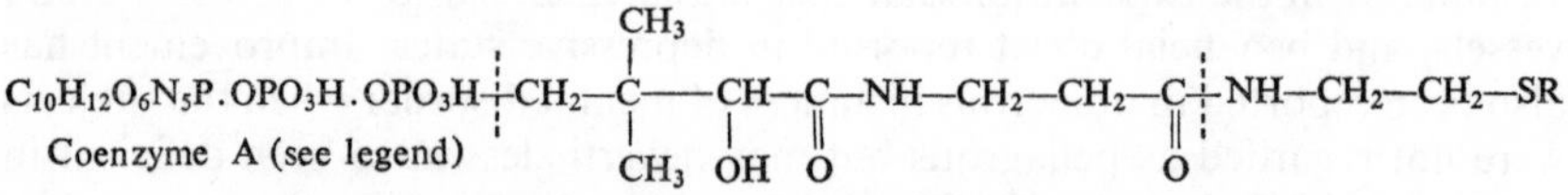
CH₃
C₁₀H₁₂O₆N₅P.OPO₃H.OPO₃H—CH₂—C——CH—C—NH—CH₂—CH₂—C—NH—CH₂—CH₂—SR
Coenzyme A (see legend)
CH₃ OH O
O

FIG. 10.9. Pyridoxine, riboflavin and pantothenate derivatives. Coenzyme A: R = H; acetylcoenzyme A: R = $COCH_3$. Hydrolysis of coenzyme A at the dotted bonds would yield an adenosine phosphate, pantothenic acid and β-mercaptoethylamine.

phate preponderate in animal tissues including those of the brain. The three compounds appear equivalent on feeding to higher animals, pyridoxol being the form normally administered under the generic name of vitamin B_6 or pyridoxine hydrochloride. Human requirements for pyridoxine have been emphasized by deficiency signs, including convulsions, in over fifty normal infants fed a manufactured food deficient in the vitamin (Coursin, 1954; *Conference*, 1960). Improvement on administering the vitamin was dramatic; abnormal electroencephalograms became normal a few minutes after its injection. The adult human need for substances of vitamin B_6 activity is normally met by about 1·5 mg. of pyridoxine per day.

Requirements for vitamin B_6 are unusually high in a small proportion of the population (Hunt *et al.*, 1954; Coursin: *Conference*, 1960; Tower, 1960). Normal reserves and needs are such that children have continued on a B_6-deficient diet for 8 weeks before developing seizures. In a few cases of extreme pyridoxine dependency, however, new-born infants have developed intractable seizures which did not respond to ordinary anticonvulsant drugs but which were controlled by large doses of pyridoxine, e.g. of 15 mg. daily for a period of many years. In other instances, pyridoxine requirement appears to be only one factor involved in cerebral abnormality. Thus among infants found at 2–12 months to be suffering spasms, mental retardation and convulsions, a proportion showed abnormal urinary excretion of tryptophan metabolites; to some of these infants vitamin B_6 was beneficial. Tryptophan metabolites, especially xanthurenic and kynurenic acids, which need pyridoxal-dependent enzymes for their further metabolism, were also measured in an adult mentally-retarded population after administering a test-dose of tryptophan (O'Brien & Jensen, 1963). Abnormally high excretion was found in a few individuals and was diminished by pyridoxine, but without improvement in mental status.

Experience with other metabolic abnormalities (Chapter 8) suggests that if the relationship to pyridoxine is a causal one, its administration might have been more successful earlier in life. It is thus significant that Hagberg *et al.* (1964) found a group of children who at 3–8 years of age were suffering epilepsy of unknown origin with intellectual regression, emotional disturbance and EEG abnormality and whose condition was ameliorated by giving vitamin B_6. Their urinary excretion of xanthurenic acid, moreover, was previously high and was diminished towards normal values by the vitamin B_6. In a further group of 70 children with convulsions, and the majority also with mental retardation, about one-third were abnormal in tryptophan metabolism (Heeley *et al.*, 1968). Although administration of 30 mg. of pyridoxine a day modified their tryptophan metabolism, the clinical abnormalities were not ameliorated. It is to be noted, however, that maternal pyridoxine deficiency in the rat can lead to congenital deficiencies in the offspring, and that subsequently these may not be made good by pyridoxine (Dakshinamurti & Stephens, 1969).

Pyridoxine and Cerebral Metabolism

The general metabolic involvement of pyridoxine-requiring enzymes is very considerable, for they include in various organisms some 17 aminotransferases, 22 transferases or lyases acting on C—C bonds and 11 on C—O bonds. Over half of these enzymes act on amino acids, and it is to be noted that the metabolism of sphingosine (q.v.) is also involved. Pyridoxal phosphate is coenzyme in the decarboxylase which yields serotonin from 5-hydroxytryptophan (Weissbach *et al.*, 1957; see Chapter 14).

Specific information about changes in the brain itself are thus needed in understanding the deficiency signs recounted above. Two of the major cerebral reactions in glutamic acid are depressed in vitamin B_6-deficient rats (Schlenk & Snell, 1945; Roberts *et al.*, 1951). The first of these is the transamination with oxaloacetate yielding asparate and α-oxoglutarate, which in the brain was depressed some 40 % on a deficient diet but recovered with administered vitamin. The other reaction is the decarboxylation of glutamic acid, which in deficiency was lowered to an even greater extent. The development of this

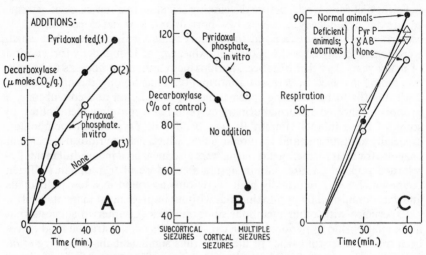

FIG. 10.10. Metabolic consequences of pyridoxine deficiency, and restoration: A and B, glutamic decarboxylase; C, respiration.

A. Rats were maintained on a pyridoxine deficient diet without (curves 2 and 3) or with (curve 8) added pyridoxol. After 8 weeks, cerebral tissues were sampled and assayed for glutamic acid decarboxylase. Curves (2) and (3) were obtained from the same cerebral dispersions, adding 1 mg. pyridoxal phosphate/g. tissue to samples (2) (Roberts *et al.*, 1951).

B. Deficiency induced in normal cats by thiosemicarbazide. Samples of cerebral cortex were taken at different stages during the development of seizures and their glutamate decarboxylase assayed in presence and absence of added pyridoxal phosphate (Killam, 1957).

C. Cats were maintained on pyridoxine-deficient diets until seizures developed, and slices of cerebral cortex examined *in vitro* with and without additions of γ-aminobutyrate or of pyridoxal phosphate (McKhann *et al.*, 1961). Respiration is given as μmoles O_2/g.hr.

defect in the brain of pyridoxine-deficient rats is shown in Fig. 10.10, together with its restoration: by pyridoxol given *in vivo*, or alternatively by addition of pyridoxal phosphate to the experimental vessels *in vitro*. As the decarboxylase in cerebral tissues could be made good by pyridoxal phosphate, the quantity of the protein part of enzyme was thus normal. Pyridoxal phosphate as coenzyme proved readily dissociable when the decarboxylase was prepared from normal mouse brain by precipitating with acetone; only a fraction of the decarboxylase of the tissue was exhibited until pyridoxal phosphate was added. This system could also be activated by pyridoxal and adenosine triphosphate, suggesting synthesis of the phosphate in cerebral tissues themselves. The product of decarboxylation of glutamic acid is γ-aminobutyric acid, whose properties are further described in Chapters 8 and 14.

The cerebral pyridoxine-requiring systems appear to offer the most sensitive site in the body to several hydrazides and oximes, of which a number are convulsive agents (*Conference*, 1960; Medina *et al.*, 1962; Minard, 1967). One of these, 1,1-dimethylhydrazine, was demonstrated to deplete rat brain of pyridoxal phosphate within 10 days, the depletion being correlated in time with the occurrence of convulsions. Again, glutamate decarboxylase is a major target for such compounds as exemplified in Fig. 10.10 with respect to thiosemicarbazide: $NH_2 . CS . NH . NH_2$. In these experiments (**B**, Fig. 10.10) cats were treated with the drug while the electrical activity of several parts of the brain was under observation. Tissues from different cerebral sites were sampled during the development of convulsions, and assayed for glutamate decarboxylase. The decarboxylase of the cerebral cortex is seen to be normal at the first development of seizure patterns, which was however subcortical. As seizure activity developed in the cortex, its decarboxylase activity fell. Examination of cerebral extracts showed γ-aminobutyrate to be the only amino acid of those assayed, whose content changed; a diminution of 40% was observed.

Further involvement of γ-aminobutyrate in the effects of pyridoxine deficiency is indicated by the experiments of **C**, Fig. 10.10. Here, cats suffering dietary pyridoxine deficiency were used as source of cerebral tissue for measurement of respiration in oxygenated glucose salines. Respiratory rates were depressed some 20% in the deficient animals, and increased to normal by added pyridoxal phosphate. γ-Aminobutyrate, however, could replace pyridoxal phosphate in this respect. Neither compound significantly affected the respiration of cerebral tissues from normal cats, nor did they affect the respiration of hepatic tissue from the deficient animals. These observations can be interpreted in terms of the oxidative route involving γ-aminobutyrate (Chapter 8) for which enzyme systems exist at adequate level in the brain but not in the liver. A related phenomenon has been shown in one instance in man, in the child first characterized as suffering extreme pyridoxine-dependency. After 6 years, the child's seizures recommenced three days following withdrawal of pyridoxine; a cerebral respiratory rate of 3·3 ml. $O_2/100$ g./min. was then found by methods described in Chapter 2. On administering pyridoxine, the seizures and associated electroencephalographic abnormalities ceased in 18 min., and cerebral respiratory rate rose to 4·4 ml. $O_2/100$ g./min. This is a value closer to normal for subjects of the child's age; she remained, however, mentally retarded (Sokoloff *et al.*, 1959).

Another inhibitor of cerebral pyridoxine-dependent enzymes, hydroxylamine, has also proved to be related in its action on γ-aminobutyrate. Hydroxylamine 5 min. after intraperitoneal injection to rats led to convulsions. Extraction of different parts of the brain then showed them to have increased in γ-aminobutyrate content by 30–85% (Baxter & Roberts, in *Conference*, 1960). Hydroxylamine was found to have its greater *in vitro* effect not on decarboxylases, but on transamination, and especially on the system involving γ-aminobutyrate and α-oxoglutarate. This system yields succinic semialdehyde (q.v.) and is an initial stage in the cerebral oxidation of γ-aminobutyrate. A common factor in the action of the two convulsive agents, thiosemicarbazide and hydroxylamine, is thus the inhibition of γ-aminobutyrate oxidation: though their different points of action lead in the one case to decrease and in the other to increase in the cerebral content of γ-aminobutyrate. Other possible mechanisms are referred to by Baxter & Roberts (*Conference*, 1960). The convulsions of hypoxia (see Tower, 1960) have also been examined from the point of view of an involvement of γ-aminobutyrate (Wood *et al.*, 1968). Relationships between pyridoxine-requiring systems and cerebral excitability are further appraised in Chapter 14.

Pyridoxine Derivatives in the Brain

The pyridoxine of the normal brain exists largely in its phosphorylated forms (Table 10.4) and at a total concentration several hundred times that of blood plasma. The quite low concentration of non-phosphorylated forms in the two materials (and also in cerebrospinal fluid) may, however, be of the same order of magnitude. On administering pyridoxol, the amount of the free compound in the brain increased and pyridoxol phosphate was found at appreciable level; under other circumstances, pyridoxal phosphate and pyridoxamine phosphate were the main forms of occurrence. In subcellular fractions, these two differ in location, more pyridoxamine phosphate existing in crude mitochondrial fractions from the brain (Bain & Williams, *Conference*, 1960).

The *phosphorylation* involved in producing the preponderant coenzyme forms of pyridoxine can take place in the brain itself (Killam & Bain, 1957; McCormick *et al.*, 1961); an ATP: pyridoxal-5-phosphotransferase, EC 2.7.1.35, has been measured by incubating with adenosine triphosphate, Mg salts, and pyridoxal. The brain of the rat produced 0·6 μmole pyridoxal phosphate/g. tissue/hr.; only kidney and liver of ten tissues of the animals which were examined gave higher values. The enzyme existed mainly in soluble form in a supernatant after centrifuging; it was at notably greater level in bovine cerebral hemispheres than in the medulla (1·6; 0·36 μmoles/g.hr.). Interestingly, the phosphokinase was found at slightly higher level in the brain of pyridoxine-deficient rats, which could produce 0·75 μmoles/whole brain/hr.; normal animals yielded 0·55 μmoles. A converse response to pyridoxine has been shown in a liver transaminase (Greengard & Gordon, 1963).

With development of pyridoxine deficiency in rats fed diets low in the vitamin, cerebral pyridoxine diminished; but as Table 10.4 shows, the depletion was not in parallel in the different pyridoxine components. Pyridoxal phosphate had fallen to one-third its normal level when pyridoxamine phosphate was less affected; in two strains of mice these proportions differed (Lyon *et al.*, 1962). Signs of pyridoxine deficiency can be precipitated in normal animals by structurally related compounds. Of these, 4-deoxypyridoxine (Fig. 10.9) markedly lowers the total cerebral content of pyridoxine derivatives and especially that of pyridoxal phosphate (Table 10.4); pyridoxal, however, accumulated. Isonicotinic acid hydrazide, the antitubercular drug which can produce psychotic episodes, is also seen from Table 10.4 to lower the pyridoxal phosphate of the brain; like the hydrazides discussed in a previous section, it causes convulsions in experimental animals. Enzymic basis for the action of the hydrazide (as a hydrazone derivative) and of deoxypyridoxine has been demonstrated in their inhibition of the pyridoxal phosphokinase described above (McCormick & Snell, 1961). The phosphokinase from beef brain had affinities for the inhibitors commensurate with those of its (differing) affinities for the different forms of pyridoxine.

The level of pyridoxal kinase activity in the brain proves to be conditioned also by the substrates of certain pyridoxal enzymes. This has been demonstrated

Table 10.4

Pyridoxine derivatives in animal tissues

Animal and tissue	Condition	Content (μg./g. fresh tissue)			
		Total	Pyridox-amine phosphate	Pyridoxol phosphate	Pyridoxal phosphate
Mouse brain	Normal	3·16	1·70	Trace	1·02
,, ,,	30 min. after pyridoxol[1]	4·90	1·07	0·15	0·96
,, ,,	Convulsing, 60 min. after 4-deoxypyridoxine[1]	1·8	1·0	0	0·08
,, ,,	Convulsing, 45 min. after isonicotinic hydrazide[1]	2·85[2]	1·38	0·01	0·26
Mouse liver	Normal	9·76	3·15	Trace	6·04
Dog liver	Normal	9·73	4·19	0	5·44
Dog, blood plasma	Normal	0·007[3]	–	–	–
		Content (μg./g. nitrogen)			
Mouse brain	Normal	198	105	–	51
,, ,,	Deficient diet	133	82	–	17
Mouse liver	Normal	374	140	–	106
,, ,,	Deficient diet	148	56	–	35

Data from Bain & Williams (*Conference*, 1960) and Lyon *et al.* (1962), who give values also for the non-phosphorylated compounds, for other strains and species, and after other treatments. The assay of the cerebral content of pyridoxine and its phosphates after their chromatographic separation to five fractions, is detailed by Loo & Badger (1969).

[1] Intraperitoneal administrations.
[2] Including 0·57 μg./g. as the isonicotinic acid hydrazide derivative.
[3] Mainly as pyridoxal and its phosphate; similar values of 0·7–1·8 μg./100 ml., were found in human plasma, and 1 μg./100 ml. in human cerebrospinal fluid.

in relation to cerebral aromatic amines: when in the rabbit, catecholamines and serotonin were depleted by reserpine, pyridoxal kinase activity increased from 0·18 to 0·8 μmoles phosphorylated/mg. cerebral protein/hr. (Ebadi *et al.*, 1968). This increase took place in the presence of puromycin, cyclo-heximide and other inhibitors of protein synthesis; it was ascribed to the cerebral amines inducing in the enzyme an allosteric change which lowered kinase activity. Alternatively, the aldimines formed by combination of pyridoxal phosphate with the bases, may function as inhibitors (Loo &

Whittaker, 1967): such is concluded to be the route by which pyridoxine-dependent enzymes are disturbed in phenylketonuria.

Several tissues of the body become depleted in pyridoxine coenzymes during dietary deficiency of pyridoxine, so diminishing their transaminase activity. The glutamine of the blood in deficient rats was found at about half its normal level, while blood urea was increased some 50%. Changes of this character in the body as a whole and in the brain are to be taken into account in appraising the convulsive tendency of pyridoxine deficiency. Antibody formation is also disturbed in pyridoxine deficiency, presumably through action on amino-acid metabolism.

Vitamin B_{12} (Cobalamines)

These substances, curative in pernicious anaemia, are the most recently isolated of the vitamins described here. Only provisional answers can be given to many questions concerning their functioning, but it is clearly involved in the central nervous system. The vitamins contain cobalt, co-ordinated to a 2:3-dimethyl-benzimidazole derivative with a porphyrin-like moiety, and are based on cobalamine, $C_{63}H_{88}N_{14}O_{14}P$.Co of which the structure is completely known (see Lester Smith, 1963; White, 1963; Bernhauer *et al.*, 1964; Sebrell & Harris, 1968). The daily requirement is no more than 1 μg. parentally or 5 μg. orally. In man, vitamin B_{12} deficiency usually results from defective absorption, but lack of cobalt produces in ruminants a severe wasting and anaemia which can be cured with B_{12}.

Neural Involvement in Pernicious Anaemia

Addison's description of pernicious anaemia includes: "Its approach is first indicated by a certain amount of langour and restlessness and indisposition to, or incapacity for, bodily or mental exertion." Mental confusion has frequently been reported as associated with the disorder, and some 16% of cases have been described as showing mental abnormalities amounting to a psychosis (Herman *et al.*, 1937). Knowing that a major defect in pernicious anaemia is in the red blood cells, it was understandable that cerebral respiration should be studied in explanation of these changes. Using the nitrous oxide technique (Chapter 2), cerebral respiration was in fact found to be depressed in a high proportion of cases, and thus clearly contributed to the disorder. In addition, however, the degree of disturbance of cerebral metabolism was not correlated with the degree of anaemia (Scheinberg, 1951). During recovery from the anaemia on treatment with vitamin B_{12}, cerebral respiration recovered in a proportion of subjects but not in all.

Electroencephalographic observations have also shown in some cases of pernicious anaemia a cerebral defect independent of the erythrocyte changes. Contribution to the electroencephalogram by the slower theta or delta rhythms increased in subjects showing mental abnormality and also in a proportion of subjects who did not. An approximate measure of these changes is given in Fig. 10.11 which records the average frequency of the EEG rhythms, seen to be low before administration of vitamin B_{12} to an anaemic subject and to increase after therapy. It is important that such recovery occurs in this and other subjects before any appreciable increase in red blood cells. Thus vitamin B_{12} may have an effect in cerebral metabolism which is not secondary to the anaemia. Final recovery in the central nervous system may however require a year or more.

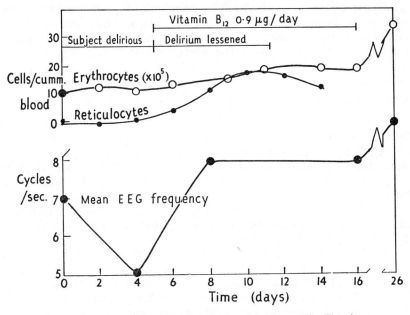

FIG. 10.11. A cerebral abnormality in pernicious anaemia. Showing the time-course of different effects of administration of vitamin B_{12} (Samson et al., 1952).

Cobalamines in Other CNS Illnesses

Some 30–70% of patients with pernicious anaemia have the neurological signs of subacute combined degeneration of the spinal cord. In this condition abnormalities are found in particular parts of the cord, peripheral nerve, and often in parts of the brain (Meyer in Blackwood et al., 1963). With the subacute combined degeneration, urinary vitamin B_{12} was low, and use of $^{60}Co\text{-}B_{12}$ showed an unusually small proportion of the compound to be absorbed and appear in urine (Bauer & Heinrich, 1961). Also, the total vitamin B_{12} of blood serum which in a normal group ranged from 80–500 pg./ml., was at 0–30 pg./ml. in both pernicious anaemia and in the subacute combined degeneration: abnormality in vitamins B_{12} and in a further factor are presumably involved in producing the subacute degeneration. The vitamin B_{12} of the cerebrospinal fluid appears to be largely uncombined and at similar level to the free B_{12} of blood plasma; a mean value of 21 pg./ml. was found in subjects with no organic lesions and also in most of a group of forty-three patients suffering various neurological disorders (Kidd et al., 1963).

It has been emphasized that neurological complications are frequent in cobalamine deficiency, and that some 10% of admissions to some geriatric wards showed low serum B_{12} levels (Buckle, 1966; Shulman, 1967). Certain drugs including phenobarbitone and diphenylhydantoin may have deleterious mental side-effects through disturbance of B_{12} metabolism (Reynolds, 1967). In surveying 150 patients admitted to a mental hospital during a few months (Hunter et al., 1967) two were found to be suffering B_{12}-deficiency syndromes, with recent mental deterioration and depression. These illnesses cleared gradually on B_{12} administration. Subsequent surveys have shown higher incidence of B_{12} deficiency in mental hospital patients (Hällström, 1969; Reynolds et al., 1970).

Cerebral Cobalamines

Rat brain contains per g. some 32 ng. of vitamin B_{12} derivatives determined by microbiological assay: quantities many times those of blood plasma (see above). Examination of six parts of the central nervous system of the dog showed relative uniformity of vitamin B_{12} content of 12–22 ng./g., except that the pituitary had the unusually high level of 3–400 ng./g.; the pituitary was indeed greater in B_{12} concentration than any other organ examined, and was comparably high in four mammalian species including man (Cooperman et al., 1960). Rat brain can be markedly depleted in vitamin B_{12} in dietary B_{12}-deficiency (Arnstein, 1959).

On subcellular fractionation of rat brain, more than half of the vitamin B_{12} was found in a crude mitochondrial fraction and was not removed by washing (Newman et al., 1962). Its turnover was appraised by giving to the rats 30–60 ng. of ^{58}Co-vitamin B_{12} intramuscularly, which represented about half the daily B_{12} intake. The proportion of the added compound found in the brain increased from 0·16% at 6 hr. to 0·47% at 22 days after injection; this corresponded to about 1% of the B_{12} of the brain, and equilibrium with the pre-existing cerebral B_{12} required at least 8 days. The cerebral ^{58}Co was demonstrated chromatographically to be present as vitamin B_{12} derivatives. After administering simple salts of ^{60}Co to animals under a variety of conditions, the brain acquired less ^{60}Co than did other organs of the body; it contains about 1 ng. Co/g. (Lester Smith, 1962).

Metabolic roles of vitamin B_{12} include its functioning in coenzyme forms which are adenosine derivatives of vitamin B_{12}, in the isomerization of methylmalonyl CoA to succinyl CoA. Patients with B_{12} deficiency excrete increased quantities of methylmalonic acid, and also of propionic and acetic acids which are metabolically related to methylmalonic acid (White, 1963; Cox et al., 1968; see Chapter 8).

Pantothenic Acid

Pantothenic acid (see Novelli, 1953) owes its name to its wide distribution in living organisms, and such distribution makes it understandable that well-defined deficiency is very rare in man though lack of pantothenate may colour the symptoms of other nutritional deficiencies. In a number of species of experimental animals, signs of malfunctioning of the nervous system appear relatively late in the deficiency, involving paralysis, coma or convulsions; after death, demyelination has been observed in peripheral nerves and in the spinal cord. Well-defined lesions occur in the adrenal especially in rats, together with failure in the formation of adrenal hormones. This leads to a lower fasting blood glucose, an increased sensitivity to insulin, and lowered resistance to anoxia. Deficiency reported to be induced in man experimentally included neural symptoms (Bean & Hodges, 1954) and in dogs, behavioural changes have been found.

Although the central nervous system is not easily depleted in pantothenate, other techniques have shown the vitamin to be of great importance in cerebral metabolism. The level in the brain is relatively high, at 15–26 μg. (70–120 nmoles)/g. and almost all of this is in a combined form which has the properties of coenzyme A, and has been determined by its acting as catalyst in acetylation. The function of this coenzyme (Fig. 10.9) in the main energy-yielding reactions of the brain is described in Chapter 6 and its functioning in synthesis of acetylcholine in Chapter 14. Acetylcoenzyme A was found in rat brain at 4–5 nmoles/g., about 1/20 of its content in coenzyme A (Schuberth et al., 1965, 1966). An acetyl CoA synthetase was responsible for its formation from acetate, coenzyme A and ATP and occurred in nerve-ending particles and mitochondria. The content of acetyl CoA in rat brain was examined after administration of drugs associated in action with acetylcholine, and found to be relatively little affected; some 25 % increase was, however, found in hypoxia (Schuberth et al., 1966).

Pantothenate is involved, as coenzyme A, in many synthetic processes in the body as a whole; noting only a few of those concerned with the central nervous system or its functioning, the processes involve the formation of C—C links in sterols as well as citrate; the C—O link in acetylcholine; and it has also been implicated in formation of amide or peptide linkages. Thus it was first assayed by its catalysis of the acetylation of sulphanilamide, and more recently benzoylation of glycine to hippuric acid in preparations from liver has been found to be coenzyme-A dependent and depressed in pantothenate deficiency. Further, antibody formation is depressed in the pantothenate-depleted animals.

It would appear probable that cerebral tissues synthesize coenzyme A from a simpler substance such as pantothenate, for coenzyme A has not been detected in blood plasma and substances with properties of pantothenate exist there. Some 10 nmoles of coenzyme A are found/g. of erythrocytes.

Riboflavin

Neural tissues are not the most sensitive to lack of riboflavin (vitamin B_2). Changes are commonly first seen in the skin, mouth and eyes but there occurs in man and experimental animals in riboflavin deficiency, a lowered physical activity and appetite which may be followed by sudden collapse and coma. Dogs deficient to varying degrees were found lacking in specific tests of performance; the deficiencies led ultimately to demyelination especially in peripheral nerves and in the posterior columns of the spinal cord (Street et al., 1941). In man, riboflavin deficiency is found as an entity in itself, and also in association with lack of nicotinamide or of thiamine.

Cerebral riboflavin levels in mouse, rat and man are about 2·5–5 µg. (7–14 nmoles)/g., about a tenth of those of liver or of heart muscle and comparable to those of skeletal muscle. The riboflavin exists largely as flavin-adenine dinucleotide presumably in different flavoproteins of which some have been noted as functioning in the main respiratory chain and in amino acid metabolism; about a fifth occurs as the mononucleotide (Chapter 6; Lowry, 1952) and a trace as riboflavin itself. Increase in the total cerebral flavines has been followed during growth of the brain in the rat (Kuzuya & Nagatsu, 1969); it followed a time-course different from that of its increase in other organs but paralleled that of the cerebral monoamine oxidase, which probably carries a flavin coenzyme.

The cerebral riboflavin derivatives probably originate from circulating riboflavin. On systemic injection of precursors to rats, the mono- and dinucleotides had little effect on cerebral flavin content (Nagatsu et al., 1967) while riboflavin itself caused considerable increase, from 9 to 14–20 nmoles/g. fresh brain. A similar conclusion was afforded by ^{14}C-labelled precursors; most of the cerebral ^{14}C from [2-^{14}C]riboflavin was found as the dinucleotide and persisted in this form with little if any loss during 15 hr.

Vitamin A

In its role as precursor of the light-sensitive pigments of the eye, vitamin A is connected with an extremely sensitive and specific neural mechanism. Thus the visual pigment rhodopsin is formed from retinaldehyde, $C_{19}H_{27}$.CHO, and the specific lipoprotein opsin, and is contained in the outer segments of retinal rods in quantities perhaps 50% of their dry weight (see Graymore, 1970). Metabolic participation of vitamin A in the functioning of the brain itself has not been observed. Deficiency in growing animals does, however, lead to degeneration of cells and fibres in the central nervous system, especially in the spinal cord and medulla. The changes are sufficiently clear and regular to be employed as a biological assay for vitamin A (Coetzee, 1949). They appear to arise mechanically through differential effects of the vitamin on growth. Skeletal growth is restricted in avitaminosis-A to a much greater extent than is that of other parts of the body, including the brain; this leaves the cranial cavity and spinal canal smaller than are required by the growing central nervous system. The loss of cells and demyelination which follow are similar to those which occur after nerve fibres are crushed. Vitamin A in excess is toxic and can change cell permeability, causing e.g. release of proteases from the cartilage of limb-bones. This property and the effects of the vitamin in normal doses, are considered to be due to actions at lipoprotein membrane-structures. Vitamin A alcohol penetrates and expands lipid monolayers, including those of lecithin and cholesterol; among structurally related compounds, specificity for this action is similar to the specificity for action as a vitamin (Fell & Dingle, 1963; Bangham et al., 1964). Electron microscopy has shown disorganization of the laminae in retinal rods of vitamin A-deficient animals (Wald, 1960).

The retinal functioning of vitamin A has been concluded to be a phenomenon of membrane reorganization (Abrahamson, 1969; Blaurock & Wilkins, 1969;

Cone & Cobbs, 1969; Duncan, 1969). Illumination of a suspension of retinal outer rod segments caused prompt entry to them of Na^+ from the surrounding solution, and efflux of K^+. Similar efflux was caused by retinal, the aldehyde derived from vitamin A. The rod segments contain 11-*cis* retinal in Schiff-base linkage with phosphatidylethanolamine which is part of a lipoprotein complex oriented in the membrane; indeed about 20–25% of the protein of these segments consists of the specific protein of rhodopsin. Light was concluded to cause the retinal to enter a new combination with the ε-amino group of a lysine residue of the protein, and this change to alter membrane structure sufficiently to allow the changes in Na^+ and K^+ which generate a receptor potential; cyclic AMP (q.v.) was involved in the membrane-change (Bitensky *et al.*, 1971).

Other Vitamins

Small quantities of sterols of vitamin-D activity have been reported in the brain, but cerebral changes are not prominent in avitaminosis-D. Vitamin-D intoxication can however involve fatigue, vertigo, psychoses and stupor (Kushner, 1956). The skeletal effects of vitamins D and their neural actions appear likely to have calcium compounds as a common factor; a vitamin D-dependent Ca-binding protein has been characterized and may have transport functions (Wasserman *et al.*, 1968).

Lack of vitamin E in most experimental animals but not in the chick, usually causes a muscular degeneration without affecting the nervous system. Some 60% of chicks on vitamin-E deficient diets develop after a month, a disorder of the central nervous system for which histological basis is seen in lesions of the cerebellum, cerebrum, and medulla. These appear to be due to obstruction of cerebral blood vessels. α-Tocopherol, the major component of vitamin E, occurs in rat brain at about 6 μg./g. and in peripheral nerve at five times this concentration; in both tissues its quantity is diminished by vitamin E deficient diets (Edwin *et al.*, 1961). The ubiquinone (coenzyme Q) of the tissues also decreased in vitamin E deficiency; this compound may have a function in connection with the respiratory chain (Morton, 1961 and see Chapter 6).

Ascorbic acid is normally present in the brain in relatively high concentration, especially in parts of the pituitary, and is also present in the cerebrospinal fluid. In the guinea pig brain Damron *et al.* (1952) found its level to be 0·8 μmole/g., second only to that of the adrenal, and to be decreased to 0·35 μmole/g. on a scorbutigenic diet. Levels of the related diketogulonic acid and ascorbone in the brain also fell. Diet also affects the cerebral ascorbate of the rat, which synthesizes the compound (Rajalakshmi *et al.*, 1967). Deficiency in ascorbic acid leads to a depressed oxidation of tyrosine in tissues from the liver, and ascorbic acid itself can under some conditions increase the oxygen uptake of cerebral tissues, as with pentobarbital *in vitro* (Greig, 1947; cf. Lin & Cohen, 1960); a search for cerebral systems oxidizing glutathione by ascorbone gave negative results (Thomson, unpublished). An ascorbate-dependent oxidation of nicotinamide–adenine dinucleotide occurs in systems of the eye, being at relatively high level in microsomal preparations from the retina (Heath & Fiddick, 1965).

Ascorbic acid has been found lower in the blood plasma of patients of certain mental hospitals than in normal subjects; when however comparison was made of normal and mentally ill persons, especially schizophrenic, maintained under similar conditions, no difference was found in plasma levels nor in their response to a dose of ascorbic acid (McDonald *et al.*, 1961; Milner, 1963). Findings here and with nicotinamide emphasize the continuing need for application of existing nutritional knowledge.

Biotin deficiency has been induced in man by diets containing a large proportion of egg-white, which carries a biotin-binding component. Neural symptoms were not prominent but mild depression, lassitude and anorexia resulted and were relieved by administered biotin (Sebrell & Harris, 1968).

Notes on Nutritional Requirements

Description of nutritional factors which affect the central nervous system has thus displayed a considerable proportion of its known metabolic machinery. Partly, this is because the substances required preformed as vitamins for any successful organism will be widely distributed in foodstuffs and it is the more important substances which are so distributed and whose functions are best known. The bloodstream probably also supplies to the brain other substances as yet unknown which are equally important for its functioning (Chapter 2).

Reasons for a dietary deficiency affecting first a given organ of the body can be formally stated to include: utilization of the vitamin by the organ at an unusually high rate; possession by the organ of only a small margin of the vitamin or of its functioning form, or inadequacies in their interconversion, assimilation from the bloodstream or retention; unusual sensitivity of the organ to the deficiency in its own vitamin content or to disturbance arising elsewhere from deficiency; or unusual importance of the organ itself in comparison with others in the body. Statement of the relative importance of these factors in the cerebral effects of the deficiencies just outlined can be adumbrated in a few cases only. Thus with thiamine there is little margin of the vitamin in the brain, and also sensitivity to abnormal metabolites from other organs. One or other of the different factors can evidently predominate as a deficiency progresses or when it arises in different circumstances.

Relations between an organ and a dietary essential include not only the factors listed above, but also others; assimilation of the vitamin from foodstuffs, and contributions by its synthesis. The multiplicity of these factors as a whole makes understandable the variations reported in nutritional requirements between different individuals or species. Individual variations in experimental animals and in man are clearly attested as involving five-fold differences in requirements and in isolated cases the difference may be forty-fold. The amino acid or vitamin requirements usually quoted are average values implying in a large population many individuals with much larger or much smaller needs. The examples of Hartnup disease and pyridoxine-dependency have shown how individual or inherited metabolic anomalies contribute to this variation.

Many instances are reported of improvement in mental and emotional disorders by administration of vitamins. Nutritional deficiencies have major effects on mental attitudes and behaviour in man and in experimental animals

(*Symposium*, 1957), but except under poor nutritional conditions, it is not to be expected that the vitamins would ordinarily act as therapeutic agents in these disorders. The small proportion of subjects who appear to be receiving an adequate diet, and yet are improved by further vitamins, may nevertheless represent the proportion who from the normal distribution of vitamin requirements would be anticipated to be more exacting in this respect. Regrettably little quantitative information about the distribution in a normal population is available (Williams *et al.*, 1950, 1956) and emotional and mental disorders can be seen as causally related to nutritional disturbance when they involve changes in intestinal functioning, important in relation to assimilation or synthesis of vitamins, or changes in appetite and feeding habits. For an experimental study of emotional modification of intestinal functioning, see Sadler & Orten (1968). The fashion in which therapeutic agents can have side-effects related to nutritional intake became prominent through the disastrous effects of eating cheese while receiving amine oxidase inhibitors (q.v.; Blackwell & Marley, 1966). As several nutritional deficiencies themselves can lead to mental and emotional changes, many opportunities are afforded for interaction of the two very different categories of disorder.

REFERENCES

ABRAHAMSON, E. W. (1969). *Second Internat. Neurochem. Meeting*, p. 65. Milan: Tamburini.

ALEXANDER, L. (1940). *Amer. J. Path.* **16**, 61.

ALEXANDER, L., PIJOAN, M., SCHUBE, P. J. & MOORE, M. (1938). *Arch. Neurol. Psychiat.* **40**, 58.

AMERINE, M. A., PANGBORN, R. M. & ROESSLER, E. B. (1965). *Principles of Sensory Evaluation of Food*. New York: Academic Press.

ARNSTEIN, H. R. V. (1959). *Biochem. J.* **73**, 23P.

AXELROD, A. E., SPIES, T. D. & ELVEHJEM, C. A. (1941). *J. biol. Chem.* **138**, 667.

BANGA, I., OCHOA, S. & PETERS, R. A. (1939). *Biochem. J.* **33**, 1980.

BANGHAM, A. D., DINGLE, J. T. & LUCY, J. A. (1964). *Biochem. J.* **90**, 133.

BAUER, H. & HEINRICH, H. C. (1961). *Proc. Internat. Neurochem. Sympos.* **3**, 120.

BAUMGARTEN, R. VON, BLOOM, F. E., OLIVER, A. P. & SALMOIRAGHI, G. C. (1963). *Pflug. Archiv.* **277**, 125.

BEAN, W. B. & HODGES, R. E. (1954). *Proc. Soc. exp. Biol.* **86**, 693.

BEHER, W. T. & ANTHONY, W. L. (1953). *J. biol. Chem.* **203**, 895.

BERNARD, R. A., HALPERN, B. P. & KARE, M. R. (1961). *Proc. Soc. exp. Biol. Med.* **108**, 784.

BERNHAUER, K., MULLER, O. & WAGNER, F. (1964). *Advanc. Enzymol.* **26**, 233.

BHAGAT, B. & LOCKETT, M. F. (1962). *J. Pharm. Pharmacol.* **14**, 37.

BITENSKY, M. W., GORMAN, R. E. & MILLER, W. H. (1971). *Proc. natl. Acad. Sci., Wash.* **68**, 561.

BLACKWELL, B. & MARLEY, E. (1966). *Brit. J. Pharmacol.* **26**, 120.

BLACKWOOD, W., MCMENEMEY, W. H., MEYER, A., NORMAN, R. M. & RUSSELL, D. S. (1963). Greenfield's Neuropathology. London: Arnold.

BLAUROCK, A. E. & WILKINS, M. H. F. (1969). *Nature*, **223**, 906.

BRIN, M., SHOHET, S. S. & DAVIDSON, C. S. (1958). *J. biol. Chem.* **230**, 319.

BROWN, R. R. & PRICE, J. M. (1956). *J. biol. Chem.* **219**, 985.

BROŽEK, J. & GRANDE, F. (1960). Neurophysiology, Vol. 3, p. 1891. Washington: American Physiological Society.

BROŽEK, J. & VAES, G. (1961). *Vitamins & Hormones*, **19**, 43.

BUCKLE, R. M. (1966). *Clin. Sci.* **31**, 181.

BURCH, H. B., BRADLEY, M. E. & LOWRY, O. H. (1967). *J. biol. Chem.* **242**, 4546.

BURCH, H. B., LOWRY, O. H. & VON DIPPE, P. (1963). *J. biol. Chem.* **238**, 2838.

CHICK, H., EL SADR, M. M. & WORDEN, A. N. (1940). *Biochem. J.* **34**, 595.
CHICK, H., MACRAE, T. F., MARTIN, A. J. P. & MARTIN, C. J. (1938). *Biochem. J.* **32**, 2207.
CLAYTON, B. E., DOBBS, R. H. & PATRICK, A. D. (1967). *Arch. Dis. Child.* **42**, 467.
COETZEE, W. H. K. (1949). *Biochem. J.* **45**, 628.
CONE, R. A. & COBBS, W. H. (1969). *Nature*, **221**, 820.
Conference (1960). Inhibition in the Nervous System and γ-Aminobutyric Acid. Ed. E. Roberts & C. F. Baxter. New York: Pergamon.
Conference (1962). Thiamine. *Ann. N.Y. Acad. Sci.* **98**, 383.
COOPER, J. R. (1968). *Biochim. Biophys. Acta*, **156**, 368.
COOPER, J. R., ITOKAWA, Y. & PINCUS, J. H. (1969). *Science*, **164**, 72 and personal communication.
COOPER, J. R., PINCUS, J. H., ITOKAWA, Y. & PIROS, K. (1970). *New England J. Med.* **283**, 795.
COOPERMAN, J. M., LUHBY, A. L., TELLER, D. N. & MARLEY, J. F. (1960). *J. biol. Chem.* **235**, 191.
COPER, H. & HERKEN, H. (1963). *Deut. Med. Wochschr.* **88**, 2025.
COPER, H. & NEUBERT, D. (1963). *J. Neurochem.* **10**, 513.
COURSIN, D. B. (1954). *J. Amer. med. Ass.* **154**, 406.
COX, E. V., ROBERTSON-SMITH, D., SMALL, M. & WHITE, A. M. (1968). *Clin. Sci.* **35**, 123.
DAKSHINAMURTI, K. & STEPHENS, M. C. (1969). *J. Neurochem.* **16**, 1515.
DAMRON, C. M., MONIER, M. M. & ROE, J. H. (1952). *J. biol. Chem.* **195**, 599.
DANN, W. J. (1941). *J. biol. Chem.* **141**, 803.
DASTOLI, F. R. (1968). *Amer. Perf. Cosm.* **83**, 37.
DASTOLI, F. R. & PRICE, S. (1966). *Science*, **154**, 905.
DAVIDSON, S. & PASSMORE, R. (1966). *Human Nutrition & Dietetics*. Edinburgh: Livingston.
DEGUCHI, T., ICHIYAMA, A., NISHIZUKA, Y. & HAYASHI, O. (1968). *Biochim. Biophys. Acta*, **158**, 382.
DEUTSCH, J. A. & DEUTSCH, D. (1966). Physiological Psychology. Illinois: Dorsey.
DICKENS, F., RANDLE, P. J. & WHELAN, W. J. (1968). Carbohydrate Metabolism and its Disorders. London: Academic Press.
DREYFUS, P. M. (1959). *J. Neurochem.* **4**, 183.
DREYFUS, P. M. (1961). *J. Neurochem.* **8**, 139.
DREYFUS, P. M. (1962). *Acta Neurol. Scand.* **38**, Suppl. **1**, 69.
DREYFUS, P. M. & VICTOR, M. (1961). *Amer. J. clin. Nutr.* **9**, 414.
DUNCAN, G. (1969). Second Internat. Neurochem. Meeting, p. 159. Milan: Tamburini.
DUNCAN, R. B. & BRIGGS, M. (1962). *Arch. Otolaryngol.* **75**, 116.
EBADI, M. S., RUSSELL, R. L. & McCOY, E. E. (1968). *J. Neurochem.* **15**, 659.
EBELS, E. J., BLOKZIJL, E. J. & TROELSTRA, J. A. (1965). *Helv. Pediat. Acta*, **20**, 310.
EDWIN, E. E., DIPLOCK, A. T., BUNYAN, J. & GREEN, J. (1961). *Biochem. J.* **79**, 91.
EDWIN, E. E. & JACKMAN, R. (1970). *Nature, Lond.* **228**, 772.
FELL, H. B. & DINGLE, J. T. (1963). *Biochem. J.* **87**, 403.
FITZSIMMONS, J. T. (1969). *J. Physiol.* **201**, 349.
FOLLIS, R. H. (1963). Deficiency Disease. Springfield: Thomas.
GARCIA-BUNUEL, L., McDOUGAL, D. B., BURCH, H. B., JONES, E. M. & TOUHILL, E. (1962). *J. Neurochem.* **9**, 589.
GORE, M., IBBOTT, F. & McILWAIN, H. (1950). *Biochem. J.* **47**, 121.
GRAYMORE, C. N. (1970). (Ed.). Biochemistry of the Eye. London: Academic Press.
GREENGARD, O. & GORDON, M. (1963). *J. biol. Chem.* **238**, 3708.
GREENGARD, P., KALINSKY, H., MANNING, T. J. & ZAK, S. B. (1968). *J. biol. Chem.* **243**, 4216.
GREGORY, I. (1955). *J. ment. Sci.* **101**, 85.
GREIG, M. E. (1947). *J. Pharmacol.* **91**, 317.
GRUBER, M. (1953). *Biochim. biophys. Acta*, **10**, 136.
GUBLER, C. J. (1961). *J. biol. Chem.* **236**, 3112.
HAGBERG, B., HAMFELT, A. & HANSON, O. (1964). *Lancet* **i**, 145.

HÄLLSTRÖM, T. (1969). *Acta Psychiat. Scand.* **45**, 19.

HARDMAN, J. M., ALLEN, L. W., BAUGHMAN, F. A. & WATERMAN, D. F. (1968). *Arch. Neurol.* **18**, 478.

HARDWICK, S. W. (1943). *Lancet*, **ii**, 43.

HARPER, R., BATE-SMITH, E. C. & LAND, D. G. (1968). Odour Description and Odour Classification. London: Churchill.

HARRIS, R. S. (1951). In The Enzymes, Vol. 1, p. 1186. Ed. Sumner & Myrbäck. New York: Academic Press.

HAYASHI, R. (1957). *Nutr. Rev.* **15**, 65.

HEALD, P. J. (1956). *Biochem. J.* **63**, 242.

HEATH, H. & FIDDICK, R. (1965). *Biochem. J.* **94**, 114.

HEELEY, A. F., PRESOWICZ, A. T. & McCUBBING, D. G. (1968). *Clin. Sci.* **35**, 381.

HERMAN, M., MORT, H. & JOLLIFFE, N. (1937). *Arch. Neurol. Psychiat.* **38**, 348.

HERSOV, L. A. (1955). *J. ment. Sci.* **101**, 878.

HERVEY, G. R. (1969). *Nature*, **222**, 629.

HOLOWACH, J., KAUFFMAN, F., IKOSSI, M. G., THOMAS, C. & McDOUGAL, D. B. (1968). *J. Neurochem.* **15**, 621.

HORWITT, M. K. (1948). *Bull. Natl. Res. Council, Washington*, **116**, 12.

HUNT, A. D., STOKES, J., McCRORY, W. W. & STROUD, H. H. (1954). *Pediatrics*, **13**, 140.

HUNTER, R., JONES, M., JONES, T. G., & MATTHEWS D. M. (1967). *Brit. J. Psychiat.* **113**, 1291.

ITOKAWA, Y. & COOPER, J. R. (1968). *Biochim. Biophys. Acta*, **158**, 180.

ITOKAWA, Y. & COOPER, J. R. (1969). *Biochem. Pharmacol.* **18**, 545.

IUPAC–IUB Commission (1970). *Biochem. J.* **119**, 1.

JOHNSON, L. R. & GUBLER, J. (1968). *Biochim. Biophys. Acta*, **156**, 85.

JOLLIFFE, N., GOODHART, R., GENNIS, J. & CLINE, J. K. (1939). *Amer. J. med. Sci.* **198**, 198.

JOLLIFFE, N., WORTIS, H. & FEIN, H. D. (1941). *Arch. Neurol. Psychiat.* **46**, 569.

KAMOSHITA, S., AGUILAR, M. J. & LANDRING, B. H. (1968). *Amer. J. Dis. Child.* **116**, 120.

KAPLAN, N. O. (1960). In the Neurochemistry of Nucleotides and Amino Acids, p. 70. Ed. Brady & Tower. New York: Wiley.

KAPLAN, N. O. *et al.* (1956). *J. biol. Chem.* **219**, 287.

KARE, M. R. & MULLER, O. (1967). (Ed.). The Chemical Senses and Nutrition. Baltimore: Johns Hopkins Press.

KIDD, H. M., GOULD, C. E. G. & THOMAS, J. W. (1963). *Canad. Med. Assoc. J.* **88**, 876.

KIESSLING, K-H. (1961). *Biochim. Biophys. Acta*, **46**, 603.

KILLAM, K. F. (1957). *J. Pharmacol.* **119**, 263.

KILLAM, K. F. & BAIN, J. A. (1957). *J. Pharmacol.* **119**, 255.

KINNERSLEY, H. W. & PETERS, R. A. (1929). *Biochem. J.* **23**, 1126.

KOEDAM, J. C. (1958). *Biochim. Biophys. Acta*, **29**, 333.

KOHN, H. I., KLEIN, J. R. & DANN, W. J. (1939). *Biochem. J.* **33**, 1432.

KOYAMA, N. & KURIHARA, K. (1971). *J. gen. Physiol.* **57**, 297.

KURIHARA, K. & BEIDLER, L. M. (1969). *Nature, Lond.* **222**, 1178.

KURIHARA, K. & BEIDLER, L. M. *Science*, **161**, 1241.

KUSHNER, D. S. (1956). *Amer. J. clin. Nutr.* **4**, 561.

KUZUYA, H. & NAGATSU, T. (1969). *J. Neurochem.* **16**, 123.

LEGGE, K. F., RANDIC, M. & STRAUGHAN, D. W. (1966). *Brit. J. Pharm.* **26**, 87.

LEHMANN, H. (1952). In Biology of Mental Health & Disease. London: Cassell.

LEIGH, D. (1951). *J. Neurol. Neurosurg. Psychiat.* **14**, 216.

LEIGH, D. (1952). *J. ment. Sci.* **98**, 130.

LESTER SMITH, E. (1962). In Mineral Metabolism, Vol. II B, p. 348. Ed. C. L. Comar & F. Bronner. New York: Academic Press.

LIN, S. & COHEN, H. P. (1960). *Arch. Biochem. Biophys.* **88**, 256.

LOO, Y. H. & BADGER, L. (1969). *J. Neurochem.* **16**, 801.

LOO, Y. H. & WHITTAKER, V. P. (1967). *J. Neurochem.* **14**, 997.

LOWRY, O. H. (1952). *Physiol. Rev.* **32**, 431.

LYON, J. B., BAIN, J. A. & WILLIAMS, H. L. (1962). *J. biol. Chem.* **237**, 1989.

306   NUTRITIONAL FACTORS AND THE CNS

MANN, P. J. G. & QUASTEL, J. H. (1941). *Biochem. J.* **35**, 502.
MARTIN, J. & LISSAK, K. (1950). *Z. Vitamin-, Hormon- u Fermentforsch.* **3**, 494.
MCCORMICK, D. B., GREGORY, M. E. & SNELL, E. E. (1961). *J. biol. Chem.* **236**, 2076.
MCCORMICK, D. B. & SNELL, E. E. (1961). *J. biol. Chem.* **236**, 2085.
MCDONALD, R. K., WEISE, V. K., EVANS, F. T. & PATRICK, R. W. (1961). *Proc. Internat. Neurochem. Sympos.* **3**, 404.
MCILWAIN, H. (1950). *Biochem. J.* **46**, 612.
MCILWAIN, H. & GRINYER, I. (1950). *Biochem. J.* **46**, 620.
MCILWAIN, H. (1968). *Brit. Med. Bull.* **24**, 174.
MCKHANN, G. M., MICKELSEN, O. & TOWER, D. B. (1961). *Amer. J. Physiol.* **200**, 34.
MEDINA, M. A., BRAYMER, H. D. & REEVES, J. L. (1962). *J. Neurochem.* **9**, 307.
MILNE, M. D. (1968). *Clin. Pharmacol. Therapeutics* **9**, 484.
MILNER, G. (1963). *Brit. J. Psychiat.* **109**, 294.
MINARD, F. N. (1967). *J. Neurochem.* **14**, 681.
MINARD, F. N. & HAHN, C. H. (1963). *J. biol. Chem.* **238**, 2474.
MONTPETIT, V. A. J., ANDERMANN, F., CARPENTER, S., FAWCETT, J. S., ZBOROWSKA-SLUIS, & GIBERSON, H. R. (1971). *Brain*, **94**, 1.
MORTON, R. A. (1961). *Vitamins & Hormones*, **19**, 1.
NAGATSU, T., NAGATSU-ISHIBASHI, I., OKUDA, J. & YAGI, K. (1967). *J. Neurochem.* **14**, 207.
NEMETH, A. M. & DICKERMAN, H. (1960). *J. biol. Chem.* **235**, 1761.
NEWMAN, G. E., O'BRIEN, J. R. P., SPRAY, G. H., WILLIAMS, D. L. & WITTS, L. J. (1962). *Biochim. Biophys. Acta*, **64**, 438.
NOVELLI, G. D. (1953). *Physiol. Rev.* **33**, 525.
O'BRIEN, D. & JENSEN, C. B. (1963). *Clin. Sci.* **24**, 179.
OCHOA, S. & PETERS, R. A. (1938). *Biochem. J.* **32**, 1501.
OOMURA, Y., ONO, T., OOYAMA, H. & WAYNER, M. J. (1969). *Nature, Lond.* **222**, 283.
OTTOSON, D. & SHEPHERD, C. M. (1967). *Progr. Brain Res.* **23**, 83.
PETERS, R. A. (1963). Biochemical Lesions and Lethal Synthesis. Oxford: Pergamon.
PILL, A. H., DAVIES, E. T., COLLINGS, D. F. & VENN, J. A. J. (1966). *Vet. Rec.* **78**, 737.
PRATT, O. E. (1953). *Biochem. J.* **55**, 140.
PROCOPIS, P. G., TURNER, B. & SELBY, G. (1967). *J. Neurol. Neurosurg. Psychiat.* **30**, 349.
RAJALAKSHMI, R., MALATHY, J. & RAMAKRISHNAN, C. V. (1967). *J. Neurochem.* **14**, 161.
REINAUER, H. & HOLLMAN, S. (1969). *Hoppe-Seyl. Z. Physiol. Chem.* **350**, 40.
REYNOLDS, E. H. (1967). *Brit. J. Psychiat.* **113**, 911.
REYNOLDS, E. H., PREECE, J. M., BAILEY, J. & COPPEN, A. (1970). *Brit. J. Psychiat.* **117**, 287.
RINDI, G., PERRI, V. & DECARO, L. (1961). *Experientia*, **17**, 546.
ROBERTS, E. & FRANKEL, S. (1951). *J. biol. Chem.* **188**, 789; **190**, 505.
ROBERTS, E., YOUNGER, F. & FRANKEL, S. (1951). *J. biol. Chem.* **191**, 277.
RUSSELL, G. F. M. (1967). *J. Psychosom. Res.* **11**, 141.
SADLER, H. H. & ORTEN, A. U. (1968). *Amer. J. Psychiat.* **124**, 1375.
SALEM, H. M. (1954). *Biochem. J.* **57**, 227.
SAMSON, D. C., SWISHER, S. N., CHRISTIAN, R. M. & ENGEL, G. L. (1952). *Arch. int. Med.* **90**, 4.
SARETT, H. P. & GOLDSMITH, G. A. (1950). *J. biol. Chem.* **182**, 679.
SCHALLENBERGER, R. S., ACREE, T. E. & LEE, C. Y. (1969). *Nature, Lond.* **221**, 555.
SCHEINBERG, P. (1951). *Blood*, **6**, 213.
SCHLENK, F. & SNELL, E. E. (1945). *J. biol. Chem.* **157**, 425.
SCHUBERTH, J., SOLLENBERG, J., SUNDWALL, A. & SÖRBO, B. (1965). *J. Neurochem.* **12**, 451.
SCHUBERTH, J., SOLLENBERG, J., SUNDWALL, A. & SÖRBO, B. (1966). *J. Neurochem.* **13**, 819.
SCRIMSHAW, N. S. & GORDON, J. E. (1968). Malnutrition, Learning and Behaviour. Cambridge, Mass.: M.I.T. Press.

SEBRELL, W. H. & HARRIS, R. S. (1968). The Vitamins. New York: Academic Press.

SHULMAN, R. (1967). *Brit. J. Psychiat.* **113**, 241, 252.

SINCLAIR, H. M. (1939). *Biochem. J.* **33**, 2027.

SINGAL, S. A., SYDENSTRICKER, V. P. & LITTLEJOHN, J. M. (1948). *J. biol. Chem.* **176**, 1069.

SOKOLOFF, L., LASSEN, N. A., McKHANN, G. M. & TOWER, D. B. (1959). *Nature, Lond.* **183**, 751.

SPIES, T. D., ARING, C. D., GELPERIN, J. & BEAN, W. B. (1938). *Amer. J. med. Sci.* **196**, 461.

STEWART, R. J. C. & PLATT, B. S. (1967). In Scrimshaw & Gordon (1967), q.v., p. 164.

STOCKLIN, W. (1967). *Helv. Chim. Acta*, **50**, 491.

STOCKLIN, W., WEISS, E. & REICHSTEIN, T. (1967). *Helv. Chim. Acta*, **50**, 474.

STREET, H. R., COWGILL, G. R. & ZIMMERMAN, H. M. (1941). *J. Nutrition*, **22**, 7.

Study Group (1967). Thiamine Deficiency: Biochemical Lesions and their Chemical Significance. Ed. G. E. W. Wolstenholme & M. O'Connor. London: Churchill.

SWISLOCKI, N. I. & KAPLAN, N. O. (1967). *J. biol. Chem.* **242**, 1083.

Symposia (1943, 1953). *Res. Publ. Ass. nerv. ment. Dis.* **22**, **32**.

Symposium (1956, 1957). *Amer. J. clin. Nutr.* **4**, 309; **5**, 103.

Symposium (1956a). Nutrition Sympos. Series No. 13. New York: National Vitamin Foundation.

Symposium (1961). *Amer. J. clin. Nutr.* **9**, 379, 414.

Symposium (1964). *Ann. N.Y. Acad. Sci.* **116**, 357.

Symposium (1965). *Canad. J. Biochem.* **43**, 1549.

Symposium (1967). Nutrition Society. *Fed. Proc.* **26**, 134.

Symposium (1969). *Biochem. J.* **111**, 40P.

SZOLCÁSNYI, J., JOÓ, F. & JANCSÓ-GÁBOR, A. (1971). *Nature, Lond.* **229**, 116.

TAYLOR, A., POLLACK, M. A. & WILLIAMS, R. J. (1942). Studies of the Vitamin Content of Tissues: Univ. Texas. Publ. 4237.

TERRIS, M. (1964). Goldberger on Pellagra. Baton Rouge: Louisiana State University Press.

THOMPSON, R. H. S. & CUMINGS, J. N. (1964). In Biochemical Disorders in Human Disease. London: Churchill.

TOWER, D. B. (1960). Neurochemistry of Epilepsy. Springfield: Thomas.

VICTOR, M. & ADAMS, R. D. (1961). *Amer. J. Clin. Nutr.* **9**, 379.

VILLELA, G. G., DIAS, M. V. & QUEIROGA, L. T. (1949). *Arch. Biochem.* **23**, 81.

WALD, G. (1960). *Proc. Nat. Acad. Sci.* **46**, 587.

WASSERMAN, R. H., CORRADINO, R. A. & TAYLOR, A. N. (1968). *J. biol. Chem.* **243**, 3978, 3987.

WEISSBACH, H., BOGDANSKI, D. F., REDFIELD, B. G. & UDENFRIEND, S. (1957). *J. biol. Chem.* **227**, 617.

WESTENBRINK, H. G. K., STEYN-PARVÉ, E. P. & GOUDSMIT, J. (1943). *Enzymologia*, **11**, 26.

WHITE, A. M. (1963). *Ann. Rep. Chem. Soc.* **59**, 400.

WILLIAMS, R. J. (1956). Biochemical Individuality. New York: Wiley.

WILLIAMS, R. J., EAKIN, R. E., BEERSTECHER, E. & SHIVE, W. (1950). The Biochemistry of B-Vitamins. New York: Reinhold.

WILLIAMS, R. R. (1961). Forward the Conquest of Beriberi. Harvard: University Press.

WINDMUELLER, H. G. & KAPLAN, N. O. (1962). *Biochim. Biophys. Acta*, **56**, 388.

WOOD, J. D., WATSON, W. J. & DUCKER, A. J. (1968). *J. Neurochem.* **15**, 603.

WOOLLEY, D. W. (1952). A Study of Antimetabolites. London: Chapman & Hall.

WORSLEY, H. E., BROOKFIELD, R. W., ELWOOD, J. S., NOBLE, R. L. & TAYLOR, W. H. (1965). *Arch. dis. Child.* **40**, 492.

YAMAMOTO, C. & McILWAIN, H. (1966). *J. Neurochem.* **15**, 1333.

YUDKIN, J. (1951). *Biochem. J.* **48**, 608.

YUDKIN, W. H. (1949). *Physiol. Rev.* **29**, 389.

ZOTTERMAN, Y. (1967). (Ed.). Sensory Mechanisms. Amsterdam: Elsevier.

11   Cerebral Lipids

Lipids comprise about half the dry matter of the brain and include substances found in lesser quantities if at all in other parts of the body. It is thus understandable that a large part of the earlier chemical studies of the brain were concerned with the fractionation and characterization of its lipid components (Chapter 1). This is not an easy subject and is still in progress, but has already given a basis for the metabolic studies, especially of biosynthetic routes, which occupy much of this chapter; such studies in a wider range of biological systems are well illustrated by the *Proceedings* (1964).

The main groups of cerebral lipids are shown in Table 11.1 in the order in which they will be discussed; two alternative classifications are given in footnotes to the table. Structural formulae are given with the different groups of lipids and also in Chapter 12, when the composition of grey matter and white is considered in more detail; see also Hanahan (1960) and McIlwain & Rodnight (1962). Very large differences between the lipid content of blood plasma and the brain are evident from Table 11.1, and still greater differences exist between brain and cerebrospinal fluid. The total lipid content of the fluid is normally only about 1–2 mg./100 ml., or 1/400 of that in plasma. Very small quantities of cholesterol, simple glycerides and sphingolipids have been determined in human cerebrospinal fluid (Curtis & Seipel, 1961), and almost all the cerebral lipids, as recounted below, are synthesized in the brain itself from water-soluble precursors.

The structures of cerebral lipids are diverse, but all except cholesterol contain long-chain aliphatic acids and in some cases also a long-chain alcohol or base. These components give the lipids their collective name and their similarity in physical properties which made separation difficult until the recent development of special partition, chromatographic, ion exchange and gas chromatographic methods. These methods depend to differing degrees on the nature of the hydrocarbon and the polar parts of constituent molecules, and the cerebral lipids differ markedly in each of these respects. It is indeed in such characteristics that their functions as well as their classification and separation are to be understood. The polar groups of the lipids condition the main categories of Table 11.1; and range from the single hydroxyl group of cholesterol through the six of the cerebrosides to some 20–40 in the gangliosides. The lipids may carry no net charge, as in simple fats or in cerebrosides, or may be negatively charged through phosphoric, carboxylic or sulphuric acid anions. These three differ markedly in acidic strength and in the phosphoinositides and gangliosides further variation is introduced through the presence of components with one, two or three such groups. In lecithins, kephalins and sphingomyelins a basic centre is also present.

A separation of cerebral lipids which takes advantage of such properties is shown in Fig. 11.1. Using column chromatography, the least polar lipids are eluted first with chloroform-rich solvents and the more polar with increasing proportions of methanol or, finally, with acetic acid and with basic solvents

Table 11.1

Lipid content of the adult mammalian brain

Group	Substances	Approximate content, % fresh weight		
		Grey matter	White matter	Blood plasma
	Total Lipids	5·9	19	0·4–0·7
Cholesterol	Cholesterol	1·0	4	0·05–0·09
	Cholesterol esters	<0·51[1]		0·12–0·18
Glycerides	Simple fats	0·03	0·11	0·07–0·17
	Diphosphatidylglycerol[2]	0·051		—
	Lecithins[2]	1·1	1·4	
	Phosphatidylethanolamines[2,3]	0·6	0·4	
	Phosphatidylserines[2,3]	0·6	1·5	0·15–0·25
	Kephalin B[2,3]	0·2	0·5	
	Plasmalogens[2]	0·7	3·3	
	Phosphoinositides[2,3]	0·15	0·3	
Sphingolipids	Sphingomyelin[2]	0·3	1·3	–
	Cerebrosides[4]	0·3	3·8	0·004–0·006
	Sulphatides[4]	0·2	1·2	–
	Gangliosides[4]	0·3	0·15	–
Prostaglandins[5]		<0·0001		—

Values from those compiled by Sloane-Stanley & McIlwain (1956); McIlwain (1963; a comparison of man and other mammalian species is included); Collins & Shotlander (1961); Davison & Wajda (1962), Thompson & King (1964) and Ansell & Hawthorne (1964); see also Adams & Davison, 1965; Dickerson, 1968.
[1] Content in whole brain. [2] Phosphatides. [3] These and possibly other components constitute "kephalin". [4] Glycolipids, as determined by the quantity of reducing sugar in lipid extracts, include cerebrosides, sulphatides and part of the ganglioside content. [5] Wolfe, 1970.

which give the most polar and acidic components. The account of individual lipids which follows is in approximately this order. It includes additional compounds not specifically indicated in Fig. 11.1 and also individual members of many of the categories of the figure.

Cholesterol

Cholesterol, separated crystalline from the brain, was shown by Gmelin's early study (1826; see Cook, 1958) to be indeed the same substance as that from gall-stones. It is present in the brain in greater quantity than is any other single constituent apart from water, comprising 4–5 % of the fresh weight of cerebral

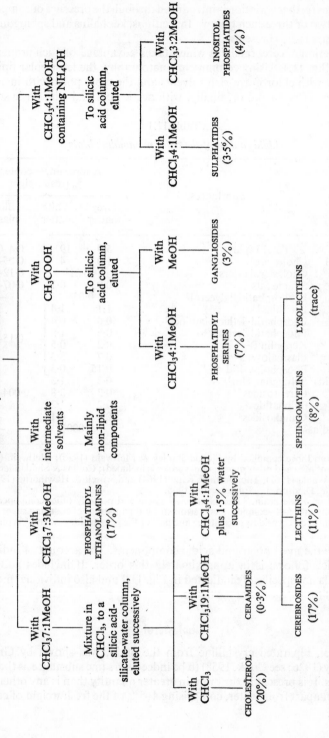

Fig. 11.1. A fractionation of cerebral lipids to their major categories by column chromatography (Rouser *et al.*, 1961; Rouser, Symposium, 1962*a*). Materials were handled at −20° to 10° in nitrogen and the contents of numerous small samples from the columns were examined, using silica-impregnated paper, in order to control elution. Values in parentheses give the proportions of the different components calculated to be present in the original extract.

white matter or of the spinal cord, and spinal cord from slaughterhouses forms a commercial source of cholesterol. In the normal adult brain it exists almost entirely as free cholesterol, apart from the associations which are described below with other lipids and with proteins, and in distinction to its occurrence in many other organs of the body where cholesterol esters preponderate. During development of the brain in growing animals, however, the proportion of cholesterol esters can rise to 20% of the concomitant cholesterol (Adams & Davison, 1959). Their maximum value, in man and the chick, was at the commencement of myelination. The esters also appear in cerebral tissues in certain abnormal conditions, for instance in the areas of demyelination in disseminated sclerosis (Cumings, 1953; Rodnight, 1957). The esterified cholesterol in human brain was analysed by a combination of thin-layer and gas-liquid chromatography. The total cholesterol esters contributed only 0·1–0·2% of the total cholesterol; fatty acids present in the esters were oleic, palmitic, palmitoleic and especially arachidonic acids (Alling & Svennerholm, 1969).

The adult human brain contains about 25 g. of cholesterol, or with the remainder of the nervous system some 33 g., which is about a quarter of the total bodily content. Over 50% of the cholesterol in the whole brain is found in nerve myelin sheaths. At birth the cerebral content is 2 g. and the most rapid increase is a three-fold one during the first year of life when myelination is proceeding relatively rapidly. Some derivatives and isomerides of cholesterol, and also non-steroid hydrocarbons, exist in very small quantities in the brain. A quite small proportion of cerebrosterol, the C_{24}-hydroxylated derivative, has been found in the brain, and a cholestane triol observed to constitute 0·5% of cholesterol specimens made from the brain (Fieser & Bhattacharyya, 1953). The general picture of cerebral steroids is, however, of a large preponderance of cholesterol present as the free compound.

Synthesis in the Brain

The greater part of cerebral cholesterol is synthesized *in situ*, as is demonstrated by administering isotopically labelled compounds and by the use of isolated tissues. Dietary ^{14}C-cholesterol contributed negligible amounts of isotope to the brain of rats, though after intraperitoneal administration some ^{14}C-cholesterol reached the brain. Investigating rabbits in their third and fourth weeks of life, during which their cerebral cholesterol increased from about 60 to about 90 mg., ^{14}C-cholesterol given intravenously or intraperitoneally appeared to a small extent only in the brain (Dobbing, 1963; Morris & Chaikoff, 1961; Clarenburg *et al.*, 1963). The amount deposited corresponded to 2·5 mg. or 0·6% of that administered. Entry of ^{14}C-cholesterol to the adult human brain from the blood has been sought and found very small (Chobanian & Hollander, 1962). Turnover of ^{14}C-cholesterol once deposited in the brain of experimental animals has also been found small, and mostly in grey matter; in white matter, ^{14}C given as cholesterol was found in the same form 6 months later in the chick and a year later in the rabbit (Davison *et al.*, 1958, 1959). From the liver or blood plasma the labelled compound was lost in 10–20 days.

In growing animals, ^{14}C given as fatty acids or glucose appears in the cholesterol of the brain, as well as in that from other parts of the body. Glucose is the precursor most rapidly incorporated into brain cholesterol if given intraperitoneally. Synthesis *in vivo* and *in vitro* of labelled cholesterol has been

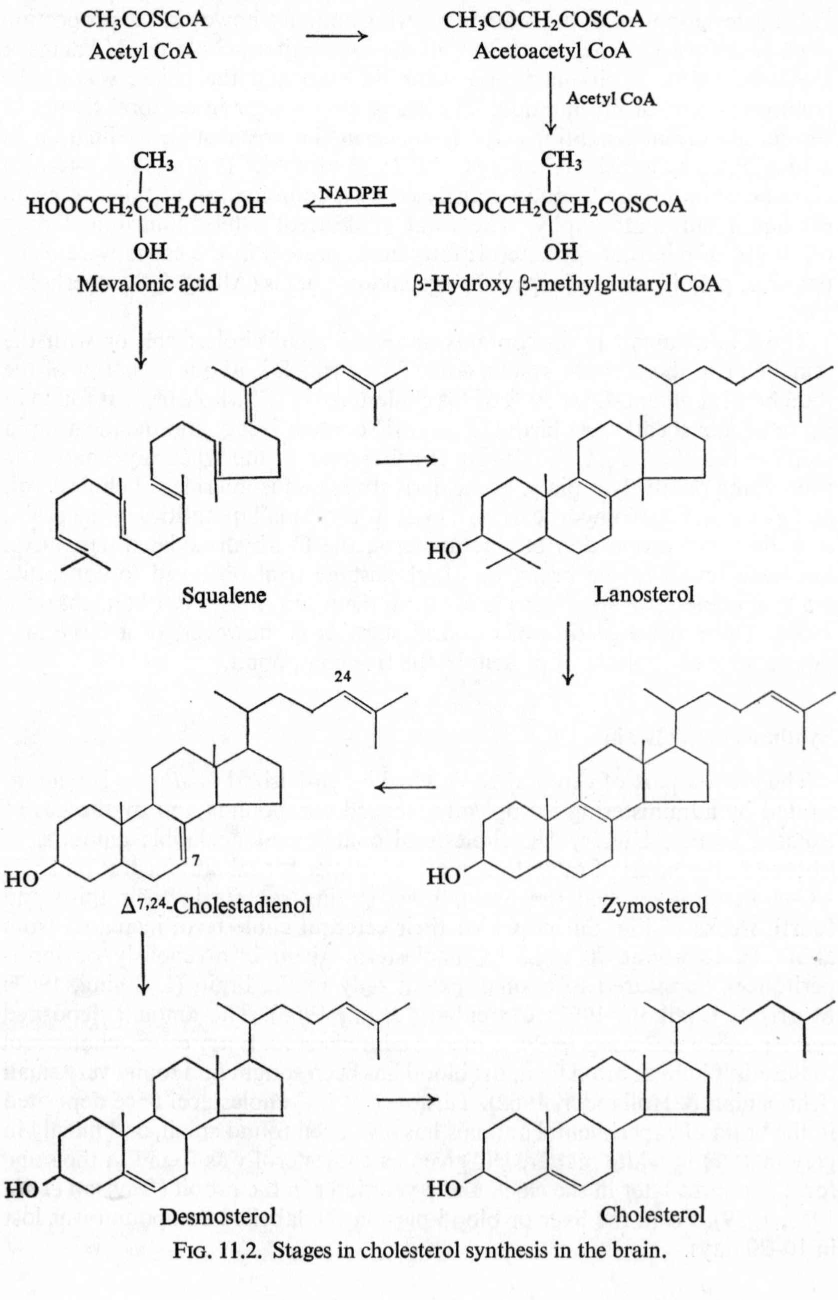

FIG. 11.2. Stages in cholesterol synthesis in the brain.

observed using ^{14}C-labelled glucose, acetate or mevalonate and proceeds through sterol precursors (Paoletti *et al.*, 1969). A day after ^{14}C-acetate was given to incubating chick embryos, labelled cholesterol and desmosterol, the C-24 dehydro-derivative of cholesterol, were readily isolated from the brain; on continued incubation, the desmosterol diminished and cholesterol increased (Fish *et al.*, 1962). *In vivo*, extent of incorporation of [2-^{14}C]-mevalonic lactone into cholesterol depends on the route of injection; in the brain cholesterol was labelled most rapidly after intraventricular administration of precursor, while in the spinal cord intracisternal injection proved more effective (Chevallier & Gautheron, 1969). With cerebral tissue-sections from rats, mevalonate as well as glucose gave detectable ^{14}C-cholesterol on 0·2–2 hr. incubation *in vitro*. An inhibitor of cholesterol synthesis, Triparnol, when given intraperitoneally to young rats for some days before their cerebral tissues were examined *in vitro* caused the tissues to form ^{14}C-desmosterol from acetate; little ^{14}C-cholesterol was produced, and the desmosterol could be isolated in crystalline form, constituting 60% of the sterols of the tissue (Scallen *et al.*, 1962; Korey & Stein, 1961). $\triangle^{7, 24}$-Cholestadienol and zymosterol ($\triangle^{8, 24}$-cholestadienol) have been detected as other precursors of cholesterol synthesis in the developing rat brain (Holstein *et al.*, 1966). Desmosterol has also been found in human foetal brain and in certain cerebral tumours (Fumagalli *et al.*, 1964). Cell-free extracts of adult rat brain also incorporate ^{14}C-mevalonate to squaline and cholesterol; Mg^{2+} was an essential requirement and ATP, NADH, glutathione and glucose-6-phosphate, though not essential, were required for optimal sterol synthesis (Kelley *et al.*, 1969).

The pathway of biosynthesis of cholesterol in the brain (Fig. 11.2) is thus similar to that shown to operate in other mammalian tissues. Turnover study with ^{14}C-labelled precursors in the developing rat brain indicated the rate limiting step to be at the stage of conversion of zymosterol to $\triangle^{7, 24}$-cholestadienol (Holstein *et al.*, 1966). Cholesterol biosynthesis is maintained in the mature brain; precursors of the sterol in adult human brain were found mainly as desmosterol (15·5 µg./g.) and cholestanol (54·8 µg./g.); the cholesterol content was 18·7 mg./g. Cholesterol and these precursors were labelled in homogenates of a sample of adult human brain incubated with ^{14}C-mevalonate (Galli *et al.*, 1968). Chemical aspects of cholesterol biosynthesis are reviewed by Clayton (1965).

In the normal brain, cholesterol once formed has not been found to undergo appreciable further metabolism. When after damage to the brain lipid components are removed by scavenging cells some cholesterol esters are found. This emphasizes that cholesterol normally functions as such, as is described more fully in Chapter 12.

Simple Fats; Fatty Acids

The brain contains only trace amounts of free fatty acids and a smaller proportion of simple glycerides than do other major tissues of the body. The content of simple fats in liver, kidney and skeletal muscle can reach some 6% of their dry weight, and in the brain the value is 3%. The brain in mammals and chicks however contains a number of esterases, apart from cholinesterase,

11

and certain of these hydrolyse glycerides. Tributyrin yields some 200 μmoles fatty acid/g. fresh rat brain/hr. Electrophoresis and differential actions of inhibitors have shown the presence of eight cerebral esterases in the rat; and in the chick cerebral esterases which are inhibited by triaryl phosphates appear to represent the point at which these compounds exert their action as neurotoxic agents (Myers, 1956; Barron *et al.*, 1961; Poulsen & Aldridge, 1963). Little hydrolysis of long-chain glycerides is catalysed except under specific conditions, but on addition of sodium oleate to cerebral suspensions incubated with triolein quite rapid hydrolysis ensues; the oleate apparently acts by presenting the substrate in an appropriate micellar form.

Occurrence and Synthesis of Fatty Acids

Fatty acids exist in most of the cerebral lipids, those present in appreciable amount ranging from C_{16} to C_{24}, often unsaturated and sometimes hydroxylated. Thus α-hydroxystearic acid and many unsaturated acids have been identified among the fatty acids from sphingolipid fractions of mammalian brain and spinal cord (Skipski *et al.*, 1959; Kishimoto & Radin, 1963). The preponderant fatty acids differ in different groups of cerebral lipids, and also in different subcellular fractions separated from the brain of a given species, as is indicated below. Different areas of the brain, however, were similar in the mixture of fatty acids yielded, and distinct in their content from sciatic nerve (Baker, 1961).

Free fatty acids have been isolated from mouse brain, rapidly frozen *in situ*. The total content was 1·3 μmoles/g. of whole brain, of which myristate (0·56), pentadecanoate (0·52) and palmitate (0·15 μmoles/g.) were preponderant. Fresh brain contained considerably less fatty acid (0·3 μmoles/g.); no myristate or pentadecanoate was detected even after incubation of cerebral cortex slices, when the total free fatty acid content increased to 0·8 μmoles/g. The free fatty acids of the slices were labelled by incubation in the presence of [1-^{14}C]-acetate. The rates were more rapid than into esterified fatty acids of complex lipids (Lunt & Rowe, 1968). Incorporation of ^{14}C or ^{3}H into the free fatty acids of rat brain has also been demonstrated when *N*-acetylaspartate was used as precursor. The incorporation was from the acetyl group of the precursor. Study of the incorporation during myelination and maturation led to the suggestion of *N*-acetylaspartate involvement in the transport of acetyl groups for extramitochondrial lipid synthesis in the brain (D'Adamo *et al.*, 1968).

Cerebral fatty acids have thus been demonstrated to arise both by synthesis *in situ* and by assimilation as such. The mixture of fatty acids obtainable from cerebral lipids of a given species is relatively constant, being markedly less dependent on moderate changes of diet than is the mixture obtainable from several other organs of the body. Incorporation of dietary fatty acids to the lipids of the brain nevertheless occurs, both during growth and in adult animals beyond the period of myelination. It was found just detectable in normal rats 10–48 hr. after feeding fats containing deuterium. In animals previously maintained on a fat-free diet, however, clearer evidence has been obtained, showing that incorporation of cod-liver oil in the diet led to increase in the highly unsaturated acids in a number of tissues including those of the brain. More specifically, increased dietary arachidonate and linolenate led to increased cerebral arachidonate, linolenate and related compounds, identified and estimated by gas chromatography (Rieckeholt *et al.*, 1949; Mohrhauer & Holman, 1963).

Synthesis of new, long-chain fatty acids in the brain has been demonstrated by using ^{14}C-acetate as substrate. When added to solutions perfusing monkey brain, the acetate and also ^{14}C-octanoate became incorporated in cerebral lipids, especially in sphingolipids. When fed to young rats ^{14}C-acetate yielded significant amounts of both saturated and unsaturated ^{14}C-acids in the lipids of the brain, and on its intracerebral administration markedly higher yields resulted (Weiss, 1956; Nicholas & Thomas, 1959). Moreover, isolated tissues were capable of the synthesis and important aspects of its enzymic basis were demonstrated by use of fatty acid–coenzyme A derivatives (Brady, 1960; Robinson *et al.*, 1963). The supernatant from centrifuged sucrose dispersions of young rat brain was fractionated to yield one of the enzymes concerned. This when incubated with malonyl-CoA, butyryl-CoA, the reduced form of nicotinamide adenine dinucleotide phosphate and a dithiol, formed long-chain fatty acids at a rate corresponding to 2·5 μmoles/hr. g. original tissue. The requirements for the synthesis did not include a fatty acyl-CoA and thus *de novo* synthesis occurs. This is in contrast to preparations of mitochondria or microsomes which incorporate malonyl-CoA and acetyl-CoA into saturated and unsaturated fatty acids but the process was concluded to be one of elongation rather than of complete synthesis (Aeberhard & Menkes, 1968).

Certain of the long-chain hydroxylated fatty acids of the brain have been demonstrated by ^{14}C-acetate administration to be synthesized in the growing animal; α-hydroxylation of the corresponding fatty acid occurs and an α-hydroxy acid decarboxylase has been characterized in cerebral microsomal fractions (Fulco & Mead, 1961; Mead & Levis, 1962, 1963; Levis & Mead, 1964). This with a soluble fraction, adenosine triphosphate and nicotinamide adenine dinucleotide yielded CO_2 and the fatty acid of one less carbon atom, e.g. heptadecanoic acid from α-hydroxystearic acid. The data are discussed more fully in considering cerebrosides; see reaction sequences *xxiv* to *xxvi* below.

Oxidation of Fatty Acids

Apart from the oxidation and decarboxylation just described, cerebral tissues can oxidize several fatty acids, but to a limited extent only (Vignais *et al.*, 1958; Geyer *et al.*, 1949; Weinhouse *et al.*, 1950). Butyric and crotonic acids do not appreciably increase the respiration of the separated tissue, but octanoic acid labelled in its carboxyl group and incubated with slices from the brain of rats, yielded labelled carbon dioxide. The yield was approaching maximal at 1 mM substrate, when the labelled carbon dioxide was being formed at about 0·6 μmole/g. hr. In contrast, the yield from kidney was still increasing at 6·6 mM-octanoate and was some twenty times that from the cerebral tissue. Similarly, labelled lauric acid employed as trilaurin also yielded a small proportion of carbon dioxide with preparations from rat brain, and a small yield has also been observed from palmitic acid. Carnitine, which can increase the oxidation of fatty acids by mitochondria, occurs in the brain and its acetyl derivative increased the respiration of cerebral mitochondria incubated with succinate as substrate (Bremer, 1962); the increase corresponded to about 8 μmoles O_2/g. tissue, and was concluded to represent oxidation of the acetyl group. Conditions for the oxidation of octanoate and palmitate by cerebral mitochondria (q.v.) have been examined (Beattie & Basford, 1965).

Oxidation of fats or fatty acids in the brain cannot however replace carbohydrate metabolism in supporting cerebral functioning. Several fatty acids of which decanoate was most active, first stimulated and later inhibited the respiration of cerebral tissues with glucose as substrate: actions concluded to be on processes controlling glucose metabolism, and not implying appreciable oxidation of the fatty acid (Ahmed & Scholefield, 1961). For the special rôle of β-hydroxybutyrate see Chapters 2 and 6.

Phospholipids: Components; ^{32}P Incorporation

The phosphorus-containing lipids of the central nervous system include lecithins, kephalins, plasmalogens and sphingomyelins, all of which through variation in their fatty acids or in other components represent groups of substances rather than individual compounds (Fig. 11.3). Collectively the

$CH_2.O.CO.R'$
|
$CH.O.CO.R''$
|
$CH_2.O.CO.R'''$

Simple fats:
  in this and other
  formulae, R'' and R'''
  are long hydrocarbon
  chains unless otherwise
  stated.

$CH_2.O.PO_3^-.R'$
|
$CH.O.CO.R''$
|
$CH_2.O.CO.R'''$

Phosphatidic acid: $R' = H$
Lysophosphatides: $R'' = H$
Phosphatides:
  lecithin, $R' = CH_2CH_2NMe_3^+$
  phosphatidylethanolamine, $R' = CH_2CH_2NH_3^+$
  phosphatidylserine, $R' = CH_2CH(NH_2).COOH$
Diphosphatidylglycerol: $RO.CH_2.CHOH.CH_2OR$
  where R is a phosphatidic
  acid residue.

$CH_2.O.PO_3^-.R'$
|
$CH.O.CO.R''$
|
$CH_2.O.R'''$

Glycerol ether phospho-
lipids (kephalin B)

$CH_2.O.PO_3^-.R'$
|
$CH.O.CO.R''$
|
$CH_2.O.CH = CH.R'''$

Plasmalogens:
  phosphatidalethanolamine, $R' = CH_2CH_2NH_3^+$

FIG. 11.3. Cerebral Glycerides. The phosphoinositides, which also are glycerides, are described in Fig. 11.4.

phospholipids constitute by weight about half the lipids of the brain. Their chemical investigation is still in progress; notable are recent applications of chromatographic methods to their fractionation and characterization. Separations based on such methods are included in Fig. 11.1, and a general account of phospholipids has been given by Ansell & Hawthorne (1964).

Phospholipids of Subcellular Fractions

The phospholipids of various subfractions of the mammalian cerebral cortex are listed in Table 11.2; the membranes of the different particles contain characteristic distributions of lipids. Thus phosphatidic acid has not been detected in purified mitochondria or microsomes; sphingomyelin is barely detectable in the mitochondria. Myelin is characteristically rich in phospholipid and cholesterol but apparently contains no cardiolipin. Of the plasmalogens, only ethanolamine plasmalogen occurs in detectable amounts in all fractions of the cerebral cortex save myelin in which traces of serine and choline plasmalogens have also been observed. Cardiolipin is characteristic of mitochondria in the brain, as in other mammalian organs (see also Chapter 12).

^{32}P-Incorporation to Lipids Generally

First will be recounted certain metabolic studies in which the cerebral phospholipids have been examined collectively, without allocating to particular compounds the change observed (Table 11.3; Ansell & Marshall, 1963). After administering isotopically-labelled inorganic phosphate or phospholipids these substances have been found in the lipids of the brain. Entry of inorganic phosphate to the brain itself is limited (Chapter 2); some 2 hr. are required for the simpler, acid-soluble, phosphates of the mouse brain to reach 10% of the activity of those of the bloodstream. Nevertheless, by comparing the concentration of newly incorporated phosphate of the cerebral lipids with the concomitant concentration of inorganic or acid-soluble phosphates in the brain, considerable incorporation to the lipids has been shown. The rate of entry to the lipids was about 0·3 μmole phosphorus/g. tissue/hr., which would correspond to replacement of the phospholipids as a whole each 70 hr., but actually the turnover in different fractions varies considerably.

Many observations in living animals connect phospholipid metabolism and cerebral functioning. Thus phospholipid turnover in the experiments just described was found to depend on the age of the animals (Chapter 13) and also on their condition, being lowered greatly in insulin coma and to a lesser extent in anaesthesia and in excitement. Actual loss of phospholipids from the brain has been found to follow long courses of insulin hypoglycaemia (McGhee *et al.*, 1951) and also to occur in some cases of Tay-Sachs' disease. The cerebral content of phospholipids has also been found to be decreased in disseminated sclerosis, in some cases before much change could be detected histologically (Cumings, 1953; Rodnight, 1957; Knauff *et al.*, 1961); for changes in other lipidoses, see *Symposium* (1957).

Many of the individual steps of cerebral phospholipid metabolism are open to examination in separated cerebral tissues, for with such tissues both incorporation and loss of the inorganic phosphate of phospholipids have been demonstrated (Table 11.3). In preparations from young and from adult rats, the cell-containing tissues were capable of forming labelled phospholipids with labelled inorganic phosphate and the quantity was greatly increased by providing glucose or related substrates. Oxygen was also required. The

Table 11.2

Lipids of subcellular fractions of the mammalian cerebral cortex

	Homogenate	Nuclei	Myelin	Mitochondria	Nerve ending particles	Microsomes
Total phospholipid	63·5	11·5	17·6	3·2	10·7	4·5
Phosphatidic acid	0·6	0·1	0·3	–	0·1	–
Phosphatidyl choline	21·0	4·3	5·1	1·3	4·2	1·9
Phosphatidyl ethanolamine	8·5	1·6	2·0	0·8	1·9	0·6
Phosphatidyl serine	7·8	1·3	2·5	0·2	1·4	0·55
Inositol phosphatides	1·9	0·3	0·55	0·2	0·45	0·2
Sphingomyelin	5·3	0·8	2·0	0·1	0·6	0·35
Gangliosides (as NANA)	1·3, 1·7*	0·3, 0·1*	1·6, 0·8*	0·3, 0·2*	0·3, 0·3*	0·2, 0·8*
Ethanolamine plasmalogen	11·5, 9·1*	2·3, 1·9*	4·1, 2·1*	0·3, 0·4*	1·6, 1·4*	0·7, 2·9*
Cerebrosides	12·0, 11·0*	1·4, 3·1*	7·5, 3·1*	0·1, 0·4*	0·2, 0·4*	0·4, 1·8*
Cholesterol	43·0, 46·5*	6·7, 7·2*	16·6, 10·0*	0·5, 0·2*	4·5, 0·5*	2·2, 1·0*
Diphosphatidyl glycerol (cardiolipin)	0·9	0·25	–	0·35	0·2	–

Values are μmoles/g. fresh weight of guinea pig forebrain (Eichberg *et al.*, 1966). *Values for rat cerebral cortex (Seminario *et al.*, 1964). The nuclei and mitochondrial fractions were purified by density-gradient centrifugation; the value for myelin is a combination of heavy myelin fragments from the crude nuclear fraction and light myelin fragments from the crude mitochondrial fraction. Analysis of lipids in the subcellular fractions from human and bovine brain are given by Rouser & Yamamoto (1969).
Some loss of individual lipids occurred during extraction and purification.

different conditions employed did not greatly affect the tissue's content of inorganic or total phosphate, but those under which greatest incorporation was observed were those which would be expected (Chapter 4) to favour resynthesis of energy-rich phosphates in the tissue.

In salines adequate for incorporation of phosphate to the phospholipids of cell-containing tissues, very little was incorporated by ground, cell-free cerebral preparations (Table 11.3). When such preparations were made from rats previously treated with labelled phosphate so that the phospholipids

Table 11.3

Incorporation of inorganic phosphate to cerebral phospholipids

Conditions	Compounds examined	Specific activity (counts/min./ unit P)
(1) Rat; brain extracted 3 hr. after intra-peritoneal $^{32}PO_4^{3-}$	Total phospholipid	3·0
	Phosphatidylcholine	2·1
	Phosphatidylserine	0·4
	Phosphatidic acid	8·8
	Phosphatidylinositol	22·4
(2) As (1); animal treated with chlorpromazine	Total phospholipid	2·2
	Phosphatidylinositol	16·8
(3) Rat, cerebral tissue sections incubated 2 hr. in oxygenated glucose media	Total phospholipid	2·9
(4) As (3) but no glucose	,,	0·6
(5) As (3) but no oxygen	,,	0·2
(6) Guinea pig cerebral dispersion in glycylglycine saline	Total phospholipid	2·2
(7) As (6) plus pyruvate, fumarate, cyto-chrome c, adenylate and Mg^{2+}	,,	12·8
(8) As (7) plus 0·1 mM-2·4-dinitrophenol	,,	6·8
(9) As (7) plus 43 mM-malonate	,,	7·0

Specific activities are comparable under conditions (1) and (2), (3)–(5), and (6)–(9). Data from Ansell & Marshall (1963) who give other effects of chlorpromazine; cf. also Strickland & Noble, *Symposium* 1961; Magee *et al.* (1963); Dawson (1953, 1960); Fries *et al.* (1942) and Schachner *et al.* (1942). Rats were aged 6–20 days and guinea pigs were young adults. For effects of different substrates in tissues from cats, see Strickland (1954). For relative activities of a number of phospholipids comparable to those of conditions (1), and from different parts of the brain, see Smirnov *et al.* (1961).

already contained the isotope, incubation caused loss of the isotope at a rate suggesting breakdown of some 10% of the phospholipid per hour. However, suitable metabolic conditions could again result in incorporation of labelled phosphate in the ground tissue. For this, additions were needed including oxygen, pyruvate, fumarate, adenylic acid, cytochrome c and magnesium salts: requirements similar to those for optimal oxidative phosphorylation (Chapter 6). In accordance with this similarity, incorporation was inhibited by cyanides and by 2:4-dinitrophenol. Its optimal rate exceeded that observed *in vivo*, reaching about 1 μmole of phospholipid/g. hr.

32P-Incorporation to Specific Lipids

After experiments in which ^{32}P has become incorporated into cerebral lipids fractionation of tissue extracts can yield information about the incorporation to individual phospholipids. It is then evident that the compounds have very different rates of turnover (Table 11.3). Inositol phosphatides prove particularly rapid in phosphate incorporation, both *in vivo* and also when tissue slices are incubated under conditions (3) of Table 11.3. The specific activity of the phosphoinositides, collectively, can reach 50–100 times that of phosphatidylserine extracted from the same tissue. Added compounds can inhibit or diminish the incorporation, occasionally showing selectivity to different phospholipids.

The synthesis and breakdown of different phospholipids are indeed differently conditioned, as will be evident below in considering individual compounds. Heterogeneity in this regard is also shown in experiments carried out under conditions (7) of Table 11.3. By preparing cerebral dispersions in water and providing specific, labelled intermediates, it was found that cytidine triphosphate and coenzyme A, catalysed the incorporation of isotopic inorganic phosphate to phospholipids (McMurray *et al.*, 1957). The two coenzymes proved to have their greatest effects in different systems. Cytidine triphosphate promoted especially the conversion of choline to lecithin, which is understandable for the synthesis proceeds through cytidine diphosphate choline (see below). Coenzyme A promoted especially the incorporation of α-glycerophosphate to phosphatidic acids, the fatty acid esters of α-glycerophosphate which are common to most of the phosphatides (Fig. 11.3 and 11.4), but not to sphingomyelins. Under some conditions the ^{32}P-labelling of phosphoinositides and phosphatidic acids in partly separated cerebral dispersions is affected by 0·1 mM-acetylcholine (Hokin & Hokin, 1958; Durell & Sodd, 1964). The stimulation by acetylcholine of cerebral phosphoinositide synthesis is inhibited by gammexane which has no effect on synthesis in the absence of acetylcholine. Interaction is thought to occur with diglyceride kinase (Hokin & Brown, 1969).

Noradrenaline at 0·1 mM also increased labelling into phosphatidic acids and phosphoinositides but not into other phospholipids. Some decrease in labelling into phospholipids generally was observed with 1 to 10 μM-dopamine (Hokin, 1969, 1970). ^{32}P-labelling of phosphoinositides in sympathetic ganglia is increased also by stimulation (Larrabee *et al.*, 1963; Larrabee, 1968). In the intact brain and in cerebral tissues, the incorporation is susceptible to chlorpromazine and azacyclonol (Table 11.3; Magee *et al.*, 1963), and ouabain markedly increased the ^{32}P-labelling of several phospholipid fractions (Nicholls *et al.*, 1962).

Reactions and Intermediates Common to more than one Phospholipid

The findings recounted contribute to indicating that phospholipid synthesis in cerebral tissues proceeds by routes including reactions (*i*) to (*iii*):

(*i*)   *Choline kinase (EC 2.7.1.32):*

$$HO.CH_2.CH_2.\overset{+}{N}(CH_3)_3 + ATP \rightleftharpoons HO.\overset{O}{\underset{OH}{\underset{|}{P}}}O.CH_2.CH_2.\overset{+}{N}(CH_3)_3 + ADP$$

Choline   Phosphoryl choline

(*ii*)   *Phosphorylcholine cytidyl transferase (EC 2.7.7.15):*

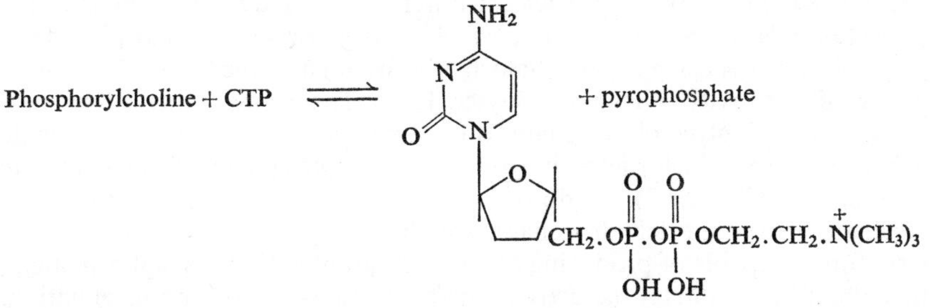

Phosphorylcholine + CTP $\rightleftharpoons$ + pyrophosphate

$$CH_2.O\overset{O}{\underset{OH}{\underset{|}{P}}}.O\overset{O}{\underset{OH}{\underset{|}{P}}}.OCH_2.CH_2.\overset{+}{N}(CH_3)_3$$

CDP-choline

(*iii*)   *Choline phosphotransferase (EC 2.7.8.2):*

$$CDP\text{-choline} + D\text{-}\alpha,\beta\text{-diglyceride} \rightleftharpoons
\begin{array}{l} CH_2O.CO.R^1 \\ | \\ R''.OC.OCH \\ | \\ CH_2O.\overset{O}{\underset{OH}{\underset{|}{P}}}O.CH_2.CH_2.\overset{+}{N}(CH_3)_3 \end{array} + CMP$$

Lecithin

This sequence, originally shown to occur in rat liver mitochondria, has been detected also in neural tissues (Rossiter, 1966); of its stages, (*i*) is potentially involved also in sphingolipid synthesis, while formation of the diglyceride linkages is common to many lipid syntheses. It will be realized that specific demonstration is needed to show whether reactions (*i*) to (*iii*) constitute the only route to lecithins in the brain, for assembly of the five components of the molecule gives fourteen possible reaction sequences. Similar problems arise in the comparable sets of reactions involved in synthesis of the inositol or sphingo-sine lipids, and it is rare that all possible routes to a given compound have been quantitatively appraised. At specific sites or periods of cerebral development, concentrations of intermediates and relative enzyme activities differ and may thus favour different sequences. In the following accounts, the reactions discussed have frequently been demonstrated by isotope incorporation, with observations suggesting that some of the alternative routes are less favoured; in a few instances the enzymes concerned have been purified. Reaction rates have been quoted when possible, and are important in appraising the reactions (see McIlwain, 1963).

Glycerol Intermediates; Phosphatidic Acids

Cerebral tissues incubated in oxygenated glucose salines containing ^{14}C-glycerol incorporate the ^{14}C to lipid-soluble material. Fractionation of the extracts from rat cerebral cortex showed the ^{14}C in lecithins, phosphatidylethanolamine, and also the serine and inositol lipids; on hydrolysis almost all the ^{14}C was recovered as glycerol (Pritchard, 1958). Both oxygen and glucose were needed for maximal incorporation, and 2:4-dinitrophenol or iodoacetate inhibited it. Glycerol-3-phosphate might be suggested as intermediate, but when isolated from the tissues was of lower specific activity than most of the phospholipids. A glycerol kinase, which in liver or kidney phosphorylates glycerol with adenosine triphosphate, has been sought in the brain but reported at negligible activity (Wieland & Suyter, 1957). The normal route for cerebral production of glycerolphosphate thus appears to be glycerolphosphate dehydrogenase, which yields it from the triosephosphate of carbohydrate degradation (Chapter 5). To do this it must effectively compete with glyceraldehyde-phosphate dehydrogenase. Cerebral dispersions from young rats were found capable of producing about 1400 μmoles of glycerolphosphate/g. tissue/hr.; interestingly, the activity increased four-fold during myelination, while the competing enzymes increased only slightly (Laatsch, 1962). Routes to the intermediary glycerides can thus include reactions (iv) to (vi).

(iv) *Glycerolphosphate acyltransferase:*
    L-Glycerol-3-phosphate + acyl-CoA =
                    CoA + monoglyceride phosphate (lysophosphatidic acid)

(v) *Glyceride kinase:*
    α-Monoglyceride + ATP = ADP + monoglyceride phosphate

(vi) *Monoglyceride phosphate acyltransferase:*
    L-α-Monoglyceride phosphate + acyl-CoA =
                    CoA + diglyceride phosphate (phosphatidic acid)

Evidence for the acyltransferase (iv) was obtained by isolating the phospholipids yielded by cerebral dispersions on incubating in mixtures containing glycerol 3-^{32}P-phosphate (McMurray et al., 1957). The ^{32}P was found incorporated, still as glycerophosphate, and the incorporation was increased by added CoA. The lysophosphatidic acids are also yielded by preparations from a cerebral microsomal fraction on incubation with an AT^{32}P-generating system and monopalmitin or monoolein (reaction v; Pieringer & Hokin, 1962; Martensson & Kanfer, 1968). The yield, of about 1 nmole of the monoglyceride phosphate, was characterized chromatographically; either the α- or β-monoglyceride served as substrate.

The lysophosphatidic acids act as substrates for several reactions in cerebral systems. Both the α- and β-acids undergo deacylation and dephosphorylation. They also, however, can be further acylated by reaction (vi) to yield phosphatidic acids (Pieringer & Hokin, 1962). With palmityl-CoA and an enzyme preparation from guinea pig brain, the diglyceride phosphate accumulated at about 0·06 μmole/g. original tissue/hr. in the presence of magnesium salts and fluorides. A different route to phosphatidic acids is provided by a diglyceride kinase. By a reaction analogous to (v), α,β-diglycerides incubated in a mixture which included a cerebral preparation and a source of AT^{32}P, formed a phosphatidic acid at rates corresponding to 0·09 μmoles/g. original tissue/hr. (Hokin & Hokin, 1958; see McIlwain, 1962). Cerebral dispersions in reaction mixtures allowing glycolysis formed phosphatidic acid from added $^{32}PO_4^{3-}$ and α,β-diglycerides, a process concluded to involve the diglyceride kinase (Strickland, 1962). As substrate, a diglyceride from spinal-cord lecithin was most effective; D-α,β-diolein was more active than the L-compound or distearin.

Table 11.4

Some enzymes of phospholipid metabolism in the brain

Enzyme	EC number (if assigned)	Substrate	Activity (μmole/hr. g. fresh brain)
Synthetic			
Choline kinase	2.7.1.32	Choline	15–20
P-choline cytidyl transferase	2.7.7.15	P-choline	8–12
Choline phosphotransferase	2.7.8.2	CDP-choline	1
Glycerol-P acyl transferase	2.3.1.15	Glycerol-P	0·4
Phosphatidic acid transferase	2.7.8	CDP-diglyceride	5
MPI kinase	–	MPI	0·4
DPI kinase	–	DPI	9
Degradative			
Phosphatidate phosphatase	3.1.3.4	Phosphatidic acid	80
Phospholipase A	3.1.1.4	Lecithin	2–3
Phospholipase B	3.1.1.5	Lysolecithin	1–3
Phospholipase C	3.1.4.3	Lecithin	1
Neuraminidase	3.2.1.18	Gangliosides	1
TPI phosphodiesterase	–	TPI	500–1000
TPI phosphomonoesterase	–	TPI	200–270
DPI phosphomonoesterase	–	DPI	200
Plasmalogenase	–	Ethanolamine plasmalogen	2–3

Values are for reactions maximally activated, usually by detergents, and are approximate only, as many were calculated from observed data in the brains of several mammalian species (Ansell & Spanner, 1965, 1968; Kai *et al.*, 1966, 1968; McCaman *et al.*, 1965; McCaman & Cook, 1966; Martensson & Kanfer, 1968; Marples & Thompson, 1960; Thompson & Dawson, 1964; Gatt, 1968; Leibovitz & Gatt, 1968; Benjamins & Agranoff, 1969; Keough & Thompson, 1970).

Phosphatidic acid is susceptible to hydrolysis by a relatively specific phosphatidic acid phosphatase, which forms α,β-diglyceride and inorganic phosphate. The enzyme is particulate and in the mammalian brain is more active than the enzymes which synthesize phosphatidic acid (Table 11.4). Highest activity of the phosphatase was observed in grey matter, especially dorsal root ganglia and area postrema (McCaman, 1962; McCaman *et al.*, 1965; McCaman & Cook, 1966).

Diphosphatidylglycerol (or cardiolipin: Fig. 11.3, Table 11.2) occurs in the brain and is enriched in mitochondrial fractions (Dawson, 1960; see Chapter 12). Purified cardiolipin from ox grey matter accounts for over 1 % of the total lipid and contains a high proportion of linoleic acid. Analysis of the positions of the fatty acids in the diphosphatidylglycerol showed palmitic, stearic and linoleic acids to be located mainly on the α positions and oleic and arachidonic acids on the β positions (Yabuuchi & O'Brien, 1968).

Choline and Phosphorylcholine

Choline as a component of lecithins and sphingomyelins is a major cerebral constituent, the brain containing some 35 μmoles/g. fresh tissue. This represents 2,000–20,000 times the cerebral content of acetylcholine; uncombined choline and the intermediates to be discussed below, are also present in relatively small amounts.

The first reaction undergone by choline in lipid synthesis is probably choline kinase, reaction (i) above. This phosphorylation of choline has been observed in cerebral preparations and assayed by incubation with ^{14}C-choline, adenosine triphosphate and magnesium salts (Berry et al., 1958; McCaman, 1962). Quite high choline phosphokinase activities were found, yielding about 20 μmoles/g. tissue/hr. in the rabbit cerebral cortex and 5 in white matter. Activity was optimal at pH 10 and the enzyme was purified by salt precipitation of extracts from acetone powders; only ATP of several nucleotides acted in phosphorylation.

Phosphorylcholine separated chromatographically has been estimated to occur normally at 0·3–0·4 μmoles/g. rat brain; after intraperitoneal $^{32}PO_4^{3-}$ it underwent the most rapid cerebral turnover of seven phospholipid intermediates examined (Ansell & Spanner, 1959). Moreover choline phosphate serves as such as a substrate for lipid synthesis: injected suboccipitally, choline-^{32}P-phosphate underwent some hydrolysis but yielded specifically choline phospholipids of greater specific activity than were yielded by $^{32}PO_4^{3-}$. Cerebral tissues in vitro caused little hydrolysis of choline phosphate and ^{32}P introduced as phosphorylcholine became incorporated preponderantly in choline phospholipids (Ansell & Marshall, 1963; Kometiani et al., Symposium, 1964b). This, and evidence cited earlier, supports the sequence (i)–(iii) above, in which phosphorylcholine next undergoes reaction with cytidine triphosphate. The product, cytidine diphosphate choline, has been characterized in extracts from rat brain frozen in situ, in quantities corresponding to 0·03 μmoles/g. tissue (Ansell & Bayliss, 1961). Cytidine diphosphate choline has been found to act as intermediate in the synthesis not only of lecithins, but also of choline plasmalogens and sphingomyelin, as indicated below.

Ethanolamine Intermediates

Cerebral ethanolamine exists mainly as a constituent of two kephalins, phosphatidylethanolamine and the preponderant plasmalogen (Fig. 11.3), and in these combined forms is nearly as plentiful as choline. Free ethanolamine has been detected at 0·01–0·03 mM in cerebrospinal fluid (Knauff, 1958). Ethanolamine kinase, catalysing the reaction analogous to (i) above, yields phosphorylethanolamine which occurs in rat brain at about 1 μmole/g. tissue. Incorporation studies using $^{32}PO_4^{3-}$ show phosphorylethanolamine to undergo rapid turnover, at about half the rate of phosphorylcholine in the same experiments and at greater rates than the ethanolamine phosphatides (Ansell & Spanner, 1959; Kometiani et al., Symposium, 1964b).

Cytidine diphosphate ethanolamine, the product of a transferase reaction analogous to (ii) above, has been detected only at quite low concentrations in the brain. Glycerophosphorylethanolamine has been found at 0·1 μmoles/g. rat brain, and after intraperitoneal or intracisternal $^{32}PO_4^{3-}$ the compound reached higher specific activities in the brain than did phosphatidylethanolamine, suggesting that it was not a degradation product; it was not however regarded as an intermediate in phosphatide synthesis (Ansell & Norman, 1953). The incorporation of ^{32}P to glycerophosphorylethanolamine took place also in cerebral dispersions, without the specific additions needed for phosphatide synthesis.

Fatty acid amides of ethanolamine, which constitute a distinct class of lipid, have been found in rat brain, which carried about 0·1 μmole/g. of palmitylethanolamide (Bachur et al., 1965). This is a concentration markedly greater than was found in other organs; cerebral tissues were capable of forming the amide from ^{14}C-palmitic acid.

Lecithins

Lecithins constitute a large part of the central nervous system, forming in the adult human brain about 5·5% of its dry weight (see also Table 11.2). The dipalmityl compound (Fig. 11.3, R″ and R‴ being palmitic acid residues) has been characterized as present in the brain as elsewhere, but much oleic acid and lesser quantities of some four other saturated and unsaturated acids have

Table 11.5

Fatty acid composition of cerebral lecithins

Fatty acid[a]	Homogenate	Myelin	Mitochondria	Microsomes	Supernatant
Myristic (14.0)	0·3	0·2	0·1	0·4	0·1
Palmitic (16.0)	45·0	34·7	47·1	56·6	38·7
Stearic (18.0)	13·8	17·3	12·2	9·8	14·7
Palmitoleic (16.1)	1·4	1·1	1·0	0·8	1·5
Oleic (18.1)	32·3	42·6	30·5	26·7	35·5
Arachidonic (20.4)	5·1	2·2	5·6	3·7	7·3

[a] Values are the percentage of total fatty acid in lecithin of each fraction; figures in parenthesis are no. of C atoms and no. of double bonds. Data is from adult rat brain (Skrbic & Cumings, 1970).

also been isolated from cerebral lecithins (Thannhauser, 1950; Klenk et al., 1953). By gas chromatographic analysis of fatty acid mixtures from lecithins, already separated from rat or ox brain by solvents or column chromatography, many fatty acids between C_{13} and C_{22} were identified (Biran & Bartley, 1961; Kai et al., 1963). A simpler composition has however been found for the lecithin prepared from the grey matter of ox brain; palmitic and oleic acids in nearly equal quantities accounted for 98% of its fatty acid mixture (Gammack *et al.*, 1964). In human grey and white matter these two acids contributed 76–89% of the mixture (O'Brien *et al.*, 1964). Differences were detectable in the fatty acid mixture so derived from crude mitochondrial and microsomal fractions from rat brain, and when the fatty acids in the α and β positions in lecithin were differentiated by using phospholipase A, 75% of the unsaturated acids were found in the β-position.

The fatty acid composition of myelin lecithin differs from that of lecithin in other membrane structures of the brain. Thus myelin lecithin is richer in oleic and stearic acids and poorer in palmitic acid than the lecithin of the mitochondria or microsomes (Table 11.5). There is thus much scope for specificity in the association of a particular lecithin with a particular site or function.

Synthesis by Choline Phosphotransferase

A major synthetic route to the lecithins by reactions (*i*) to (*iii*) above has already been stated and data given regarding the choline kinase and cytidyl transferase in cerebral systems. Investigation of the final choline phosphotransferase reaction in the brain has employed cytidine diphosphate choline labelled as CMP-[^{32}P]-phosphorylcholine. The ^{32}P became incorporated to lecithins on incubation with cerebral dispersions (Ansell & Marshall, 1963). Further, using CDP-^{14}C-choline and similar cerebral preparations, incorporation of the ^{14}C to lecithin was found to be increased when certain D-α,β-diglycerides were included in the reaction mixture. The glyceride derived from a lecithin from ox spinal cord, and D-α,β-diolein, were most active in this respect; the L-isomer was inactive (Strickland *et al.*, 1963). Choline phosphotransferase (Table 11.4) is less active than choline kinase in the brain and produces lecithin at rates of about 1 μmole/hr. g. of tissue in the cerebral cortex and 0·5 in white matter (McCaman & Cook, 1966).

Lysolecithin

Lysolecithin lacks one of the fatty acid residues of lecithin and has been found in rat and human brain at about 0·1–0·2 μmoles/g. fresh tissue (Webster & Thompson, 1962). It has proved of significance in both the synthesis and degradation of lecithin, the two processes (*vii*) and (*viii*) occurring by distinct routes:

(*vii*) *Lysolecithin acyltransferase;*
Lysolecithin + acyl-CoA → lecithin + CoA

(*viii*) *Phospholipase A (EC 3.1.1.4):*
Lecithin → lysolecithin + fatty acid

(*ix*) *Phospholipase B (EC 3.1.1.5):*
Lysolecithin → glycerylphosphorylcholine + fatty acid

Acylation of ^{14}C-lysolecithin to lecithin on incubation with cerebral dispersions, oleate, MgATP and coenzyme A was shown after silicic acid chromatography of the reaction products. Also, the product was degraded by a phospholipase to yield most of the ^{14}C again as lysolecithin. The acylation was also demonstrated by using either ^{14}C-palmitate or -oleate in a similar reaction mixture containing fluoride. Over 90% of the ^{14}C-oleate added at quite low concentrations could be incorporated into lecithins; 1 mM-oleate gave maximum rates, which corresponded to formation of 8 μmoles/g. fresh tissue/hr. The reaction was concluded to proceed by the fatty acid-CoA derivatives, and ^{14}C-palmityl-CoA yielded the corresponding lecithin from lysolecithin (Webster & Thompson, 1962; Webster & Alpern, 1964). The demonstrated rates of this reaction (*vii*) are thus greater than those of the alternative route (*iv*) to (*vi*), and presumably contribute to maintaining the cerebral lysolecithin at the relatively low concentrations observed.

Cerebral tissues themselves show a small phospholipase A activity and thus (reaction *viii*) can form lysolecithin from lecithin, at possibly 0·3 μmoles/g. hr. if maximally activated by detergents. The purified enzyme from rat or calf brain was equally active against lecithin and phosphatidyl-ethanolamine but produced negligible hydrolysis of lysolecithin (Gatt, 1968). Moreover, cerebral tissues also carry phospholipase B activity and degrade lysolecithin to glycerylphosphorylcholine by removing the remaining fatty acid residue. The reaction (*ix*) proceeded at 1·7 μmoles/g. rat brain/hr.; in human brain, white matter was markedly less active than grey, which could yield 6·4 μmoles of glycerylphosphorylcholine/g. hr. (Marples & Thompson, 1960; Gallai-Hatchard *et al.*, 1962, 1965). α-Glycerylphosphorylcholine is, further, degraded to α-glycerol phosphate and choline by a diesterase which is quite active in cerebral tissues. Dispersions from several parts of the brain of species including dog and man yielded from 2 to 36 μmoles choline/g. tissue/hr. (Webster *et al.*, 1957).

The marked cytolytic properties of lysolecithin give an added interest to its formation in the brain (Webster *et al.*, 1957; McArdle *et al.*, 1960). It not only haemolyses, but also causes rapid clearing of the normal opacity of cerebral dispersions, presumably solubilizing lipid components by micelle-formation (Chapter 12). Added to cell-containing cerebral preparations it increases up to five-fold the release of some enzymes to surrounding fluids, and led to progressive fall in respiratory rate. As the venoms of cobra and certain other snakes contain phospholipase A, lysolecithin may mediate in their actions, and also in certain demyelinating conditions (Thompson, 1965).

Kephalins

Phospholipids in early studies were separated only to lecithins, soluble in ethanol, and kephalins which were insoluble in ethanol. The complexity of the cerebral kephalins was first recognized by fractional precipitation from chloroform solution with increasing quantities of ethanol (Folch, 1942) which yielded successive fractions enriched in phosphatidylinositol, phosphatidyl-serine and phosphatidylethanolamine. The structurally related plasmalogens and glycerol ether phospholipids (Fig. 11.3) are also present, and chromatographic methods have since given more quantitative separations, as is exemplified in Fig. 11.1.

A variety of fatty acids has been detected and estimated in kephalin fractions, with stearic and oleic acids preponderating. The composition of the fatty acid mixture differed in different subcellular fractions from rat brain, and was distinct from that of the lecithins isolated from the same material (Biran & Bartley, 1961). In human brain, distinctive patterns of fatty acid components were found in the ethanolamine, serine and choline phosphatides from grey and white matter (O'Brien *et al.*, 1964): values for palmitic acid ranged from 0·5–45% of the mixture, for oleic acid from 12–58%, and for hexenoic C_{22}-acids, from a trace to 25%.

Phosphatidylethanolamine and Phosphatidylserine

Phosphatidylethanolamine is the major kephalin in grey matter where it constitutes some 8–10 μmoles/g. Evidence that its synthesis proceeded by a transferase reaction similar to that of reaction (*iii*) was obtained by using CMP-[^{32}P]-phosphorylethanolamine as substrate with dispersions of rat brain; some 10% of the added compound became incorporated in ethanolamine phospholipids (McMurray *et al.*, 1957; Ansell & Chojnacki, 1962; Ansell & Marshall, 1963). This incorporation is affected by chlorpromazine, and the analogous base 2-dimethylaminoethanol, which has been used as a centrally-acting drug, can also become incorporated in cerebral phosphatides.

Using the ^{14}C-labelled compound, ethanolamine was shown to become incorporated into specifically the ethanolamine phospholipids of cerebral tissues. After incubating CDP-^{14}C-ethanolamine with dispersions from the brain of young rats, incorporation occurred into both phosphatidylethanolamine and ethanolamine plasmalogens, but phosphatidylserine was not significantly labelled (Pritchard, 1958; McMurray, 1964).

Phosphatidylserine, as indicated by Fig. 11.1 and Table 11.2, is also a major component of the cerebral kephalins. Of its precursors, serine has been noted in Chapter 8 as occurring in the brain at about 0·4 μmoles/g. Judged by $^{32}PO_4^{3-}$ incorporation *in vivo* or *in vitro*, phosphatidylserine is less rapidly metabolized in the brain than are the other phospholipids of Table 11.3. When ^{14}C-serine was added to rat cerebral tissues incubated in glucose-containing media, the ^{14}C became incorporated to the serine phospholipids, and also in lesser degree to ethanolamine lipids (Pritchard, 1958; Ansell & Spanner, 1962; Pritchard & Rossiter, 1963). The incorporation was depressed in absence of glucose or on adding 2:4-dinitrophenol.

Aqueous extracts from the grey matter of human brain, or from rat brain, catalysed the breakdown of phosphatidylethanolamine and of phosphatidyl-serine (Gallai-Hatchard *et al.*, 1962). The corresponding lyso-derivatives accumulated; reaction was at about the same rate as with lecithin.

Glycerol Ether Phospholipids

This category of lipid (Fig. 11.3; see Ansell & Spanner, 1963) was termed kephalin B after its recognition, in cerebral and certain other tissues, by a relative stability to mild acid and alkaline hydrolysis. The sphingomyelins are also stable under these conditions but on treatment with methanolic-HCl they yielded phosphorylcholine and its sphingosine derivative, whereas kephalin B was more resistant to acid hydrolysis and yielded ethanolamine. The new compound was prepared from mixed cerebral lipids by chromatography on alumina and constituted about 3% of the lipid phosphorus of the brain. It had the properties of a glycerol ether of the structure shown in Fig. 11.3, R' being $-CH_2.CH_2.NH_3^+$. On incubating CDP-^{14}C-ethanolamine with cerebral dispersions from young rats part of the ^{14}C accumulated in a compound with the properties of the glycerol ether phospholipid (Rossiter et al., 1964). Presumably a reaction analogous to (iii) above had occurred with an endogenous monoglyceride ether as second reactant. The ether phospholipids have been recognized in human and in other mammalian cerebral tissues (Svennerholm & Thorin, 1960).

Plasmalogens

Plasmalogens were recognized when Schiff's reagent for aldehydes was applied histochemically and found to give a slow, positive reaction with non-nuclear constituents of cerebral and of other tissues. The aldehydes concerned, mainly palmital and stearal, were not free but were liberated by successive treatment with alkaline and mildly acid reagents from precursors which were accordingly termed plasmalogens. These constitute 18–30% of the cerebral phospholipids and are especially enriched in the myelin of white matter; the brain is the organ richest in plasmalogens (see Chapter 12; Webster, 1960; Rapport & Norton, 1962).

The structure of a major component of the cerebral plasmalogens is given in Fig. 11.3. From this molecule, alkali liberates the fatty acid, giving a glycerophosphorylethanolamine derivative obtained in quantity in crystalline form from ox brain. This derivative was for some time itself regarded as the native plasmalogen, because it retained the aldehydogenic group. From this product, mildly acid conditions (pH 2) yielded L-α-glycerophosphorylethanolamine; the plasmalogen is thus closely related to the phosphatidylethanolamine of the kephalins. The portion of the molecule which yielded the aldehyde was identified as an α,β-unsaturated ether, which reacted as:

$$R.CH = CH.OR' + H_2O \rightarrow R.CH_2CHO + R'OH$$

(Rapport & Franzl, 1957; Klenk & Debuch, 1954).

Catalytic hydrogenation of the plasmalogen led to loss of its aldehydogenic properties and to the appearance of a normal ether linkage, stable to mild acid and alkali: that is, to a kephalin B. The ether linkage proved to be at the α-OH of glycerol, α-octadecylglyceryl ether being a major product (Debuch, 1959). In addition to phosphatidalethanolamine which is present in greatest quantity, phosphatidalserine and a small proportion of phosphatidalcholine have been found in the brain. The fatty acids of cerebral plasmalogens were almost entirely unsaturated; about half were based on C_{18}, 24% on C_{20} and 22% on C_{22}. This mixture was characteristically different from the fatty acid mixture of phosphatidylethanolamine (Debuch, 1956). An enzyme detected in acetone-dried cerebral preparations cleaved preferentially the vinyl ether linkage of ethanolamine plasmalogen. The enzyme, "plasmalogenase", which requires Mg^{2+}, hydrolysed plasmalogens at rates of 2–3 μmoles/hr. g. of whole rat brain and was more active in white than in grey matter. No activity was detected in myelin; occurrence was mainly in microsomes and in unpurified mitochondrial fractions (Ansell & Spanner, 1965, 1968).

Cerebral systems synthesize plasmalogens; evidence for a reaction analogous to (iii) above, was obtained by incubating CDP-[^{14}C]-ethanolamine with cerebral dispersions from young rats. The ^{14}C was incorporated to ethanolamine plasmalogens, presumably by reaction with an unsaturated glyceride native to the tissue. By providing additional glyceride prepared from a plasmalogen specimen, the incorporation which occurred also to other ethanolamine lipids, was increased in specifically the plasmalogen fraction (McMurray, 1964). Incorporation of ^{14}C palmitate has also been shown but ^{14}C from palmitaldehyde is not incorporated directly into cerebral plasmalogens, requiring prior oxidation to palmitate. From observations that phosphatidyl ethanolamine is labelled more rapidly than ethanolamine plasmalogen in rat brain in vivo when ^{14}C-ethanolamine was the precursor, it appears that plasmalogen synthesis may involve dehydrogenation of the saturated phosphatide. Similarly, results from use of ^{14}C-palmitate as precursor indicated that incorporation was first into phosphatidylethanolamine which was then oxidized to form the alkenyl ether (Ansell & Spanner, 1967; Bickerstaffe & Mead, 1967).

Inositol Phosphatides

The phosphoinositides include the most recently recognized and most actively metabolized of the cerebral phosphatides. Inositol itself was isolated from the brain and characterized as a non-fermentable carbohydrate over a century ago; Thudichum (1884) separated some 0·5 g./kg., which represents only part of that present. Rat brain contains about 7 μmoles/g. of uncombined inositol and nearly 9 μmoles/g. of total inositol, all of which is the L-myoinositol isomeride; it has a quite limited ability to synthesize inositol from glucose (Hauser & Finelli, 1963). Using ^{14}C-glucose, production of about 0·01 μmoles inositol/g. tissue/hr. was estimated, which is very small in comparison with rates of interconversion among the phosphoinositides. In young rats the production is more rapid; 2-^{14}C-pyruvate also yielded inositol but 1-^{14}C-acetate and 6-^{14}C-glucuronate did not (Hauser, 1963). Cerebral tissues exchange inositol with surrounding salines, or, in vivo, with the cerebrospinal fluid where inositol exists at several times its blood level. In the body as a whole inositol can take part in general carbohydrate metabolism but it is doubtful if the substance is oxidized by separated cerebral tissues.

Three major groups of phosphoinositides are separable from the brain (Fig. 11.4). Detection of a fourth, tetraphosphoinositide, has been reported in human and beef brain (Klenk & Hendricks, 1961; Santiago-Calvo et al., 1963) but none was found in another study of human brain (Hendrickson & Ballou, 1964). In the monophosphoinositides, the phosphate is present as a diester of L-myoinositol and a diglyceride. The di- and triphosphoinositides carry the additional phosphate groups on the 3- and 4-positions of the inositol moiety. Of them, only the monophosphoinositides are readily extracted from cerebral tissues by a chloroform–methanol mixture; on acidifying, the other two categories become extractable and are separable chromatographically. These properties have been used in analysis of the inositide mixture and reflect a firm but not covalent attachment of the di- and triphosphoinositides to tissue proteins (Dittmer & Dawson, 1961; LeBaron, 1963; Palmer & Rossiter, 1964). A preparative method for the inositides extracted them from human and other brain with solvents and separated the mixture by exchange chromatography using a diethylaminoethyl cellulose column (Hendrickson & Ballou, 1964). This yielded distinct fractions which were deacylated by NaOH in methanol, giving from each phosphoinositide a mixture of fatty acids. Gas chromatography showed in each mixture about 40% of stearic acid, 22% of arachidonic acid and 16% of oleic acid with much lesser amounts of some seven other fatty acids. These proportions (see also Kerr & Read, 1963) differed markedly from

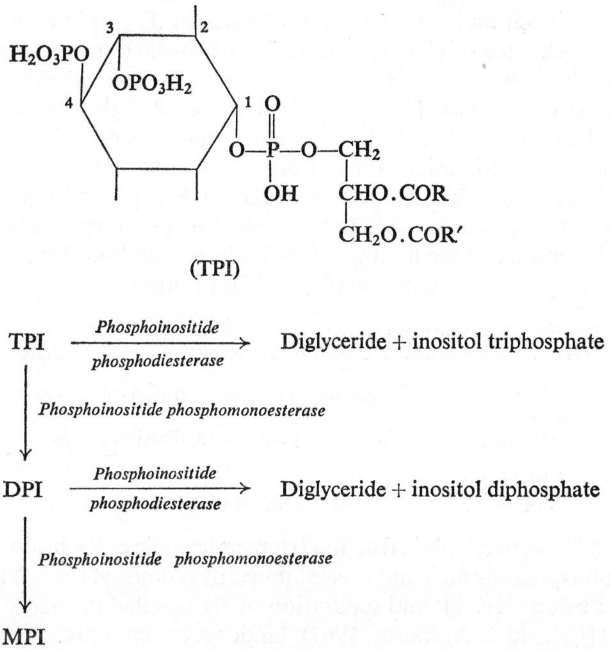

FIG. 11.4. Triphosphoinositide (TPI) and the reactions catalysed by the phosphoinositide phosphomono- and di-esterases of cerebral tissues; DPI and MPI, di- and mono-phosphoinositide (Tomlinson & Ballou, 1961; Rapport & Norton, 1962; Dawson & Thompson, 1964; Thompson & Dawson, 1964).

those of the fatty acids from the phosphatidylserine also present in the extracts, so indicating the likelihood of a common synthetic route to the three inositides. The major unsaturated fatty acids, arachidonic and oleic, have been detected mainly on the 2-position of the glycerol skeleton whereas the saturated fatty acids occur predominantly on the 1-position (Thompson, 1969).

Synthetic Routes

The rapid incorporation of $^{32}PO_4^{3-}$ to inositol phosphatides in the brain *in situ* and in cerebral preparations *in vitro* has already been noted (Table 11.3). In distinction to many other reactions in cerebral lipids, these and the following changes are prominent in the brain from adult animals. Routes by which the inositides are synthesized have been deduced by including likely cofactors in experiments similar to those of Table 11.3, and by providing other components of the molecules. With cerebral dispersions, cytidine triphosphate accelerated the $^{32}PO_4^{3-}$ incorporation. This nucleotide could also increase ten-fold the incorporation of ^3H-inositol to the inositides (McMurray *et al.*, 1957; Thompson *et al.*, 1963); a number of other nucleotides did not so act, including ATP and nicotinamide-adenine dinucleotide.

^{14}C-Glycerol was also rapidly incorporated to the inositides (Pritchard, 1958); but, examining (specifically) the incorporation of ^3H-inositol to the monophosphoinositide in the presence of excess CTP, only certain glycerol derivatives accelerated this incorporation. Distearin did not, but distearoyl-L-α-glycerophosphate was effective, as was also a natural phosphatidic acid mixture. Interaction of CTP and phosphatidic acid thus appeared likely (reaction x below) and therefore CDP-diglyceride was examined as reactant with ^3H-inositol. With microsomal fractions from rat brain, especially in reaction mixtures containing a detergent, the CDP-diglyceride increased 300-fold the incorporation of inositol to the monophosphoinositides; CTP gave a twenty-fold increase. These findings (Brockerhoff & Ballou, 1962; Thompson *et al.*, 1963) supported the reactions (x) and (xi) below:

(x) *CTP-diglyceride phosphate: cytidyl transferase*
     CTP + phosphatidic acid = CDP-diglyceride + pyrophosphate

(xi) *CDP-diglyceride: inositol diglyceride phosphate transferase* (phosphatidic acid transferase)
     CDP-diglyceride + inositol = phosphatidylinositol + CMP

(xii) *Phosphoinositide kinase*
     Phosphatidylinositol + ATP = diphosphoinositide + ADP

Reaction (x) in the particulate fraction from embryonic chick brain was shown to require phosphatidic acid and was inhibited by palmitoyl CoA. The reaction was studied using ^3H-CTP and separation of ^3H labelled products chromatographically (Petzold & Agranoff, 1967). Under some circumstances, however, labelled L-α-glycerophosphate can lead to a greater labelling of phosphoinositide than of phosphatidic acid. Conceivably, therefore, reaction of α-glycerophosphate with inositol may precede its acylation.

Routes to the di- and tri-phosphoinositides have been explored by comparing the entry of the precursors just described, to the three inositides (Brockerhoff & Ballou, 1962; Rossiter *et al.*, 1964). For these experiments, cell-containing tissues were employed, for in cerebral dispersions little of the di- and tri-phosphates accumulated: emphasizing the potency of the degrading enzymes discussed subsequently. When $^{32}PO_4^{3-}$ was incorporated to the inositides by incubating with cat or rabbit cerebral tissues, and the inositide mixture separated and hydrolysed, the phosphate of greatest activity was that derived from positions 3 and 4 (Fig. 11.4). These operations gave three samples of monophosphoinositide: that already in the tissue as MPI, that derived from DPI and that from TPI. The enrichment of ^{32}P in these compounds was in the order MPI > DPI > TPI. The phosphate liberated in hydrolysis however was of much higher activity than that remaining in the MPI, so that the inositides as extracted showed activity in the order TPI > DPI > MPI. Both these findings are consistent with synthesis by the reactions (xi), (xii) and further phosphorylation of DPI.

Specific activities of the three inositides were compared also after incorporation of ^{3}H-inositol and ^{14}C-glycerol. In some circumstances these activities were again in the order MPI > DPI > TPI but in others the order was DPI > MPI > TPI; possibly in addition to the previous sequence, inositol may first yield a monophosphate which then undergoes reactions analogous to (xi) and (xii) to yield successively DPI and TPI without intermediation of MPI.

Two phosphoinositide kinases have been demonstrated: MPI kinase and DPI kinase which phosphorylate MPI and DPI to form DPI and TPI respectively. The MPI kinase of mammalian brain produces the naturally occurring isomer of diphosphoinositide with phosphate groups at positions 1 and 4 (Fig. 11.4). The enzyme in rat brain phosphorylated MPI at rates of about 0·4 μmole/g. fresh tissue/hr. and was enriched in membrane containing fractions, particularly microsomes. Metal requirement was satisfied by Mg^{2+} or Mn^{2+} and Ca^{2+}, Cu^{2+}, Na^+ or K^+ inhibited; the enzyme required SH groups and was stimulated by detergents (Colodzin & Kennedy, 1965; Kai et al., 1966; Prottey et al., 1968; Harwood & Hawthorne, 1969).

Distribution of DPI kinase is quite different from MPI kinase as the activity is confined almost entirely to the supernatant fraction of brain homogenates prepared in sucrose. It differs also from the MPI kinase in certain of its properties: there is no SH group requirement and while Mg^{2+} is required, Ca^{2+} or Mn^{2+} are less satisfactory activators and may be inhibitory at optimum Mg^{2+} concentration. Activity in the brain is higher than that of the MPI kinase (Table 11.4). Isolation of the product of DPI kinase confirmed that the naturally occurring isomer of TPI was formed with phosphate groups at positions 1, 4 and 5 (Figs. 11.4 and 11.5) (Kai et al., 1966; 1968; Prottey et al., 1968).

Phosphoinositides as Substrates

Shortly after their recognition as cerebral constituents, phosphoinositides were found to be rapidly degraded by enzymes from the brain. Subsequent purification of both enzymes and substrates has enabled the reactions of Fig. 11.4 to be characterized (Sloane Stanley, 1953; Rodnight, 1956; Thompson & Dawson, 1964; Chang & Ballou, 1967; Salway et al., 1967; Friedel et al., 1967, 1969).

The triphosphoinositide phosphodiesterase was prepared from an acetone powder of ox brain by extraction, heating, and salt precipitation. When maximally activated it split the linkage between phosphate and glycerol, yielding inositol triphosphate and diglycerides at 1000 μmoles/hr. with material from 1 g. brain. This rate was achieved at neutral pH with added cetyltrimethylammonium bromide in quantities about equimolar with the substrate. Inositide and activator were shown electron-microscopically to form an association complex which presumably facilitated approach to the enzyme by orienting and partly neutralizing the acidic groups of the inositide. The enzyme acted also on diphosphoinositide, again yielding a diglyceride without liberation of

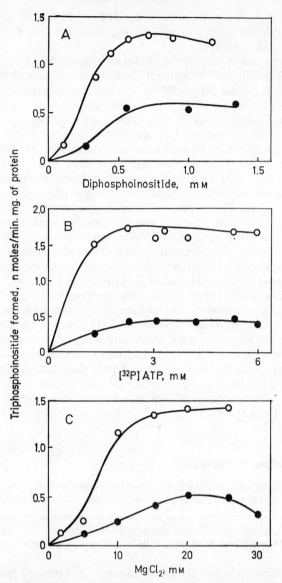

FIG. 11.5. Synthesis of triphosphoinositide by rat brain diphosphoinositide kinase.

Samples of homogenate (○) or of the supernatant fraction (●) were
obtained by high-speed centrifugation of the homogenate. Homogenates
were incubated with diphosphoinositide, [^{32}P]ATP, MgCl$_2$, EDTA, in
tris-HCl buffer, pH 7·4, at 37° for 5 min. The product was extracted and
isolated by paper-chromatography. Incubation of supernatant
fractions was similar except that glutathione replaced EDTA. In both,
the tissue fraction was added last. Assay of diphosphoinositide kinase
in the supernatant fraction gave lower rates if the substrate was added
last. Requirement is shown for diphosphoinositide (A), ATP (B) and
Mg^{2+} (C). Data from Kai et al., 1968.

inorganic phosphate, but had no effect on four other phosphatides or on diphenylphosphate.

Triphosphoinositide phosphomonoesterase catalysed an alternative break-down of the inositide by liberating inorganic orthophosphate. This enzyme was separated from an extract of acetone-dried ox brain by salt precipitation and density gradient electrophoresis. After taking to pH 5, the phosphomono-esterase needed Mg salts for activity and, again, cetyltrimethylammonium bromide or an analogous compound. It acted also on diphosphoinositide and to a lesser extent on inositol triphosphate but was without effect on glycerophos-phate, serine phosphate, or ten other phosphate esters. The enzyme occurs mainly in the supernatant fraction but not in myelin and activity is inhibited by Na^+ or K^+. Diphosphoinositide phosphomonoesterase and monophospho-inositide phosphomonoesterase activities have also been detected. Both, like the TPI esterase, are soluble enzymes but the MPI esterase requires Ca^{2+} rather than Mg^{2+} for activity.

The enzyme capacity of the phosphoinositide esterases does not appear to have been exhibited in experimental systems so far devised with intact cerebral tissues. Relationship to ion movement has received comment but not demon-stration. In the superior cervical ganglion of the rat, the monophosphoinositide was the only one of a number of phospholipids in which $^{32}PO_4^{3-}$ incorporation was altered by electrical stimulation (Larrabee et al., 1963). The stimulation resulted in a gradually increasing turnover during 4 hr., corresponding to change from a normal incorporation of 0·15 μmole/g. tissue to 0·3 μmoles. This is much below the concomitant change in Na^+ or K^+ flux, though a less direct role for the inositide is feasible. It is perhaps noteworthy that the phosphomonoesterase converts TPI and DPI which bond strongly to neural protein, into the MPI which does not. The increased $^{32}PO_4^{3-}$ incorporation indeed appears to be associated with synaptic activity (Larrabee & Leicht, 1965): it was blocked by curare and did not occur when the ganglion was stimulated antidromically.

Electrical stimulation causes change in the relative rates of incorporation of ^{32}P-phosphate into the phospholipids of cerebral cortex slices. Thus stimulation for 1 hr. at a frequency of 5 pulses/sec. increased the incorporation into inositol phosphatides by 86% but the incorporation into lecithin, ethanolamine phospholipids and cardiolipin was halved (Pumphrey, 1969). Changes in phosphoinositide metabolism with development of tolerance to morphine are described in Chapter 15.

Sphingolipids

The lipids remaining to be discussed are not glycerides and most are character-ized by their containing the base sphingosine. They comprise the four main groups of Figs. 11.6 and 11.9. Of them sphingomyelin is also a phospholipid; cerebrosides, sulphatides and gangliosides contain carbohydrate moieties and are glycolipids. The root sphingo- for a sphingolipid was adopted by Thudichum "in commemoration of the many enigmas which it presented to the enquirer".

Within the group of sphingolipids, components range from the neutral cerebrosides to the strongly acidic sulphatides and gangliosides; sphingo-myelins contain also the ionized basic group of choline. Thus they behave very differently on chromatography and do not occur together in a single subgroup in the separation of Fig. 11.1. In the following account, components which are common to more than one sphingolipid will be described first, and subsequently the main components enumerated in Table 11.1. These may not comprise all the sphingolipids: compounds in which the second hydroxyl group of dihydro-sphingosine is substituted have received preliminary characterization as sphingoplasmalogens (Kochetov *et al.*, 1963).

Sphingosine

The base sphingosine and its dihydroderivative were isolated on a large scale from hydrolysates of ox cerebral tissues in the investigations which established their accepted structure (Carter *et al.*, 1947); they were derived from the sphingolipids collectively. Some of the compounds which when

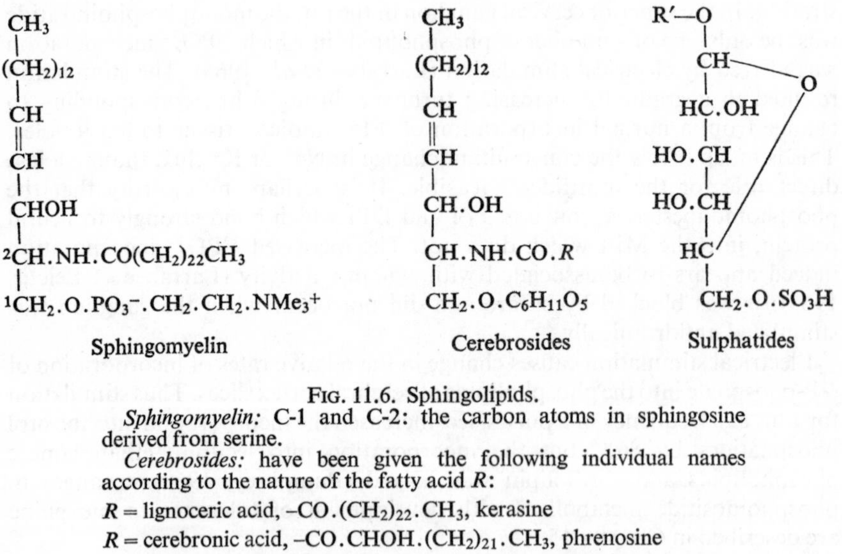

CH_3	CH_3	R'—O
$(CH_2)_{12}$	$(CH_2)_{12}$	CH—
CH	CH	HC.OH
CH	CH	HO.CH
CHOH	CH.OH	HO.CH
$^2CH.NH.CO(CH_2)_{22}CH_3$	CH.NH.CO.R	HC
$^1CH_2.O.PO_3^-.CH_2.CH_2.NMe_3^+$	$CH_2.O.C_6H_{11}O_5$	$CH_2.O.SO_3H$
Sphingomyelin	Cerebrosides	Sulphatides

FIG. 11.6. Sphingolipids.

Sphingomyelin: C-1 and C-2: the carbon atoms in sphingosine derived from serine.

Cerebrosides: have been given the following individual names according to the nature of the fatty acid R:

R = lignoceric acid, –CO.$(CH_2)_{22}$.CH_3, kerasine

R = cerebronic acid, –CO.CHOH.$(CH_2)_{21}$.CH_3, phrenosine

R = nervonic acid, –CO.$(CH_2)_{13}$CH = CH.$(CH_2)_7$.CH_3, nervone

R = hydroxynervonic acid,

   –CO.CHOH.$(CH_2)_{12}$.CH = CH.$(CH_2)_7$.CH_3, hydroxynervone

Ceramides: lack the galactose residue of cerebrosides.
Psychosine: lacks the fatty acid of the cerebrosides.
Sulphatides: R' represents a ceramide residue.

injected systemically to intact animals contribute to formation of the cerebral sphingosine have been determined by administering isotopically labelled substances which might act as precursors. In this way it was found that glycine or serine was utilized for the C-1 and C-2 positions of sphingosine (Fig. 11.6).

The carboxyl of serine was not incorporated but its amino group formed the amino group of sphingosine. The increase in sphingosine synthesis which results from *in vivo* administration of puromycin (q.v.) is thought to be due to increased availability of serine (Kanfer *et al.*, 1967). Ethanolamine was not utilized in the 1 and 2 positions of sphingosine but contributed to the remainder of the carbon chain (Sprinson & Coulon, 1954; Zabin & Mead, 1954), as did acetate and other ^{14}C precursors, in a pattern suggesting that they had entered as a single long-chain unit which provided carbon atoms 3–18 of sphingosine. Moreover, the brain itself was capable of the synthesis, for cerebral tissues or dispersions from young rats yielded ^{14}C-sphingosine when either ^{14}C-serine or ^{14}C-glucose was added to incubation media.

The enzymic systems involved in the synthesis were explored by using cerebral dispersions from young rats, or fractions derived by differentially centrifuging the dispersions (Brady *et al.*, 1958; Fujino & Zabin, 1962; Weiss, 1963); the more difficultly deposited fractions were used in experiments including those of Fig. 11.7. Palmitate-1-^{14}C yielded sphingosine containing the ^{14}C, in reaction mixtures with coenzyme A and adenosine triphosphate; alternatively these requirements were met by providing palmityl-CoA. The palmityl-CoA underwent reduction by nicotinamide adenine dinucleotide phosphate (A, Fig. 11.7; reaction *xiii* below), yielding palmitaldehyde which itself, when suitably dispersed, could be incorporated to sphingosine. For incorporation of the serine, it was necessary for reaction mixtures to include pyridoxal phosphate and manganese salts, and the Schiff base of reaction (*xiv*), detected fluorometrically was proposed as intermediate.

(*xiii*) $CH_3(CH_2)_{14}CO.S.CoA + NADPH + H^+ \rightleftharpoons CH_3(CH_2)_{14}CHO + CoASH + NADP^+$
      Palmityl-CoA   Palmitaldehyde

(*xiv*) Serine + pyridoxal phosphate + $Mn^{2+} \rightleftharpoons HOCH_2\overset{\displaystyle COO^-}{\underset{\displaystyle |}{CH}}-N = CH.R \, Mn^{2+} + H^+$

(*xv*) Palmitaldehyde + Schiff base from (*xiv*) $\rightarrow$
                                  Dihydrosphingosine + pyridoxal phosphate + CO_2 + Mn^{2+}

Ethanolamine was not as effective a reactant as serine, apparently because it did not as readily yield a Schiff base as intermediate.

The two components of the condensation reaction which follows are not firmly established; they may comprise the aldehyde and Schiff base as quoted in (*xv*), but the acyl CoA is also possible. Isolation and characterization of 3-oxodihydrosphingosine as intermediate suggested the involvement of the following reactions (*xvi, xvii*; Stoffel *et al.*, 1968; Braun *et al.*, 1970). Palmitoyl-CoA and pyridoxal phosphate were required for reaction with serine, but no requirement for metal ions could be confirmed.

(*xvi*) Palmitoyl-CoA $\xrightarrow[\text{phosphate}]{\text{pyridoxal}}$ $CH_3(CH_2)_{14}\underset{\displaystyle O}{\overset{\displaystyle ||}{C}}.\underset{\displaystyle NH_2}{\overset{\displaystyle |}{C}}H_2OH$
                                       3-Oxodihydrosphingosine

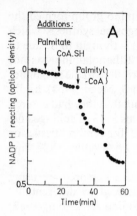

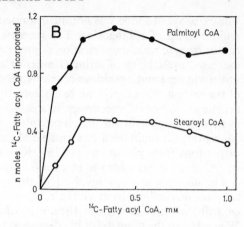

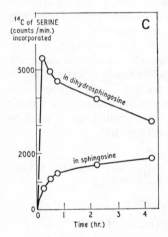

FIG. 11.7. Reactions involved in the cerebral synthesis of sphingosine.

A. Utilization of the reduced form of nicotinamide adenine dinucleotide phosphate in reducing palmityl-coenzyme A (reaction *xiii*). The reaction mixture included a differentially centrifuged fraction from rat brain, NADPH and buffer and received the additions indicated, the last two being of 30 nmoles of palmityl-CoA.

B. Formation of ^{14}C-oxodihydrosphingosine from ^{14}C-labelled fatty acyl-CoA as a function of the fatty acyl CoA concentration. Mouse brain microsomes were incubated for 10 min. with L-serine and the fatty acyl-CoA as indicated, in phosphate buffer, pH 7·4. The products were separated and identified by radio-autography.

C. Appearance of ^{14}C from L-serine-U-^{14}C in dihydrosphingosine and sphingosine. The cerebral fraction of A was used in a mixture which included NADPH, pyridoxal phosphate and MnCl$_2$.

(Data from Brady *et al.*, 1958; Braun *et al.*, 1970).

The synthesis occurs more rapidly with palmitoyl-CoA than with stearoyl-CoA (**B**, Fig. 11.7). Formation of dihydrosphingosine (reaction *xvii*) is followed by dehydrogenation to produce sphingosine (**C**, Fig. 11.7).

(*xvii*) 3-Oxodihydrosphingosine + NADPH → CH$_3$(CH$_2$)$_{14}$CH.CH.CH$_2$OH + NADP$^+$
$$\underset{\text{OH NH}_2}{\phantom{CH_3(CH_2)_{14}CH.CH.CH_2OH}}$$
Dihydrosphingosine (*erythro*)

This reaction was examined separately by adding dihydrosphingosine as such to a cerebral fraction with nicotinamide nucleotides and a methylphenazonium salt as carrier. Both the dihydrosphingosine and sphingosine produced enzymically had the *erythro*-configuration, which is that of the natural sphingolipids. Sphingosine is the preponderating long-chain base of the sphingolipids of animals, but certain sphingolipids based on dihydrosphingosine have been obtained from cerebral preparations, as is indicated below.

Ceramides

In sphingolipids the amino group of sphingosine is then acylated (reaction *xviii*). These derivatives, termed ceramides, have themselves been isolated

$$(xviii) \quad CH_3(CH_2)_{12}CH = CH.CH.CH.CH_2OH + R.CO.S.CoA \rightarrow$$
$$\text{Sphingosine} \quad \underset{OH}{|} \ \underset{NH_2}{|}$$
$$Co.ASH + CH_3(CH_2)_{12}CH = CH.CH.CH.CH_2OH$$
$$\text{Ceramide} \quad \underset{OH}{|} \ \underset{NH.CO.R}{|}$$

from the brain of a child suffering Tay-Sach's disease (see below; Gatt & Berman, 1963) and may occur in small quantities in normal brain (Fig. 11.1). The fatty acids of ceramides are often of unusually long chain and unsaturated or hydroxylated, as is indicated below in considering other sphingolipids; the non-hydroxylated fatty acids of ceramides resembled those of sphingomyelin more than they did those of other sphingolipids (O'Brien & Rouser, 1964).

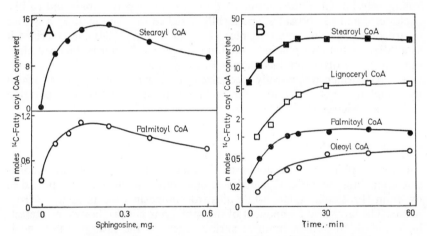

FIG. 11.8. Biosynthesis of ceramides in mouse brain microsomes. The microsomes were incubated for 10 min. in phosphate buffer, pH 7·4, with sphingosine or dihydrosphingosine, dithiothreitol (1 mM), ATP (2 mM), and ^{14}C-fatty acyl CoA (0·32 mM). Products were separated and identified by radioautography (Morell & Radin, 1970).
  A. Acylation of sphingosine with palmitoyl-CoA or stearoyl-CoA as a function of the sphingosine concentration.
  B. Acylation of dihydrosphingosine with various types of fatty acyl-CoA as a function of time. Relative rates from the log scale are, stearoyl-CoA:lignoceryl-CoA:palmitoyl-CoA:oleoyl-CoA =
60:12:3:1.

The process of acylation was catalysed by rat brain dispersions at pH 5 in presence of cholate and was detected using ^{14}C-palmitate or ^{3}H-sphingosine (Sribney, 1962, 1966; Gatt, 1963, 1966). The *acyltransferase* involved (reaction *xviii*) shows specificity towards different types of fatty acyl-CoA. Thus ceramide synthesis in mouse brain microsomes was most rapid with stearoyl-CoA; the ratios of incorporation of ^{14}C-labelled substrates were, stearoyl:lignoceryl:

palmitoyl:oleoyl $= 60:12:3:1$ (Morell & Radin, 1970; Fig. 11.8). It was suggested that the specificity of the acyltransferase may contribute to control of fatty acid distribution in sphingolipids. Ceramides are formed also from sphingomyelin (q.v.) by phosphatases, and are further hydrolysed to sphingosine by cerebral dispersions. From dispersions of young rat brain the ceramide-splitting enzyme was extracted by cholate; after salt fractionation a 100-fold purification was achieved, yielding a preparation which hydrolysed oleyl-sphingosine and certain other ceramides, but not sphingomyelin (Gatt, 1963). It seems possible that ceramides may also be synthesized by reversal of cerebral ceramidase activity (q.v., Fig. 11.11); the purified enzyme was subjected to numerous physical and chemical methods in attempts to separate the hydrolytic and synthetic activities, without success (Yavin & Gatt, 1969).

Sphingomyelin

Sphingomyelin constitutes about 10% of cerebral phospholipids and is, like cholesterol and cerebrosides, specifically enriched in white matter; it is thus regarded as a myelin lipid (Chapter 12). Thudichum (1884) characterized it as a "diamidated phosphatide containing no glycerol", purified its cadmium salt and by hydrolysis obtained the new hydroxyamine now termed sphingosine, with a base which was already recognized in other phospholipids and which gave analytical values required for choline. Current methods of preparation have been reviewed (Hanahan, 1961).

Components: Synthesis

Cerebral sphingomyelins are based almost entirely on choline and sphingosine. Small amounts of a C_{20}-analogue of sphingosine have been reported in ox brain (Proštenik, 1960), while dihydrosphingosine occurs in those from plants. The fatty-acid component of the sphingomyelins is, however, interestingly varied. In human brain at various ages, all the saturated fatty acids between C_{16} and C_{24} are represented, together with mono-unsaturated acids from C_{22} to C_{26} (Svennerholm, *Symposium*, 1963). Whereas in the foetus the C_{16} and C_{18} acids comprised 80% of the whole, a gradual increase in chain length occurred with myelination and with increasing age, until in white matter the C_{24} acids preponderated, especially the $C_{24:1}$, which formed 35% of the sphingomyelin fatty acids from the cerebral white matter of adults. In sphingomyelin from beef brain this acid and stearic preponderated, and the hydroxy acids present in cerebrosides and sulphatides were absent (O'Brien & Rouser, 1964).

Two alternative routes for sphingomyelin synthesis have been detected; only one may be relevant *in vivo* (below). The first has been characterized by following the incorporation of ^{14}C from CDP-^{14}C-choline (Sribney & Kennedy, 1958). This reaction (*xix*), catalysed by a phosphorylcholine-ceramide transferase (EC 2.7.8.3), is the analogue of reaction (*iii*) of lecithin synthesis. Cerebral dispersions from 10–20-day-old rats in a reaction mixture containing also a synthetic ceramide and a detergent gave incorporation corresponding to

0.1 μmole sphingomyelin/g. tissue/hr.: appreciably less than in renal preparations, which were however the main subject of the study.

(*xix*) $CH_3(CH_2)_{12}CH=CH.CH.CH.CH_2OH + CDP\text{-choline}$
$$\qquad\qquad\qquad\qquad\qquad\overset{|}{O}H\ \overset{|}{N}H.CO.R$$
Ceramide

$$CH_3(CH_2)_{12}CH=CH.CH.CH.CHO\overset{O}{\overset{\|}{P}}.OCH_2CH_2\overset{+}{N}(CH_3)_3 + CMP$$
$$\qquad\qquad\qquad\overset{|}{O}H\ \overset{|}{N}H\qquad \overset{|}{O}H$$
$$\qquad\qquad\qquad\qquad\quad\overset{|}{C}O.R$$
Sphingomyelin

The relevance of this route has been questioned because only the *threo* and not the *erythro* isomer of the sphingosine molecule reacts; *erythro* is the naturally-occurring form. The second alternative, reaction (*xx*), is therefore considered to be the more likely to operate *in vivo* since both *erythro* and *threo* isomers react (Brady *et al.*, 1965; Kanfer & Brady, 1967; Sribney, 1966; Fujino & Negishi, 1968). In this reaction, sphingomyelin is formed by direct acylation of sphingosine phosphorylcholine without involving ceramide as intermediate. Reaction (*xx*) is catalysed by *acyl-CoA: sphingosine N-acyl transferase*, a particulate enzyme more active in unpurified mitochondrial fractions than in microsomes and activated by Mg^{2+}.

(*xx*) Sphingosine + CDP-choline →

$$CH_3(CH_2)_{12}CH = CH.CH.CH.CH_2O\overset{O}{\overset{\|}{P}}.OCH_2CH_2\overset{+}{N}(CH_3)_3 + CMP$$
$$\qquad\qquad\qquad\overset{|}{O}H\ \overset{|}{N}H_2\qquad \overset{|}{O}H$$
Sphingosine phosphorylcholine

Fatty acyl-CoA

$$CH_3(CH_2)_{12}CH = CH.CH.CH.CH_2O\overset{O}{\overset{\|}{P}}.OCH_2CH_2\overset{+}{N}(CH_3)_3$$
$$\qquad\qquad\qquad\overset{|}{O}H\ \overset{|}{N}H\qquad \overset{|}{O}H$$
$$\qquad\qquad\qquad\qquad\overset{|}{C}O.R$$
Sphingomyelin

Enzymes degrading sphingomyelins have also been detected in the brain; a sphingomyelinase closely related to lecithinase yields ceramides and phosphorylcholine (Sribney, 1962; Roitman & Gatt, 1963; Brady, Symposium, 1970).

Sphingomyelin and Lipidoses

Sphingomyelin metabolism has a particular interest through abnormalities which occur in certain lipidoses. In one of the familial lipidoses, Niemann-Pick disease, disturbance of the nervous system is usually prominent and marked cellular changes occur in the brain. Lecithins and kephalins in the tissues are not abnormal, but sphingomyelin accumulated in abnormal amounts in the brain and in other organs, especially the liver. Cerebral sphingomyelin rose to maximum values of some 6% of the fresh weight in grey and white matter, representing a three- to twelve-fold increase (Klenk; Cumings, *Symposia*, 1957, 1962*a*). Sphingomyelin was enriched also in cerebrospinal fluids of the two cases examined by Tourtellotte *et al.* (*Symposium*, 1962*b*; 0·56 μmoles/100 ml.; normal value 0·12) but levels in blood serum were normal. In a few less typical instances, cerebral sphingomyelin and functioning may be little disturbed while sphingomyelin deposits occur elsewhere (Crocker, 1961; Ivemark *et al.*, 1963). In Tay-Sachs' disease (q.v.), a distinct sphingolipidosis, sphingomyelin was normal. In the sphingomyelin which accumulated in the brain in a case of infantile Niemann-Pick disease, C_{18}-fatty acids formed a larger proportion than usual, though C_{24}-acids also increased; the disease was considered to be due to a defect in the enzyme which normally hydrolysed sphingomyelin to produce phosphorylcholine and ceramide (Pilz and Jatzkewitz, 1964; Kampine *et al.*, 1967). Post mortem samples showed a loss of sulphatides as well as of sphingomyelin and an increase in cerebrosides and gangliosides G_{M2} and G_{M3} (q.v.) (Austin, 1965; Wallace *et al.*, 1964; Seiter & McCleur, 1970).

Sphingomyelin with other myelin lipids was greatly diminished in cerebral white matter from infants suffering the globoid-cell type of Krabbe's disease (Lees, *Symposium*, 1962*b*; Svennerholm, *Symposium*, 1963). This leucodystrophy is associated with regression of mental and motor development in the first year of life. Proteins of the cerebrospinal fluid are at three to ten times their normal value and of a pattern sufficiently characteristic to aid diagnosis (Hagberg *et al.*, 1963).

Glycolipids

The sphingolipids still to be discussed: cerebrosides, sulphatides and gangliosides, are no longer phospholipids but all carry carbohydrate residues and are thus glycolipids, a name which may also be extended to the inositides. The hydroxyl groups of the carbohydrate moiety make the glycolipids quite polar compounds as is evident in their chromatographic behaviour, when polar solvents are needed for their separation (Rouser *et al.*, 1961*b*; Rumsby, 1967). The cerebrosides and sulphatides remain, however, preponderantly fat-soluble; only the gangliosides, carrying many sugar residues, are readily soluble in water. Cerebral tissues have proved capable of most of the stages of glycolipid synthesis; the following account describes first some intermediates common to several glycolipids.

Hexose Incorporation

Galactose is the preponderant hexose of the glycolipids now to be considered, and the major cerebral deposition of lipids takes place during myelination, while mammals are ingesting much galactose in the lactose of milk. However, the brain has been found to contain normal quantities of galactolipids in two situations in which the available dietary galactose was negligible (Varma *et al.*,

1962); first, in young kittens reared on a galactose-free diet, and secondly in infants suffering galactosemia (q.v.).

After giving ^{14}C-galactose or ^{14}C-glucose intraperitoneally to young rats or mice, ^{14}C was found in cerebral glycolipids, mainly cerebrosides, in amounts which increased gradually between 1 and 6 hr. Degradation of the glycolipid showed the ^{14}C to be greatly enriched in the hexose moiety in comparison with the distribution to be expected had it been randomly incorporated (Burton et al., 1958). Also, from cerebral dispersions incubated anaerobically for 2 hr. with either of the ^{14}C-hexoses, MgATP and uridine, ^{14}C was again found in glycolipid fractions. Differential behaviour towards the hexoses was however induced by heating the dispersion to 50° before incubation: it could then incorporate ^{14}C of galactose but not of glucose. Differential centrifugation of the dispersion gave fractions of which the microsomal was most active in yielding labelled glycolipid from galactose. With this fraction and the previous reaction mixture, little ^{14}C incorporation took place without uridine; but galactose as UDP-^{14}C-galactose was still more effectively incorporated and ATP was not then required. Knowing the functions of uridine derivatives in other systems, this data led to the proposal of reactions which included:

(xxi) *Glucose-1-phosphate uridyltransferase:*
$$\text{Glucose-1-phosphate} + \text{UTP} \rightleftharpoons \text{UDP-glucose} + \text{pyrophosphate}$$

(xxii) *UDP-Glucose-4-epimerase:*
$$\text{UDP-Glucose} \rightleftharpoons \text{UDP-galactose}$$

(xxiii) *(See reactions xxvii to xxix below):*
$$\text{UDP-Galactose} + \text{acceptor} \rightleftharpoons \text{glycolipid} + \text{UDP}$$

The ^{14}C of glucose and galactose were maximally incorporated to the cerebral lipids of mice at 22 days of age, and were found in gangliosides (q.v.) as well as cerebrosides (Moser & Karnovsky, 1959).

Psychosine

This compound, sphingosine galactoside (Fig. 11.6) is the characteristic unit of the glycolipids; it was first obtained by their hydrolysis by baryta and fully characterized by Thudichum (1884). Evidence for its synthesis in the brain has been gained in the course of specifying the acceptor in reaction (xxiii) above. Using UDP-^{14}C-galactose and a microsomal fraction from the brain of young rats, no incorporation was obtained with ceramides. Thus the glycolipids were not synthesized from UDP-galactose in a single step. Sphingosine, however, acted as acceptor and psychosine was formed (Cleland & Kennedy, 1960). Incorporation was optimal with the natural *erythro*-sphingosine, and proceeded at a rate equivalent to 0·01 μmoles/hr. with microsomal material from 1 g. brain; a number of related compounds also reacted. Examination of other compounds in place of UDP-galactose showed it itself to be the primary galactose donor, but again the epimerase (reaction xxii) allowed UDP-glucose also to give psychosine. The galactosylsphingosine transferase (reaction xxvi below), was enriched in the more easily deposited microsomal fraction from guinea-pig brain; Mg^{2+}, a specific proportion of a polyoxyethylene detergent and a pH of 7–9 gave optimal reaction. The product was characterized as psychosine by a number of solvent and chromatographic distributions.

Cerebrosides

The cerebrosides also were first characterized by Thudichum in his studies of cerebral lipids; they have since been found in many other animal tissues. Cerebral white matter of many animal species remains one of the richest normal sources of cerebrosides; in adult mammals the spinal cord contains some 5·3% of its fresh weight and the brain as a whole 2·4%. Cerebrosides have been found absent from the nervous system of some but not all invertebrates (McColl & Rossiter, 1952; Varma *et al.*, 1962). Like sphingomyelin they lack glycerol but contain sphingosine; they are distinguished from other lipids in containing a carbohydrate radical, normally galactose. They contain a long-chain fatty acid as does sphingomyelin, and can be regarded as derivatives either of ceramides or of psychosine.

The bases yielded by a mixed cerebroside fraction from ox spinal cord have been found to contain 17% of dihydrosphingosine, and a cerebroside based on dihydrosphingosine has been isolated from human brain (Sweeley, 1959; Okuhara & Yasuda, 1960). The major component is C_{18}-sphingosine; only trace amounts of the C_{16}- or C_{20}-bases are present (Schwarz *et al.*, 1967). In other organs of the body and in blood plasma, cerebroside-like compounds have been found containing glucose, disaccharide or trisaccharide residues (Svennerholm & Svennerholm, 1963).

Cerebroside Fatty Acids

The fatty acids of four major cerebrosides from the mammalian brain are sufficiently distinct to have enabled the cerebroside mixture to be separated by solvents and fractional crystallization to the differently-named compounds of Fig. 11.6. Subsequent studies have confirmed the major fatty acids of cerebrosides as of C_{24}-chain length, with hydroxylated and unsaturated members, and have examined their synthesis and relationship to the many other acids present in smaller amounts (Radin & Akahori, 1961; Fulco & Mead, 1961; Mead & Levis, 1963; Klenk & Rivera, 1969).

From the brain of young rats, 1-^{14}C-acetate intraperitoneally during the four days before sampling afforded ^{14}C-glycolipids. The crude cerebroside fraction obtained on silicic acid chromatography, after methanolysis gave saturated and unsaturated fatty acids by mercuric acetate. Chromatography then gave many fractions with acids of chain length between C_{15} and C_{24}, and the C_{24} components were isolated in pure form. Stepwise degradation of the C_{24} acids showed ^{14}C almost entirely in the odd-numbered carbon atoms: suggesting synthesis by a simple repetitive process from the acetate (reactions *xxiv* and *xxv* below). In the case of the saturated acids lignoceric and cerebronic (Fig. 11.6) this occurred with very little dilution from preformed fatty acids. Moreover, lignoceric acid, the simplest and preponderating component, could be concluded by ^{14}C distribution to be the precursor of cerebronic acid. With the unsaturated acids, however, more ^{14}C was found in carbons near the carboxyl end of the molecule, and a synthetic route was postulated which involved lengthening the chain of oleic acid. The olefinic linkage is similarly placed in oleic, nervonic and hydroxynervonic acids; and again ^{14}C distribution suggested the hydroxy acid to derive from the non-hydroxylated.

The hydroxyacids of the cerebrosides appear likely, moreover, to be intermediates in the formation of some of the less usual cerebroside fatty acids, which have odd numbers of carbon atoms. These occur as minor constituents, for example the C_{19} and C_{21} components as about 1 % of the total saturated acids from several regions of two human brains; the C_{25} acid 1–8 % and the C_{23} as about 9 % (Radin & Akahori, 1961). For in rats, 5 months after 1-^{14}C-acetate administration in experiments similar to those just described, much ^{14}C remained in the cerebral sphingolipids; isolation of their C_{23}-fatty acids now showed the ^{14}C to be preponderantly in their even-numbered carbon atoms. An enzymic basis for this was demonstrated in cerebral microsomal fractions: on incubation with ATP, NAD$^+$ and ^{14}C-α-hydroxytricosanoic acid, $^{14}CO_2$ was evolved. From the corresponding non-hydroxylated acid, no $^{14}CO_2$ was obtained, but the α-keto acid yielded $^{14}CO_2$ more readily; ^{14}C-α-hydroxystearic acid also gave $^{14}CO_2$. In producing the odd-numbered acids from acetate, the following sequences are therefore suggested:

(*xxiv*) 12 Acetate $\rightarrow$ Lignoceric acid $\rightarrow$ Cerebronic acid

(*xxv*) 9 Acetate $\rightarrow$ Stearic acid $\rightarrow$ Oleic acid; + 3 Acetate $\rightarrow$ Nervonic acid

(*xxvi*) $CH_3.(CH_2)_nCHOH.COOH \rightarrow CH_3(CH_2)_nCO.COOH \rightarrow$
$$CH_3.(CH_2)_nCOOH + CO_2$$

Synthetic Routes and Breakdown

Two possible precursors of cerebrosides have been described above: ceramides and psychosine. Of these, ceramides do not readily yield cerebrosides under the experimental circumstances examined. Psychosine, however, is acylated by a microsomal fraction from the brain of young rats (Brady, 1962). Using ^{14}C-stearyl-CoA, in an anaerobic reaction mixture containing also ATP and a polyoxyethylene detergent, the ^{14}C was isolated and identified with carrier cerebroside. ^{14}C-Stearate did not so react and sphingosine in place of psychosine was less effective. This supports as synthetic route to cerebrosides a sequence of reactions (*xxi*), (*xxii*), (*xxvii*) and (*xxviii*):

(*xxvii*) *Galactosyl-sphingosine transferase:*
Sphingosine + UDP-galactose $\rightleftharpoons$ Psychosine + UDP

(*xxviii*) Psychosine + acyl-CoA $\rightleftharpoons$ Cerebroside + CoA

(*xxix*) Cerebroside + 3'-phosphoadenosine-5'-phosphosulphate $\rightleftharpoons$ sulphatide + ADP

with fatty acids produced as indicated above. That reaction (*xxviii*) is not the sole route of formation of cerebroside in the brain has recently been demonstrated; an alternative route is given by transfer of galactose from UDP-galactose to ceramide (Fujino & Nakano, 1969). The naturally occurring *erythro*-ceramides proved more reactive than *threo*-ceramides and the enzyme enriched in crude mitochondrial and particularly microsomal preparations was more active in the brain than in the liver. The methods of demonstrating

12

the two routes of cerebroside biosynthesis depend on extraction and chromato-graphic separation of isotopically-labelled products; it is not clear which of the two is the preferred pathway *in vivo*. It is of interest that these two reactions are analogous to the two alternative reactions which have been observed to lead to sphingomyelin biosynthesis (*xix* and *xx*, above). The reaction with UDP-galactose is also involved in synthesis of cerebrosides containing hydroxy-fatty acids: mouse brain microsomes were found to catalyse formation from UDP-galactose and 2-hydroxy-fatty acid ceramide. The activity was exhibited best when the ceramide was finely dispersed in diatomaceous earth in the absence of detergent and showed a high degree of specificity in that ceramides with non-hydroxylated fatty acids did not react. Optimally activated, about 3 nmoles of ^{14}C-galactose were incorporated per hr. into the microsomes from 1 g of immature mouse brain (Morell & Radin, 1969).

On continued growth of rats after ^{14}C-galactose has been incorporated to cerebrosides of the brain, the ^{14}C is gradually lost though cerebroside content increases (Radin *et al.*, 1957). Liberation of galactose from its combined form by cerebral enzymes has been observed at 2·3 μmoles/g. hr. Chemically synthesized ^{14}C-cerebrosides administered to young rats also yielded ceramides; no incorporation to ganglioside-like compounds was detected (Kanfer, 1965). The *cerebrosidase* of rat brain occurs in lysosomes and required detergent for maximal activity. Inhibition studies suggested the enzyme to be active on galactosides rather than glucosides (Bowen & Radin, 1968).

Cerebrosides and Lipidoses

In Tay-Sachs' disease, which is considered more fully below, an unusual class of cerebrosides containing glucose in place of galactose occurs in the membranous cytoplasmic bodies which are then found in cerebral cells (Samuels *et al.*, 1963). Such glucocerebrosides had been found previously to accumulate in several organs of the body in the infantile form of Gaucher's disease (Thannhauser, 1953; Banker *et al.*, *Symposium*, 1962a). Involvement of the central nervous system is prominent in infantile Gaucher's disease; glucosylceramide accumulates in the grey matter and in peripheral tissues as a result of virtual absence of glucocerebrosidase (β-glucosidase; *e*, Fig. 11.11). Partial deficiency of the enzymic activity (15% of normal) has been observed in the tissues of patients with the adult form of the disease (Brady; Jatzkewitz *et al.*, Symposium, 1970).

In the globoid-cell type of Krabbe's disease, cerebrosides with other myelin lipids are found in diminished amounts in the white matter of the brain (Lees, *Symposia*, 1962a, 1962b). Cerebrosides are diminished also in the metachro-matic leucodystrophy discussed below.

Ceramide trihexoside (galactosyl-galactosyl-glucosyl-ceramide) is a neutral glycolipid which accumulates in the tissues of patients suffering from Fabry's disease. Cerebral dysfunction is prominent in this sex-linked inherited disease; deposition of glycolipid occurs in neurons as well as in many non-neural sites in the body. Activity of *ceramide trihexosidase*, which normally removes the terminal galactose from the glycolipid, has been shown to be decreasd in many tissues examined, and to be absent from the blood, of Fabry's patients

(Brady et al., 1967; Gatt & Berman, 1963; Sweeley & Klionsky, 1966; Mapes et al., 1970). The ceramide trihexoside has been found elevated in the plasma of patients and of female relatives but the erythrocyte content remained normal (Vance et al., 1969). The use of leucocytes also has been recommended as diagnostic material for a range of lipidoses. Good correlation of activities of glucocerebrosidase, sphingomyelinase and arylsulphatase A was found with Gaucher's disease, Niemann-Pick disease and metachromatic leucodystrophy respectively (Snyder & Brady, 1969).

Sulphatides

Thudichum (1884) found fractions from the brain which contained sulphur as well as phosphorus, which he attributed to "sulphocerebrosides". Sulphatides as now recognized with equimolar quantities of galactose, sphingosine and sulphur but no phosphorus were characterized by Blix (1933) and given the structure of Fig. 11.6 by Thannhauser et al. (1955), with cerebronic acid as the main fatty acid. Sulphatides based on lignoceric acid and possibly on nervonic acid have since been separated by partition chromatography and counter-current distribution, and the main components synthesized by chlorosulphonic acid sulphonation of phrenosine and kerosine (Jatzkewitz, 1960). Sulphatides are separable from cerebrosides on silicic acid columns and by chromatography with silica-impregnated paper, which also gives several fractions among the sulphatides as also does thin-layer chromatography (Long & Staples, 1961; Rouser et al., 1961b; O'Brien et al., 1964).

Formation of Sulphatides

In young rats, $^{35}SO_4^{2-}$ becomes incorporated to cerebral lipids and could still be detected in the brain, as sulphatides, many months later; much more rapid turnover of sulphatides occurred in other organs (Green & Robinson, 1960; Davison, 1961). Incorporation was most rapid during myelination, and sulphatides are enriched in white matter (Table 11.1). The incorporation still occurred in older rats though at much diminished rate and cerebral tissues from adult guinea pigs yielded ^{35}S-sulphatides from $^{35}SO_4^{2-}$ in vitro (Bakke & Cornatzer, 1961; Heald & Robinson, 1961). For maximum incorporation oxygen and an oxidizable substrate were needed; no breakdown of the sulphatides, once formed, was detected in these experiments (see below). This is in keeping with the persistence of ^{35}S and ^{14}C-galactose in the sulphatides of the brain in vivo (Radin et al., 1957, and Chapter 13). The time-course of ^{14}C-galactose incorporation was consistent with cerebrosides yielding sulphatides in vivo, and in vitro sulphonation was indeed demonstrated with 3'-phosphoadenosine-5'-phosphosulphate (reaction xxix above; Goldberg, 1961), catalysed by a cerebral preparation.

The fatty acid mixture from the sulphatides of ox brain resembled that from the cerebrosides but was distinct from that of other sphingolipids (O'Brien & Rouser, 1964). The similarity extended to both the hydroxylated and the non-hydroxylated fatty acids and again suggested cerebrosides and sulphatides to have synthetic routes in common.

Sulphatide Lipidosis

Some 25 years after their characterization, the sulphatides were realized to represent the main chemical peculiarity of an inherited disorder of lipid metabolism. In this condition, a late infantile metachromatic leucodystrophy or Scholz's leucodystrophy, the first symptoms are seen in apparently normal children at 1–2 years and are of motor weakness which increases and becomes associated with optic atrophy and dementia before death at about 5 years. Lesions are then evident macroscopically in white matter of the spinal cord and brain which also shows atrophy. Lipid deposits are seen microscopically in the affected areas and these stain metachromatically (see Chapter 12) with basic dyes including cresyl violet and toluidine blue. By extraction and fractionation, the constituent responsible for this staining was shown to be a sulphatide (Austin; Svennerholm; Lees in *Symposium*, 1963). Accumulation in the brain of heparan sulphate may occur in variants of the disease (Bichel *et al.*, 1966).

Analysis of cerebral tissues from normal infants of 1–5 years of age then showed sulphatides in grey matter to range from 0·4–0·8% of the dry weight, and in white matter, from 2 to 4·1%. In specimens from infants who had suffered the metachromatic leucodystrophy values were 2% in grey and 16% in white matter. Especially characteristic was the ratio of cerebroside to sulphatide content, of 4:1 in normal infant brain, becoming 1:4 in the leucodystrophy. The sulphatides accumulate not only in the brain but also in peripheral nerve and in the kidney, and biopsy specimens of a few mg. of tissue from each of these sources have been found to yield sufficient sulphatides to afford a chemical diagnosis of the leucodystrophy. Minute quantities only of the sulphatides were detectable in cerebrospinal fluid, normal or from the patients; urinary sediments by extraction and chromatography yielded sulphatides, but afforded less secure diagnosis than did the tissue samples (Hagberg, *Symposium*, 1963; Austin, Lees, *Symposium*, 1962a; Evans & McCleur, 1969).

Cerebral samples taken post mortem from two children suffering metachromatic leucodystrophy showed several enzymes relevant to sulphatide metabolism to be at normal levels. The formation of 4-nitrocatechol from its sulphuric ester on incubating with a cerebral extract, however, occurred at rates equivalent to about 0·1 μmole/g. tissue/hr., whereas tissues from normal subjects gave values of about 2–4 (Austin *et al.*, 1963). Enzymes normally active on sulphatides (arylsulphatase A and cerebroside sulphatase) were deficient in the white matter of such post-mortem samples (Jatzkewitz & Meyl, 1969) and in the leucocytes of patients and their female relatives (Snyder & Brady, 1969).

Gangliosides

Gangliosides are the most hydrophilic of the fatty acid derivatives of the brain. The name comes from their enrichment in cerebral grey matter ("ganglia") and was given when they were known to contain stearic acid, sphingosine, galactose and a specific acidic component newly named neuraminic acid (Klenk, 1941, 1942). Klenk had observed a red colour given with Bial's reagent by cerebral lipids from cases of Tay-Sachs' disease. The reagent (orcinol-HCl-

FeCl$_3$) is still valuable in recognizing N-acetylneuraminic acid; gangliosides were soon detected in normal brain but are indeed greatly increased in amount in Tay-Sach's disease (see below). Later N-acetylgalactosamine was recognized in gangliosides and they were extracted by much simpler processes which gave about 2 μmoles of lipid N-acetylneuraminic acid/g. of normal cerebral grey matter (Blix *et al.*, 1950; Folch *et al.*, 1951). By chromatographic methods, these extracts from normal and abnormal cerebral tissues have been shown to contain a group of lipids, related in structure as is shown in Fig. 11.9 (Klenk & Gielen, 1963; Kuhn & Wiegandt, 1963; Svennerholm, 1963; Wolfe & Lowden, 1964).

Gangliosides have been found in the brain of birds, fishes, and a number of mammalian species; they were present in all of ten cerebral regions examined and also in retina. Particular ganglioside components were also detectable in the spleen, kidney, liver and muscle of the guinea pig (Trams & Lauter, 1962; Svennerholm, 1963; Wherrett & Cumings, 1963). In the brain from several mammals, stearic acid formed 80–90% of their fatty acid component. Gangliosides determined in some 20 parts of the human brain were enriched in neuronal rather than white-matter regions (Lowden & Wolfe, 1964). Immunoelectrophoretic methods for detecting different gangliosides are now available (Pascal & Saifer, 1969).

Sialoproteins also contain N-acetylneuraminic acid and may contribute as much as 15% of the total protein of the brain; the N-acetylneuraminic acid of the glycoproteins accounts for some 30% of the total present in the brain. In addition to N-acetylneuraminic acid and protein, they contain hexoses (mannose, galactose and glucose), glucosamine, galactosamine and fucose (6-deoxygalactose; Brunngraber & Brown, 1963, 1964; Brunngraber, 1969).

Ganglioside Components

The gangliosides can be defined as acylsphingosyl oligosaccharides containing a sialic acid. In a number of chromatographic systems they separate in the order quoted in Table 11.6. Least retarded is the monosialoganglioside of smallest molecular size, followed by the intermediate compound and then by the most plentiful monosialocompound which is formulated in full in Fig. 11.9. The two disialogangliosides follow, first (*a*) which constitutes 60% of the cerebral ganglioside content and in which the two acetylneuraminic acid residues are separated by three hexose residues: and then (*b*) in which the two residues are adjacent. The trisialoganglioside follows.

Ganglioside structures have been established by detailed analyses of the different components and of derivatives, especially after methylation and hydrolysis. The components differ in their susceptibility to acid and enzymic hydrolysis (Kuhn & Wiegandt, 1963; Svennerholm, 1963). In particular, the two most abundant monosialogangliosides were resistant to a microbial sialidase which liberated N-acetylneuraminic acid from many natural products. The sialidase however converted the trisialoganglioside first to a mixture of the disialo compounds and subsequently to monosialoganglioside (1, G$_{M1}$).

Ganglioside components differ also in their reactivity towards tissue constituents. Thus the trisialoganglioside is extracted from the brain only with difficulty by the chloroform–methanol mixtures usually employed, or by tetrahydrofuran (Wolfe & Lowden 1964). The quantity of gangliosides retained in tissues so extracted, increases after they have been kept cold or under anoxic conditions (Balakrishnan & McIlwain, 1961; Thompson & McIlwain, 1961; Booth, 1962, 1963) and of tissue constituents, basic proteins were found to cause the retention. The gangliosides so retained were richer in N-acetylneuraminic acid than those extracted. Presumably salt-formation was involved, for extraction could be increased by addition of suramin, a polyacidic

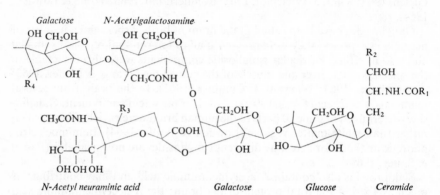

Compound[1]	Abbrev.[1]	R_3	R_4	Other change
Monosialoganglioside (1)	G_{M1}	OH	OH	—
Monosialoganglioside (2)	G_{M2}	OH	OH	Lacks terminal galactose
Monosialoganglioside (3)	G_{M3}	OH	OH	Lacks terminal galactose and acetylgalactosamine
Disialoganglioside a	G_{D1a}	OH	N-AN	–
Disialoganglioside b	G_{D1b}	N-AN	OH	–
Trisialoganglisode	G_{T1}	N-AN	N-AN	–
Tetrasialoganglioside	G_{Q1}	N-AN	N-AN-N-AN	–

FIG. 11.9. Cerebral gangliosides.
R_1 is preponderantly stearic acid and the carbon chain terminating in R_2, preponderantly sphingosine. See Kuhn & Wiegandt (1963); [1] nomenclature of Svennerholm (1963). N-AN: N-acetylneuraminic acid.

antitrypanosomal drug. These interactions could condition tissue excitability (McIlwain, 1961 and see Chapter 12).

Body fluids contain very little ganglioside-like material (Tourtellotte *et al.*, *Symposium*, 1962b; Booth, 1964). In cerebrospinal fluid no more than 0·1 nmole/ml. was found, close to the limits of the methods available; the total phosphorus-free sphingolipids were about 1 nmole/ml. Much more N-acetyl-neuraminic acid occurred in non-lipid combined forms: about 50 nmoles/ml. In blood plasma, again, any ganglioside-like compounds were barely detectable and the phosphorus-free sphingolipids, some 0·3 nmoles/ml. Erythrocytes, however, from normal or schizophrenic subjects, yielded about 5 nmoles/ml. of ganglioside-like substances.

Metabolism of Ganglioside Constituents

Synthesis, interconversion and degradation of ganglioside constituents are as yet only partly investigated. Available data indicate moderate metabolic rates: among acidic cerebral lipids, ganglioside components show rates of turnover much below those of the phosphoinositides but greater than found in the sulphatides. Aminosugars and N-acetylneuraminic acid are considered first in the account which follows; it is to be noted that these compounds form part of mucoproteins and of mucopolysaccharides as well as of gangliosides.

Aminosugars

Isotope incorporation studies (see below) indicate the formation of ganglio-sides to proceed by routes which in other systems involve some or all of the N-acetyl and uridine diphosphate derivatives of glucosamine, galactosamine and mannosamine. The numerous relevant reactions in the brain itself have been most fully explored in relation to glucosamine. Investigation of the metabolism of glucosamine derivatives in the body as a whole suggests glucos-amine to be preferred for further synthetic routes rather than N-acetylglucos-amine (Kohn *et al.*, 1962). Presumably phosphorylation occurs before acetylation; the sugar phosphates are readily available, and, as noted above a route has been demonstrated in the brain between glucose- and galactose-1-phosphates through uridine diphosphate derivatives (Chapters 5 and 8; Burton, *Symposium*, 1960). Cerebral hexokinase has been considered to catalyse the phosphorylation of glucosamine, but a distinct acetylglucosamine kinase which brings about the phosphorylation of N-acylated aminosugars has been purified from sheep brain (Pattabiraman & Bachhawat, 1961).

Commencing with fructose-6-phosphate, available as an intermediate in glycolysis, the initial stage of amination is catalysed by buffered extracts from human cerebral cortex (Pattabiraman & Bachhawat, 1961; reaction *xxx* below). After salt precipitation and heat treatment which together gave a 70-fold enrichment, the yield of glucosamine-6-phosphate from fructose-6-phosphate and ammonium salts was markedly accelerated by small amounts of N-acetyl-glucosamine-6-phosphate. Galactose and mannose-6-phosphates did not serve as substrates; in other systems, it may be noted, distinct enzymes have been suggested as responsible for interconversion among the aminosugars or their derivatives.

Acetylation of glucosamine-6-phosphate (reaction *xxxi*) by acetyl CoA was catalysed by an aqueous extract of grey matter from sheep brain, forming per hr. with material from 1 g. brain about 0·1 μmoles of N-acetylglucosamine-6-phosphate. Salt precipitation and adsorption gave a 75-fold enrichment of the enzyme, which then needed MgATP and cysteine as well as the major reactants. Its product can be converted by a cerebral mutase to N-acetyl-glucosamine-1-phosphate which acts as substrate for a uridyl transferase (reaction *xxxii*; Burton, *Symposium*, 1960; Pattabiraman & Bachhawat, 1962):

(*xxx*) Fructose-6-phosphate + NH_3 ⇌ Glucosamine-6-phosphate

(*xxxi*) Glucosamine-6-phosphate + acetyl-CoA →
$$N\text{-Acetylglucosamine-6-phosphate} + CoA$$

(xxxii) N-Acetylglucosamine-1-phosphate + UTP $\rightleftharpoons$

UDP-Acetylglucosamine + pyrophosphate

Uridine diphosphate acetylglucosamine was demonstrated in rat brain, and the uridyltransferase in an extract from sheep brain, which was purified by ethanol and salt fractionations.

N-Acetylneuraminic Acid

The component which most clearly differentiates the gangliosides from other sphingolipids is the sialic acid, which in all instances examined has been N-acetylneuraminic acid. Neuraminic acid itself is unstable and synthetic routes have proved to involve the N-acyl derivatives or sialic acids; gangliosides comprise about half the sialic acid derivatives of human brain, the remainder being mainly as sialoproteins, and from both these sources crystalline N-acetylneuraminic acid has been isolated and characterized (Svennerholm, 1956). Any free N-acetylneuraminic acid which may exist in cerebrospinal fluid is at quite low concentration; the value found for total dialyzable N-acetylneuraminic acid and derivatives in human cerebrospinal fluid was 15 nmoles/ ml. (Booth, 1964).

Synthesis of N-acetylneuraminic acid in the brain itself has been observed and the system responsible, extracted by buffered salines from sheep brain, purified 20-fold by salt precipitation (Joseph & Bachhawat, 1964). From about 1 mM-N-acetylmannosamine-6-phosphate and phosphoenolpyruvate, with glutathione and Mg^{2+}, 0·1 μmole N-acetylneuraminic acid was produced per hour with material from 1 g. tissue. N-Acetylmannosamine or pyruvate did not substitute for the phosphorylated derivatives in the condensation, but the product, measured and characterized, was N-acetylneuraminic acid itself. Two reactions, xxxiii and xxxiv, were presumably involved:

(xxxiii) N-Acetyl-D-mannosamine-6-phosphate + phosphoenolpyruvate $\rightarrow$

N-Acetylneuraminic acid-9-phosphate + PO_4^{3-}

(xxxiv) N-Acetylneuraminic acid-9-phosphate $\rightarrow$ N-Acetylneuraminic acid + PO_4^{3-}

(xxxv) N-Acetylneuraminic acid $\rightarrow$ N-Acetylmannosamine + pyruvate

The rate of formation of N-acetylneuraminic acid by this route in some fifteen parts of the brain, though low, was greater than in other tissues rich in sialic acid derivatives. The equilibrium of reaction xxxiii is markedly in favour of formation of N-acetylneuraminic acid phosphate (Warren & Felsenfeld, 1962). Cleavage of N-acetylneuraminic acid to N-acetylmannosamine and pyruvate (reaction xxxv) has been observed in preparations from a number of animal organs including the brain of some but not all mammals (Brunetti et al., 1962). In guinea pig it corresponded to about 2 μmoles/g. brain/hr. Reversal of reaction xxxv had been thought a possible route to N-acetylneuraminic acid, but the irregular distribution reported makes this less likely. It is probable that N-acetylneuraminic acid is incorporated to gangliosides or mucoproteins as its cytidine monophosphate derivative, formed by a reaction in part analogous to (ii) above. In mixtures with CTP, Mg^{2+} and thiols a cerebral extract equivalent to 1 g. sheep brain catalysed the formation of about 0·5 μmoles of cytidine monophosphate-N-acetyl neuraminic acid per hour (Shoyab et al., 1964).

By adsorption and salt fractionation forty-fold enrichment of the enzyme was obtained; other nucleotides did not replace CTP and the reaction was inhibited by excess pyrophosphate.

Incorporation of Precursors to Gangliosides

Ganglioside synthesis occurs in the brain as indicated by the incorporation of a number of isotopically-labelled compounds to cerebral ganglioside fractions. Thus after perfusing the brain of a monkey with solutions containing $1\text{-}^{14}C$-acetate or $1\text{-}^{14}C$-octanoate, the ^{14}C became widely distributed in cerebral lipids, and greatest activity among sphingolipids was found in a crude fraction containing gangliosides; long-chain fatty acids were incorporated in other experiments (Weiss, 1956; Berman & Gatt, *Symposium*, 1962a). In young rats, $1\text{-}^{14}C$-galactose given intraperitoneally on one day sufficiently labelled the sphingolipids for change in ^{14}C in several fractions to be followed in subsequent weeks. The exchange which followed resulted in loss of half the ^{14}C from gangliosides in 8 days, which was a more rapid change than in cerebrosides; in sulphatides no change was detected (Radin *et al.*, 1957).

When ^{14}C-glucose and ^{14}C-galactose were compared as lipid precursors after intraperitoneal injection to young mice (Moser & Karnovsky, 1959), ganglioside fractions became labelled to a degree below that of lipids generally but above that of cholesterol. The incorporation was greatest in mice of 5–20 days of age, falling in adults to one-quarter of the maximal value. When $6\text{-}^{14}C$-glucose was used, all the ^{14}C in the glucose of the gangliosides remained in the 6 position; ^{14}C was found also in the galactose and galactosamine residues, and of this 20–40% was in the 6-position. Direct incorporation of glucose to gangliosides was thus indicated, and relatively little unspecified change during the conversion to and incorporation as galactose. Use of pure labelled precursors and a particulate fraction from embryonic chicken brain has led to elucidation of some of the intermediate stages (Basu *et al.*, 1968; Kaufman *et al.*, 1968). Two UDP-hexosetransferases and three sialyl transferases participate in the reaction sequence of Fig. 11.10. The first stages (*a, b*) involve the stepwise transfer of UDPG and UDP-galactose to ceramide to produce ceramide lactose (**A**, Fig. 11.10). Stage **A** is sequential: galactosyl transferase (*b*) reacts only with ceramide–glucose. Three types of sialyl transferase (CMP-NANA-monosialoganglioside transferase) are thought to occur and require detergents for activity *in vitro* (*c, d* and *e* of **B** and **C**, Fig. 11.10).

Net increase in the ganglioside content of rat brain takes place after birth, the lipid-soluble N-acetylneuraminic acid increasing from 0·12 to 1 μmole/ brain and from 0·3 to 0·7 μmole/g. fresh brain in the first 30 days. The mixture of ganglioside components appeared similar during this time (Burton *et al.*, 1963). The incorporation of several labelled precursors administered intraperitoneally 1 day before cerebral samples were taken occurred at greatest rate in animals about 10–12 days old. Isolation and degradation of the gangliosides showed different precursors to have labelled different parts of the ganglioside molecules. Glucosamine gave much more ^{14}C to galactosamine and N-acetylneuraminic acid than to other components. $3\text{-}^{14}C$-Serine contributed to sphingosine as well as to carbohydrates including N-acetyl-neuraminic acid. The ^{14}C from D-1-^{14}C-glucose and -galactose appeared in all the carbohydrate components; it could be concluded that the precursor

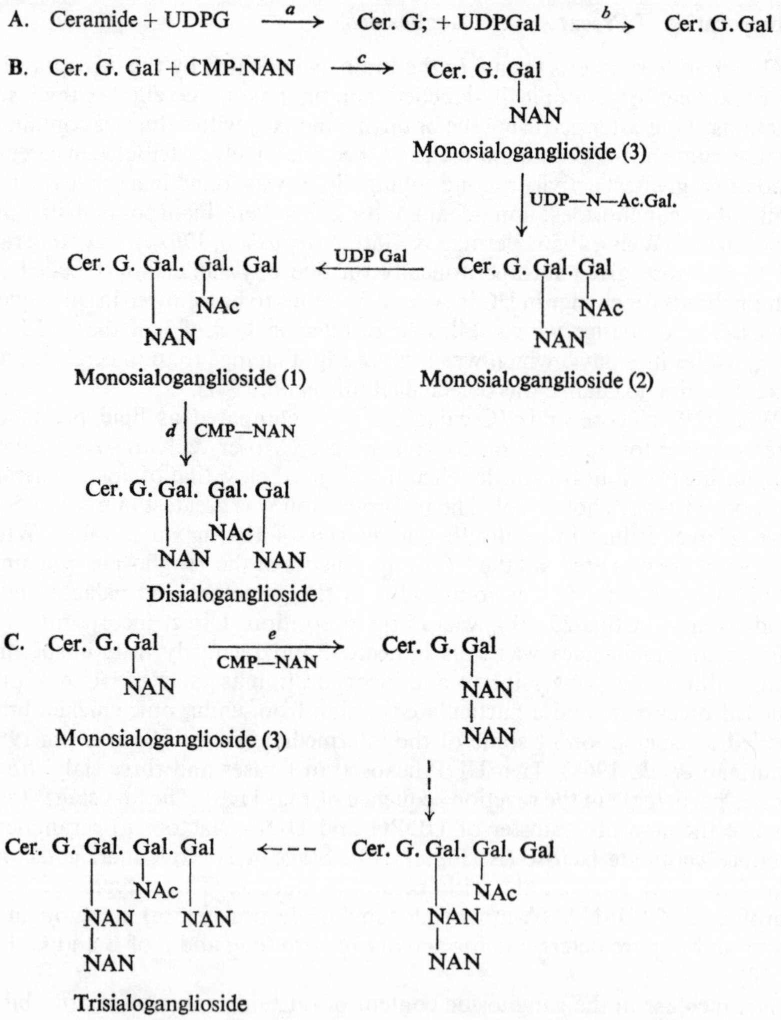

A. Ceramide + UDPG $\xrightarrow{a}$ Cer. G; + UDPGal $\xrightarrow{b}$ Cer. G. Gal

B. Cer. G. Gal + CMP-NAN $\xrightarrow{c}$ Cer. G. Gal
  |
  NAN

Monosialoganglioside (3)

| UDP—N—Ac.Gal.

Cer. G. Gal. Gal. Gal $\xleftarrow{\text{UDP Gal}}$ Cer. G. Gal. Gal
  | |
  NAc   NAc
NAN   NAN

Monosialoganglioside (1)   Monosialoganglioside (2)

d | CMP—NAN

Cer. G. Gal. Gal. Gal
  |
  NAc |
NAN   NAN

Disialoganglioside

C. Cer. G. Gal $\xrightarrow[\text{CMP—NAN}]{e}$ Cer. G. Gal
  | |
  NAN   NAN
                                     |
Monosialoganglioside (3)   NAN

Cer. G. Gal. Gal. Gal $\xleftarrow{---}$ Cer. G. Gal. Gal. Gal
  | |
  NAc | NAc
NAN   NAN   NAN
  | |
NAN   NAN

Trisialoganglioside

FIG. 11.10. Biosynthesis of gangliosides.
For chemical structures, see Fig. 11.7. Cer, Ceramide; G, glucose; Gal, galactose; NAN, N-acetylneuraminyl; NAc, N-acetyl-. a: glucosyl transferase; b: galactosyl transferase; c, d, e: different sialyl transferases. The dotted lines represent stages involving more than one enzymic reaction.

pools for synthesis of galactosamine and N-acetylneuraminic acid were small. When the mono-, di- and tri-sialogangliosides were obtained from young rats receiving ^{14}C-glucose and were degraded, the N-acetylneuraminic acid in each was found to contain ^{14}C, but the monosialo compound did not appear to act as precursor for the others (Suzuki & Korey, 1964). N-Acetylneuraminic acid, injected intracisternally, is itself incorporated directly to the gangliosides of the brain but to a lesser extent than is glucosamine. Only 0·3% of the ^{14}C from labelled N-acetylneuraminic acid was found in the ganglioside fraction compared with 2 to 3% of the ^{14}C from glucosamine (DeVries & Barondes, 1971).

Cerebral Sialidases

Cerebral dispersions catalyse a slow liberation of N-acetylneuraminic acid from native or added gangliosides (Carubelli et al., 1962; Booth, 1963, 1964). The reaction can proceed at about 0·5 μmoles/g. tissue/hr. and was found maximal at pH 5·2; it ceased before all the ganglioside-N-acetylneuraminic acid had been released, and in this resembled the action of the microbial sialidase mentioned above. The cerebral reaction was not inhibited by D-glucurono-lactone and thus was not likely to represent activity of a glucuronidase. It contributed partly to the loss of extractable ganglioside which occurred when cerebral tissues or dispersions were incubated anaerobically (Korey, *Symposium*, 1963: Lowden & Wolfe, 1963; Booth, 1963); combination with tissue constituents also contributes, as noted above.

The neuraminidase of calf brain hydrolyses di- and tri-sialogangliosides but is inactive against mono-sialogangliosides. Extraction from acetone powders required detergents; rates of about 1 μmole/hr. g. of original tissue were reported (Leibovitz & Gatt, 1968; Tettamanti & Zambotti, 1968). Full degradation of the cerebral gangliosides requires enzymes other than neuraminidase (a), shown in Fig. 11.11. Two β-galactosidases have been detected: one (b) active on monosialogangliosides, the other (d) on lactosylceramide. A β-glucosidase (e) hydrolyses the glucosylceramide produced from lactosylceramide degradation. All of these enzymes are particulate and require detergents for maximal activity. The same seems true for N-acetylhexosaminidase (c) which forms N-acetylneuraminyl-lactosylceramide from monosialoganglioside (2; G_{M2}). The final stage of ganglioside degradation is catalysed by ceramidase (f) which splits ceramide to form sphingosine and free fatty acid (Gatt, 1965; 1966; Gatt & Rapport, 1966; Frohwein & Gatt, 1967; Gatt, 1970).

Mild acid hydrolysis can liberate all the N-acetylneuraminic acid from gangliosides, yielding "asialogangliosides": ceramide-sugar derivatives which have proved of value in understanding the structure of gangliosides. The neuraminidase activity of human and bovine cerebral cortex was found highest in grey matter and in synaptosomal subfractions; half-maximal activity of bovine brain preparations was obtained with 8×10^{-5} M ganglioside (Schengrund & Rosenberg, 1970; Öhman, 1971; Öhman & Svennerholm, 1971).

Gangliosidoses

Tay-Sachs' Disease

This disease (*Symposia*, 1959, 1962a, b), in the infantile form first recognized, begins in the first few months of the life of those who have inherited the recessive factors involved. Muscular weakness and blindness develop, and mental development stops or regresses; death occurs at 1–5 years. The head and brain often increase in size, the increase being especially in white matter of the cerebral hemispheres. Microscopically, increased extracellular space is evident and cellular changes are seen, especially the occurrence among the normal organelles, of abundant granules 0·5–2 μ in diameter. These are found electron microscopically after osmic acid treatment to consist almost entirely of concentric layers of membranes, closely and regularly packed. By dispersing biopsy specimens of the affected tissue in ethylenediamine tetraacetate solution, differentially centrifuging and then collecting material between 0·75 and 1·2 M-sucrose, preparations were obtained in which the granules formed over 90 % (Korey et al., 1963; Samuels et al., 1963). These contained 92 % of lipid and

Table 11.6

Distribution of cerebral gangliosides

Ganglioside component	Abbrev.	R_f, n-propanol-water, thin-layer silica gel	Distribution (%) in the brain of infants	
			Normal	Tay-Sach's
Monosialo-3	G_{M3}	0·47	0·7	0
2	G_{M2}	0·42	5·7	90*
1	G_{M1}	0·37	25·2	5
Disialo- a	G_{D1a}	0·27	60	+
b	G_{D1b}	0·22	3·3	+
Trisialo-	G_{T1}	0·19	4·8	+

R_f values give the distribution on chromatographic analysis; the cerebral composition was obtained from samples from the whole brain of infants, normal and suffering Tay-Sach's disease (Svennerholm, 1962, 1963). For structures, see Fig. 11.9.

* Wherrett & Cumings (1963) found 83% and Booth (1964), 87% ; + : component detectable.

8 % protein, and, remarkably, of their dry weight 35 to 50% consisted of gangliosides; cholesterol and phospholipid were also present.

Direct analysis of the brain in Tay-Sachs' disease shows an accumulation of gangliosides, which increase to two to three times their normal value in grey matter and five to six times in white matter (Korey et al., 1963; Svennerholm, 1963). Moreover, a single ganglioside component now preponderates: the monosialoganglioside (2, G_{M2}). Table 11.6 shows that this is usually only a minor constituent of the cerebral gangliosides; it lacks the terminal galactose residue found in the gangliosides which normally are most plentiful. By contrast, the cerebral grey matter in Tay-Sachs' disease has normal content of cholesterol, sphingomyelins, and other phospholipids collectively (Crocker, 1961); but its glycolipids are increased not only among hydrophilic compounds which would include gangliosides but also in less hydrophilic compounds. Changes in white matter followed a different course; after initially normal values almost all categories of lipids diminished between 20–40 months of age, when active myelination is normally in progress. Biopsy specimens from the brain soon after the appearance of Tay-Sachs' disease have been found normal in respiratory rate but to retain an amino acid content below normal; with progress of the disease, respiratory rate diminished (Korey *et al.*, 1963).

Total *N*-acetylhexosaminidase activity (*b* of Fig. 11.11) seems to be unchanged in Tay-Sach's disease. However, the enzyme occurs in two forms (A and B); hexosaminidase A activity is deficient in the disease. The ganglioside which accumulates is the substrate for the enzyme when present. Prenatal diagnosis of the disease has proved possible by estimation of hexosaminidase A activity in foetal cells cultured from samples of amniotic fluid from the mother (Schneck *et al.*, 1970).

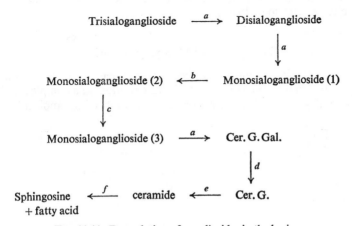

FIG. 11.11. Degradation of gangliosides in the brain.
a: Neuraminidase; *b*: β-galactosidase I; *c*: *N*-acetylhexosaminidase; *d*: β-galactosidase II; *e*: β-glucosidase; *f*: ceramidase.
For ganglioside structures, see Fig. 11.9; abbreviations are as in Fig. 11.10.

Generalized Gangliosidosis

A form of infant amaurotic idiocy or "late infantile lipidosis", distinct from Tay-Sachs' disease, has recently been detected and given a variety of names (see O'Brien, 1969). It is caused by deficiency of β-galactosidase (*b* of Fig. 11.11) and characterized by accumulation in the brain of ceramide tetrahexoside and G_{M1}-ganglioside, and in the urine of an undersulphated keratan sulphate. The enzyme has been shown to be deficient in the brains, leucocytes and cultured fibroblasts from the diseased infants. Two forms of the disorder are known and differ in time of onset and in enzymic properties. In Type I the symptoms are similar to those of Hurler's syndrome (see below) and become apparent within the first 5 months of life; death occurs by 2 years of age. The β-galactosidase activity in cultured fibroblasts was about 5% of normal and its pH optimum and thermostability were abnormal. In Type II, the symptoms appear later, within 1 year, and death occurs usually by 5 years of age. The β-galactosidase activity was lower than in Type I (less than 1% of normal) and its properties were similar to that of the normal fibroblasts. It has been suggested that the 2 types of G_{M1}-gangliosidosis involve 2 different isoenzyme forms of β-galactosidase. (Derry *et al.*, 1968; Klibansky *et al.*, 1970; O'Brien, 1969; O'Brien *et al.*, 1965; Pinsky *et al.*, 1970; Suzuki & Chen, 1967; Suzuki *et al.*, 1969; Wolfe *et al.*, 1970).

In gangliosidoses, it can be pictured that the accumulation of gangliosides disorganizes neuronal activities; whether the abnormality is only in ganglioside metabolism or also involves factors which condition membrane organization is not at present known, and Tay-Sachs' disease receives only supportive therapy. Gangliosides may function in relation to synaptic vesicles (q.v.). Analysis of cerebral samples for glycolipids has been reported also in other forms of amaurotic idiocy and in Niemann-Pick disease (Jatzkewitz *et al.*, 1965; Seiter & McCluer, 1970).

Gargoylism and Mucopolysaccharides

Gargoylism (Hurler's syndrome) receives comment here as an inherited enzymic defect in metabolism of carbohydrate residues of a complex molecule, which like Tay-Sachs' disease, results in deposition of the molecules in the

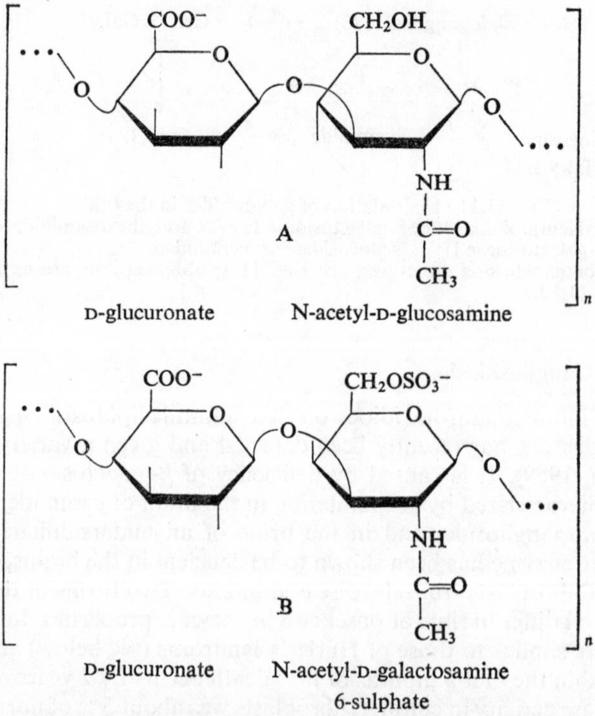

FIG. 11.12. Repeating disaccharide subunits of hyaluronic acid (A) and chondroitin 6-sulphate (B). Chondroitin 4-sulphate is as B, except that the ester sulphate group is on the 4-position of the galactosamine.

brain. The compounds concerned are however not lipids but mucopoly-saccharides. The basic structure of this group of heterologous polymers consists essentially of repeating disaccharide units, usually containing a hexur-onic acid residue and a hexosamine, which may be N-acetylated. Those which have been shown to occur normally in the brain are hyaluronic acid, chondroitin 4-sulphate (chondroitin sulphate A) and chondroitin 6-sulphate (chondroitin sulphate B); the repeating units of these are illustrated in Fig. 11.12. The polymers are usually isolated in association with varying amounts of protein, probably bound in covalent linkage; papain digestion disrupts the protein–carbohydrate linkage in cerebral hyaluronic acid. Total mucopoly-saccharide of the normal brain may be as high as 1·7 mg./g. of fresh tissue; gray matter contains approximately twice the concentration of white matter (Szabo & Roboz-Einstein, 1962; Stary et al., 1964; Singh & Bachhawat, 1965; Margolis, 1967).

The precise sites of mucopolysaccharide occurrence in the brain have not been clearly established. Histochemical examination suggests that the acidic polymers are found mainly in the extracellular space. Any which exists intracellularly is thought to be in the neurons and neuronal processes rather than in glial cells. None has been detected in myelin (Young & Abood, 1960; Pease, 1966; Bondareff, 1967; Adams & Bayliss, 1968).

In gargoylism, mental retardation is accompanied by a 10- to 14-fold increase in urinary excretion of mucopolysaccharides. The molecules excreted consist mainly of dermatan sulphate and heparan sulphate. These two muco-polysaccharides are barely detectable in the normal brain but are found in appreciable amount in the brain in gargoylism. The disorder is thought to be due, not to synthesis of abnormal molecules, but to defective degradation of molecules normally produced so that accumulation results (Dorfman, 1966; Knecht et al., 1967; Baker, 1968; Fratantoni et al., 1968).

Prostaglandins

This group of cyclic and hydroxylated carboxylic acids is distinct from the fatty acids of the glycerides and accordingly receives separate description. Prosta-glandins comprise a group of biologically-active acidic lipids and have usually been detected as a result of their effect in producing slow contractions of smooth muscle, often requiring concentrations as low as 10^{-9} to 10^{-8} M. They are unsaturated hydroxy fatty acids, with the structures illustrated in Fig. 11.13. The name "prostaglandin" comes from the richest source of these lipids, human seminal plasma, and was given by von Euler who first detected them. In the 35 years which have since elapsed, some 13 types have been identified. Prostaglandins found in the brain all contain hydrocarbon chains of 20 carbons with a hydroxyl substituent on C 15 and either a hydroxyl or carbonyl group on C 9. They may also vary in the position of double bonds. The prosta-glandin type present in the highest amount in the brain is type $F_{2\alpha}$ (Fig. 11.13); types E_1, E_2 and $F_{1\alpha}$ also are found, in lower concentrations.

Biosynthesis in seminal vesicles requires tetrahydrofolate or tetrahydropteri-dine cofactor and arachidonic acid is a precursor. Little is known of prosta-glandin metabolism in the brain; arachidonic acid is involved here also. The major type in the brain (F2α) occurs in amounts of about 0·3 μg./g. fresh weight of ox brain.

Analysis of subcellular fractions showed these lipids to be enriched in microsomes and in nerve ending particles (Samuelsson, 1964; Kataoka *et al.*, 1967).

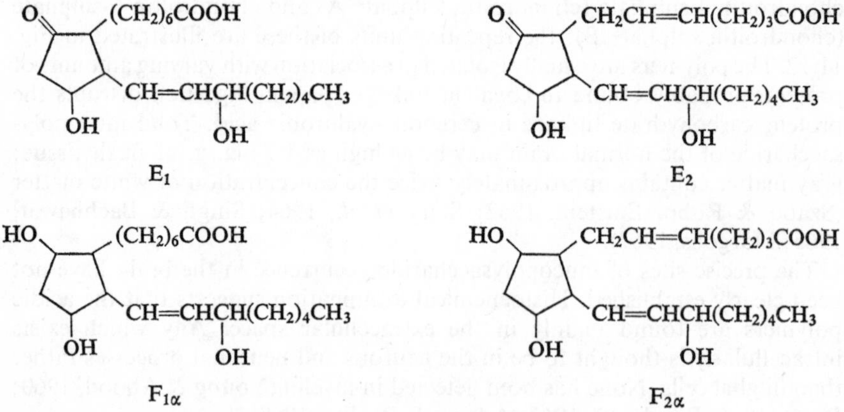

E_1

E_2

$F_{1\alpha}$

$F_{2\alpha}$

FIG. 11.13. Structure of prostaglandins found in the brain.

The pharmacological effects of prostaglandins on neural systems and their role in the brain have been reviewed (Horton & Main, 1967; Pickles, 1967; Bergstrom *et al.*, 1968, Wolfe, 1970).

Comment

The many reaction sequences described in this chapter represent only a part of those whose activities are normally coordinated, in place and time, in producing and maintaining cerebral lipids. They make a notable contribution to understanding how the individual brain becomes as it is, and their failure can disorganize cerebral functioning. But the reactions in themselves do not explain many important aspects of lipid economy: the specificity of particular lipids to particular parts of cells, or the initiation and cessation of synthesis or breakdown according to conditions of growth or maturity. Moreover, the unusual richness of the brain in lipids leads to querying how this is connected with the characteristic behaviour of the brain as an excitable organ showing continuous electrical activity. Such questions lead to the subjects of membrane phenomena, of cytochemistry and of the development of the brain, which are considered in the following two chapters.

REFERENCES

ADAMS, C. W. M. & BAYLISS, O. B. (1968). *J. Histochem. Cytochem.* 16, 119.
ADAMS, C. W. M. & DAVISON, A. N. (1959). *J. Neurochem.* 4, 282.
ADAMS, C. W. M. & DAVISON, A. N. (1965). Neurohistochemistry, p. 332. Ed. C. W. M. Adams. Amsterdam: Elsevier.
AEBERHARD, E. & MENKES, J. H. (1968). *J. biol. Chem.* 243, 3834.

AGRANOFF, B. W. (1962). *J. Lipid. Res.* **3**, 190.
AHMED, K. & SCHOLEFIELD, P. G. (1961). *Biochem. J.* **81**, 37.
ALLING, C. & SVENNERHOLM, L. (1969). *J. Neurochem.* **16**, 751.
ANSELL, G. B. & BAYLISS, B. J. (1961). *Biochem. J.* **78**, 209.
ANSELL, G. B. & CHOJNACKI, T. (1962). *Nature, Lond.* **196**, 545.
ANSELL, G. B. & HAWTHORNE, J. N. (1964). Phospholipids. Chemistry, Metabolism & Function. Amsterdam: Elsevier.
ANSELL, G. B. & MARSHALL, E. F. (1963). *J. Neurochem.* **10**, 875, 883.
ANSELL, G. B. & NORMAN, J. M. (1953). *Biochem. J.* **55**, 768.
ANSELL, G. B. & SPANNER, S. (1959). *J. Neurochem.* **4**, 325.
ANSELL, G. B. & SPANNER, S. (1962). *Biochem. J.* **84**, 12P.
ANSELL, G. B. & SPANNER, S. (1963). *Biochem. J.* **88**, 56.
ANSELL, G. B. & SPANNER, S. (1965). *Biochem. J.* **94**, 252.
ANSELL, G. B. & SPANNER, S. (1967). *J. Neurochem.* **14**, 873.
ANSELL, G. B. & SPANNER, S. (1968). *Biochem. J.* **108**, 207.
AUSTIN, J. H. (1965). *J. Neuropath. exp. Neurol.* **24**, 170.
AUSTIN, J. H., BALASUBRAMANIAN, A. S., PATTABIRAMAN, T. N., SARASWATHI, S., BASU, D. K. & BACHHAWAT, B. K. (1963). *J. Neurochem.* **10**, 805.
BACHUR, N. R., MASEK, K., MELMON, K. L. & UDENFRIEND, S. (1965). *J. biol. Chem.* **240**, 1019.
BAKER, J. R. (1968). Some Recent Advances in Inborn Errors of Metabolism, p. 143. Ed. K. S. Holt & V. P. Coffey. London: Livingstone.
BAKER, R. W. R. (1961). *Biochem. J.* **79**, 642.
BAKKE, J. E. & CORNATZER, W. E. (1961). *J. biol. Chem.* **236**, 653.
BALAKRISHNAN, S. & MCILWAIN, H. (1961). *Biochem. J.* **81**, 72.
BARRON, K. D., BERNSOHN, J. I. & HESS, A. (1961). *J. Histochem. Cytochem.* **9**, 656.
BASU, S., KAUFMAN, B. & ROSEMAN, S. (1968). *J. biol. Chem.* **243**, 5802.
BEATTIE, D. S., & BASFORD, R. E. (1965). *J. Neurochem.* **12**, 103.
BENJAMINS, J. A. & AGRANOFF, B. W. (1969). *J. Neurochem.* **16**, 513.
BERGSTROM, S., CARLSON, C. A. & WEEKS, J. R. (1968). *Pharmacol. Revs.* **29**, 1.
BERRY, J. F., MCPHERSON, C. F. & ROSSITER, R. (1958). *J. Neurochem.* **3**, 65.
BICHEL, M., AUSTIN, J. H. & KEMENY, M. (1966). *Arch. Neurol.* **15**, 13.
BICKERSTAFFE, R. & MEAD, J. F. (1967). *Biochemistry, Easton.* **6**, 655.
BIRAN, L. A. & BARTLEY, W. (1961). *Biochem. J.* **79**, 159.
BLIX, G. (1933). *Z. physiol. Chem.* **219**, 82.
BLIX, G., SVENNERHOLM, L. & WERNER, I. (1950). *Acta Chem. Scand.* **4**, 717.
BONDAREFF, W. (1967). *Anat. Rec.* **157**, 527.
BOOTH, D. A. (1962). *J. Neurochem.* **9**, 265.
BOOTH, D. A. (1963). *Biochim. Biophys. Acta*, **70**, 486.
BOOTH, D. A. (1964). Thesis: Sialolipids in Mammalian Brain and Body Fluids. University of London.
BOWEN, D. M. & RADIN, N. S. (1968). *Biochim. Biophys. Acta*, **152**, 587, 599.
BRADY, R. O. (1960). *J. biol. Chem.* **235**, 3099.
BRADY, R. O. (1962). *J. biol. Chem.* **237**, PC2416.
BRADY, R. O., BRADLEY, R. M., YOUNG, O. M. & KALLER, H. (1965). *J. biol. Chem.* **240**, PC 3693.
BRADY, R. O., FORMICA, J. V. & KOVAL, G. J. (1958). *J. biol. Chem.* **233**, 1072.
BRADY, R. O., GAL, A. E., BRADLEY, R. M., MARTENSSON, E., WARSHAW, A. L. & LASTER, L. (1967). *New Engl. J. Med.* **276**, 1163.
BRADY, R. O. & KOVAL, G. J. (1958). *J. biol. Chem.* **233**, 26.
BRAUN, P. E., MORELL, P. & RADIN, N. S. (1970). *J. biol. Chem.* **245**, 335.
BREMER, J. (1962). *J. biol. Chem.* **237**, 2228.
BROCKERHOFF, H. & BALLOU, C. E. (1962). *J. biol. Chem.* **237**, 49, 1764.
BRUNETTI, P., JOURDAIN, G. W. & ROSEMAN, S. (1962). *J. biol. Chem.* **237**, 2447.
BRUNNGRABER, E. G. (1969). Abstr. 2nd I.S.N. Conf. Milan, p. 109.
BRUNNGRABER, E. G. & BROWN, B. D. (1963). *Biochim. Biophys. Acta*, **69**, 581.
BRUNNGRABER, E. G. & BROWN, B. D. (1964). *Biochim. Biophys. Acta*, **83**, 357.
BURTON, R. M., GARCIA-BUNUEL, L., GOLDEN, M. & BALFOUR, Y. McB. (1963). *Biochemistry*, **2**, 580.

BURTON, R. M., SODD, M. A. & BRADY, R. O. (1958). *J. biol. Chem.* **233**, 1053.
CARTER, H. E., NORRIS, W. P., GLICK, F. J., PHILLIPS, G. E. & HARRIS, R. (1947). *J. biol. Chem.* **170**, 269.
CARUBELLI, R., TRUCCO, R. E., & CAPUTTO, R. (1962). *Biochim. Biophys. Acta*, **60**, 196.
CHANG, M. & BALLOU, C. E. (1967). *Biochem. Biophys. Res. Communs.* **26**, 199.
CHEVALLIER, F. & GAUTHERON, C. (1969). *J. Neurochem.* **16**, 323.
CHOBANIAN, A. & HOLLANDER, W. (1962). *J. clin. Invest.* **41**, 1732.
CLARENBURG, R., CHAIKOFF, I. L. & MORRIS, M. D. (1963). *J. Neurochem.* **10**, 135.
CLAYTON, R. B. (1965). *Quart. Rev. Chem. Soc.* **19**, 168.
CLELAND, W. W. & KENNEDY, E. P. (1960). *J. biol. Chem.* **235**, 45.
COLODZIN, M. & KENNEDY, E. P. (1965). *J. biol. Chem.* **240**, 3771.
COLLINS, F. D. & SHOTLANDER, V. L. (1961). *Biochem. J.* **79**, 316.
COOK, R. P. (1958). Cholesterol: Chemistry, Biochemistry and Pathology. New York: Academic Press.
CROCKER, A. C. (1961). *J. Neurochem.* **7**, 69.
CUMINGS, J. N. (1953). *Brain*, **76**, 551.
CURTIS, W. C. & SEIPEL, J. H. (1961). *J. Neurochem.* **6**, 318.
D'ADAMO, A. F., GIDEZ, L. I. & YATSU, F. M. (1968). *Exp. Brain Res.* **5**, 267.
DAVISON, A. N. (1961). *Biochem. J.* **78**, 28P.
DAVISON, A. N. (1968). Applied Neurochemistry, p. 178. Ed. A. N. Davison & J. Dobbing. Oxford: Blackwell.
DAVISON, A. N., DOBBING, J., MORGAN, R. S. & PAYLING WRIGHT, G. (1958). *J. Neurochem.* **3**, 89.
DAVISON, A. N., DOBBING, J., MORGAN, R. S. & PAYLING WRIGHT, G. (1959). *Lancet*, i, 658.
DAVISON, A. N. & WAJDA, M. (1962). *Biochem. J.* **82**, 113.
DAWSON, R. M. C. (1953). *Biochem. J.* **55**, 507.
DAWSON, R. M. C. (1960). *Biochem. J.* **75**, 45.
DAWSON, R. M. C. & THOMPSON, W. (1964). *Biochem. J.* **91**, 244.
DEBUCH, H. (1956). *Z. physiol. Chem.* **304**, 109.
DEBUCH, H. (1959). *Z. physiol. Chem.* **314**, 49.
DERRY, D. M., FAWCETT, J. S., ANDERMANN, F. & WOLFE, L. S. (1968). *Neurology*, **18**, 340.
DEVRIES, C. H. & BARONDES, S. H. (1971). *J. Neurochem.* **18**, 101.
DICKERSON, J. W. T. (1968). Applied Neurochemistry, p. 48. Ed. A. N. Davison & J. Dobbing. Oxford: Blackwell.
DITTMER, J. C. & DAWSON, R. M. C. (1961). *Biochem. J.* **81**, 535.
DOBBING, J. (1963). *J. Neurochem.* **10**, 739.
DORFMAN, A. (1966). The Metabolic Basis of Inherited Disease, 2nd ed., p. 963. Ed. J. B. Stanbury, J. B. Wyngaarden & D. S. Fredrickson. New York: McGraw-Hill.
DURRELL, J. & SODD, M. A. (1964). *J. biol. Chem.* **239**, 747.
EICHBERG, J., WHITTAKER, V. P. & DAWSON, R. M. C. (1964). *Biochem. J.* **92**, 91.
EVANS, J. E. & McCLUER, R. H. (1969). *J. Neurochem.* **16**, 1393.
FIESER, L. & BHATTACHARYYA, B. K. (1953). *J. Amer. Chem. Soc.* **75**, 4418.
FISH, W. A., BOYD, J. E. & STOKES, W. M. (1962). *J. biol. Chem.* **237**, 334.
FOLCH, J. (1942). *J. biol. Chem.* **146**, 35.
FOLCH, J., ARSOVE, S. & MEATH, J. A. (1951). *J. biol. Chem.* **191**, 819.
FRATANTONI, J. C., HALL, C. W. & NEUFELD, E. F. (1968). *Proc. natn. Acad. Sci. U.S.A.* **60**, 699.
FRIEDEL, R. O., BROWN, J. D. & DURRELL, J. (1967). *Biochim. Biophys. Acta*, **144**, 684.
FRIEDEL, R. O., BROWN, J. D. & DURRELL, J. (1969). *J. Neurochem.* **16**, 371.
FRIES, B. A., SCHACHNER, H. & CHAIKOFF, I. L. (1942). *J. biol. Chem.* **144**, 59.
FROHWEIN, Y. Z. & GATT, S. (1967). *Biochemistry, Easton*, **6**, 2783.
FUJINO, Y. & NEGISHI, T. (1968). *Biochim. Biophys. Acta*, **152**, 428.
FUJINO, Y. & NAKANO, M. (1969). *Biochim. Biophys. J.* **113**, 573.
FUJINO, Y. & ZABIN, I. (1962). *J. biol. Chem.* **237**, 2069.
FULCO, A. J. & MEAD, J. F. (1961). *J. biol. Chem.* **236**, 2416.

FUMAGALLI, R., GROSSI, E., PAOLETTI, P. & PAOLETTI, R. (1964). *J. Neurochem.* **11**, 561.

GALLAI-HATCHARD, J., MAGEE, W. L., THOMPSON, R. H. S. & WEBSTER, G. R. (1962). *J. Neurochem.* **9**, 545.

GALLAI-HATCHARD, J. I., & THOMPSON, R. H. S. (1965). *Biochim. Biophys. Acta*, **98**, 128.

GALLI, G., PAOLETTI, E. G. & WEISS, J. F. (1968). *Science*, **162** 1495.

GAMMACK, D. B., PERRIN, J. H. & SAUNDERS, L. (1964). *Biochim. Biophys. Acta*, **84**, 576.

GATT, S. (1963). *J. biol. Chem.* **238**, PC 3131.

GATT, S. (1965). *Biochim. Biophys. Acta*, **137**, 192.

GATT, S. (1966). *Biochem. J.* **101**, 687: *J. biol. Chem.* **241**, 3724.

GATT, S. (1968). *Biochim. Biophys. Acta*, **159**, 304.

GATT, S. (1970). *Chem. Phys. Lipids.* **5**, 235.

GATT, S. & BERMAN, E. R. (1963). *J. Neurochem.* **10**, 43, 65, 75.

GATT, S. & RAPPORT, M. M. (1966). *Biochem. J.* **101**, 680.

GEYER, R. P., MATTHEWS, L. W. & STARE, F. J. (1949). *J. biol. Chem.* **180**, 1037.

GOLDBERG, I. H. (1961). *J. Lipid Res.* **2**, 103.

GREEN, J. P. & ROBINSON, J. D. (1960). *J. biol. Chem.* **235**, 1621.

HAGBERG, B., SOURANDER, P. & SVENNERHOLM, L. (1963). *J. Neurol. Neurosurg. Psychiat.* **26**, 195.

HANAHAN, D. J. (1960). Lipid Chemistry. New York: Wiley.

HANAHAN, D. J. (1961). *Biochem. Preparations*, **8**, 121.

HARWOOD, J. L. & HAWTHORNE, J. N. (1969). *J. Neurochem.* **16**, 1377.

HAUSER, G. (1963). *Biochim. Biophys. Acta*, **70**, 278.

HAUSER, G. & FINELLI, V. N. (1963). *J. biol. Chem.* **238**, 3224.

HEALD, P. J. & ROBINSON, M. (1961). *Biochem. J.* **81**, 157.

HENDRICKSON, H. S. & BALLOU, C. E. (1964). *J. biol. Chem.* **239**, 1369.

HOKIN, L. E. & HOKIN, M. R. (1958). *J. biol. Chem.* **233**, 800, 822.

HOKIN, M. R. (1969). *J. Neurochem.* **16**, 127.

HOKIN, M. R. (1970). *J. Neurochem.* **17**, 357.

HOKIN, M. R. & BROWN, D. F. (1969). *J. Neurochem.* **16**, 475.

HOLSTEIN, T. J., FISH, W. A. & STOKES, W. M. (1966). *J. Lipid Res.* **7**, 734.

HORTON, E. W. & MAIN, I. H. M. (1967). *Brit. J. Pharmacol. Chemotherap.* **30**, 568, 582.

IVEMARK, B. I., SVENNERHOLM, L., THOREN, T. & TUNNELL, R. (1963). *Acta Pediat.* **52**, 391.

JATZKEWITZ, H. (1960). *Z. physiol. Chem.* **320**, 134.

JATZKEWITZ, H. & MEHL, E. (1969). *J. Neurochem.* **16**, 19.

JATZKEWITZ, H., PILZ, H. & SANDHOFF, K. (1965). *J. Neurochem.* **12**, 135.

JOSEPH, R. & BACHHAWAT, B. K. (1964). *J. Neurochem.* **11**, 517.

KAI, M., JOSHITA, J. & SAGA, M. (1963). *J. Biochem. (Jap.),* **54**, 403.

KAI, M., SALWAY, J. G. & HAWTHORNE, J. N. (1968). *Biochem. J.* **106**, 791.

KAI, M., SALWAY, J. G., MITCHELL, R. H. & HAWTHORNE, J. N. (1966a). *Biochem. Biophys. Res. Communs.* **22**, 370.

KAI, M., WHITE, G. L. & HAWTHORNE, J. N. (1966b). *Biochem. J.* **101**, 328.

KAMPINE, J. P., BRADY, R. O., KANFER, J. N., FELD, M. & SHEPIRO, D. (1967). *Science*, **155**, 86.

KANFER, J. (1965). *J. biol. Chem.* **240**, 609.

KANFER, J. N., BRADLEY, R. M. & GAL, A. E. (1967). *J. Neurochem.* **14**, 1095.

KANFER, J. N. & BRADY, R. O. (1967). 3rd Int. Sympos. Cerebral Sphingolipidoses; Inborn Errors of Sphingolipids Metabolism, p. 187. Ed. N. Aronson & B. W. Volk. Oxford: Pergamon.

KATAOKA, K., RAMWELL, P. & JESSUP, S. (1967). *Science*, **157**, 1187.

KAUFMAN, B., BASU, S. & ROSEMAN, S. (1968). *J. biol. Chem.* **243**, 5804.

KELLEY, M. T., AEXEL, R. T., HERNDON, B. L. & NICHOLAS, H. J. (1969). *J. Lipid. Res.* **10**, 166.

KEOUGH, K. M. W. & THOMPSON, W. (1970). *J. Neurochem.* **17**, 1.

KERR, S. E. & READ, W. W. C. (1963). *Biochim. Biophys. Acta*, **70**, 477.

KISHIMOTO, Y. & RADIN, N. S. (1963). *J. Lipid Res.* **4**, 437.
KLENK, E. (1941). *Hoppe-Seyl. Z.* **268**, 50.
KLENK, E. (1942). *Hoppe-Seyl. Z.* **273**, 76.
KLENK, E. & DEBUCH, H. (1954). *Hoppe-Seyl. Z.* **296**, 179.
KLENK, E., DEBUCH, H. & DAHN, H. (1953). *Hoppe-Seyl. Z.* **292**, 241.
KLENK, E. & GIELEN, W. (1963). *Hoppe-Seyl. Z.* **330**, 218.
KLENK, E. & HENDRICKS, U. W. (1961). *Biochim. Biophys. Acta*, **50**, 602.
KLENK, E. & RIVERA, M. E. (1969). *Z. Physiol. Chem.* **350**, 1589.
KLIBANSKY, C., SAIFER, A., FELDMAN, N. I., SCHNECK, L. & VOLK, B. W. (1970). *J. Neurochem.* **17**, 339.
KNAUFF, H. G. (1958). *Z. Physiol. Chem.* **312**, 264.
KNAUFF, H. G., MARX, D. & MAYER, G. (1961). *Z. Physiol. Chem.* **326**, 220, 227.
KNECHT, J., CIFONELLI, J. A. & DORFMAN, A. (1967). *J. biol. Chem.* **242**, 4652.
KOCHETOV, H. K., ZHUKOVA, I. G. & GLUKHODED, I. S. (1963). *Biochim. Biophys. Acta*, **70**, 716.
KOHN, P., WINZLER, R. J. & HOFFMAN, R. C. (1962). *J. biol. Chem.* **237**, 304.
KOREY, S. R., GONATAS, J. & STEIN, A. (1963). *J. Neuropath. exper. Neurol.* **22**, 56.
KOREY, S. R. & STEIN, A. (1961). *Proc. Internat. Neurochem. Sympos.* **4**, 175.
KUHN, R. & WEIGANDT, H. (1963). *Chem. Ber.* **96**, 866; *Z. Naturforsch*, **18b**, 541.
LAATSCH, R. H. (1962). *J. Neurochem.* **9**, 487.
LARRABEE, M. G. (1968). *J. Neurochem.* **15**, 803.
LARRABEE, M. G., KLINGMAN, J. D. & LEICHT, W. S. (1963). *J. Neurochem.* **10**, 549.
LARRABEE, M. G. & LEICHT, W. S. (1965). *J. Neurochem.* **12**, 1.
LEBARON, F. N. (1963). *Biochim. Biophys. Acta*, **70**, 658.
LEIBOVITZ, Z. & GATT, S. (1968). *Biochim. Biophys. Acta*, **152**, 136.
LEVIS, G. M. & MEAD, J. F. (1964). *J. biol. Chem.* **239**, 77.
LONG, C. & STAPLES, D. A. (1961). *Biochem. J.* **78**, 179; **80**, 557.
LOWDEN, J. A. & WOLFE, L. S. (1963). *Nature, Lond.* **197**, 771.
LOWDEN, J. A. & WOLFE, L. S. (1964). *Canad. J. Biochem.* **42**, 1587.
LUNT, G. G. & ROWE, C. E. (1968). *Biochim. Biophys. Acta*. **152**, 681.
MAGEE, W. L., BERRY, J. F., STRICKLAND, K. P. & ROSSITER, R. J. (1963). *Biochem. J.* **88**, 45.
MAPES, C. A., ANDERSON, R. L. & SWEELEY, C. C. (1970). *FEBS Letters*, **7**, 180.
MARGOLIS, R. U. (1967). *Biochim. Biophys. Acta*, **141**, 91.
MARPLES, E. A. & THOMPSON, R. H. S. (1960). *Biochem. J.* **74**, 123.
MARTENSSON, E. & KANFER, J. N. (1968). *J. biol. Chem.* **243**, 497.
MCARDLE, B., THOMPSON, R. H. S. & WEBSTER, G. R. (1960). *J. Neurochem.* **5**, 135.
MCCAMAN, R. E. (1962). *J. biol. Chem.* **237**, 672.
MCCAMAN, R. E. & COOK, K. (1966). *J. biol. Chem.* **241**, 3390.
MCCAMAN, R. E., SMITH, M. & COOK, K. (1965). *J. biol. Chem.* **240**, 3513.
MCCOLL, J. D. & ROSSITER, R. J. (1952). *J. exp. Biol.* **29**, 196, 203.
MCGHEE, E. C., PAPAGEORGE, E., BLOOM, W. L. & LEWIS, G. T. (1951). *J. biol. Chem.* **190**, 127.
MCILWAIN, H. (1961). *Biochem. J.* **78**, 24.
MCILWAIN, H. (1962). *Proc. Assoc. Res. Nerv. Ment. Dis.* **40**, 43, 364.
MCILWAIN, H. (1963). Chemical Exploration of the Brain: a Study of Cerebral Excitability and Ion Movement. Amsterdam: Elsevier.
MCILWAIN, H. & RODNIGHT, R. (1962). Practical Neurochemistry. London: Churchill.
MCMURRAY, W. C. (1964). *J. Neurochem.* **11**, 287, 315.
MCMURRAY, W. C., STRICKLAND, K. P., BERRY, J. F. & ROSSITER, R. J. (1957). *Biochem. J.* **66**, 621, 634.
MEAD, J. F. & LEVIS, G. M. (1962). *Biochem. Biophys. Res. Commun.* **9**, 231.
MEAD, J. F. & LEVIS, G. M. (1963). *J. biol. Chem.* **238**, 1634; *Biochim. Biophys. Res. Comm.* **11**, 319.
MOHRHAUER, H. & HOLMAN, R. T. (1963). *J. Neurochem.* **10**, 523.
MORELL, P. & RADIN, N. S. (1969). *Biochemistry, Easton*, **8**, 506.
MORELL, P. & RADIN, N. S. (1970). *J. biol. Chem.* **245**, 342.
MORRIS, M. D. & CHAIKOFF, I. L. (1961). *J. Neurochem.* **8**, 226.

MOSER, H. W. & KARNOVSKY, M. L. (1959). *J. biol. Chem.* **234**, 1990.
MYERS, D. K. (1956). *Biochem. J.* **64**, 740.
NICHOLLS, D., KANFER, J. & TITUS, E. (1962). *J. biol. Chem.* **237**, 1043.
NICHOLAS, H. J. & THOMAS, B. E. (1959). *J. Neurochem.* **4**, 42.
O'BRIEN, J. S. (1969). *J. Pediat.* **75**, 167.
O'BRIEN, J. S., FILLERUP, D. L. & MEAD, J. F. (1964). *J. Lipid Res.* **5**, 109, 329.
O'BRIEN, J. S. & ROUSER, G. (1964). *J. Lipid Res.* **5**, 339.
O'BRIEN, J. S., STERN, M. B., LANDING, B. H., O'BRIEN, J. K. & DONNELL, G. N. (1965). *Amer. J. Dis. Child.* **109**, 338.
ÖHMAN, R. (1971). *J. Neurochem.* **18**, 89.
ÖHMAN, R. & SVENNERHOLM, L. (1971). *J. Neurochem.* **18**, 79.
OKUHARA, E. & YASUDA, M. (1960). *J. Neurochem.* **6**, 112.
PALMER, F. B. & ROSSITER, R. J. (1964). See Rossiter *et al.*, 1964.
PAOLETTI, R., GROSSI-PAOLETTI, E. & FUMAGALLI, R. (1969). Handbook of Neuro-chemistry, Vol. 1, p. 195. Ed. A. Lajtha. New York: Plenum.
PASCAL, T. A. & SAIFER, A. (1969). *J. Neurochem.* **16**, 301.
PATTABIRAMAN, T. N. & BACHHAWAT, B. K. (1962). *Biochim. Biophys. Acta*, **59**, 681.
PEASE, D. C. (1966). *J. Ultrastruct. Res.* **15**, 555.
PETZOLD, G. C. & AGRANOFF, B. W. (1967). *J. biol. Chem.* **242**, 1187.
PICKLES, V. R. (1967). *Biol. Revs.* **42**, 614.
PIERINGER, R. A. & HOKIN, L. E. (1962). *J. biol. Chem.* **237**, 653, 659.
PILZ, H. & JATZKEWITZ, H. (1964). *J. Neurochem.* **11**, 603.
PINSKY, L., POWELL, E. & CALLAHAN, J. (1970). *Nature, Lond.* **228**, 1093.
POULSON, E. & ALDRIDGE, W. N. (1963). *Biochem. J.* **86**, 4P.
PRITCHARD, E. T. (1958). *Canad. J. Biochem. Physiol.* **36**, 1211.
PRITCHARD, E. T. & ROSSITER, R. J. (1963). *Canad. J. Biochem. Physiol.* **41**, 341.
Proceedings (1964). Metabolism and Physiological Significance of Lipids. Ed. Dawson & Rhodes. London: Wiley.
PROSTENIK, M. (1960). *Naturwiss.* **47**, 399.
PROTTEY, C., SALWAY, J. G. & HAWTHORNE, J. N. (1968). *Biochim. Biophys. Acta*, **164**, 238.
PUMPHREY, A. M. (1969). *Biochem. J.* **112**, 61.
RADIN, N. S. & AKAHORI, Y. (1961). *J. Lipid Res.* **2**, 335.
RADIN, N. S., MARTIN, F. B. & BROWN, J. R. (1957). *J. biol. Chem.* **224**, 499.
RAPPORT, M. M. & FRANZL, R. E. (1957). *J. Neurochem.* **1**, 303.
RAPPORT, M. M. & NORTON, W. T. (1962). *Ann. Rev. Biochem.* **31**, 103.
RIECKEHOLT, I. G., HOLMAN, R. T. & BURR, G. O. (1949). *Arch. Biochem.* **20**, 331.
ROBINSON, J. D., BRADLEY, R. M. & BRADY, R. O. (1963). *J. biol. Chem.* **238**, 528.
RODNIGHT, R. (1956). *Biochem. J.* **63**, 223.
RODNIGHT, R. (1957). *J. Neurochem.* **1**, 207.
ROITMAN, A. & GATT, S. (1963). *Israel. J. Chem.* **1**, 190.
ROSSITER, R. J. (1966). Nerve as a Tissue, p. 175. Ed. K. Rodahl & B. Issekutz. New York: Harper.
ROSSITER, R. J., MCMURRAY, W. C. & PALMER, F. B. (1964). *Abstr., Internat. Congr. Biochem.* **6**, 541.
ROUSER, G., BAUMAN, A. J. & KRITCHEVSKY, G. (1961a). *Amer. J. clin. Nutr.* **9**, 112.
ROUSER, G., BAUMAN, A. J., NICOLAIDES, N. & HELLER, D. (1961b). *J. Amer. Oil Chem. Soc.* **38**, 565.
ROUSER, G. & YAMAMOTO, A. (1969). Handbook of Neurochemistry, Vol. 1, p. 121. Ed. A. Lajtha. New York: Plenum.
RUMSBY, M. G. (1967). *J. Neurochem.* **14**, 733.
SALWAY, J. G., KAI, M. & HAWTHORNE, J. N. (1967). *J. Neurochem.* **14**, 1013.
SAMUELS, S., KOREY, S. & GONATAS, J. (1963). *J. Neuropath. exp. Neurol.* **22**, 81.
SAMUELSSON, B. (1964). *Biochim. Biophys. Acta*, **84**, 218.
SANTIAGO-CALVO, E., MUTE, S. J. & HOKIN, L. E. (1963). *Biochim. Biophys. Acta*, **70**, 91.
SCALLEN, T. J., CONDIE, R. M. & SCHROEPFER, G. J. (1962). *J. Neurochem.* **9**, 99.
SCHACHNER, H., FRIES, B. A. & CHAIKOFF, I. L. (1942). *J. biol. Chem.* **146**, 95.
SCHENGRUND, C.-L. & ROSENBERG, A. (1970). *J. biol. Chem.* **245**, 6196.

366 CEREBRAL LIPIDS

SCHNECK, L., FRIEDLAND, J., VALENTI, C., ADACHI, M., AMSTERDAM, D. & VOLK, B. W. (1970). *Lancet*, **i**, 582.
SCHWARZ, H. P., KOSTYK, I., MARMOLEJO, A. & SARAPPA, C. (1967). *J. Neurochem.* **14**, 91.
SEITER, C. W. & McCLUER, R. H. (1970). *J. Neurochem.* **17**, 1525.
SEMINARIO, L. M., HREN, N. & GOMEZ, C. J. (1964). *J. Neurochem.* **11**, 197.
SHOYAB, M., PATTABIRAMAN, T. N. & BACHHAWAT, B. K. (1964). *J. Neurochem.* **11**, 639.
SINGH, M. & BACHHAWAT, B. K. (1965). *J. Neurochem.* **12**, 519.
SKIPSKI, V. P., ARFIN, S. M. & RAPPORT, M. M. (1959). *Arch. Biochem. Biophys.* **82**, 487.
SKRBIC, T. R. & CUMINGS, J. N. (1970). *J. Neurochem.* **17**, 85.
SLOANE STANLEY, G. H. (1953). *Biochem. J.* **53**, 613.
SLOANE STANLEY, G. H. & McILWAIN, H. (1956). Handbook of Biological Data. Washington: National Research Council.
SMIRNOV, A. A., CHIRKOVSKAYA, E. V. & MANUKYAN, K. G. (1961). *Biokhimiya*, **26**, 1027.
SNYDER, R. A. & BRADY, R. O. (1969). *Clin. Chim. Acta.* **25**, 331.
SPRINSON, D. B. & COULON, A. (1954). *J. biol. Chem.* **207**, 585.
SRIBNEY, M. (1962). *Fed. Proc.* **21**, 280.
SRIBNEY, M. (1966). *Biochim. Biophys. Acta*, **125**, 542.
SRIBNEY, M. & KENNEDY, E. P. (1958). *J. biol. Chem.* **233**, 1315.
STARY, Z., WARDI, A. & TURNER, D. (1964). *Biochim. Biophys. Acta*, **83**, 242.
STOFFEL, W., LeKIM, D. & STICHT, G. (1968). *Hoppe-Seyl. Z. Physiol. Chem.*, **349**, 664, 1637.
STRICKLAND, K. P. (1954). *Canad. J. Biochem. Physiol.* **32**, 50.
STRICKLAND, K. P. (1962). *Canad. J. Biochem. Physiol.* **40**, 247.
STRICKLAND, K. P., SUBRAHMANYAM, D., PRITCHARD, E. T., THOMPSON, W. & ROSSITER, R. J. (1963). *Biochem. J.* **87**, 128.
SUZUKI, K. (1970). *J. Neurochem.* **17**, 209.
SUZUKI, K. & CHEN, G. C. (1967). *J. Lipid Res.* **8**, 105.
SUZUKI, K. & KOREY, S. R. (1964). *J. Neurochem.* **11**, 647.
SUZUKI, K., SUZUKI, K. & KAMOSHITA, S. (1969). *J. Neuropath. exp. Neurol.* **28**, 25.
SVENNERHOLM, E. & SVENNERHOLM, L. (1963). *Nature, Lond.* **198**, 688.
SVENNERHOLM, L. (1956). *Acta Chem. Scand.* **10**, 694.
SVENNERHOLM, L. (1962). *Biochem. Biophys. Res. Comm.* **9**, 436.
SVENNERHOLM, L. (1963). *J. Neurochem.* **10**, 612; *Acta Chem. Scand.* **17**, 239.
SVENNERHOLM, L. & THORIN, H. (1960). *Biochim. Biophys. Acta*, **41**, 371.
SWEELEY, C. C. (1959). *Biochim. Biophys. Acta*, **36**, 268.
SWEELEY, C. C. & KLIONSKY, B. (1966). The Metabolic Basis of Inherited Disease, 2nd ed., p. 618. Ed. J. B. Stanbury, J. B. Wyngaarden & D. S. Fredrickson. New York: McGraw-Hill.
Symposium (1957). Cerebral Lipidoses. Ed. Cumings & Lowenthal. Oxford: Blackwell.
Symposium (1959). *A.M.A. J. Dis. Child.* **97**, 655.
Symposium (1960). The Neurochemistry of Nucleotides and Amino acids. Ed. R. O. Brady & D. B. Tower. New York: Wiley.
Symposia (1961, 1964a). *Proc. Internat. Neurochem. Sympos.* **3, 5**.
Symposium (1962a). Cerebral sphingolipidoses. Ed. S. M. Aronson & B. W. Volk. New York: Academic Press.
Symposium (1962b). Ultrastructure and Metabolism of the Nervous System. *Proc. Assoc. Res. nerv. ment. Dis.* **40**.
Symposium (1963). Brain Lipids and Lipoproteins and the Leucodystrophies. Ed. J. Folch-Pi & H. Bauer. Amsterdam: Elsevier.
Symposium (1964b). Problems of the Biochemistry of the Nervous System. Ed. A. V. Palladin, H. H. Hillman & R. Woodman. Oxford: Pergamon.
Symposium (1970). Catabolism of Complex Lipids of the Brain. *Biochem. J.* **117**, 4P.
SZABO, M. M. & ROBOZ-EINSTEIN, E. (1962). *Arch. Biochem. Biophys.* **98**, 406.
TETTAMANTI, G. & ZAMBOTTI, V. (1968). *Enzymologia*, **35**, 61.

THANNHAUSER, S. J. (1950). The Lipidoses. Oxford: University Press.

THANNHAUSER, S. J. (1953). *Res. Publ. Ass. Nerv. ment. Dis.* **32**, 238.

THANNHAUSER, S. J., FELLIG, J. & SCHMIDT, G. (1955). *J. biol. Chem.* **215**, 211.

THUDICHUM, J. W. L. (1884). Chemical Constitution of the Brain. London: Baillière, Tindall & Cox.

THOMPSON, C. G. & McILWAIN, H. (1961). *Biochem. J.* **79**, 342.

THOMPSON, W. (1969). *Biochim. Biophys. Acta.* **187**, 150.

THOMPSON, R. H. S. (1965). *Sci. Basis Med.,* **58**.

THOMPSON, R. H. S. & KING, E. J. (1964). Biochemical Disorders in Human Disease. London: Churchill.

THOMPSON, W. & DAWSON, R. M. C. (1964). *Biochem. J.* **91**, 233, 237.

THOMPSON, W., STRICKLAND, K. P. & ROSSITER, R. J. (1963). *Biochem. J.* **87**, 136.

TOMLINSON, R. V. & BALLOU, C. E. (1961). *J. biol. Chem.* **236**, 1902.

TRAMS, E. G. & LAUTER, C. J. (1962). *Biochim. Biophys. Acta,* **60**, 350.

VANCE, D. E., KRIVIT, W. & SWEELEY, C. S. (1969). *J. Lipid. Res.* **10**, 188.

VARMA, S. N., SCHWARTZ, V. & SIMPSON, I. M. N. (1962). *Biochem. J.* **85**, 546.

VIGNAIS, P. M., GALLAGHER, C. H. & ZABIN, I. (1958). *J. Neurochem.* **2**, 283.

WALLACE, B. J., ARONSON, S. M. & VOLK, B. W. (1964). *J. Neurochem.* **11**, 367.

WARREN, L. & FELSENFELD, H. (1962). *J. biol. Chem.* **237**, 1421.

WEBSTER, G. R. (1960). *Biochim. Biophys. Acta,* **44**, 109.

WEBSTER, G. R. & ALPERN, R. N. (1964). *Biochem. J.* **90**, 35.

WEBSTER, G. R., MARPLES, E. A. & THOMPSON, R. H. S. (1957). *Biochem. J.* **65**, 375.

WEBSTER, G. R. & THOMPSON, R. H. S. (1962). *Biochim. Biophys. Acta,* **63**, 38.

WEINHOUSE, S., MILLINGTON, R. H. & VOLK, M. E. (1950). *J. biol. Chem.* **185**, 191.

WEISS, B. (1956). *J. biol. Chem.* **223**, 523.

WEISS, B. (1963). *J. biol. Chem.* **238**, 1953.

WHERRETT, J. R. & CUMINGS, J. N. (1963). *Biochem. J.* **86**, 378; *Trans. Amer. Neurol. Assoc.* **88**, 108.

WIELAND, O. & SUYTER, M. (1957). *Biochem. Z.* **329**, 320.

WOLFE, L. S. (1970). Handbook of Neurochemistry, Vol. 4, p. 149. Ed. A. Lajtha. New York: Plenum.

WOLFE, L. S., CALLAHAN, J., FAWCETT, J. S., ANDERMANN, F. & SCRIVER, C. R. (1970). *Neurology,* **20**, 23.

WOLFE, L. S. & LOWDEN, J. A. (1964). *Canad. J. Biochem.* **42**, 1041.

YABUUCHI, H. & O'BRIEN, J. S. (1968). *J. Neurochem.* **15**, 1383.

YAVIN, E. & GATT, S. (1969). *Biochemistry, Easton,* **8**, 1692.

YOUNG, J. & ABOOD, C. G. (1960). *J. Neurochem.* **6**, 89.

ZABIN, I. & MEAD, J. F. (1954). *J. biol. Chem.* **211**, 87.

12 Membrane Structure and Cytochemistry

This chapter outlines investigations in which chemical and biochemical studies of the brain have been coordinated with cell structure, especially at microscopic and electron-microscopic levels. It necessarily describes only briefly, aspects which are primarily biophysical or morphological, and emphasizes those in which biochemical studies have been most enlightening. Cellular components selected on this basis are listed in Table 12.1 in the order in which they will receive comment below. In describing myelin and other membrane-structures, opportunity has been taken to describe lipid–lipid and lipid–protein associations. The protein content of the components of Table 12.1 was given in Chapter 9 (Table 9.6).

The heterogeneity of cell types and structures in the brain renders purification of components and localization of individual activities more difficult than is the case with less complex tissues. Identification of cellular constituents in a separated preparation from the brain comes partly from electron-microscopic examination and partly from estimation and detection of "marker" chemicals and enzymes. Association of markers with specific sub-cellular components derives from a combination of histochemical study of tissue sections and of biochemical study on rigorously purified components. Thus 5′-nucleotidase activity in the brain appeared only in nerve sheaths on histochemical study (Naidoo & Pratt, 1952; Naidoo, 1962) and was found enriched, but not exclusively in myelin, during biochemical study of cerebral subfractions (Keough & Thompson, 1970). These results are in contrast to those obtained with the liver, where the enzyme has been concluded to be a marker for the plasma cell membrane (Coleman & Finean, 1966; Coleman et al., 1967). Yet 5′-nucleotidase is sometimes incorrectly cited as a plasma membrane marker in cerebral studies. Other examples of different localization of enzymes in different tissues occur; for example, glucose-6-phosphatase is a marker for the endoplasmic reticulum of liver cells but has not been demonstrated to occur in cerebral microsomal preparations. Again, NADH-cytochrome c reductase activity is used for identification of membranes of the endoplasmic reticulum in the liver; in the brain its localization is less specific (Koch & Lindall, 1966).

Nevertheless a number of markers, chemical or enzymic, can now be listed for cerebral sub-cellular components (Table 12.2). For example succinate

Table 12.1

Cellular components and the centrifugal methods used in their preparation

Component; centrifugal methods	Some constituents	Some activities
1. Myelin sheath: Density-gradient from grey or white matter	Enrichment in cholesterol, cerebrosides, sphingo-myelin; proteolipids	Electrical insulation Barrier to water-soluble substances
2. Microsomal membrane structures: Differential, from grey matter dispersion	Enrichment in cholesterol, gangliosides, Na-K-Mg-adenosine triphosphat-ase, cholinesterases	Exchange between cell and environment. Lipid synthesis
3. Mitochondria: Differential and gradient, from grey matter dispersion	Lipids; Krebs-cycle and respiratory-chain en-zymes and cofactors	Oxidative phosphoryla-tion
4. Nucleus: As 3	The genetic apparatus; deoxyribonucleoprotein	Production of specific ribonucleic acids
5. Ribosomes: As 3	Ribonucleoprotein	Protein synthesis
6. Lysosomes: As 3	Hydrolytic enzymes	Storage and release of degradative enzymes
7. Nerve terminals: As 3	Synaptic vesicles, mito-chondria, synaptic structure, entrapped cytoplasm; portion of pre- and post-synaptic cells	Storage and release of neurohumoural agents
8. Synaptic vesicles: Density-gradient from lysed terminals	Acetylcholine or other neurohumoural agent	Release of contents at synaptic cleft

dehydrogenase and monoamine oxidase are valid mitochondrial markers and $2'3'$-cyclic nucleotidase activity provides evidence for the presence of myelin.

Myelin

The obvious division of the brain and spinal cord to grey matter and white, early gave occasion for a combination of chemical and cytological studies. "Myelin" became the name for the material seen microscopically around typical white-matter fibres, both in its cytological and chemical senses (*Symposium*, 1959). Its composition was first approached by two indirect methods. (1) Analyses such as those of Table 11.1 show most categories of lipid to occur throughout the brain but to be enriched on average by three-fold in white matter. Certain components, however, are still further enriched: especi-ally cholesterol, sphingomyelin and plasmalogens, four- to five-fold; cerebro-sides and sulphatides, six- to twelve-fold. These lipids were therefore correctly regarded as myelin components. (2) Moreover, the enrichment in these lipids occurs during the period of growth when white matter takes on its character-istic appearance (Chapter 13), as also does enrichment in proteolipid-protein, a specific type of protein extractable from the tissue by organic solvents. Estimation of the proteolipid content of isolated myelin (below) and of white matter suggests that between 40 and 50 % of the dry weight of cerebral white matter is myelin (Norton & Autilio, 1965, 1966; Cuzner et al., 1965). Specifically associated with myelin in the brain is 2′3′-cyclic nucleotide 3′-phosphohydrolase (Table 12.2). It was first noted to be 10 times more active in white than in grey matter and then to be localized in the myelin sheath. Confidence in the enzyme as a myelin marker was increased by a finding of very low activity in strains of

Table 12.2

"Markers" for cerebral sub-cellular components

Component	Marker chemicals	Marker enzymes
1. Nuclei	DNA	RNA polymerase Nicotinamide mono- nucleotide-adenyl transferase
2. Myelin	Lipid ratios; high cerebroside	2′3′-Cyclic nucleotidase 5′-Nucleotidase*
3. Mitochondria		Succinate dehydrogenase Monoamine oxidase
4. Membrane fragments from:		
a. Endoplasmic reticulum	Gangliosides	Acetyl cholinesterase NADH-cytochrome c reductase*
b. Plasma membrane	Gangliosides	5′-Nucleotidase*
c. Nerve endings		Acetyl cholinesterase
5. Ribosomes	RNA:DNA ratio	
6. Lysosomes		β-Glucuronidase Cathepsin

* Enzymes used as markers, but of doubtful validity (see text).

mice in which deficient myelination occurs (Kurihara & Tsukada, 1967; Kurihara et al., 1970). Leucine aminopeptidase also appears to be enriched in myelin (Adams et al., 1963; Beck et al., 1968). An esterase, active in hydrolysing β-naphthylacetate, has been shown to be present in myelin and was retained in the myelin after rigorous purification which included osmotic shock and repeated density-gradient centrifugation (Riekkinen & Rumsby, 1969; Rumsby et al., 1970). Preparation of myelin has now given more direct information about its composition.

Separation of Myelin

Myelin was isolated and identified as an entity in cerebral tissue dispersions by techniques which included density-gradient centrifugation (Patterson &

Finean, 1961; August *et al.*, 1961). By careful choice of conditions some 40% of the myelin of cerebral white matter has been prepared with minimal admixture of other materials (Autilio *et al.*, 1964). Dispersions of corpus callosum and adjacent white matter of ox brain were repeatedly centrifuged between sucrose of density 1·04 and 1·085; subsequent washing and gradient centrifugation gave two major fractions with the morphological characteristics of the myelin sheath: its regular, concentric layers seen electron-microscopically. The preparations were soluble to the extent of 95–99% in $CHCl_32:1CH_3OH$, and consisted almost entirely of lipids together with the proteolipid-protein.

The lipid content of the myelin preparation was such as to approximate to simple stoichiometric ratios: cholesterol, 4; galactolipids, 2; phospholipids, 3 of which plasmalogens formed 1. Similar ratios were a feature also of the composition of myelin as deduced indirectly by methods (1) and (2) above, but the actual composition is more complex (Table 12.3). The remainder of

Table 12.3

Major components of myelin

Component	% of total dry weight
Protein	25
Cholesterol	34
Phospholipids (25%):	
Ethanolamine phospholipids	12
Lecithins	6
Sphingomyelin	4
Minor acid phospholipids	3
Glycolipids (16%):	
Cerebrosides	13·5
Cerebroside sulphates	2
Gangliosides	1

Data from the text and Norton & Autilio, 1965.

the white matter lipids, separated in obtaining the myelin preparation, constituted rather more than half of the original white matter content and contained more phospholipid, but less cholesterol and galactolipid, than did the myelin. The proteolipid-protein formed 22% by weight and contributed about fifteen amino acid residues for each nine equivalents of the lipids. Myelin lipids showed marked differences from those of the microsomes, in a number of vertebrate species (Cuzner *et al.*, 1965; McIlwain, 1963; Suzuki *et al.*, 1968).

From the whole forebrain of guinea pigs, presumably with preponderance of grey matter, fractions enriched in small and large myelin fragments were obtained (Eichberg *et al.*, 1964). These differed in composition but contained the same major components as the more extensively-washed white-matter preparation just described. Myelin preparations can be taken to solution by lysolecithin, and physical examination of the resulting micelles has given indications of the manner of association between myelin components (Gent *et al.*, 1964).

Structure of Myelin

When examined optically and by X-ray diffraction, the myelin sheath in specimens of peripheral nerve and of cerebral white matter showed striking regularities in structure. These indicated a radial arrangement of units, in concentric layers some 85 Å apart. The dimensions of lipid molecules permitted structures to be suggested including those of **A** to **D**, Fig. 12.1.

These perspicacious conclusions, arrived at some 30 years ago, have been confirmed by electron-microscopy. More recently some evidence for a globular unit in membranes, including myelin, has appeared as illustrated by **D**, Fig. 12.1. Electron-microscopy has also shown how the myelin arises. Each lipid bilayer with its associated protein is a unit membrane which has been an outer cell membrane of satellite cells: Schwann cells or an equivalent which in the central nervous system may be oligodendroglia. Most neurons, myelinated or not, are associated with a form of satellite cell; in myelination these become wrapped round the axon but lose much of their cell contents, and the process leaves the concentric array of membranes with minimal other material. Small quantities of ribonucleic acid, and of protein other than proteolipid-protein, however, persist in the myelin prepared as described above and indicate its cellular origin.

The proteolipid-protein, defined according to its solubility in chloroform–methanol mixtures, accounts for some 60% of the total protein of myelin (Autilio, 1966; Mokrasch, 1967). Myelin protein fractions also contain basic protein with encephalitogenic antigenic properties, demonstrated using fluorescent immunochemical techniques and subsequently isolated from the myelin of white matter (Kies et al., 1965, 1966; Martenson & LeBaron, 1966). These and other proteins specific to neural systems are described in Chapter 9. Triphosphoinositide and other lipids of myelin are described in the preceding Chapter.

The importance of the myelin sheath appears to lie in its acting as an electrical insulator and allowing rapid saltatory conduction over sections of nerve fibre about a mm. in length (*Symposium*, 1959; *Reviews*, 1959). Although some movement of cations through the myelin sheath has been observed (Singer & Solpeter, 1966), ion exchange between axon and environment is confined by the sheath mainly to narrow nodes and clefts where the covering is interrupted; these can be of complex structure, with the surrounding cells and the axon rich in mitochondria.

Withdrawal of cytoplasm from most of the myelin sheath makes understandable the metabolic stability of many of the cerebral lipids. The myelin lipids can be seen to have structural rather than metabolic functions and are stable in circumstances when lipids in several other parts of the body undergo change, as in starvation or in inositol or choline deficiencies. Contribution to this stability is probably made by the particular lipids which occur in the sheath: thus myelin carries only one-fifth of the proportion of unsaturated fatty acids found in the grey matter of the brain, but ten times its quantity of fatty acids with chain-lengths of C_{20} or greater (O'Brien, 1965). Cerebral myelination in young animals can proceed during partial starvation. The reverse process of demyelination is a prominent sequel to many types of damage

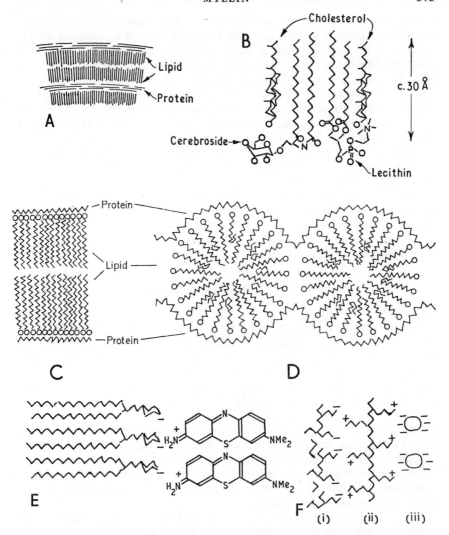

FIG. 12.1. Membrane structures and oriented lipid arrays (see *Reviews*, 1959; *Symposia*, 1959, 1964).

A. Myelin, shown as part of a cross-section of a myelinated fibre (Schmidt, see Frey-Wyssling, 1948).

B. Suggested arrangement of lipids in myelin (Finean & Robertson, 1958).

C. Membrane structure as a continuous lipoprotein bilayer (Davson & Danielli, 1943; Finean, 1965).

D. Membrane structure as subunits of globular lipoproteins, possibly co-existing with C (Sjöstrand, 1963; Gent *et al.*, 1964; Wolman, 1970).

E. Oriented array of acidic lipids prompting the association of molecules of a basic dyestuff, which is suggested as the basis for metachromasy; the example quoted is a ganglioside (full formula, Fig. 11.9) with toluidine blue (see text and McIlwain, 1963).

F. Suggested relationship between (i) acidic groups of tissue components, (ii) basic polypeptides which inhibit excitability and (iii) polyacidic agents which restore excitability (McIlwain, 1964).

to the central nervous system in which nerve cells or their fibres are destroyed or their functioning severely impaired. Thus it follows mechanical injury, deprivation of glucose or oxygen, and occurs in many avitaminoses, intoxications and allergic reactions in which cerebral tissues are involved. Of demyelinating processes those described as primary, which leave the sheath-cells relatively intact though without myelin, appear most likely to have direct metabolic basis. In other, secondary, demyelination the cells of the sheath with which the myelin has been associated are lost, the myelin breaks up and is absorbed by other cells. In this process in peripheral nerve several metabolic changes appear to reflect the proliferation and activities of the scavenging cells: deoxypentose nucleic acid increases as also does an acid phosphomonoesterase and 5'-nucleotidase (q.v.) acting on adenylic acid (Hollinger et al., 1952). In the central nervous system the appearance of cholesterol esters during demyelination can also be pictured as due to the activity of the cells newly invading the damaged tissue. The loss of myelin which occurs in subacute sclerosing panencephalitis is thought to be due to damage to oligodendrocytes (Allen, 1969).

Lipid and Lipid-protein Associations

Structures such as those of Fig. 12.1 are based not only on examination of myelin but also on knowledge of the oriented associations which are formed spontaneously by most naturally-occurring lipids, in aqueous solutions or at interfaces (Davies & Rideal, 1961; Bangham, 1963; Staehelin, 1968). The association is due to an interplay of attractive forces: on the one hand, among long aliphatic parts of the molecules, and on the other, between water and the polar parts of the molecules. Natural membranes are much more complex than this picture implies. Thus although bimolecular leaflets represent the state of lowest free energy for most cerebral lipids in aqueous solutions, other lipids including gangliosides form spheroidal micelles. Transformations between lamellar and micellar phases of natural membranes may contribute to membrane reorganization in different functional states (Kavanau, 1965). Though much remains unknown about such changes, relevant properties may be noted in several membrane-constituents.

Thus the manner in which many phospholipids dissolve is unusual: lecithin specimens swell when placed in water, spontaneously yielding twisting cylindrical shapes which were called "myelin forms" because they resembled the neural sheath (see Nageotte, 1936; Elworthy & Saunders, 1956). The resemblance is real, for the myelin forms show birefringence and a layered structure as does myelin. That the myelin forms are transitory under conditions in which myelin is stable, presumably reflects the particular lipid composition of myelin, and the function of the proteolipid-protein. Ultrasonic dispersion yields from the dissolving lecithin, bimolecular leaflets some 70 Å thick; such sols can be stabilized by small quantities of soaps or lysolecithins, are non-dialysable and have apparent molecular weights of some millions.

Gangliosides are unusual among the cerebral lipids in being very readily water-soluble; but these solutions also are non-dialysable and show apparent molecular weights of about 300,000 (see Gammack, 1963; McIlwain, 1963).

This represents an aggregation of some 200 molecules of the structures quoted in Chapter 11, the values constituting particle weights.

Lipid-lipid Associations

Cholesterol will be recalled as the major lipid of myelin as well as of the brain itself. Although its molecule is largely saturated, the fashion in which its rings are fused gives it rigidity and it forms coherent, incompressible films at a water surface, when its single hydrophilic group, the hydroxyl, is at the aqueous phase and the remainder of the molecule vertical. It is now important to note that cholesterol markedly alters the surface and micellar properties of a number of other lipids, in fashions which can suggest its role in membrane structure (see Adam, 1941; Finean & Robertson, 1958; Goldup *et al.*, 1970).

Thus, long-chain fatty acids themselves form relatively loose surface films, but with cholesterol present in a ratio of 20 % or more, the films formed are more rigid and of smaller area than their components. These associations exist not only with free fatty acids which are rare in the brain, but also with the plentiful aliphatic chains of the other lipids. Thus cholesterol alters markedly the properties of lecithin sols and films (below); associations are formed in cholesterol: lecithin ratios of 1:3 and 3:1. Although cholesterol is normally almost insoluble in water, clear aqueous sols can be obtained containing about 1 g. cholesterol and 2 g. lecithin/10 ml. (Saunders *et al.*, 1962; Staehelin, 1968). Such solubilizing can be brought about also by synthetic detergents, for example the long-chain alkyl sulphates, which disorganize a cholesterol film and take cholesterol to solution as a stable micellar complex. Penetration of lipid arrays by detergents and perhaps the formation of micelles, give reasons for the frequent inclusion of detergents in reaction mixtures concerned with lipids, as was exemplified in Chapter 11.

Lipid-protein Associations

One such association has been mentioned above: the proteolipid of myelin. Its amino acids are, interestingly, relatively poor in both acidic and basic residues, and rich in the less polar amino acids: which contributes to explaining its insolubility in water, the solubility of the proteolipid in $CHCl_3$-CH_3OH, and also the association between the two classes of components in the proteolipid (Folch, *Symposium*, 1963).

Evidence of varied lipid and protein interactions has been given by surface-film techniques. Thus a monolayer of a simple fatty acid, as stearate, can be penetrated spontaneously by serum albumin added to the aqueous solution below, and cholesterol films are similarly penetrated by haemoglobin (Doty & Schulman, 1949; Sobotka, 1956). Association with a protein may be necessary for enzymic reaction in a lipid: a lipoprotein lipase hydrolyses triglycerides rapidly only with protein addition. Many reactions of Chapter 11 inherently involve lipid-protein associations and can be conditioned in unusual fashions: for example action of a phospholipase on lecithin sols or films is promoted by relatively small additions of cationic lipids (Bangham & Dawson, 1962). The cation was concluded to condition the approach of the enzyme to the phospholipid by giving an appropriate charge to the surface or micelle carrying the substrate; diglycerides which are of opposite charge, by contrast inhibited the phosphatase.

Charged groups of cerebral lipids can themselves come to be arranged in specific patterns when the lipids form films or micelles. This gives a basis for the phenomenon of metachromasy, used histochemically for characterizing lipid deposits (Sylvén, 1954; Harris & Saifer, 1960). The term is applied when a dye produces in staining a colour different from that of the dye itself: for example when toluidine blue colours gangliosides red-purple. The arrays of acid groups of a ganglioside micelle (Fig. 12.1) occur at intervals suitable for promoting association, with change of colour, among the dye molecules. Fluorescence may similarly be modified; the combination with gangliosides is interrupted by certain bases including protamines and histones (McIlwain, 1961; Albers & Koval, 1962). The basic proteins themselves interact with gangliosides, both in aqueous solution and when attached to cerebral tissues, as adumbrated in Fig. 12.1. Interactions at the tissues affect ion movements between the tissues and surrounding fluids, and also their response to electrical stimulation: protamine inhibits potassium uptake after excitation and added gangliosides remove the inhibition (McIlwain et al., 1961; McIlwain, 1963).

Lipid interactions are likely to be involved in the effects of tetanus toxin, which are primarily on the central nervous system. The toxin acts in minute amounts and was recognized in 1898 to become attached to an emulsion of cerebral tissue; lipid fractions were implicated, especially crude cerebroside mixtures. Fractionation of these showed two components, individually less active, to become fully active in fixing the toxin when they were present together (van Heyningen, 1959; van Heyningen & Miller, 1961). Phrenosine or a mixture of cerebrosides formed one component; the other was enriched in grey matter and by solubility characteristics was judged to be a ganglioside. Purified ganglioside components indeed acted, their potency increasing with increasing sialic acid content. Ultracentrifugally, gangliosides were shown to combine with the tetanus toxin yielding a complex from which the ganglioside could be recovered unchanged. Such combination presumably contributes to the transport or action of the toxin; in producing tetanus, inhibitory pathways are blocked near synaptic junctions in the spinal cord (Eccles, 1964). On examining subcellular fractions for their ability to combine with tetanus toxin, fractions containing nerve terminals showed marked activity (Mellanby et al., 1965).

Approaches to Reconstructing Membranes from Cerebral Constituents

The understanding of lipid and lipo-protein associations which has been outlined, has inspired attempts to place such materials as layers of molecular dimensions between two aqueous solutions. Thicker membranes in such situations can show much specificity in the size and charge of compounds which are allowed to pass across: for example, the sheets of synthetic polymers carrying charged groups at pores or interstices, which can allow or block the passage of chloride ions or small cations (Symposium, 1955a).

By applying lipid extracts from cerebral tissues to apertures of a few mm. between aqueous solutions, the lipid drop, initially thick, drains away to leave paucimolecular films, ultimately only a bilayer (Mueller *et al.*, 1962, 1963; Huang *et al.*, 1964; *Symposium*, 1968; Goldup *et al.*, 1970). The process is akin to the formation of "black"_soap films in air, and leaves in the film a minute quantity only of the original lipid, as a layer 60–90 Å thick. Remarkably, the film was of capacity about 1 μF/cm.^{2} and resistance 10^7-10^8 ohm/cm^2; it supported a potential difference of up to 0·15–0·2 v. The film contains only about 10^{13} molecules and therefore may differ in composition from the mixture applied, which in the first experiments still contained a significant amount of protein. Comparable films were however obtained from lecithin specimens with tetradecane in $CHCl_3$-CH_3OH solution, so minimizing adventitious materials. Their refractive index and susceptibility to reagents suggested the lecithin to be present in the final film; when made in 0·1 M-NaCl, ^3HOH showed it was quite permeable to water despite a high electrical resistance, of 10^6 ohms/cm^2. Light reflection gave a thickness of 61 Å, corresponding to a lecithin bilayer; a lecithin–cholesterol–decane mixture also yielded stable films (Simons, 1968).

Artificial membrane bilayers made from lecithin–cholesterol mixtures in water or 20% glycerol were freeze-etched; the preparations then presented an appearance in the electron microscope similar to natural membranes, similarly treated (Moor & Muhlethaler, 1963; Branton & Moor, 1964; Staehelin, 1968). Selective cation permeability of bilayers made from cholesterol–phospholipid–benzene mixtures was decreased by Ca^{2+}, which lowers the density of fixed negative charges. The number of negative charges was decreased further by La^{3+}, which changed the artificial membrane from a cation exchanger to an anion exchanger (Tobias *et al.*, 1962; van Breeman, 1968). Basic proteins, acting as large cations, may cause profound changes in membrane preparations formed from lecithin–squalene–decane mixtures or from 1% oxidized cholesterol, 0·25% dodecyl acid phosphate, 0·42% cholesterol mixtures in octane–dodecane, 1:3 (Mueller & Rudin, 1968). The basic protein protamine, or spermine, were added in trace amounts with less than 1 μg./ml. of alamethicin, a cyclic peptide. The treatment caused depolarization of the artificial membranes in the presence of applied pulses and cation gradients. The depolarizations were of amplitude 30–60 mv and had an appearance similar to the action potentials evoked from natural neural systems. Valinomycin, a cyclic dodecadepsipeptide with antibiotic activity and known to have selective actions on cation movements in biological systems, affects also the selective permeability to monovalent cations of synthetic membrane bilayers. These were prepared from solutions of phospholipid and cholesterol in chloroform-decane mixtures and bathed in media containing varying concentrations of cations and of valinomycin. Membrane permeability for the cations was in the ratio 18,000:4:1 for K^+:Na^+:Li^+, μM valinomycin decreased the specific conductivity of the artificial membrane for K^+ to one-third and for Na^+ to one-sixth of their original values (Gotlib *et al.*, 1968; see also Pinkerton *et al.*, 1969).

Membranes with protein components have been made by placing above an albumin sol, one of cholesterol–lecithin, each containing about mM-$CaCl_2$ (Saunders, 1960, 1963). Elastic interfacial films formed, of appreciable electrical

13

resistance; resistance, interestingly, was diminished by choline. It will be attractive if either of these methods can display relevant differences in the behaviour of lipid components or extracts from the particular membranes, very different in function, found in different situations in the brain. The preponderance of unsaturated fatty acids and of unusually long-chain acids in distinct subcellular fractions, was noted above.

Microsomal Membrane-structures

Reverting now to membrane-structures pre-existing in the brain, the next group of components to be discussed, numbered 2 to 4 in Table 12.1, are all obtained after disrupting the cell structure of cerebral grey matter. Their cellular origin is indicated in Fig. 12.2. The material most difficult to deposit on

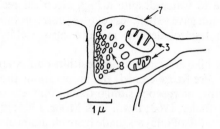

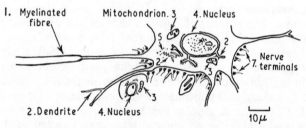

Fig. 12.2. Parts of a cortical neuron and of surrounding structures (based on Gray, 1958, 1959; De Robertis, 1964) drawn to indicate the origins suggested for material separated by centrifuging after dispersing mammalian cerebral cortex in isotonic solutions. The numbers are those of the fractions of Table 12.1.
    1. Myelin fractions derive not only from large myelinated fibres of the type indicated, but also from smaller fibres. 2. Microsomal fractions include material from the endoplasmic reticulum and also outer cell membranes of dendrites and other parts of neurons; the cell membrane and endoplasmic reticulum from other cells also contribute. 3. Mitochondria of various sizes derive from neurons, and associated cells. 4. Nuclei. 5. Ribosomes may be attached to the endoplasmic reticulum or free, and again derive from each cell-type. 7. A nerve-terminal is shown further enlarged in the upper diagram, containing mitochondria and (8) synaptic vesicles.

centrifuging the resulting suspension is termed a microsomal fraction and contains the membrane-structures, synaptic vesicles from disrupted nerve endings, lysosomes, ribosomes and probably other components, in proportions depending on conditions of dispersion and centrifugation. By selecting the conditions for repeated differential or density-gradient centrifugation and controlling separations by electron-microscopy and analysis, a lighter fraction of membrane-structures is obtained.

These microsomal membrane-structures are empty, rounded bodies 500–5000 Å across, bounded by a single membrane 40–60 Å thick (Toschi, 1959; Hanzon & Toschi, 1959; see also Sellinger et al., 1966); they are concluded to be derived from part of the endoplasmic reticulum and outer cell membranes of the different cell types of the cortex. The endoplasmic reticulum probably contributes to the Golgi apparatus, shown histochemically to contain both lipids and proteins. It is presumably across such membrane-structures, collectively, that the greater part of the exchange between cerebral cells and their environment takes place. Thus neurosecretory granules are often seen to be concentrated in the immediate vicinity of the cisternae of the Golgi apparatus. Autoradiography of nerve cells suggests this region to be an important site of incorporation of ^{3}H-labelled glucosamine and galactose to glycoprotein. Proteins of the Golgi region are labelled also when ^{3}H-leucine is used as precursor (Droz & Koenig, 1970), but the label appears more slowly there than in the Nissl substance (q.v.). Enzyme histochemical study has shown the Golgi apparatus to be enriched in nucleoside diphosphatase and thiamine pyrophosphatase activities, in contrast to the Nissl substance, which is apparently devoid of these enzymes. Damage to the Golgi zone has been observed as a result of anoxia or post-mortem autolysis of the brain (Cohen, 1970). Preparations of membrane-structures more defined in cellular origin receive comment subsequently.

Lipids, especially cholesterol and gangliosides, are enriched in the microsomal membrane-structures in comparison with the grey matter from which they originated (Wolfe, 1961; Wherrett & McIlwain, 1962; Bradford et al., 1964); dry matter contents are approximately 10% cholesterol, 5% gangliosides, 24% phospholipid and 40% protein. Gangliosides represent the most characteristic of these components and might serve as chemical marker (Table 12.2). The protein, in contrast to that of myelin, is to a considerable extent insoluble in $CHCl_3$-CH_3OH, and was described in Chapter 9. A large proportion of both lipids and protein can be taken to solution by detergents. Studies with NaCl and KCl indicate that the membrane-structures are not sufficiently intact to retain differential concentrations of Na^+ or K^+ (Swanson et al., 1964); membrane-disruption is necessarily involved in their preparation.

The membrane fragments which derive from the endoplasmic reticulum or the outer cell membranes have not been clearly distinguished from one another, though much research has been devoted to this purpose. Some indications have appeared; acetylcholinesterase is found in the endoplasmic reticulum and in synaptic membranes but not in the plasma cell membrane. NADH-Cytochrome c reductase, while relatively widely-spread, seems to be enriched in membranes of the endoplasmic reticulum rather than the plasma membrane or nerve ending membranes. 5′-Nucleotidase can be used in identification of the plasma membrane, provided myelin is absent. Thus from a combination of various enzyme determinations, identification of the source of membrane fragments may be possible (Table 12.2). Care should also be exercised in ensuring that the vesicles, which form from membrane fragments during tissue dispersion and fractionation, do not contain entrapped cyto-plasm. Lactate dehydrogenase activity is often used as a cytoplasmic marker.

The Na–K–Mg Adenosine Triphosphatase

The microsomal membrane structures would be expected to retain systems concerned with transport of the many substances to which cerebral tissues stand in special relationship. Of these, Na and K ions are of outstanding importance and for maintenance of their normal tissue content require metabolically-derived energy, deployed as phosphocreatine or adenosine triphosphate (Chapter 4). After pioneering investigations with erythrocytes (Clarkson & Maizels, 1952; Dunham & Glynn, 1961; Post et al., 1960) and with a crab nerve (Skou, 1957, 1960) a potent enzyme system which degraded Mg^{2+} adenosine triphosphate maximally only in the presence of Na^+ and K^+ was recognized in the cerebral microsomal fraction (Deul & McIlwain, 1961; McIlwain, 1963). The following data connect this enzyme with active cation transport.

1. In comparison with other subcellular fractions, the microsomal mem-brane-structures are indeed a most active site of the enzyme; their increment in adenosine triphosphatase on adding Na^+ to otherwise adequate media is about 800 μmoles reacting/g. tissue/hr. This is commensurate with the most rapid rates of active Na and K movement in cerebral tissues (Chapter 4).

2. Requirement of the adenosine triphosphatase for both Na and K is to be compared with the requirement of Na^+ for K^+ uptake, and of K^+ for Na^+ extrusion from cerebral tissues. The concentrations of Na^+ and K^+ required for near-maximal adenosine triphosphatase activity are, significantly, compar-able to intracellular $[Na^+]$ and extracellular $[K^+]$: i.e. those relevant to the active movement of the ions (A, Fig. 12.3).

3. The adenosine triphosphatase is inhibited by concentrations of ouabain and digitoxin which disturb energy-assisted Na^+ and K^+ movements at cerebral tissues (B, Fig. 12.3).

4. A number of properties connect the cerebral Na^+–K^+–Mg^{2+}–ATPase with comparable systems in other tissues, including erythrocytes and giant nerve fibres to which reagents can be applied inside or out. Here it is found that Na^+ and ATP are required within the cell; outside, K^+ is required and ouabain inhibits. The cerebral enzyme is firmly attached to microsomal structures and modification of these structures by surface-active agents can enhance their ATPase activity (Swanson, Bradford & McIlwain, 1964; Pull & McIlwain, 1970); the sodium-dependence of the reaction remained or was increased.

Elucidating the mechanism of such ATPases is of major importance in understanding active cation movements. Several phosphate intermediates have been proposed and attention should also be given to the sodium affinities of adenosine triphosphate itself (McIlwain, 1963; Post et al., 1965; Stahl et al., 1965). One intermediate was proposed on finding that cerebral microsomes catalyzed the exchange of ^{14}C-ADP with ATP at a rate comparable to that of their ATPase, which could imply an energy-rich intermediate in the ATPase. Most of this exchange activity proved to be separable; it has received prelim-inary purification (C, Fig. 12.3). Evidence for a further intermediary com-

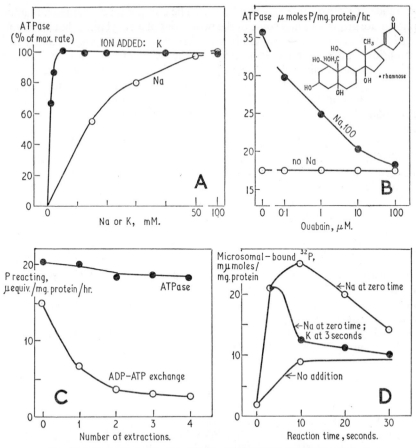

FIG. 12.3. Properties of the Na–K–Mg-adenosine triphosphatase system of microsomal membrane-structures from the brain (Schwartz *et al.*, 1962, Swanson *et al.*, 1964; Swanson & McIlwain, 1965).

A. Dependence of phosphate liberation on concentration of Na+ and K+; except for the ion specified, reaction mixtures contained 3 mM-MgATP, 30 mM-KCl, 100 mM-NaCl, and tris buffer of pH 7·4.

B. Inhibition by ouabain (structure given as inset): complete reaction mixtures were of the composition just specified; others contained ouabain in the concentrations shown; Na+ omitted from those indicated.

C. Separation of ADP-ATP exchange activity from the Na, K-ATPase of cerebral microsomal fractions. The successive extractions were with a mM-solution of NaATP and MgCl₂, and assay of the exchange was by the incorporation of ¹⁴C-ADP into ATP.

D. Formation of an intermediate compound between MgATP (20 μM) and a cerebral microsomal fraction. The intermediate, measured by ³²P, is seen to be increased by 15 mM-Na+ and its breakdown to be accelerated by 0·5 mM-K+.

Stahl, Sattin & McIlwain, 1966; Hems & Rodnight, 1965; see Post *et al.*, 1965.

pound in the transport system has come from the attachment of ³²P from ATP to microsomal fractions on a few second's incubation (**D**, Fig. 12.3). For formation of the intermediate, Na+ was necessary while the additional presence of K^+ prompted its breakdown. The compound contained a reactive phosphate group and had some of the properties of an acyl phosphate (Nagano et al., 1965). Its phosphate could be transferred to hydroxyl groups under acid conditions, non-enzymically; in this way the serine of phosphoproteins may appear to be implicated secondarily (Rodnight & Lavin, 1964), while the acylphosphate proves to be the intermediate of functional significance. The mechanism connecting the ATPase with Na^+ and K^+ movement is still under investigation; proposals involve interaction between acidic groups of the membrane structure, basic groups of the enzyme centre, and the different affinities of ATP, ADP, and the enzyme for Na^+ and K^+ (see McIlwain, 1963; Caldwell, 1968). The mechanism may involve intermediation of free radicles; this seems possible from the results of electron spin resonance spectroscopy of brain microsomal preparations (Kometiani & Cagan, 1967). Characterization of the phosphorylated intermediate as an acyl phosphate has depended partly on its sensitivity to hydroxylamine; identification of the acyl group involved has been achieved using $[2,3-^3H]$-N-(n-propyl)hydroxylamine. Enzyme preparations were treated with the propylhydroxylamine after peptic digestion and the labelled peptides produced were digested further with pronase. Chromatographic and electrophoretic separations resulted in isolation and identification of L-glutamyl-γ-N-(n-propylhydroxamate) which was more highly labelled after isolation from the phosphorylated than from the non-phosphorylated enzyme. The acylphosphate intermediate of the Na,K-ATPase was concluded to be at a L-glutamyl-γ-phosphate residue (Kahlenberg et al., 1968).

Relationships between the Na,K-ATPase preparations and their metal cofactors are open to investigation in purely chemical fashions. The preparations bind Na^+, K^+ and Mg^{2+} quite firmly but repeated washing with mM-ethylene diaminetetraacetic acid diminished the Na content to 24, the K to 7 and the Mg to 3 nmoles/mg. protein (Goldfarb & Rodnight, 1970). Moreover, the treated preparations showed increased dependence on the three cations for Na,K-ATPase activity. Preparations of the Na,K-ATPase made after extracting cerebral microsomal fractions with an NaI-reagent were of high activity, liberating about 100 μequiv. P/mg. protein/hr. They were enriched in lipid, containing about $1 \cdot 1$ mg. of cholesterol plus phospholipid per mg. of protein. Dissociation of lipid from the ATPase preparation by various reagents diminished Na,K-ATPase activity, often reversibly; and activity could be enhanced by various micelle-forming reagents: by synthetic detergents as well as phospholipids of natural occurrence. Thus the ATPase activity was diminished by a number of amino acids at about 1 M concentration, an action probably due to lipid-protein dissociation; arginine was the most effective, and ATPase activity was regained on dilution. Preparations also lost their Na,K-ATPase activity on exposure to urea but were protected from this inactivation by specifically the Na salt of ATP. In attempts to specify the groupings involved, compounds were examined which inactivated by forming covalent linkages under mild conditions. Of these compounds methylmaleic anhydride caused 50% inactivation when 5% of the amino groups of the preparation had been acylated; these groups were both lipid and protein in nature. Again, NaATP partly protected the enzyme from the methylmaleic anhydride (Cooper & McIlwain, 1967; Pull & McIlwain, 1970; Pull, 1970). The Na,K,-

Mg-ATPases of excitable tissues have been comprehensively reviewed (Bonting, 1970) and from the brain, require cholesterol (Noguchi & Freed, 1971).

Cholinesterases; Other Microsomal Systems

Of the different subcellular fractions obtained by differential centrifuging, the microsomal showed greatest enrichment in cholinesterase, hydrolysing some 50–60 μmoles acetylcholine/hr. with material from 1 g. cerebral tissue. It is especially interesting that examination of the substrate specificity of the systems showed the acetylcholinesterase to preponderate, for histochemical studies have shown this enzyme at neurons while a non-specific cholinesterase occurs in glial and vascular elements (see Chapter 14; Aldridge & Johnson, 1959; Holmstedt & Toschi, 1959).

Presumably the systems concerned with the ion movements of the nerve impulse, which are in some instances triggered by acetylcholine, are also present in the microsomal membrane-fractions. Several enzymes concerned with the synthesis of cerebral lipids have been found in microsomal fractions, as is noted in Chapter 11. The association of microsomes with protein synthesis is discussed in detail in Chapter 9. Cerebral microsomes share with similar preparations from other mammalian tissues the presence of 5'-nucleotidase and NADH-cytochrome c reductase activities (Table 12.2).

Mitochondria

Mitochondria from the brain are similar in structure and in most properties to those from other tissues, attractively described by Lehninger (1964) and Slater *et al.* (1967). Their outstandingly important characteristics in relation to respiration and oxidative phosphorylation have been described in Chapter 6.

Distribution and Metabolism

Mitochondria can be seen as rods or rounded granules in the cell body of living neurons. Normally they are probably mobile and are distributed fairly uniformly in the cytoplasm around the nucleus. They are sparser in the axons of the central nervous system and of peripheral nerve, but can be seen throughout the length of the axons. In peripheral nerve small mitochondria have been reported in axons. The more vascular parts of the central nervous system contain most mitochondria (Sinden & Scharrer, 1949; Friede & Pax, 1961), which of course are present in the tissue's non-neuronal as well as in its neuronal elements. Electron micrographs of fine sections of the brain, less than 0·1 μ across, have shown mitochondria *in situ* with defined outer membranes and considerable internal structure. A variety of different arrangements of cristae have been found in the mitochondria which are of varied shape and size from different parts of the nervous system. The number of mitochondria per cell includes those of the cellular cytoplasm; about 1,100 were estimated to be present per cell in rat brain (Samson *et al.*, 1961). In addition, the numerous nerve endings attached to the neuronal surface may contribute many thousands, since each contains one or two mitochondria; mitochondria are also found within the axoplasm of neuronal processes.

Separation of dispersions of cerebral tissues from the rat or rabbit by differential centrifugation yields as one of the more difficultly sedimenting fractions, rod-like or spherical mitochondria of about 1 μ by 2·5 or 4 μ in size. These, like the mitochondria from other tissues, stain with dilute Janus green B (an aminophenazine) to a much greater extent than do other cell components. This staining is seen also in the mitochondria of cerebral tissues treated by normal histological techniques, and also when the dye is added to slices of cerebral tissue during their *in vitro* metabolism (McIlwain & Grinyer, 1950). Electron-microscopic control of subcellular fractions has emphasized the care needed to obtain suspensions of cerebral mitochondria free from contamination and damage (Løvtrup *et al.*, 1961, 1963; Tanaka & Abood, 1963; Eichberg *et al.*, 1964). In particular, contamination with nerve-terminal fractions (q.v.) has led to several incorrect conclusions on the metabolic activities and responses of cerebral mitochondria. It is probable that the mitochondria themselves do not convert glucose to lactate, nor do they oxidize glucose or γ-aminobutyrate at appreciable rates, participation of other parts of the cell being needed for these activities.

Purification of cerebral mitochondria requires separation from the elements (nerve terminals and myelin fragments) which sediment with mitochondria during differential centrifugation. This is achieved by one of two methods. Centrifugation of primary mitochondrial preparations through a density gradient of sucrose or of Ficoll (a polysaccharide) results in partial separation of constituents and is the method most generally adopted (Gray & Whittaker, 1960; de Robertis *et al*, 1961). A preparation of purified mitochondria which are better preserved biochemically, has been claimed from the application of simpler techniques. Thus mitochondria, prepared by rapid passage through dense sucrose solutions of the "tan" fraction which partially separates during differential centrifugation, showed more tightly coupled oxidative phosphorylation than mitochondria produced by density-gradient centrifugation.

The rapidly-purified mitochondria, from enzymic analysis, compared favourably with those from density-gradient centrifugation in extent of contamination by other components (Løvtrup & Svennerholm, 1964; see also Brunngraber *et al.*, 1963; Milstein *et al.*, 1968; Ozawa *et al.*, 1966). It should be noted that while the latter method may offer advantages in the quality of the separated mitochondria, the former density gradient method becomes the method of choice if nerve ending particles (q.v.) are also required.

Oxidative phosphorylation is a major property of mitochondrial fractions from cerebral as from other tissues. With suitable reaction mixtures (Chapters 6 and 7) and pyruvate as substrate, oxygen uptake proceeded at 5–12 μmoles O_2/mg. nitrogen/hr. for some 20 min. at 37° or for 45 min. at 30°C. At the same time inorganic phosphate was esterified at 24–56 μmoles/mg. nitrogen/hr. The cerebral mitochondrial preparations were distinct from those from kidney or liver in the substances which served as oxidizable substrates. Neither alanine nor aspartic acid performed this role with mitochondria from rat or rabbit cerebral hemispheres; glutamic acid as well as most acids of the tricarboxylic cycle did however do so to varying degrees. These factors, important in respiratory control, are described in Chapters 6 and 7. Octanoate, again in distinction to findings in other mitochondrial preparations, is oxidized only in the particular circumstances and to the extent indicated in Chapter 11. In such metabolic characteristics the mitochondria thus parallel the intact cerebral tissue. Of individual enzymes, those concerned with the pathways of electron transport and oxidative phosphorylation and many known to be involved with the synthesis of fatty acids have been described (see Chapters 6, 7 and 11). The occurrence of succinic dehydrogenase and monoamine oxidase in sub-cellular fractions from cerebral as from other tissues, has been taken as indi-cating the presence of mitochondria (Table 12.2).

Mitochondrial Constituents

Lipids constitute about half the dry weight of mammalian cerebral mito-chondrial fractions, and proteins some 40%. Of the lipids, phospholipids preponderate. Cerebrosides and gangliosides were sparse or almost absent (Eichberg et al., 1964), which markedly differentiated the mitochondrial lipids from those of myelin or microsomes. Of the phospholipids lecithins formed 40%, based on lipid-P, phosphatidylethanolamine 23% and phosphatidal-ethanolamine, 9%. Cardiolipin at 11% was markedly enriched in the mito-chondria; comparable values are found in mitochondria from other mam-malian sources. Mitochondrial lipids in other tissues show some associations with the oxidative enzymes, e.g. cardiolipin in liver mitochondria (Lehninger, 1964; see Giuditta & Strecker, 1963). With cerebral mitochondrial fractions, a non-ionic detergent was particularly effective in solubilizing constituent enzymes including fumarate hydratase, the condensing enzyme forming citrate, malate dehydrogenase and aspartate transaminase (Brunngraber & Aguilar, 1962); not all of these may have come from the mitochondria. Cerebral mitochondria contain over 50% of the cellular hexokinase, in contrast to many other tissues in which the enzyme is mainly extramitochondrial. The mitochondrial hexo-kinase, extracted by non-ionic detergents, remains soluble after removal of detergent from the extracts (Thompson & Bachelard, 1970; see also Chapter 5). The mitochondria from the brain also contain β-hydroxybutyrate dehydro-genase which may vary in activity according to the age of the animal, as described in Chapters 2, 6 and 7. Lysolecithin, of detergent properties, also markedly inhibited oxidative phosphorylation (Aravindakshan & Braganca, 1961). Certain effects of thyroxine may be associated with release of a fatty acid, and mitochondrial swelling: a change to which liver but not cerebral mito-chondrial preparations were susceptible (see Tata, 1964). In appraising these and many other data, the purity of the cerebral mitochondrial preparation needs careful consideration.

Nuclear Components and Cellular Control

Sufficient is known of events in the brain to indicate that, as in other biological systems, cellular growth and maintenance involve specific reactions of deoxy-ribonucleic and of ribonucleic acids. Description of these reactions commenced in Chapter 9 and continues in Chapter 13 in relation to cerebral development.

The present account describes briefly some of the cytological components involved: nucleus, nucleolus, and ribosomes. Neurons exhibit a greater array of cell components than the majority of other adult cells of the animal body. In fully-developed neurons nuclear components persist which in most cells are to be seen only at certain stages of their growth or division, and which do not appear in the fully grown cells. This characteristic of neurons is probably related to the relatively enormous volume of cytoplasm associated with a given nucleus; in one sense the nerve cell body is continually growing constituents of its axon and cell processes.

Nucleus

This, the most prominent component of the cell body, and the site of nucleic acid synthesis (Chapter 9), is seen in neuroblasts to display the usual complement of chromosomes on cell division, but by birth in most mammals net increase in the number of cells is proceeding at a much diminished rate in the brain (Chapter 13). The nucleus is then typically large and spherical, of diameter 15–20 μ in a motor cell of diameter 40–50 μ. Analysis after their separation or by histochemical methods has shown in nerve cell nuclei much protein, little lipid, and the relatively high content of deoxyribose nucleic acid typical also of other nuclei. The nucleus, easily stained by basic dyes, is in the normal state of the cell approximately at its centre, but becomes displaced during the changes which take place in neurons after intense activity or loss of the axon. Abnormality in chromosome complement of bodily cells is a fundamental defect in mongolism (see Chapter 13). In normal neurons, electron microscopy shows the nucleus surrounded by a membrane which has numerous pores and deep infoldings, which allow contact with the cytoplasm.

As such nuclei are themselves large structures susceptible to mechanical damage, disintegration of neural tissues to liberate nuclei needs controlled conditions for which particular apparatus and suspending and washing solutions have been devised (Emanuel & Chaikoff, 1960; Rappoport et al., 1963). A number of glycolytic enzymes have been described in some cerebral nuclear preparations, but further investigation would be needed to establish these as nuclear enzymes. Oxidative phosphorylation has not been detected in cerebral nuclei and any ATP produced there is thought to result from glycolysis.

Cerebral nuclear fractions often contain non-nuclear elements, in particular large myelin fragments, cell debris and whole cells which have escaped intact from the tissue disruption process. By techniques similar to those applied in purification of mitochondria, cerebral nuclei have been separated from contaminants by sucrose density-gradient centrifugation; Mg^{2+} of about 1 mM was required for optimal preservation of nuclear structure. Some success has also been achieved in separating different types of nuclei on discontinuous sucrose gradients. Morphological examination indicated partial separation of neuronal nuclei from glial nuclei (Løvtrup-Rein & McEwen, 1966; Kato & Kurokawa, 1967).

The characteristic nuclear constituents, deoxyribonucleic acids and histones, have received study in nuclei from cerebral tissues (Chapter 9). They occur in the nuclei from chicken brain in quantities nearly equal in weight, with a slight preponderance of DNA, as is observed also in other organs (Dingman & Sporn, 1964). After washing the nuclei in isotonic solutions, addition of NaCl to 1–2 M causes a gel of nucleoprotein to form. From this, dilute acid extracts the histones and precipitates the deoxyribonucleic acid; nuclei from chick brain have been reported to contain rather less histone per unit deoxyribonucleic acid phosphorus (266 μg/mole P) than nuclei from other organs of the chick. Conceivably such differences are related to the different expression given in different tissues to a common genetic complement. It is also to be noted that migration of histones can occur from cerebral nuclei to other parts of the cell (Wolfe & McIlwain, 1961; McIlwain et al., 1961; Sporn & Dingman, 1963). The histone mixture from cerebral grey matter is separable by ethanol precipitation to lysine-rich and arginine-rich fractions; in the latter, electrophoresis suggested nine components.

Histones purified from cerebral nuclei were similar in amino acid composition and electrophoretic and ultracentrifugal behaviour to nuclear histones from liver and kidney. These results supported the view that total nucleohistones from different cells are similar (Piha et al., 1966). It has been argued that cell specificity of histones may be due, not to the content and sequence of amino acids, but to the presence of phosphate ester groups or of N-methyl groups at specific sites. The occurrence of such substituents in cerebral nuclear histones has not been systematically studied, but convincing evidence for cell specificity of one purified brain histone has been produced (Tomasi & Kornguth, 1967, 1968). The histone (molecular weight 27,000) contained 24 arginine and 20 lysine residues per molecule. It behaved more like a "lysine-rich" histone during separation and exhibited antigenic properties in the rabbit; antibodies so produced were used in a fluorescent immunochemical study. Specific reaction was observed with the neuronal nuclei of many mammals and amphibia, but not with the nuclei of non-neural tissues from the same animals.

Deoxyribonucleic acid from ox brain contained adenine, guanine, cytosine and thymine in quantities such that the total pyrimidine content was nearly equimolar with the total purine: a relationship involved in the spiral structure for deoxyribonucleic acid (Chapter 9). Cerebral nuclei share with the nuclei of other tissues, the capacity for RNA synthesis; RNA polymerase is particularly active in the immature brain (Chapters 9 and 13). Use of the DNA content of the tissue to provide a basis for cell numbers is based on the assumption that the DNA content/cell is constant. This is valid if all cells are diploid. However there is evidence that some of the cells are tetraploid, i.e. they contain twice the amount of DNA in the nucleus. This is discussed more fully in Chapter 13. Cerebral nuclei also contain nicotinamide mononucleotide-adenyltransferase, which forms NAD^+ from the mononucleotide (Kurokawa et al., 1966; Kato & Kurokawa, 1967). The enzymic activity appeared to be higher in glial than in neuronal nuclei.

Inclusion of virus particles in cerebral nuclei is seen in virus diseases affecting the central nervous system. Examples are given by the nuclear inclusions seen in the brains of patients who died from subacute sclerosing panencephalitis (Allen, 1969) and in the brain of a child who died of virus encephalitis. In this case fragmentation of the nuclei subsequent to invasion by virus particles was described (Hughes, 1969).

Nucleolus and Associated Regions

The nucleolus is a well-defined round central body in the nucleus of neurons. It may be 0·5 to 2 μ in diameter, which is large in comparison with nucleoli of other cells. Again in distinction to most other cells, the nucleolus in neurons is always present, whereas in for example the nucleus of hepatic cells it is seen only during a particular stage of cell division. Staining and spectrophotometric methods show the nucleolus in neurons as in other cells to be rich in polynucleotides and in basic proteins. The ultraviolet light absorbing material of neuronal nucleoli consists of 15% nucleic acid and 85% of protein (Watson, 1968). The nucleotides are predominantly of ribosomal type more characteristic of the cytoplasm, and these are suggested as synthesized at the nucleolus in analogous fashion to other systems where synthesis of ribosomal RNA has been described as occurring in the nucleolus (Perry, 1966). Nucleolar ribonucleic acids increase in motor cells of the spinal roots during proliferation of the poliomyelitis virus. In the rhinencephalic cortex of mice infected with a rodent encephalitis virus, regular crystalline aggregates were found (Nelson *et al.*, 1960). Although biochemical analysis of isolated brain nucleoli has received little attention (Rappoport *et al.*, 1969), the nucleolus has been shown histochemically to be more active in liberating phosphate from thiamine pyrophosphate, adenosine triphosphate and from glycerophosphate than is the remainder of the nucleus.

A region within the nucleus of neurons, adjoining the nucleolus and of similar size to it, can be recognized as containing basic material by its staining with acid dyes. The region has been shown spectrophotometrically to contain nucleoprotein termed nucleolus-associated chromatin, which in distinction to that of the nucleolus itself is of deoxyribose type. The nucleolus appears to arise from the chromatin. Acid phosphatase activity is evident in the chromatin region.

Associated also with the nucleolus in larger neurons is a site with basic protein and relatively small quantities of pentose nucleic acids, which is possibly analogous to the chromocentre seen in neuroblasts and in other cells during a particular stage of cell division. The chromocentre substances increase in sensory neurons after stimulation, and in anterior horn cells after ischaemia and during the beginning of poliomyelitis infection.

During periods of very active growth in cells of the nervous system and in other cells (Hydén, 1960; Caspersson, 1950) the nucleolus increases in size, often enormously, and spectrophotometric evidence shows it to contain both ribonucleic acids and proteins rich in diamino acids. Nucleolar material appears to be absent during cell division when the cell is not growing, and to be reduced in other non-growing periods. It is indeed found in other cells that production of nuclear ribonucleic acid is an early stage in the synthetic activity initiated at the nucleus. The nuclear ribonucleic acid from the brain differs in base-composition from that of the ribosomes (Chapter 9), which are now described.

Ribosomes and Nissl Bodies

The synthetic processes which are linked to the genetic apparatus and which have commenced in the nucleus, now continue elsewhere in the cell. Messenger ribonucleic acid and transfer ribonucleic acid are involved between the nucleus and the ribosomes which are the main site of protein synthesis (Chapter 9). Relationships between ribonucleic acid and cellular activities in neurons were first suggested by observation of Nissl bodies, differentiated microscopically after staining with methylene blue or toluidine blue. The Nissl bodies were normally found in the cell body and in some larger dendrites, but not in the axon. They were observed in spinal ganglion cells to be displaced by centrifugal forces. During development, they appeared after the period of rapid cell division and growth, and have been taken as marking the transition of the embryonic neuroblast to the adult neuron. An early deduction that Nissl bodies contain nucleoprotein has been confirmed by spectrophotometric methods and the nucleic acids recognized as of ribonucleic type by Feulgen's reaction. Moreover, on treatment with a pure ribonuclease the affinity for basic dyes was lost although protein still remained at the sites of the Nissl bodies. These were clearly the first sites of incorporation of ^{3}H-leucine seen on autoradiographic examination and were concluded to be the main sites of protein synthesis in nerve cells (Droz & Koenig, 1970). They thus corresponded to the ribosomes of other cells.

Ribosomes

When dispersions of cerebral tissues are differentially centrifuged and the resulting fractions analysed for ribonucleic acid, a major part but not all of the acid is found in the microsomal fraction. Here it is separable by density gradient centrifugation from lighter fractions containing the membrane-structures already described; heavier fractions bear the ribonucleic acid. Electron-microscopically, these contain dense particles, 150–250 Å across and staining throughout their cross-section. In the original tissue such granules are seen in a region corresponding to that occupied in neurons by the Nissl bodies, occasionally attached to the endoplasmic reticulum and then constituting a "rough" reticulum, and also free. They are sparser in glial cells. After separation by centrifuging from the brain of the rat, guinea pig or goat, the granules can be freed from associated membrane-structures by deoxycholate to which they are resistant; they are however dispersed by ethylenediamine tetraacetic acid (Hanzon & Toschi, 1959; Datta & Ghosh, 1963; Yamagami et al., 1963) and are separable to numerous particle-types, the polyribosomes, which consist of aggregates of various numbers of monoribosomes (Chapter 9).

Ribosomes so prepared contained 30% of their dry weight as ribonucleic acid, and almost all the remainder as protein; in particular, no deoxyribonucleic acid, lipid or hexose derivatives were found. Ribonucleoprotein still in the ribosomes was attacked by a crystalline pancreatic ribonuclease, but at a rate markedly slower than ribonucleic acid which has been extracted from the ribosomes by a method using phenol and water. Enzyme activities are associated with the ribosomes, in particular the protein-synthesizing systems described in Chapter 9; ribosomes prepared with deoxycholate were still capable of incorporating ^{14}C-leucine to protein. On keeping in simple salt solutions, the granules gradually released a number of constituents, including a phosphomonoesterase and ribonuclease. The ribonuclease yielded 3'-

mononucleotides from the ribonucleic acid of the granules themselves and also from soluble ribonucleic acids (Datta *et al.*, 1964). The ribonuclease had no action on deoxyribonucleic acid, which was inhibitory, and was pictured to contribute to the changes in cell content of ribonucleic acid which are noted below; liberation of phosphate from a number of other substrates was also catalysed by the ribosomes.

Changes in Nissl Bodies and in Ribonucleic Acid

Since Nissl described changes in these basophilic bodies in ganglion cells of the dog on cutting their axons, many studies of their change during cell degeneration and regeneration have been made. In cells of the spinal cord, decrease in Nissl bodies is evident within a day of axon section and proceeds for about a week; both protein and nucleotide components diminish. In cells serving peripheral axons recovery of the Nissl bodies roughly parallels that of the axon. The positions in which Nissl bodies are found during such recovery have suggested that the bodies are formed by the nucleus or nucleolus. Degeneration of Nissl bodies occurs also at an early stage of infection with neurotropic viruses, for example in the motoneurons of rhesus monkeys during poliomyelitis. In view of the association of nucleoprotein with both virus and Nissl body, it is significant that regenerating neurons, undergoing changes in Nissl substances, are markedly more resistant to invasion by the virus (Howe & Bodian, 1941). By microchemical determination of ribonucleic acid, association has been shown in certain instances between the quantity present in neurons and their presumed level of protein synthesis (Edström *et al.*, 1961; see also Chapter 9). Thus when nerve regeneration was in progress after nerve section, the neuron body increased in ribonucleic acid; similar increase accompanied the hypothalamic production of a pituitary hormone.

Increase in the ribonucleic acid of cerebral neurons of rabbits was caused by administering 1,1,2-tricyano-2-amino-1-propene; existing differences in base-composition between the ribonucleic acids of their neurons and glial cells were accentuated (Egyházi & Hydén, 1961).

Lysosomes

Lysosomes (*Symposium*, 1963a; Koenig, 1969) have proved interesting biological entities, present in most cells and carrying enzymes capable at acid pH of hydrolysing many structural materials. The lysosomes are pictured to release such enzymes on appropriate occasions, but normally to retain them in a relatively inactive state. A group of such enzymes has been found to occur in the brain, in association with particles bearing resemblance to other lysosomes.

From dispersions of rat brain, made with minimal abrasion in isotonic sucrose, differential and density gradient centrifuging enriched the following enzymes together in a dense fraction (Koenig *et al.*, 1964): acid phosphatase observed with either β-glycerophosphate or *p*-nitrophenol phosphate as substrate; β-glucuronidase observed with phenolphthalein glucuronide as substrate; cathepsin; and enzymes degrading ribonucleic acid and deoxyribonucleic acid. All five enzymes were active at pH 5 and their enrichment was accompanied by increasing evidence of particles seen microscopically as the site of acid phosphatase; this was revealed by the use of lead salts, the insoluble phosphate being converted to PbS. Other enzymes, also active at pH 5, and concluded to occur in cerebral lysosomes include β-galactosidase, sialidase, N-acetyl-β-D-glucosaminidase, arylsulphatase and cerebroside galactosidase. Many of these have also been demonstrated to occur within the lysosomal particles by the use of cytochemical techniques (Koenig, 1969). Aldehyde-fixation of cerebral tissues not only activates lysosomal enzymes, but also fixes them by rendering them insoluble within the lysosomal particle. Acid phosphatase, acid RNase and DNase, acid esterase, β-glucuronidase, N-acetyl-β-D-glucosaminidase and arylsulphatase are among those demonstrated histochemically after aldehyde-fixation. Lysosomal particles were detected also by unusual fluorescence after exposing suspensions to dilute acridine orange, a metachromatic (q.v.) phenomenon probably indicating specific acidic substances in the lysosomes. Electron microscopy after osmium tetroxide staining showed the lysosomes as rounded but rather irregular, dense, granular bodies variable in size but with many about 0·5 μ across.

A feature of lysosomal enzymes is their facile activation or release. Attachment of acid phosphatase to the cerebral preparation was examined in suspensions which contained the lysosomes with other particles. A detergent rapidly released the enzyme, as also did a few minutes' grinding, and treatment with water. The phosphatase as well as N-acetyl-β-D-glucosaminidase were also released by temperature manipulation, mechanical treatment, and digitonin (Sellinger et al., 1964); this was again attributed to occurrence in lysosomes. In other respects, release of acid phosphatase and of β-glucuronidase activities were sufficiently different to suggest distinct forms of occurrence. Cerebral lysosomal enzymes are also released by extremes of pH or by addition of small (mM) amounts of heavy metal cations without causing perceptible change in the structure of the particles (Koenig, 1967, 1969). Release by such manipulations, which affect electrostatic bonds, suggests an involvement of electrostatic forces in the structural latency of the lysosomal enzymes. When fractions enriched in lysosomes were prepared from the brain of mice infected with the virus-like scrapie-agent, several of the lysosomal enzymes were released unusually easily, but acid phosphatase was not; this could be of diagnostic value. The scrapie-agent may contain deoxyribonucleic acid, and it induces nuclear changes in cerebral cells of the infected animals (Millson, 1965; Mordoh, 1965; Hunter, 1969).

Many of the enzymes concerned with catabolism of complex lipids in the brain have pH optima below pH 5·5, but in contrast to the findings for liver or kidney, have not been confirmed as truly lysosomal (Koenig, 1969). It is therefore uncertain at present whether these lipid-degrading enzymes of the brain are lysosomal; it has been suggested that their absence from the lysosomes is responsible for the deposits seen in lysosome-like particles (Symposium, 1963a). Such deposits, termed lipofuscin, increase with age in the large motor cells of the human brain. The accumulation of macromolecules in various storage diseases, such as gangliosides in Tay-Sachs', cerebroside in Gaucher's and in metachromatic leucodystrophy, and acid-mucopolysaccharides in

Hurler's disease, may possibly occur within lysosomal-like particles. Some, if not all, of the defective enzymes are normally present as lysosomal enzymes; their absence would be expected to lead to accumulation of substrate within the particle. The role of lysosomes is thus seen as scavengers in that they comprise a means of intracellular digestion of endogenous material. Compelling evidence for this role has been obtained from electron microscopic examination of the pituitary, where mature secretory granules were observed within dense bodies, suggested by enzyme histochemistry to be lysosomal particles. The lysosomes were concluded to provide a mechanism for control by removing the results of overproduction of secretory substances in the pituitary (Smith & Farquhar, 1966). That mechanisms for disposal of neuronal material are needed is emphasized by the phenomena of axonal flow which are described in the following section.

Neuronal Regions

Neurons of the central nervous system of fully-grown mammals are often enormously elongated. A cell body some 30 μ across, of volume 10^4 cu. μ and mass 10^{-8} g., may have an attached axon 7 μ diameter and some centimetres or decimetres long. Its length is thus some 10^4–10^5 times its diameter, and its total volume about 10^7 cu. μ, or 1,000 times that of the cell body. Metabolic relationship between different parts of neurons thus present special problems and experimental opportunities not found to the same degree in other cells.

Within the cerebral cortex it is estimated that the cell bodies of the neurons themselves occupy only some 3% of the total volume, though with their processes the neuronal volume may be 50%. The remainder of the volume comprises extracellular fluid (possibly 25%; see Chapter 3), glial cells and fibres and dendritic processes from neurons. In the grey matter of the spinal cord, the large motoneuron cell bodies contribute some 5% of the total volume. That these enormously elongated structures nevertheless remain single cells emphasizes the importance of the cell as the unit of structure in the animal body. It is not surprising, however, that neurons are unusual among cells and include biochemical among their other peculiarities. Thus, supply of material from the nucleus involves its transportation over distances enormous in relation to ordinary cell magnitudes. Yet evidence is available by study of peripheral nerve that such translocation occurs. Material accumulates between an experimentally-made constriction and the nucleus; and isotopically-marked materials move relatively rapidly, at some mm./hr., in the endoneural fluid and more slowly in the axon itself (Weiss, *Symposium*, 1961; Ochs, 1965).

Translocation in Neurons

Interesting attempts have been made to characterize material supplied by the normal cell-nuclei of spinal ganglia to axons of spinal roots and of the sciatic nerve (Samuels *et al.*, 1951; Ochs *et al.*, 1962). Isotopic inorganic phosphate was injected to guinea pigs and the concentration and isotopic content determined of different phosphorus-containing fractions of the brain, cord, and peripheral nerve. Analyses at intervals during 30 days showed labelled phosphate to be incorporated in the acid-soluble phosphates, nucleo-protein, and in most phospholipids of the nerve. Incorporation in these substances was uniform along the length of the nerve; but this was not the case with a fraction containing phosphoproteins and probably also a phosphoinosi-tide (Chapter 11). This fraction in the first 10 days was found to contain more of the isotope at the part near the cell body, and later to contain more in the distal portion. By such measurements, the rate of migration of this fraction along the axon was judged to be about 2·5 mm./day, which is similar to the rate of initial outgrowth of an axon, and also to movements of neurosecretory granules in some special neurons in which they occur (Chapter 16). More detailed examination of the rate of flow was made after injecting $^{32}PO_4^{3-}$ to ven-tral horn regions of the spinal cord of cats. Some 3–4 cm. of the spinal roots up to the point at which they left the cord were removed at chosen times and their ^{32}P measured at 3 mm. intervals, giving initially an exponential fall with

Table 12.4

Axoplasmic flow: slow and fast rates

System studied	Metabolite	Rate (mm./day)
Rat hypoglossal nerve:		
Immature	^{3}H-leucine	2·2
Mature	^{3}H-leucine	0·6
Cat dorsal root nerve	^{3}H-leucine	1–2, 100–500
Cat sciatic nerve	^{3}H-leucine	400
	^{32}P-phosphate	4–5
Guinea pig peripheral nerves	^{32}P-phosphate	2·5
Rabbit hypoglossal nerve	^{32}P-phosphate (as phospholipid)	40–70
Rat and cat sciatic nerves	Noradrenaline	100–250

Data were derived from autoradiographic study, fluorescence microscopy and counts of radioactive isotopes in tissue extracts; details are given in the text.

distance from the site of injection. After 20 days maximal ^{32}P had moved peripherally by 10–20 mm., this spread possibly indicating different move-ments of different ^{32}P derivatives. Migration was slower at 30° than at 37°, and was diminished in quantity and rate by damage caused a week earlier to the region containing the neurons concerned; it was thus unlikely to represent passive movement along channels provided by neural structures.

Rates of axonal migration of amino acids also were found to vary for different amino acids under different conditions; rates of 2–11 mm./day have been recorded (Koenig, 1958; Waelsch, 1958; Droz & LeBlond, 1963; see Table 12.4 and Fig. 12.4). Considerably higher rates of axonal flow have been observed for a variety of substances, including amino acids, phospholipids and catecholamines; these were measured at rates of up to hundreds of mm./day (Miani, 1962, 1963; Dahlström, 1967; Lasek, 1968; Lajtha, 1964; Ochs &

Ranish, 1969). Evidence has thus accumulated in support of the occurrence of slow and fast rates of axonal flow. Confirmation that the protein which so migrates originates in the neuronal perikarya has come from careful studies

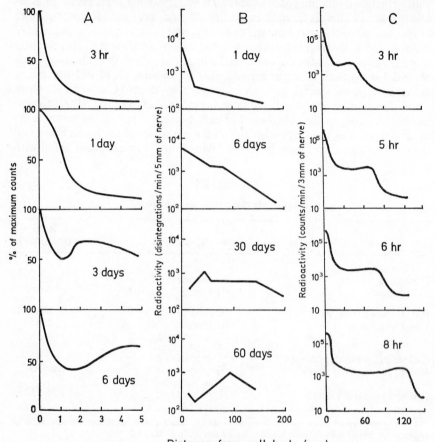

Distance from cell body (mm)

FIG. 12.4. Axoplasmic flow.

A. Silver grains were counted on autoradiographs of sections of mouse optic nerve, from 3 hr. to 6 days after injection of ³H-leucine. The rate of movement of the peak was approximately 1 mm./day (Taylor & Weiss, 1965).

B. Tritium was counted in segments of cat sciatic nerve, 1–60 days after injection of ³H-leucine. A rate of flow of 11 mm/day is indicated by the change in radioactivity between 1 and 6 days; this is followed by a slower rate of 2 mm./day, seen between 30 and 60 days (Lasek, 1968).

C. A rapid rate of axoplasmic flow of some 400 mm./day was observed in cat sciatic nerve examined within the first 8 hr. after injection of ³H-leucine (Ochs et al., 1969).

with puromycin and cycloheximide (Ochs et al., 1970). Kinetic studies indicate that the mechanism is unlikely to be due to simple diffusion: time-lapse photography provides good evidence for pulsation in the axon and the movement of molecules through the axon is regarded as a peristaltic or contractile process (Ochs, 1966). The underlying differences between the fast and slow types of transport are not understood but some relevant observations have been made. Thus the slow type carries most but not all of the constituent soluble proteins; among the exceptions is the highly acidic S100 protein (q.v.). The rapid type, measured by the transport at 400 mm/day of labelled protein, was observed to be dependent on oxidative metabolism: the transport *in vitro* was inhibited when the O_2 supply was replaced by N_2. Cyanide and dinitrophenol both inhibited in the presence of O_2 but tetrodotoxin (q.v.) had no effect (McEwen & Grafstein, 1968; Karllson & Sjöstrand, 1971; Ochs & Hollingsworth, 1971).

The axoplasm contains *neurofilaments*, visible microscopically, running longitudinally along the length of the axon. The filaments are about 100 Å in diameter and consist of helically-coiled protein. The microtubules, or *neurotubules*, seen in fixed and stained sections of cerebral tissue, occur less frequently and were earlier suspected of being artefacts of preparation. They are now known to occur *in situ* throughout the tissue, particularly in cellular processes, axons and dendrites. They have been isolated from disrupted axons as elements some 200–250 Å in diameter, composed of globular proteins which are characterized by specific binding of colchicine (Maxfield, 1953; Schmitt, 1968; Schmitt & Samson, 1968). The number of neurotubules, visible electron-microscopically in the axon, was decreased to 40% of normal by the application *in vitro* of 10 mM colchicine (Hinkley & Green, 1971). It is these colchicine-binding proteins which are thought to be associated with axonal transport. After injection of colchicine (10 μg) to the ventral horn of chick spinal cord the slow axonal flow in sciatic nerve of labelled protein (2 mm/day) was inhibited more than the fast, estimated to be about 300 mm/day (James & Austin, 1970; James *et al.*, 1970). It was concluded therefore that in sciatic nerve, the colchicine-binding proteins affect primarily the slow type of axonal flow. However, such may not be the case for all systems: intracisternal injection of colchicine (50–100 μg) to the rabbit affected the rapid axonal flow of proteins (*ca* 300–400 mm/day) in the hypoglossal and vagus nerves more profoundly than the slow (5–255 mm/day) which included measurement of translocation of labelled proteins and acetylcholine metabolizing enzymes (Sjöstrand *et al.*, 1970). The fast component may also be essentially particulate in nature, involving participation of intracellular organelles. Neurons in tissue culture show movement of cytoplasmic particles, 0·1–1 μ in size, at rates of some hundreds of mm./day (McEwan & Grafstein, 1968).

The occurrence of retrograde flow (i.e. flow in a centripetal direction) is shown from accumulation of metabolites also on the distal side of the injury after nerve crush. This reverse flow is thought to be slow rather than of fast type, but no assessment of the proportion of retrograde flow to proximo-distal flow has as yet proved feasible (Lubinska, 1964; Dahlström, 1965, 1967).

It is clear from the description of Chapter 9 that axonal transport mechanisms cannot account for renewal of all material in the nerve at sites far removed from the perikaryon. It is now generally accepted that a local axonal mechanism of protein synthesis, independent of the neuronal nucleus, must operate even though ribonucleic acid granules are apparently absent from the axon.

Nerve Terminals

At the points of a neuron most distant from its nucleus are its characteristic terminal structures. In the brain these usually impinge on another neuron, constituting the synaptic junctions at which neurons make functional contact. These are extremely numerous in the brain; up to 1,500 occur at a neuron and the terminals from numerous cells may cover nearly 40% of the surface of the postsynaptic cell body. The synaptic junctions at neuronal dendrites occur frequently at projections from the dendrites, which form the postsynaptic components of the junctions. The dendrites of the Purkinje cells of the cerebellum and of the pyramidal cells of the cerebral cortex are covered with these projections, or *dendritic spines*. They are seen electron-microscopically to project from the apical and basal dendrites, but not from the perikaryon, the adjacent dendritic stumps or the axon. Some 40,000 spines may be present on the dendrites of each Purkinje cell. Deafferentation causes loss of the spines, including those in the visual cortex (Whittaker & Gray, 1962; Eccles, 1964; Valverde, 1967). Electron microscopy of the nerve terminal shows the structure outlined in Fig. 12.2; presynaptically, the terminal swells to a bouton $1 \cdot 2$–$1 \cdot 5 \mu$ in diameter containing mitochondria and the synaptic vesicles described below. Where it meets the postsynaptic cell or dendrite is a synaptic cleft of about 200–300 Å. This is a real discontinuity between the cells, though stainable material may appear there. In the postsynaptic cell a special thickening exists at the junction. The shearing forces involved in making cerebral dispersions usually tear these structures away by breaking the postsynaptic cell membrane just beyond the synaptic cleft, and breaking the presynaptic dendrite just beyond the terminal bouton. The resulting relatively artificial structures have been termed synaptosomes; they are usually deposited with mitochondrial fractions on differential centrifugation but can then be separated by density gradient centrifuging (De Robertis & Bennett, 1955; Gray & Whittaker, 1962; De Robertis, 1964).

The synaptic vesicles (q.v.) are the characteristic component of the nerve ending and some thousands may be present per ending, often distributed somewhat in favour of the synaptic cleft. Electron micrographs very occasionally show in this region an infolding which appears to represent a vesicle fusing with the outer membrane of the nerve ending so that the contents of the vesicle are in communication with the synaptic cleft (De Robertis, 1964). This is pictured to be an important unit of action in neural transmission: the release of the vesicle's content of transmitting agent at a point where it acts on the postsynaptic cell (see Chapter 14).

Separation of Nerve-endings and their Components

From a preparative point of view, the vesicles and other components have been found difficult to release by further mechanical disruption of the ending but have been obtained after resuspending in water the nerve-ending fraction prepared in sucrose. Density gradient centrifugation then yields new fractions variously enriched in relation to the vesicles, mitochondria, the nerve-ending outer membrane or ghost, and other membrane-fragments (De Robertis, 1964; Whittaker et al., 1964).

Of these components, the mitochondria have been characterized by succinate dehydrogenase as well as morphologically. The membrane fractions give an opportunity of examining the properties of outer cell membranes from this specific site; thus they have been found rich in the Na^+, K^+-adenosine triphosphatase which is absent from the vesicles (Hosie, 1964). Also, the nerve-ending fractions carry through the different stages of their preparation not only the organelles described but also entrapped cytoplasm. Thus they carry K^+ and soluble enzymes, which appear in solution after treating the sucrose suspension of endings with water. This content of cytoplasm in the endings has contributed to several incorrect statements about the properties of cerebral mitochondria and other components which have been obtained with nerve-ending admixture. Thus the cerebral mitochondria have been wrongly credited with performing glycolysis and carrying much lactate dehydrogenase but these are properties of the nerve endings, which release lactate dehydrogenase on treatment with water. However these properties have proved useful in identification of nerve endings in subcellular fractions. Thus occurrence of Na^+,K^+-ATPase and acetylcholinesterase activities, together with occluded lactate dehydrogenase activity, provides good biochemical evidence for the presence of nerve-endings. Detection of occluded lactate dehydrogenase depends on release of enzymic activity by treatment with detergent, usually Triton X-100; without such treatment, the occluded activity is not detected (Marchbanks, 1967).

The full complement of glycolytic enzymes, together with one or more mitochondria, enclosed within a complete external membrane provide the pinched-off nerve ending with properties analogous to a small, independent, non-nucleated cell. Many of the studies of Chapter 4, cation movement, respiration and oxidative phosphorylation have now been reproduced using purified nerve ending preparations, which may therefore be regarded as unique neural systems for metabolic study (Bradford, 1969; Bradford & Thomas, 1969; Whittaker, 1969; Abdel-Latif et al., 1970; Bradford, 1970).

Relationship of the nerve-endings to substances which are or may be transmitting agents is of outstanding importance. On suspending the fraction in water containing eserine, about half its acetylcholine appears in solution and half, as noted below, in the vesicles. The choline acetyltransferase system which synthesizes acetylcholine is also present in the endings, and appears largely in solution under these circumstances: unless, therefore, the water is leaching it from a normal attachment, it also is presumably free in the cytoplasm. The nerve ending fraction carries also γ-aminobutyrate, 5-hydroxytryptamine and noradrenaline (q.v.), which are suspected to be in different populations of nerve endings. Indeed centrifugation can yield the endings in two fractions which show some morphological differences; one of these shows greater enrichment in the glutamate decarboxylase and γ-aminobutyrate transaminase which are concerned in formation and removal of the aminobutyrate, but the enrichment is not great (Chapter 14). Partial separation of cholinergic from adrenergic or other non-cholinergic nerve endings has been reported (de Robertis et al., 1962b; deLorez Arnaiz et al., 1968).

Synaptic Vesicles

In electron micrographs from intact cerebral cortex, the vesicles are seen in nerve terminals as small bodies, spherical or oval in profile and about 0·05 μ in diameter, bounded by a membrane 40–50 Å thick. They have also been seen free or in ordered array in some axons, possibly attached to or associated with neurofilaments, and suspected to take part in the translocation of materials from the cell body. On disrupting the cortex by grinding in isotonic fluids, the vesicles are obtained either free or still within broken-off nerve terminals, according to conditions employed. They can be freed from the terminals by suspending in water; when free, the vesicles can be separated by differential and density gradient centrifuging (De Robertis *et al.*, 1962, 1963; Whittaker *et al.*, 1964). A preparation of synaptic vesicles from rat brain contained 45% of its dry weight as lipids, with a high proportion of gangliosides (Burton & Gibbons, 1964). Earlier reports that the vesicles were the main site of gangliosides in the brain have been re-assessed; it is now thought that synaptic vesicles and microsomes are enriched to a similar extent in gangliosides (Whittaker, 1966, 1969; Weigandt, 1967). Purified synaptic vesicles seem to contain only one identifiable enzyme: a MgATPase probably involved in transmitter-release (Poisner, 1970).

A major importance of the synaptic vesicles is their containing substances recognized as involved in neural transmission, and described in Chapter 14. The vesicles prepared as described above retained about half the acetylcholine of nerve-endings from which they were derived. The acetylcholine of the vesicle suspension was inactive pharmacologically and not affected by cholinesterase, but was released by quite mild conditions: incubation at 35° for 30 min., or in 1–2 min. at 0° and pH 4. Filled, empty and annular types have been recognized among the vesicles and their contents suspected to differ. Thus, in addition to the 500 Å smooth rounded vesicles, granular, dense-core vesicles, elongated vesicles and larger vesicles of 1,000 Å diameter have been described; the differences in morphology are suspected to be associated with the presence of different transmitters. There is some evidence that the dense-core vesicles contain monoamine transmitters and that elongated vesicles may occur in nerve endings of inhibitory pathways (Whittaker, 1968).

Comments on Microdissection and Histochemistry

In the preceding description, those cellular entities which have been separated from the central nervous system on a scale sufficient for detailed biochemical study, have necessarily received most attention. The account is not an inclusive one; for example the neuroglial fibrils seen in the brain can only be noted (Gray, 1958, 1959; Davison & Taylor, 1960), as also can the application of spectro-photometric methods to localized cell-regions (*Symposia*, 1955, 1961); see also David (1964). Certain histochemical techniques based on deposition of Pb salts by phosphatase action have been demonstrated to give almost quantitative appraisal of reaction rate within cerebral cells (Naidoo & Pratt, 1952; Pratt, 1953). Cell-bodies, usually shorn of longer processes, have also been separated individually or after crushing or sieving cerebral tissues (see Chapter

4; Edström *et al.*, and Hydén, *Symposium*, 1961; Roots & Johnston, 1965; Rose, 1969).

Unless the properties to be measured demand the relatively undisturbed intact cell, it is often easier to handle minute quantities of tissues after freeze-drying them. Valuable technical details, many specific to cerebral tissues, have been described by Lowry (1953). The frozen tissue is cut to sections about 20 μ in thickness, which are dried while frozen and may then be stored for considerable periods. Histological elements can be recognized microscopically in the dried sections and small areas dissected from them and weighed to 0·01 μg. The methods include several for determining individual constituents and

Table 12.5

Analysis of Ammon's horn in the rabbit, after microdissection

Layers (outermost first):	Alveus		Oriens		Pyramidal cell	
Thickness (μ):	200		250		50	
			Non-myelinated			
Major components:	Myelinated fibres		axons and dendrites		Cell bodies	
Dry wt. (mg./ml.)	303	± 11	204	± 8	170	± 3
Protein (mg./g. dry wt.)	308	± 18	510	± 14	660	± 13
Chloride (μequiv./g. dry wt.)	195	± 4	189	± 7	238	± 2
Cholesterol (μmoles/g. protein)	841	± 23	308	± 18	93	± 10
Adenosine triphosphatase (μmoles reacting/mg. protein/hr.)	5·53 ±	0·1	10·62 ±	0·27	7·61 ±	0·26
Fumarase (μmoles reacting/mg. protein/hr.)	20·6 ±	1·1	27·9 ±	1·3	38·7 ±	1·9

Data from Lowry *et al.* (1954), who quote values also for other estimations and for other layers of Ammon's horn, a region of the hippocampus. From 3 to 20 samples of 5–20 μg. were used; values quoted are for the mean followed by its standard error. For application of the methods to other enzymes and metabolites and to other parts of the brain, see Robins *et al.* (1956); Gatfield *et al.* (1966) and Folbergrova *et al.* (1970).

enzyme activities in fragments of a few μg. in weight. The remarkably reproducible data which can be obtained are illustrated in Table 12.5 with analyses of different parts of a small area of cortex of the rabbit. The dendritic layers were in general as active metabolically as those in which cells preponderated, and occupied a large part by volume of the cortex.

Fluorescent techniques have been widely applied in histochemical study of the brain. One involves the use of fluorescent antibodies in detection of proteins specific to the brain; examples of these are given in Chapter 9. Another has proved of particular value in detection and localization of monoamines in specific regions of neural tissues; use is made of the formation of fluorescent molecules when amines are treated with formaldehyde (Falk, 1962; Falk *et al.*, 1962). Freeze-dried tissue sections are caused to react with moist formaldehyde vapour; the products fluoresce at different wavelengths on excitation with U.V. light. 3,4-Dihydro-β-carboline, formed from 5-hydroxytryptamine, emits a yellow fluorescence and the quinonoid forms of

3,4-dihydroxyisoquinolines, formed from catecholamines, fluoresce with a green light. Noradrenaline and dopamine can be distinguished by treatment with HCl: the fluorescence of the product from noradrenaline changes but not that from dopamine (Bjorklund, 1968). The techniques which depend on fluorescent molecules are at present limited to the level of resolution of the light microscope. They have contributed greatly to identification of specific monoamines in neurons and their processes; elucidation of the main mono-amine transmitter pathways in the brains and spinal cords of various mammals and invertebrate species has followed their use (Dahlström & Fuxe, 1964; Dahl et al., 1966; Kerkut et al., 1967).

The components of demonstrable function now characterized biochemically in the central nervous system, afford interesting evolutionary contrasts. They include some relatively standard units, as mitochondria, minimally adapted from their form of occurrence elsewhere in higher organisms. They include also the much more specialized myelin, excitable membrane and synaptic structures. It is encouraging that many of these can be separated for metabolic study; the processes of assembly of their component molecules into a function-ing organelle become more susceptible to examination. The extent to which ease of assembly conditions the structure of enzyme, organelle and membrane-constituent is as yet little explored. Evolutionary and developmental matters considered from a different viewpoint form the subject of the following chapter.

REFERENCES

ABDEL-LATIF, A. A., SMITH, J. P. & HEDRICK, N. (1970). *J. Neurochem.* **17**, 391.
ADAM, N. K. (1941). The Physics and Chemistry of Surfaces. London: Oxford Univ. Press.
ADAMS, C. W. M., DAVISON, A. N. & GREGSON, N. A. (1963). *J. Neurochem.* **10**, 383.
ALBERS, R. W. & KOVAL, G. J. (1962). *Biochim. Biophys. Acta*, **60**, 359.
ALDRIDGE, W. N & JOHNSON, M. K. (1959). *Biochem. J.* **73**, 270.
ALLEN, I. (1969). In Whitty et al., 1969, p. 157.
ARAVINDAKSHAN, I. & BRAGANCA, B. M. (1961). *Biochem. J.* **79**, 84.
AUGUST, C., DAVISON, A. N. & MAURICE-WILLIAMS, F. (1961). *Biochem. J.* **81**, 8.
AUTILIO, L. (1966). *Feder. Proc.* **25**, 764.
AUTILIO, L. A., NORTON, W. T. & TERRY, R. D. (1964). *J. Neurochem.* **11**, 17.
BANGHAM, A. D. (1963). *Advanc. Lipid Res.* **1**, 65.
BANGHAM, A. D. & DAWSON, R. M. C. (1962). *Biochim. Biophys. Acta*, **59**, 103.
BARONDES, S. H. (1968). *J. Neurochem.* **15**, 699.
BECK, C. S., HASINOFF, C. W. & SMITH, M. E. (1968). *J. Neurochem.* **15**, 1297.
BJORKLUND, A., EHINGER, B. & FALK, B. (1968). *J. Histochem. Cytochem.* **16**, 263.
BONTING, S. L. (1970). Membranes and ion transport, p. 257. Ed. E. E. Bittar. New York: Wiley.
BRADFORD, H. F. (1969). *J. Neurochem.* **16**, 675.
BRADFORD, H. F. (1970). *Brain Res.* **19**, 239.
BRADFORD, H. F., SWANSON, P. D. & GAMMACK, D. B. (1964). *Biochem. J.* **92**, 247.
BRADFORD, H. F. & THOMAS, A. J. (1969). *J. Neurochem.* **16**, 1495.
BRANTON, D. & MOOR, H. (1964). *J. Ultrastruct. Res.* **11**, 401.
BRUNNGRABER, E. G. & AGUILAR, V. (1962). *J. Neurochem.* **9**, 451.
BRUNNGRABER, E. G., AGUILAR, V. & OCCOMY, W. G. (1963). *J. Neurochem.* **10**, 433.
BURTON, R. M. & GIBBONS, J. M. (1964). *Biochim. Biophys. Acta* **84**, 220.
CALDWELL, P. C. (1968). *Physiol. Rev.* **48**, 1.
CASPERSSON, T. (1950). In Cell Growth and Cell Function. New York: Norton.

CLARKSON, E. M. & MAIZELS, M. (1952). *J. Physiol.* **116**, 112.

COHEN, S. R. (1970). *Handbook of Neurochem.* **3**, 87.

COLEMAN, R. & FINEAN, J. B. (1966). *Biochim. Biophys. Acta*, **125**, 197.

COLEMAN, R., MICHELL, R. H., FINEAN, J. B. & HAWTHORNE, J. N. (1967). *Biochim. Biophys. Acta*, **135**, 573.

COOPER, J. R. & MCILWAIN, H. (1967). *Biochem. J.* **102**, 675.

CUZNER, M. L., DAVISON, A. N. & GREGSON, N. A. (1965). *J. Neurochem.* **12**, 469.

DAHL, E., FALK, B., VON MECKLENBERG, C., MYHRBERG, H. & ROSENGREN, E. (1966). *Z. Zellforsch. mikrosk. Anat.* **74**, 464.

DAHLSTRÖM, A. (1965). *J. Anat.* **99**, 677.

DAHLSTRÖM, A. (1967). *Acta physiol. Scand.* **69**, 158, 167.

DAHLSTRÖM, A. & FUXE, K. (1964). *Acta physiol. Scand.* **62**, suppl. 232, 1.

DATTA, R. K. & GHOSH, J. J. (1963). *J. Neurochem.* **10**, 363, 611.

DATTA, R. K., BHATTACHARYYA, D. & GHOSH, J. J. (1964). *J. Neurochem.* **11**, 87, 779.

DAVID, G. B. (1964). *Proc. Internat. Neurochem. Sympos.* **5**, 59.

DAVIES, J. T. & RIDEAL, E. K. (1961). Interfacial Phenomena. London: Academic Press.

DAVISON, P. F. & TAYLOR, E. W. (1960). *J. gen. Physiol.* **43**, 801.

DAVSON, H. & DANIELLI, J. F. (1943). The Permeability of Natural Membranes. London: Cambridge Univ. Press.

DELOREZ ARNAIZ, G. R., ALBERICI, M. & DE ROBERTIS, E. (1968). *J. Neurochem.* **14**, 215.

DE ROBERTIS, E. (1964). Histophysiology of Synapses and Neurosecretion. London: Pergamon.

DE ROBERTIS, E., ARNAIZ, G. R. DE L., DE IRALDI, A. P. (1962). *Nature, Lond.* **194**, 794.

DE ROBERTIS, E., ARNAIZ, G. R. DE L., SALGANICOFF, L., DE IRALDI, A. P. & ZIEHER, L. M. (1963). *J. Neurochem.* **10**, 225.

DE ROBERTIS, E. & BENNETT, H. S. (1955). *J. Biophys. Biochem. Cytol.* **1**, 47.

DE ROBERTIS, E., DE IRALDI, A. P., DE LOREZ ARNAIZ, G. R. & GOMEZ, G. (1961). *J. Biophys. Biochem. Cytol.* **9**, 229.

DE ROBERTIS, E., DE IRALDI, A. P., DE LOREZ ARNAIZ, G. R. & SALGANICOFF, L. (1962b). *J. Neurochem.* **9**, 23.

DEUL, D. H. & MCILWAIN, H. (1961). *J. Neurochem.* **8**, 246; *Biochem. J.* **80**, 19P.

DINGMAN, C. W. & SPORN, M. B. (1964). *J. biol. Chem.* **239**, 3483.

DOTY, P. & SCHULMAN, J. H. (1949). *Farad. Soc. Disc.* **6**, 21.

DROZ, B. & LEBLOND, C. P. (1963). *J. comp. Neurol.* **121**, 325.

DROZ, B. & KOENIG, H. L. (1970). In Protein Metabolism of the Nervous System, p. 92. Ed. A. Lajtha. New York: Plenum.

DUNHAM, E. T. & GLYNN, I. M. (1961). *J. Physiol.* **156**, 274.

ECCLES, J. C. (1964). The Physiology of Synapses. Berlin: Springer.

EDSTRÖM, J-E., EICHNER, D. & SCHOR, N. (1961). *Proc. Internat. Neurochem. Sympos.* **4**, 274.

EGYHÁZI, E. & HYDÉN, H. (1961). *Biophys. Biochem. Cytol.* **10**, 403.

EICHBERG, J., WHITTAKER, V. P. & DAWSON, R. M. C. (1964). *Biochem. J.* **92**, 91.

ELWORTHY, P. H. & SAUNDERS, L. (1956). *J. Pharm. Pharmacol.* **8**, 1001.

EMANUEL, C. F. & CHAIKOFF, I. L. (1960). *J. Neurochem.* **5**, 236.

FALK, B. (1962). *Acta physiol. Scand.* **56**, suppl. 197, 1.

FALK, B., HILLARP, N.-A., THIEME, G. & TORP, A. (1962). *J. Histochem. Cytochem.* **10**, 345.

FINEAN, J. B. (1965). *Ann. N.Y. Acad. Sci.* **122**, 51.

FINEAN, J. B. & ROBERTSON, J. D. (1958). *Brit. Med. Bull.* **14**, 267.

FOLBERGROVA, J., LOWRY, O. H. & PASSONNEAU, J. V. (1970). *J. Neurochem.* **17**, 1155.

FREY-WYSSLING, A. (1948). Submicroscopic Morphology of Protoplasm and its Derivatives. Amsterdam: Elsevier.

FRIEDE, R. L. & PAX, R. A. (1961). *Histochimie*, **2**, 186.

GENT, W. L. G., GREGSON, N. A., GAMMACK, D. B. & RAPER, J. H. (1964). *Nature, Lond.* **204**, 553.

GAMMACK, D. B. (1963). *Biochem. J.* **88**, 373.

GATFIELD, P. D., LOWRY, O. H., SCHULZ, D. W. & PASSONNEAU, J. V. (1966). *J. Neurochem.* **13**, 185.
GIUDITTA, A. & STRECKER, H. J. (1963). *Biochim. Biophys. Acta*, **67**, 316.
GOLDFARB, P. S. G. & RODNIGHT, R. (1970). *Biochem. J.* **120**, 15.
GOLDUP, A., OHKI, S. & DANIELLI, J. F. (1970). *Rec. Progr. Surface Sci.* **3**, 193.
GOTLIB, V. A., BUZHINSKII, E. P. & LEV, A. A. (1968). *Biophysics*, **13**, 675.
GRAY, E. G. (1958). *J. Physiol.* **145**, 25P.
GRAY, E. G. (1959). *J. Biophys. Biochem. Cytol.* **6**, 121.
GRAY, E. G. & WHITTAKER, V. P. (1960). *J. Physiol.* **153**, 25.
GRAY, E. G. & WHITTAKER, V. P. (1962). *J. Anat. Lond.*, **96**, 79.
HANZON, V. & TOSCHI, G. (1959). *Exp. Cell. Res.* **16**, 256.
HARRIS, A. F. & SAIFER, A. (1960). *J. Neurochem.* **5**, 218.
HEMS, D. A. & RODNIGHT, R. (1965). *Biochem. J.* **96**, 57P.
HINKLEY, R. E. & GREEN, L. S. (1971). *J. Neurobiol.* **3**, 97.
HOLLINGER, D. M., ROSSITER, R. J. & UPMALIS, H. (1952). *Biochem. J.* **52**, 652.
HOLMSTEDT, B. & TOSCHI, G. (1959). *Acta Physiol. Scand.* **47**, 280.
HOSIE, R. J. A. (1964). *Biochem. J.* **93**, 13P.
HOWE, H. A. & BODIAN, D. (1941). *Johns. Hopk. Hosp. Bull.* **69**, 92.
HUANG, C., WHEELDON, L. & THOMPSON, T. E. (1964). *J. mol. Biol.* **8**, 148.
HUGHES, J. T. (1969). In Whitty *et al.*, 1969, p. 29.
HUNTER, G. D. (1969). In Whitty *et al.*, 1969, p. 123.
HYDÉN, H. (1960). In The Cell, Vol. 4, p. 215. Ed. Brachet & Mirsky. New York: Academic Press.
JAMES, K. A. C. & AUSTIN, L. (1970). *Biochem. J.* **117**, 773.
JAMES, K. A. C., BRAY, J. J., MORGAN, I. G. & AUSTIN, L. (1970). *Biochem. J.* **117**, 767.
KAHLENBERG, A., GALSWORTHY, P. R. & HOKIN, L. E. (1968). *Arch. Biochem. Biophys.* **126**, 331.
KARLLSON, J. O. & SJÖSTRAND, J. (1971). *J. Neurobiol.* **2**, 135.
KATO, T. & KUROKAWA, M. (1967). *J. cell. Biol.* **32**, 649.
KAVANAU, J. L. (1965). Structure and Function in Biological Membranes. San Francisco: Holden-Day.
KEOUGH, K. M. W. & THOMPSON, W. (1970). *J. Neurochem.* **17**, 1.
KERKUT, G. A., SEDDON, C. B. & WALKER, R. J. (1967). *Comp. Biochem. Physiol.* **21**, 687.
KIES, M. W., ALVORD, E. C., MARTENSON, R. E. & LeBARON, F. N. (1966). *Science*, **151**, 821.
KIES, M. W., THOMPSON, E. B. & ALVORD, E. C. (1965). *Ann. N. Y. Acad. Sci.* **122**, 148.
KOCH, R. B. & LINDALL, A. W. (1966). *J. Neurochem.* **13**, 1231.
KOENIG, H. (1958). *Trans. Amer. Neurol. Assoc.* **83**, 162.
KOENIG, H. (1967). *J. Histochem. Cytochem.* **15**, 767.
KOENIG, H. (1969). Handbook of Neurochemistry Vol. 2, p. 255. Ed. A. Lajtha. New York: Plenum.
KOENIG, H., GAINES, D., McDONALD, T., GRAY, R. & SCOTT, J. (1964). *J. Neurochem.* **11**, 729.
KOMETIANI, Z. & CAGAN, R. H. (1967). *Biochim. Biophys. Acta*, **135**, 1083.
KURIHARA, T. & TSUKADA, Y. (1967). *J. Neurochem.* **14**, 1167.
KURIHARA, T., NUSSBAUM, J. L. & MANDEL, P. (1970). *J. Neurochem.* **17**, 993.
KUROKAWA, M., KATO, T. & IMAMURA, H. (1966). *Proc. Japan. Acad.* **42**, 1217.
LAJTHA, A. (1964). *Internat. Rev. Neurobiol.* **6**, 1.
LASEK, R. J. (1968). *Brain Res.* **7**, 360.
LEHNINGER, A. L. (1964). The Mitochondrion. Amsterdam: Benjamin.
LØVTRUP, S. & SVENNERHOLM, L. (1963). *Exp. Cell. Res.* **29**, 298.
LØVTRUP, S. & SVENNERHOLM, L. (1964). *Exp. Cell. Res.* **29**, 298.
LØVTRUP, S. & ZETLANDER, T. (1961). *Exp. Cell. Res.* **27**, 468.
LØVTRUP-REIN, H. & McEWEN, B. S. (1966). *J. cell. Biol.* **30**, 405.
LOWRY, O. H. (1953). *J. Histochem. Cytochem.* **1**, 420.
LOWRY, O. H., ROBERTS, N. R., LEINER, K. Y., WU, M-L., FARR, A. L. & ALBERS, R. W. (1954). *J. biol. Chem.* **207**, 39.
LUBINSKA, L. (1964). *Progr. Brain Res.* **13**, 1.

McEwen, B. S. & Grafstein, B. (1968). *J. cell. Biol.* **38**, 494.

McIlwain, H. (1961). *Biochem. J.* **78**, 24.

McIlwain, H. (1963). Chemical Exploration of the Brain: A Study of Cerebral Excitability and Ion Movement. Amsterdam: Elsevier.

McIlwain, H. (1964). *Biochem. J.* **90**, 442.

McIlwain, H. & Grinyer, I. (1950). *Biochem. J.* **46**, 620.

McIlwain, H., Woodman, R. J. & Cummins, J. T. (1961). *Biochem. J.* **81**, 79.

Marchbanks, R. M. (1967). *Biochem. J.* **104**, 148.

Martenson, R. E. & LeBaron, F. N. (1966). *J. Neurochem.* **13**, 1469.

Maxfield, M. (1953). *J. Gen. Physiol.* **37**, 201.

Mellanby, J., van Heyningen, W. E. & Whittaker, V. P. (1965). *J. Neurochem.* **12**, 77.

Miani, N. (1962). *Nature*, **193**, 887.

Miani, N. (1963). *J. Neurochem.* **10**, 859.

Millson, G. C. (1965). *J. Neurochem.* **12**, 461.

Milstein, J. M., White, J. G. & Swaiman, K. F. (1968). *J. Neurochem.* **15**, 411.

Mokrasch, L. C. (1967). *Life Sci.* **6**, 1905.

Moor, H. & Muhlethaler, K. (1963). *J. cell. Biol.* **17**, 609.

Mordoh, J. (1965). *J. Neurochem.* **12**, 505.

Mueller, P. & Rudin, D. O. (1968). *Nature*, **217**, 713.

Mueller, P., Rudin, D. O., Ti Tien, H. & Westcott, W. C. (1962, 1963). *Nature*, **194**, 979; *J. Phys. Chem.* **67**, 534.

Nagano, K., Kanazawa, T., Mizuno, N., Tashima, Y., Nakao, T. & Nakao, M. (1965). *Biochem. Biophys. Res. Comm.* **19**, 759.

Nageotte, J. (1936). Morphologie des gels lipoides. Paris: Hermann.

Naidoo, D. (1962). *J. Histochem. Cytochem.* **10**, 421.

Naidoo, D. & Pratt, O. E. (1952). *J. Neurol. Neurosurg. Psychiat.* **15**, 164.

Nelson, E., Hager, H. & Kovaks, E. (1960). *J. Biophys. Biochem. Cytol.* **8**, 825.

Noguchi, T. & Freed, S. (1971). *Nature New Biol.* **230**, 148.

Norton, W. T. & Autilio, L. A. (1965). *Ann. N.Y. Acad. Sci.* **122**, 77.

Norton, W. T. & Autilio, L. A. (1966). *J. Neurochem.* **13**, 213.

O'Brien, J. S. (1965). *Science*, **147**, 1099.

Ochs, S. (1965). Elements of Neurophysiology. New York: Wiley.

Ochs, S. (1966). Macromolecules and Behaviour, p. 20. Ed. J. Gaito. Amsterdam: North-Holland.

Ochs, S., Dalrymple, D. & Richards, G. (1962). *Exper. Neurol.* **5**, 349.

Ochs, S. & Hollingsworth, D. (1971). *J. Neurochem.* **18**, 107.

Ochs, S. & Ranish, N. (1969). *J. Neurobiol.* **1**, 247.

Ochs, S., Sabri, M. I. & Johnson, J. (1969). *Science*, **163**, 686.

Ochs, S., Sabri, M. I. & Ranish, N. (1970). *J. Neurobiol.* **1**, 329.

Ozawa, K., Seta, K., Takeda, H., Ando, K., Handa, H. & Araki, C. (1966). *J. Biochem. Japan*, **59**, 501.

Patterson, J. D. & Finean, J. B. (1961). *J. Neurochem.* **7**, 251.

Perry, R. P. (1966). *Natn. Cancer Inst. Monogr.* **23**, 527.

Piha, R. S., Cuenod, M. & Waelsch, H. (1966). *J. biol. Chem.* **241**, 2397.

Pinkerton, M., Steinrauf, L. K. & Dawkins, P. (1969). *Biochem. biophys. Res. Commun.* **35**, 512.

Poisner, A. M. (1970). *Advances in Biochem. Psychopharmacol.* **2**, 95.

Post, R. L., Merritt, C. R., Kinsolving, C. R. & Albright, C. D. (1960). *J. biol. Chem.* **235**, 1796.

Post, R. L., Sen, A. K. & Rosenthal, A. S. (1965). *J. biol. Chem.* **240**, 1437.

Pratt, O. (1953). *Biochem. J.* **55**, 140.

Pull, I. (1970). *Biochem. J.* **119**, 377.

Pull, I. & McIlwain, H. (1970). *Biochem. J.* **119**, 367.

Rappoport, D. A., Fritz, R. R. & Morazewski, A. (1963). *Biochim. Biophys. Acta* **74**, 42.

Rappoport, D. A., Maxcy, P. & Daginawala, H. F. (1969). *Handbook of Neurochem.* **2**, 241.

Reviews (1959). Biophysical Science—A Study Program. Ed. J. L. Oncley, in *Rev. mod. Physics*. New York: Wiley.

RIEKKINEN, P. J. & RUMSBY, M. G. (1969). *Brain Res.* **14**, 772.

ROBINS, E., SMITH, D. E. & EYDT, K. M. (1956). *J. Neurochem.* **1**, 54, 77.

RODNIGHT, R. & LAVIN, B. E. (1964). *Biochem. J.* **91**, 24P.

ROOTS, B. I. & JOHNSTON, P. V. (1965). *Biochem. J.* **94**, 61.

ROSE, S. P. R. (1969). Handbook of Neurochemistry Vol. 2, p. 183. Ed. A. Lajtha. New York: Plenum.

RUMSBY, M. G., RIEKKINEN, P. J. & ARSTILA, A. V. (1970). *Brain Res.* **24**, 495.

SAMSON, F. E., BALFOUR, W. M. & JACOBS, R. J. (1961). *Amer. J. Physiol.* **199**, 693.

SAMUELS, A. J., BOYARSKY, L. L., GERARD, R. W., LIBET, B. & BRUST, M. (1951). *Amer. J. Phys.* **164**, 1.

SAUNDERS, L. (1960, 1963). *J. Pharm. Pharmacol.* **12**, 253T; **15**, 155, 348.

SAUNDERS, L., PERRIN, J. & GAMMACK, D. (1962). *J. Pharm. Pharmacol.* **14**, 567.

SCHMITT, F. O. (1968). *Proc. natl. Acad. Sci. U.S.A.* **60**, 1092.

SCHMITT, F. O. & SAMSON, F. E. (1968). *Neurosciences Res. Prog. Bull.* **6**, 113.

SCHWARTZ, A., BACHELARD, H. S. & McILWAIN, H. (1962). *Biochem. J.* **84**, 626.

SELLINGER, O. Z., DE BALBIAN VERSTER, F., SULLIVAN, R. J. & LAMAR, C. (1966). *J. Neurochem.* **13**, 501.

SELLINGER, O. Z., RUCKER, D. L., VERSTER, F. DE B. (1964). *J. Neurochem.* **11**, 271.

SIMONS, R. (1968). *J. mol. Biol.* **36**, 287.

SINDEN, J. A. & SCHARRER, E. (1949). *Proc. Soc. exp. Biol. Med.* **72**, 60.

SINGER, M. & SOLPETER, M. M. (1966). *Nature*, **210**, 1225.

SJÖSTRAND, F. S. (1963). *J. Ultrastruct. Res.* **9**, 340.

SJÖSTRAND, J., FRIZELL, M. & HASSELGREN, P.-O. (1970). *J. Neurochem.* **17**, 563.

SKOU, J. C. (1957). *Biochim. Biophys. Acta*, **23**, 394.

SKOU, J. C. (1960). *Biochim. Biophys. Acta*, **42**, 6.

SLATER, E. C., KANUGA, Z. & WOJTCZAK, L. (1967). Biochemistry of Mitochondria. New York: Academic Press.

SMITH, R. E. & FARQUHAR, M. G. (1966). *J. cell. Biol.* **31**, 319.

SOBOTKA, H. (1956). *Biochem. Probl. Lipids*, **2**, 108.

SPORN, M. B. & DINGMAN, C. W. (1963). *Science*, **140**, 316.

STAEHELIN, L. A. (1968). *J. ultrastruct. Res.* **22**, 326.

STAHL, W. E., SATTIN, A. & McILWAIN, H. (1966). *Biochem. J.* **99**, 404.

SUZUKI, K., PODUSLO, J. F. & PODUSLO, S. E. (1968). *Biochim. Biophys. Acta.* **152**, 578.

SWANSON, P. D., BRADFORD, H. F. & McILWAIN, H. (1964). *Biochem. J.* **92**, 235.

SWANSON, P. D. & McILWAIN, H. (1965). *J. Neurochem.* **12**, 877.

SYLVÉN, B. (1954). *Quart. J. Micros. Sci.* **95**, 327.

Symposium (1955a). Electrochemistry in Biology & Medicine. Ed. T. Shedlovsky. New York: Wiley.

Symposia (1955, 1961). *Proc. Internat. Neurochem. Sympos.* **1, 4**.

Symposium (1959). The Biology of Myelin. Ed. S. R. Korey. London: Cassell.

Symposium (1963). Brain Lipids and Lipoproteins and the Leucodystrophies. Ed. Folch-Pi & Bauer. Amsterdam: Elsevier.

Symposium (1963a). Lysosomes. Ed. deReuck & Cameron; Ciba Foundation. London: Churchill.

Symposium (1964). Cellular Membranes in Development. Ed. M. Locke. New York: Academic Press.

Symposium (1968). Models and model membranes. *J. Gen. Physiol.* **52**, 125.

TANAKA, R. & ABOOD, L. G. (1963). *J. Neurochem.* **10**, 571.

TATA, J. R. (1964). *Ann. Rep. Chem. Soc.* **60**, 501.

TAYLOR, A. C. & WEISS, P. (1965). *Proc. natl. Acad. Sci. U.S.A.* **54**, 1521.

THOMPSON, M. F. & BACHELARD, H. S. (1970). *Biochem. J.* **118**, 25.

TOBIAS, J. M., AGIN, D. P. & PAWLOWSKI, R. (1962). *J. gen. Physiol.* **45**, 989.

TOMASI, L. G. & KORNGUTH, S. E. (1967). *J. biol. Chem.* **242**, 4933.

TOMASI, L. G. & KORNGUTH, S. E. (1968). *J. biol. Chem.* **243**, 2507.

TOSCHI, G. (1959). *Exper. Cell. Res.* **16**, 232.

VALVERDE, F. (1967). *Expl. Brain Res.* **3**, 337.

VAN BREEMAN, C. (1968). *Biochem. Biophys. Res. Commun.* **32**, 977.

VAN HEYNINGEN, W. E. (1959). *J. gen. Microbiol.* **20**, 301, 310.
VAN HEYNINGEN, W. E. & MILLER, P. A. (1961). *J. gen. Microbiol.* **24**, 107.
WAELSCH, H. (1958). *J. Nerv. Ment. Dis.* **126**, 33.
WATSON, W. E. (1968). *J. Physiol.* **196**, 655.
WEIGANDT, H. (1967). *J. Neurochem.* **14**, 671.
WHERRETT, J. R. & MCILWAIN, H. (1962). *Biochem. J.* **84**, 232.
WHITTAKER, V. P. (1966). *Ann. N. Y. Acad. Sci.* **137**, 982.
WHITTAKER, V. P. (1968). *Biochem. J.* **106**, 412, *Proc. natl. Acad. Sci. U.S.A.* **60**, 1082.
WHITTAKER, V. P. (1969). *Handbook of Neurochemistry*, **2**, 327.
WHITTAKER, V. P. & GRAY, E. G. (1962). *Brit. med. Bull.* **18**, 223.
WHITTAKER, V. P., MICHAELSON, I. A. & KIRKLAND, J. A. (1964). *Biochem. J.* **90**, 293.
WHITTY, C. W. M., HUGHES, J. T. & MACCALLUM, F. O. (1969). Virus Diseases and the Nervous System. Oxford: Blackwell.
WOLFE, L. S. (1961). *Biochem. J.* **79**, 348.
WOLFE, L. S. & MCILWAIN, H. (1961). *Biochem. J.* **78**, 33.
WOLMAN, M. (1970). *Rec. Progr. Surface Sci.* **3**, 261.
YAMAGAMI, S., MASUI, M. & KAWAKITA, Y. (1963). *J. Neurochem.* **10**, 849.

13 Chemical and Enzymic Make-up of the Brain During Development

Reasons for the mammalian brain being as it is, biochemically or otherwise, relate not only to its adult structure and functioning but also to its origins. It is impressive to trace this development through different phyla or in an individual species. Principles regarding the development of living organisms generally, apply to the brain: critical stages in development are irreversible; their timing and nature are partly intrinsic and partly dependent on environmental factors. Progression from DNA, to RNA species, to proteins and to the great variety of cerebral constituents proceeds by routes the description of which commenced in Chapter 9. In one sense the building of nutrients to an adult organ is entirely a matter of biosynthesis. But the sequence of time and place in such syntheses is so intricate and has aspects so little understood chemically that the process and product of biosynthesis, when the product has the complexity of the brain, are to be described first in embryological and histological terms. So much which is biochemical is involved, however, that these aspects also can be seen to be gradually becoming a major part of neurochemistry.

Cell Differentiation and Proliferation in the Brain

In the present Chapter, cerebral growth will be considered first from the point of view of cellular differentiation and proliferation, and subsequently in relation to the accretion of material and the flux of metabolic systems.

Chemical Factors in Differentiation

The cells which constitute the central nervous system normally have the same complement of genes as most other cells of the body; their metabolic specialization has occurred during growth in parallel with other aspects of differentiation. An organ-specific masking of deoxyribonucleic acid (DNA) has been shown in differentiated cells from organs of the rabbit; transcription from 90% of the DNA may be blocked in comparison with transcription in the embryo. Histones were concluded to repress the functioning of DNA non-specifically, but the existence of more specific repressors, protein in nature, was demonstrated. After differentiation has occurred in mammals, neurons

406

as other cells typically breed true and do not revert; much differentiation is concluded to occur by the cumulative effect of numerous stages at each of which is taken one of two possible types of development. Quite simple compounds, as an amino acid, may condition the resulting cell-type. Hormones are also important among the compounds which can act in this switch-like fashion in determining routes of development (Bellamy, 1967; Paul & Gilman, 1968; Weiss, 1968; Wigglesworth, 1967). For details of the cell types of the brain other books must be consulted.

Differentiation of the cells of the neural tube takes place early, before the stages at which most chemical data are available. Of the major ectodermal components, spongioblasts which form glial cells become differentiated from neuroblasts which form the neurons; the microglia are of mesodermal origin. The interaction of cells which in the developing organism results in tissue differentiation is in part chemical (see Needham, 1942; *Symposia*, 1956, 1959; Brachet, 1960; Yamada, 1967; Barondes, 1969). Thus the formation of the neural tube can be brought about in suitable embryos by heated tissue extracts and by certain added substances, including minute amounts of a dibenzanthracene derivative or of polynucleotides. The neural tube itself at or before its first closure has a complex pattern of regional differences which is open to chemical modification. Not only growth and differentiation, but also migration of cell groups in the developing central nervous system, is governed by factors which include chemical ones. Distinct factors condition the tendency to migrate, the direction and the distance of migration, in elements of the neural crest. In vertebrate embryos, the neural crest gives rise to several types of cells and tissues; contributing to their identification have been experiments in which ^{3}H-thymidine has been applied to the crest at chosen times, and its subsequent location determined (Weston, 1970 and see below).

While migration from the neural crest is in progress, and for a variable but usually only short time afterwards, the form of the vertebrate central nervous system is open to experimental modification. More nerve fibres will appear in a ganglion and possibly in the primary motor areas if an additional limb- or wing-bud is grafted to a chick or rat embryo, and fewer will appear if limbs are extirpated. Fibres from a transplanted portion of the central nervous system may also in some cases reach their normal nuclei by new, circuitous routes. Inhibitors, e.g. iodoacetate or antimycin A, affect differentially the growth of the brain, the heart or other organs in chick embryos. A particular fraction from an embryo-dispersion was found to promote especially the growth of the hind-brain of chick embryos; the fraction contained ribonucleoprotein (Tiedemann *et al.*, 1963).

The initial growth of an axon involves chemically conditioned processes not involved in its maintenance (*Symposia*, 1959, 1961, 1964; Filogamo, 1969). After a given stage, however, specific connections are essential for orderly development in the brain, especially of dendrites (Szentágotai & Hámori, 1969). This was displayed in the lateral geniculate body of the dog or rat, where spine development in optic terminals was prevented by visual deprivation. Also, after cell-damage by X-irradiation, dendrites in the cerebellum of kittens appeared to "explore" an available region for fresh connections; the orderly development of a dendritic tree depended on the availability of potentially postsynaptic structures. The tip of a growing axon is highly active, with almost amoeboid pseudopodia which may be protruded, moved and retracted. In tissue culture the neurons appear unable to extend to a homogeneous medium but tend to grow along interfaces. Choice among interfaces can be conditioned by their chemical and physical nature and by electric fields. The rate of growth of axon tips has been observed microscopically in tissue culture or sometimes *in vivo*, and progresses at about 3–4 mm. per day. Chemotropism in the sense of growth towards distant sites by virtue of their chemical nature does not appear to occur, though this is debated. It is impressive to realize that parts of the brain, such as the optic lobes in birds, have been formed by migration of groups of cells which originally were elsewhere in the central nervous system. Much development of the brain appears to be intrinsic and independent of peripheral connections, though in their absence degeneration may later occur and, as indicated above, hyperplasia can be induced by providing an unusually large nerve input.

Time-Course of Cell Proliferation

Cell proliferation in the mammalian brain continues throughout life; it is widespread in embryo and becomes gradually more restricted in site and cell-type during maturation. Histological and cytological techniques employed in showing this have included the use of colchicine and related compounds to arrest cell-division and allow the enumeration of dividing cells; for other aspects of their neural action, see Chapter 9. Also, administration of ^{3}H-thymidine and subsequent autoradiography has been used to show the formation of new DNA and the subsequent fate of the cells so labelled; for appraisal of the technique in neural studies, see Altman (1969). A dose of about 1 μCi of ^{3}H-thymidine/g. body weight has been found to be cleared from the blood of small laboratory animals in about 30 min. but to sufficiently label the nuclei into which it has become incorporated to be detected still after several cell-divisions and the passage of several months.

Cells of the neuroepithelium of embryonic mice are shown by these methods to undergo cell-division about each 11 hr. (A, Fig. 13.1). For about half this time, between cell-divisions, the cells were in a "synthetic" phase during which they incorporated ^{3}H-thymidine to DNA (see Chapter 9). Subsequent cell-divisions distributed the DNA among increasing numbers of cells. This process is seen in operation in young rats 13 days after birth in **B**, Fig. 13.1: division of the labelled cells is still in progress in the brain of 19-day-old animals. At this time a high proportion of subependymal cells of the lateral ventricle were labelled, indicating rapid regional proliferation: but the majority of the labelled cells migrated. It was concluded that they proceeded by the corpus callosum to the neocortex. Some 36% of cells in dorsal regions of the neocortex in rats 3 months of age, were concluded to have been produced postnatally, as shown by ^{3}H-thymidine injections during the first week of life (Altman, 1969); the majority of these were glia, but a proportion of small neurons of the upper layers of the cortex were also labelled.

Examining cell proliferation in the mouse cerebellum, Fujita (1967) found at 10–11 days of age a generation time of 19 hr. during 8 hr. of which DNA synthesis was in progress. Neuroblasts differentiated from matrix cells and migrated to the molecular and granular layers during a few days; such cell formation continued until the animals were 18 days old. Cells still in the course of formation in adult mice, rats and cats included neurons of the

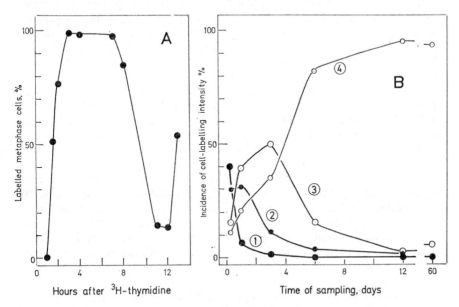

FIG. 13.1. Cell proliferation in the brain shown by injection of ³H-thymidine and subsequent autoradiography (Altman, 1966; Langman & Welch, 1967).
A. Measurements in the neuroepithelium of mouse embryos at 15 days. The ordinate gives the proportion of cells in metaphase, which are found to be labelled with thymidine at different periods after the ³H-thymidine was administered.
B. Measurements in the subependymal layer of the lateral ventricle of rats, on injecting ³H-thymidine at 13 days of age and sampling after the stated intervals. Cell categories: 1, intensely labelled; 2, less so; 3, lightly and 4, very lightly labelled. Those of category 1 are presumed not to have undergone cell-division since the ³H-thymidine administration, and those of 2–4 to have increasingly divided.

hippocampus, and glial cells in many regions. In rats 3 months of age, newly-formed cells still appeared to be proceeding from periventricular structures to parts of the forebrain and to the olfactory lobe and bulb.

Chemical Factors Displayed in Cultured Tissues

In tissue culture a number of parts of the central nervous system have been grown on media containing known substances plus plasma or ascitic fluids and embryo extract (Hild; Murray, *Symposium*, 1959; Geiger, 1963; Lumsden, 1968). A medium adequate for growth of fibroblasts and containing some thirty known substances, allowed only limited aspects of growth in relatively non-exacting spinal ganglia from chicks. Plasma as only addition permitted

14

appreciable growth of both axon and soma, and embryo extract also encouraged myelination and the development of associated cells. In the enriched media, the parts of the mammalian brain which grew most readily included areas from the hypothalamus, reticular formation and cerebellum. Thus in cerebellar folia from a 4-week kitten, Purkinje cells developed and underwent myelination during 40 days in roller-tubes. By providing a fibrous support with a protein clot, dorsal root ganglia from chicks were found capable of growth and development for some weeks, initially with no Schwann cells. Such explants needed to be of a critical size; outgrowth occurred in culture at some 0·2 mm./day.

Electrical stimulation has evoked neuronal responses in suitably cultured tissues from the brain and spinal cord (Hild & Tasaki, 1962; Crain, 1963, 1964; Crain et al., 1968). Commencing with sections $2 \times 1 \times 0.5$ mm. from the cerebral cortex of mice a few days after birth, outgrowths occurred to a medium containing salts, glucose, bovine serum ultrafiltrate and placental cord serum. In 4–5 days cell bodies of neurons were found in the outgrowth, closely packed and surrounded with cell processes. Electrical stimulation then afforded simple spike discharges, recorded extracellularly with micropipette electrodes. By 2–3 weeks, myelination had occurred and synaptic junctions were found microscopically; responses to stimuli were then more complex and sustained and could be potentiated by strychnine. Procaine selectively inhibited certain of the responses. The presence during tissue growth of xylocaine or augmented Mg^{2+} sufficient to inhibit electrical activity, did not prevent the formation of synaptic contacts in explants from the brain of foetal or neonatal mice. Moreover, within a few minutes of placing in fresh media lacking the blocking agents, the tissue gave large and complex electrical responses to mild stimuli; and after 10 min. of intermittent stimuli, afterdischarges also developed. Functioning connections between explants of rat spinal cord and brainstem, and between explants of medulla and cerebrum from foetal mice have also been established and demonstrated electrophysiologically.

Neural outgrowth from sensory ganglia of chicks was slow in culture media, but was accelerated by the presence of a mouse sarcoma (Levi-Montalcini & Angeletti, 1961, 2; Levi-Montalcini, 1968). An extract from the sarcoma also accelerated outgrowth, and a survey of natural materials showed that others also carried activity. Most effective, and acting in µg. quantities, was an extract of salivary glands; the active material was non-dialysable and relatively stable to heat or proteolytic enzymes (Cohen, 1960; Shooter et al., 1969). Both this factor, and antisera to it, had remarkable properties in embryos and new-born animals in vivo: causing in the one case proliferation or in the other near-absence of a large part of the peripheral sympathetic nervous system. Purification of material derived from mouse submaxillary glands and carrying nerve growth-factor activity, showed it to occur as a multisubunit protein. The components could be dissociated by change of pH or by urea, and of them a β-subunit showed nerve-growth activity while a γ-subunit carried peptidase and esterase activity. On recombination, reconstituting "7S NGF", most of the enzymatic activity became masked.

From spinal ganglia preparations cultured in presence of ^3H- or ^{14}C-uridine, RNA has been extracted and characterized chromatographically and by sedimentation analysis (Toschi *et al.*, 1966). Salivary nerve growth factor augmented RNA labelling under these conditions, but did not appear to alter the species of RNA present.

Accretion of Material to the Mammalian Brain

With cellular differentiation and proliferation in the brain come accumulation of materials and changes in enzyme activity. Salient chemical and metabolic aspects of cerebral development are summarized in Table 13.1, and approxi-

Table 13.1

Periods in cerebral development

Period:	I	II	III	IV
Dominant characteristic:	Cell proliferation	Growth of cells, axons and dendrites	Growth; myelination	Myelination; later development
Approximate duration (days; ges.= of gestation) and weight of brain (g.) — Rat	to birth 0·25 g.	0 to 10 d. 0·86 g.	10 to 20 d. 1·28 g.	1·67 g.
— Guinea pig	to 40 d. ges.	40 to 46 d. ges.	to birth	3·5 g.
— Man	to 210 d. ges. 120 g.	to birth 250 g.	0 to 120 d. 650 g.	1,400 g.
Deoxypentose nucleic acid (μg. P/g.)*	700 to 150	110	80	60
Pentose nucleic acid (μg. P/g.)	350 to 180	160	160	170
Respiratory rate (O_2)	23	23	60	59
Respiratory rate with applied electrical pulses (O_2)	32	41	114	108
Succinoxidase (O_2)	28	28	60	60
Succinic dehydrogenase (succinate)	50	63	75	70
Cytochrome oxidase (O_2)	290	350	800	680
Acid phosphatase (P)	–	215	215	108
Cholinesterase (CH_3COOH)	18	56	130	168

Quantitative data is for the guinea pig unless indicated otherwise, and for the end of the periods named. Rates of enzymic change refer to the substance given in parentheses and are in μmoles/g. fresh weight of cerebral cortex/hr.

Values are from the sources of Fig. 13.9, Koch & Koch (1913), the *Symposium* (1955) and Himwich (1962). For a study of specifically the cerebral cortex, see Kuhlman & Lowry (1956). * Values possibly 30% high: see text.

mately correlated with cellular events. The division to four phases, I to IV, has much arbitrariness but is convenient for correlating data from animals which differ in life span and maturity at birth. In reality the development is continuous, and neither its chemical, histological or cytological aspects change at the same time in all parts of the brain; the periods thus of necessity partly overlap and are to be described in terms of some characteristics which at a given time are dominant but not the only ones in progress. Periods so characterized are as follows.

I. The initial period is of cell division, in which cell numbers reach nearly their adult values though the brain is still only a fraction of its adult weight. In the rat, this period lasts until birth when the brain has about 15% of its adult weight; in the guinea pig, pig, or man it occupies the first three-quarters of gestation. During this period there are no signs of transmission of nerve impulses in the brain.

II. A subsequent period is characterized by the growth in size of the individual cells of the brain, and especially the outgrowth of axons and dendritic connections. It is fairly well differentiated from the period of cell proliferation: at birth in the rat the brain has 94–97 % of its adult number of nerve cells, and the present period occupies the first 10 days after birth; in man it lasts until birth.

III. There follows a period in which the overall rate of growth decreases but in which some new processes commence, and outstanding among these in its effects on activity and composition is the formation of myelin sheaths around the axons. Changes in potential can then be detected at the cerebral cortex; neuromuscular control begins. This period in man occupies the first few months after birth and in the rat about the time between the 10th and 20th day. In any one part of the brain it is quite distinct from the preceding period for myelination of a given axon is not observed to commence until it has reached its end-organ or nucleus.

IV. During a fourth period myelination is still active but overall growth proceeds only very slowly to the adult size. This stage lasts much longer than those which precede it and during its latter part the size and composition of the brain are relatively stable.

Expression of Changing Composition

The stages of cerebral development just outlined were first studied extensively in relation to the chemical composition of the brain by Koch & Koch (1913) and have been adopted by several subsequent workers (MacArthur & Doisy, 1918–19; Page, 1937; May, 1945; and, in part, Brante, 1949 and Wells & Dittmer, 1967). They give also a convenient framework for expressing the enzymic composition of the developing brain. Before discussing the change in individual cerebral constituents, it is of value to consider how the changing composition of the brain in the different periods can be expressed, and for that purpose certain of Koch & Koch's results are shown graphically in Figs. 13.2 and 13.3.

The Kochs' data concern the rat and were obtained with mixed cerebral tissue derived from very many animals at the six ages indicated. The group of extractives comprises water-soluble organic substances and all the inorganic components. As proteins are determined by the N content of a residue after extracting lipids and substances soluble in hot acid, the resulting values may be too high; when a similar method was compared by Flexner & Flexner (1950) in the analysis of guinea pig cerebral tissues, with protein as determined by trichloroacetic acid precipitation, values by this latter method were lower. Koch & Koch (1913) also computed indirectly different constituents among the lipids, but values here are less certain. Values for lipid-sulphur, probably proportional to sulphatides, have been included in the present diagrams for the course of their change is interesting; values for total lipids have been recalculated.

It is probable that the composition of the human brain during development follows a course similar to that shown for the rat in Figs. 13.2 and 13.3. Results of Koch & Mann (1909), MacArthur & Doisy (1918–19), Brante (1949), and Crocker (1961) suggest that the stage reached in the rat at 10 days is reached in man at about 8 months, and that at 40 days in the rat, at about 18 months in man. Curves for the composition of human cerebral tissues similar to those of Figures 13.2 and 13.3 have been reproduced elsewhere, but they appear to be drawn by analogy to the findings with the rat, as the data with human tissues concern a few specimens only which necessarily give somewhat scattered results.

In a comprehensive study of postnatal changes in the concentration of lipids of the developing rat brain, Wells & Dittmer (1967) report on 24 classes of lipids in animals of ages similar to those quoted in Fig. 13.2 and 13.3. The account includes discussion of the expression of results and of correlation with cytological changes.

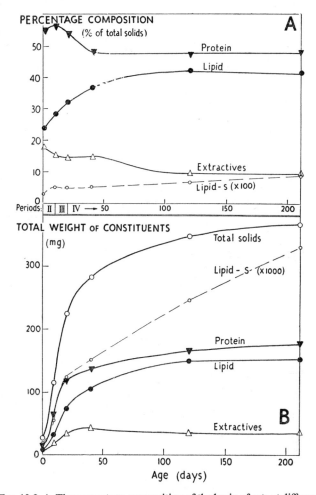

FIG. 13.2. **A,** The percentage composition of the brain of rats at different ages. **B,** The mass of material of different types in rat brain. Data calculated from Koch & Koch (1913); see also *Symposium* (1955).

The different methods of expression used in these figures are as follows.

Percentage composition (**A,** Fig. 13.2). Usually, analysis gives first the percentage composition of the tissue, as is given here with respect to components of the dry (water-free) rat brain. Although this shows the marked increase in lipids during development, it is not as revealing as the other modes of expression. Enzyme systems of the brain cannot yet be expressed in this

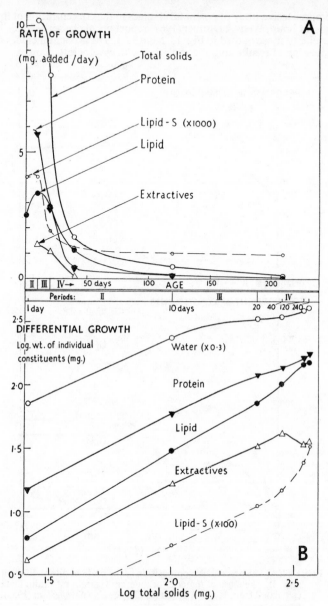

FIG. 13.3. A, Rate of growth of rat cerebral constituents. B, Differential growth of rat cerebral constituents. Periods refer to Table 13.1 and data are derived from those of Fig. 13.2.

fashion, but can be expressed in the following three ways if enzyme activity or rates of reaction are employed in place of quantity of material.

Total mass of material (**B**, Fig. 13.2). This, the most direct mode of expression, shows the total quantity of all the major groups of substances to increase in absolute quantity throughout the development of the brain to its adult size. Thereafter some may fall; there is a tendency for the extractives to fall earlier.

Rate of growth. Calculation of the same results to show the quantity of material added in unit time gives the curves of **A**, Fig. 13.3 which most clearly reveal the net synthetic activities of the organ. A very high level is shown in the first 10–20 days after birth, with a rapid fall later, so that the formation of extractives at 40 days is only some 4% of that at 10 days; lipid formation, however, is still proceeding at over 40% of its peak rate.

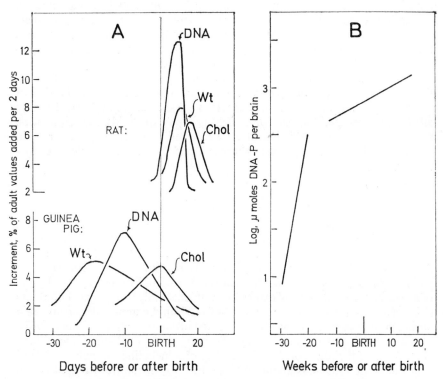

FIG. 13.4. Augmentation of cerebral DNA (Davison & Dobbing, 1968; Dobbing & Sands, 1970).
   A. In the rat and guinea pig in relation to change in total dry weight and cholesterol (Chol.).
   B. In human brain, expressed semilogarithmically. Data from regional analysis of 76 specimens were combined to give the data shown.

Proportion of adult weight added per unit time (**A**, Fig. 13.4) can be valuable also in comparing the composition of different species. Thus it is shown that in the rat, peak proportional accumulation of DNA is followed by peak accumulation of solid matter and of cholesterol. In the guinea pig, however, the peak accumulation of DNA occurs before birth and is not followed by a rise in the proportional rate of solid matter accumulation; this accumulation is, instead, more prolonged.

Relative growth. Consideration of the processes of growth (Thomson, 1942; Needham, 1942) suggests logarithmic expression of results to be most revealing of underlying principles and in **B**, Fig. 13.3 the cerebral content of several. components is expressed in terms of the concomitant dry weight of the tissue. The figure shows clearly a similarity in relative growth of all constituents between 1 and 10 days corresponding to period II (Table 13.1) during which growth of most histologically recognized components is also taking place. In this period the brain increases four-fold in weight; a further four-fold increase brings it to its adult weight, but requires some 200 days. This mode of expression also shows that different components vary appreciably in their development after 10 days. Thus between 10 and 20 days, whereas the relative formation of extractives and proteins decreases, that of lipids continues un-checked: this is the period III of growth and myelination. In the subsequent period of myelination and later development, with little change in total mass, the relative formation of lipid is at first markedly accelerated while that of other components falls below their previous values. Between 100 and 210 days all changes are small but one component group of the lipids, the sulphatides, continues to increase. This has already received comment in Chapter 11 in relation to the enzyme systems concerned, and to metachromatic leucodys-trophy.

Lipid Components

Lipids are normally the preponderating class of compound in the adult human brain, and the course of change in the total lipids of the brain of the rat, shown in Figs. 13.2 and 13.3, is paralleled in the guinea pig and in man (Mac-Arthur & Doisy, 1918–19; Brante, 1949; Flexner & Flexner, 1950). Data for 16 lipid components of normal human brain from individuals up to 98 years of age have been collated and expressed mathematically from logarithmic plots (Rouser & Yamamoto, 1969); and data for 24 lipid components of rat brain during the first year of life have been reported in detail (Wells & Dittmer, 1967).

In cerebral tissues analysed at the earliest period of growth, lipids constituted about 20 % of the total solids; in several species including rat, guinea pig and man the adult value was about 60 %, or 10–18 % of the fresh weight of the brain. The distribution is, however, highly localized: in adult man, lipids constituted 7·5 % of the fresh weight of the cerebral cortex where no con-siderable concentration of lipids can be seen microscopically but 18–22 % of white matter where the myelin sheaths are evident. In the early stages of development "white matter" in the ordinary sense is not present, but lipid accumulation is proceeding steadily; only in period III, late in myelination, does the relative rate of formation of lipid components increase; the rate of formation per unit weight of tissue is then much below its maximum value. After reaching maximum values of 12 % of the fresh weight of the brain at about 20–30 years of age in man, the lipid content declined to 9 % in old age.

The contributions made by different groups of lipids to these changes differ considerably. The part contributed by the *phosphatides* (calculated as phosphate derivatives soluble in fat solvents) is usually between 65 % (in the early stages) and 50 % of the whole; but this is a very heterogeneous group containing lecithins, kephalins, and sphingomyelin. Changes in lecithin as well as in other phospholipids were reported in rabbits (Cuarón *et al.*, 1963) and effects of methylthiouracil examined in relation to cerebral changes in cretins; a small diminution in lecithin deposition or turnover was detected.

The *cerebrosides*, on the other hand (phrenosine and kerasine; determined as fat-soluble carbohydrate), are barely detectable until myelination begins and thus their maximal rate of deposition comes in period III, later than that of the phosphatides; at this time in man, 4 months after birth, some 25 mg. are added each day to the brain (MacArthur & Doisy, 1918–19; Crocker, 1961). In mice, Folch *et al.* (*Symposium*, 1959) confirmed the trends of Figs. 13.2 and 13.3 and in addition showed the sharp increase in cerebrosides which accompanied myelination; a comparable increase in proteolipid-protein receives comment below. ^{14}C-Glucose afforded in the brain of mice ^{14}C-lipids, of which cerebrosides were most heavily labelled; computing the change as galactose incorporated per brain, it was maximal at 22 days, which was also the time of greatest net increase in cerebrosides (Karnovsky *et al.*, *Symposium*, 1959). A myelin-like fraction separated centrifugally from the brain of young rats (Agrawal *et al.*, 1970) was similar to myelin in many respects but lacked cerebrosides and basic proteins. These constituents are thus characteristic of normal, "compact", myelin.

The *sulphatides*, estimated as fat-soluble sulphur, were reported to be deposited in the brain of the rat at greatest rate during period II; with other lipids they shared the increase in relative rates of formation during period III. Chromatographic methods applied to the human brain showed a course of change in sulphatides similar to that in cerebrosides, which were present in about four times the quantity. The fatty acid components of these two lipid classes also altered with age, and here the alterations were not in parallel (Rouser & Yamamoto, 1969).

It is interesting that other glycolipids, the *gangliosides*, are present in the brain of the human newborn in greater quantities than cerebrosides, though later cerebrosides greatly preponderate (Uzman & Rumley, 1959; Rouser & Yamamoto, 1969). Cerebrosides also appear later in phylogeny: they, and sulphatides, are absent from invertebrates. A sialidase which degrades gangliosides reached its maximum activity in the human brain several years after birth, that is at a much later age than several glycosidases (Öhman & Svennerholm, 1971). Of cognate synthetic enzymes, several glycosyltransferases have been examined in the brain of the chick embryo (Den *et al.*, 1970).

Cholesterol shares the general increase in lipid constituents occurring before myelination proper, though by far the greater quantity is laid down later when myelin is visibly increasing. Thus the quantity in the human brain at birth is about 2 g. and increases to some 25 g. in the adult (Page, 1937). The smaller quantity of cholesterol esters is augmented notably in period III (see Chapter 11). In man, their maximum was reached in the spinal cord before birth and in the corpus callosum during infancy: here and also in the chick the maximum quantity of cholesterol esters occurred at the period of most rapid myelination. In the brain of chick embryos and of immature rats, about 12 steriod species were identified; in particular, precursor-product relationships were evident between desmosterol and cholesterol (Paoletti et al., 1969; see Chapter 11).

It can be judged from data of Chapter 11 that the rapid lipid deposition during myelination represents an actual increase in lipid-synthesizing enzymes. Such increase has been demonstrated in the case of cerebroside synthesis from ^{14}C-glucose, which reached a prominent peak at 22 days in the mouse (Karnovsky et al., Symposium, 1959). Sulphatide synthesis is also most active in the brain of young rats, and was demonstrated in vitro in tissues from 9- to 10-day-old animals (Pritchard, 1966); tissues from the brain stem showed greatest activity, and in vivo no depletion of ^{35}S-sulphatide formed neonatally was found after 60 days. The quantities of cerebrosides and ganglioside-like compounds have been followed also in the brain of the chick and its embryo (Garrigan & Chargaff, 1963). The most rapid increase in cerebrosides again accompanied myelination, though they were also detected in appreciable quantities at an earlier stage.

Individual fatty acids of myelin lipids collectively, have been examined in fractions separated centrifugally from the brains of rats of different ages (Banik & Davison, 1969); comparison with lipids of microsomal fractions emphasized the chemical distinctiveness of myelin, especially in its cerebrosides.

Cell Numbers, Nucleic Acids and Proteins

The cerebral content of deoxyribonucleic acid is of especial importance because of the fundamental role of DNA species in cellular events, described in respect to the brain above and in Chapters 9 and 12. Also, it was found on an empirical basis that the DNA content of most cells of the body was nearly constant, a relationship first established in lower organisms and in other tissues of the animal body (Boivin et al., 1948; Thomson et al., 1953). In the cerebral cortex of the guinea pig, also, the number of nuclei per unit volume of cortex was at first found to be directly proportional to the tissue content of deoxyribonucleic acid (Peters & Flexner, 1950; see Flexner & Flexner, 1951). These values imply a fixed content of deoxyribonucleic acid per nucleus; in many tissues of the rat the content was about 6×10^{-12} g./nucleus (Thomson et al., 1953; Heller & Elliott, 1954). Two limitations to this relationship are known to operate in the brain. (i) Mitochondria also contain DNA, though the amount is small in comparison with the nuclear content (Chapter 9). (ii) Certain cerebral neurons, especially Purkinje cells, prove to contain double the typical DNA content, or an amount corresponding to a tetraploid cell (Chapter 12). Relative constancy in the average cellular content of DNA thus depended on the preponderance of diploid cells. It is also to be noted that the cerebral tetraploid cells and their nuclei are large and are presumed to be of high metabolic activity (Lapham, 1968; Lentz & Lapham, 1969); thus much of the basis for taking the DNA content of cerebral samples as a standard of reference in relation to their biochemical status, remains valid.

Determination of DNA in cerebral tissues by otherwise standard methods, has proved subject to interference from phosphoinositides and gangliosides; methods which avoided this gave a DNA content for calf brain of 920 μg./g.

and for adult rat brain, of 700 μg./g. (Zamenhof *et al.*, 1964). Optical methods have also been applied to individual neuronal nuclei at defined wavelengths (Lentz & Lapham, 1969). The DNA content quoted implies that a rat brain of 1·25 g. contains some 140–150 × 10^6 cells. Earlier values including those of Table 13.1 are probably about 35% too high but retain some relative value, for the DNA per unit weight of brain undergoes large changes after birth. The age at which the deoxypentose nucleic acid in the brain of the rat attained its maximal value was 16 days after birth. The corresponding times, presumably those of attaining adult cell numbers, were in the guinea pig, before birth; in the rat, at 2–3 weeks; in fowls, 1 month; in several mammals, 1–5 months, and in man, about a year after birth (Mandel *et al.*, 1952, 1964; Dobbing & Sands, 1970; Fig. 13.4). In man, this maximum value was approached in two phases which have been proposed as representing periods of proliferation first of neuroblasts and subsequently of glial cells. Determination of cerebral DNA has received recent reappraisal (Penn & Suwalski, 1971).

The adult quantity of deoxyribose nucleic acids in the guinea pig brain increased little after period I when the greater part of cell division also ceased. As after this period the brain increased some ten to fifteen times in fresh or dry weight before reaching its adult mass, the content of deoxyribonucleic acid expressed as a percentage of the tissue weight greatly fell (Table 13.1). On the other hand, its content per unit volume of nucleus remained constant, for the volume of the nuclei of guinea pig cerebral cortex reached its adult value at the beginning of period II (Peters & Flexner, 1950); in these respects the nucleus was reaching maturity much earlier than the cell as a whole. The DNA-dependent DNA polymerase (q.v.) which forms DNA from a mixture of four deoxyribonucleotide triphosphates, was assayed in cerebral dispersions or extracts from chick embryos of varying age by following the incorporation of ^{3}H-thymidine (Margolis, 1969). Maximal polymerase activity was found in several regions at 15 days incubation, a period at which DNA was increased most rapidly. Shortly after hatching the polymerase was at less than 10% of its maximal value.

Ribonucleic Acids in Development and Training

The role of ribonucleic acids in protein synthesis (Chapters 9 and 12) gives specific interest to their change during development, for during this process the enzymic constitution of the brain is itself changing rapidly. Presumably the material measured as ribonucleic acid is qualitatively different at different developmental stages, corresponding to the changing proteins synthesized. Examination of RNA species in rat brain showed that short-lived RNA which hybridized with DNA, although constituting a small proportion of the total RNA was present in greater amounts in the brain of new-born animals than in the adult (Bondy & Roberts, 1968; Zomzely *et al.*, 1968). The adult animals moreover, showed a greater proportion of RNA species of rapid turnover in the brain than in the liver; this applied to both nuclear and cytoplasmic RNA.

Cerebral tissues taken from rats 1–3 days of age and examined *in vitro*, showed high rates for the incorporation of 2-^{14}C uridine into RNA. Rates with tissues from adult animals were 0·2–0·3 of those of the younger tissues; in

each case an oxidizable substrate, as glucose, was required for the incorporation and was effective in proportion to its ability to support tissue levels of
ATP (Itoh & Quastel, 1969).

Change in quantity of ribonucleic acid (RNA) during development follows
a characteristically different course from that of the deoxy compound. It will
be recalled that the RNA is largely localized outside the nucleus and that
much of it can be seen histochemically to be a component of the Nissl substance.
The appearance of Nissl bodies during period II has been taken as marking the
change of the neuroblast to the neuron, but is not accompanied by much
increase in rate of formation of RNA. Rather, an increase in the RNA formation takes place in the guinea pig some days earlier; the acid occurs in other
sites as well as in the Nissl bodies. Ribonucleic acid constitutes on the average a
remarkably steady fraction of the weight of the guinea pig cerebral cortex
after period I; during development its content per unit of DNA changes from
about 0·5 at 25 days' gestation to over 3 in the adult. These ratios are common
to many species and to most but not all tissues (Chargaff & Davidson, 1955–60).
In man, the increase in RNA appeared to be unusually delayed (Mandel
et al., 1964).

Much experimental work has examined RNA amounts or turnover with
changed environmental circumstances (Kandel & Spencer, 1968; Glassman,
1969; Rose, 1969) and long-term changes in RNA so imposed can be regarded
as an aspect of cerebral development; with appropriate measurements of
animal behaviour, the findings are relevant to mechanisms of learning and
training. Cerebral RNA of young rats was fractionated on Sephadex columns
to ribosomal and to transfer RNA (Dellweg et al., 1968). The ribosomal RNA
was present in five to six times the quantity of the transfer RNA, and both
species increased as the rats grew, especially between 30 and 60 days of age.
The ratio of ribosomal to transfer RNA remained almost constant during
normal development, but could be increased slightly by causing the rats to
undergo a training or learning procedure. During the procedure the proportion
of cerebral RNA present as polysomes also increased, and this was taken as
indicative of increased protein synthesis.

Visual deprivation in several mammalian species caused loss of neural
RNA; in the rabbit this occurred first from retinal ganglion cells and subsequently from the occipital cortex. Denervation also lowered RNA in the lateral
geniculate nucleus. Dual effects on cerebral RNA have been reported for
electrical or sensory stimulation of normal animals; in some cases an increase,
but more frequently a decrease, in cerebral RNA content or precursor-
incorporation: the decrease often with relatively intense stimulation. However, after keeping animals in the dark their return to light and sound increased
cerebral polysomes, though without affecting net RNA content. Some relevant
changes have been induced in isolated cerebral tissues (Huttunen, 1969;
Prives & Quastel, 1969): diminution in the incorporation of ^{14}C-orotate or
-uridine to RNA on electrical stimulation and an increase by 1 mM-acetylcholine.

Histological observations on individual cells of the nervous system show
considerable variations in their staining with basic dyes, to which process the
ribonucleic acids probably contribute considerably. Basophilia in the glial

cells is markedly less than in the neurons, and different neurons of a given section can be heterogeneous from this point of view; intense activity appears to cause diminution of the basophilic material of the cell (Chapter 12). These factors presumably contribute to variations found in analytical values for the total tissue-content of RNA.

The size-distribution of RNA-containing particles also changes during development (Murthy, 1966). In particular, the RNA present as polyribosomes in the brain of rats diminished during the first 6 months of their lives, while in the liver polyribosomal RNA increased. These changes were correlated with rates of protein synthesis in the two tissues, the rates diminishing with age in the brain and increasing in the liver. In these tissues also, it therefore appears that multiple ribosomal structures, held by messenger RNA, are prerequisite for synthesis of proteins (q.v.).

Proteins

Protein synthesis and breakdown, and aspects of their control which are very relevant to cerebral development, are described in Chapters 9 and 12. Regarded simply as cerebral materials, proteins in most species and at most times during development constitute about half the dry weight of the brain; only in man the adult value falls to about 35% of the solids. There are however in all species marked differences in different parts of the brain when protein is expressed as a percentage of dry weight, largely due to the very different contribution which the lipids make to the dry weight in white and in grey matter. Thus in the almost purely white matter of the corpus callosum of man or the dog, protein constituted some 30% of the dry matter when lipids formed over 60% (Koch & Koch, 1917).

The course of change in the total protein of the brain of the rat, shown in Figs. 13.2 and 13.3, is in part paralleled in the cerebral cortex of the guinea pig at comparable stages of development (Flexner & Flexner, 1950). It is, however, different from that in the liver of the same animals. In the liver the percentage of protein was greater throughout the periods of development observed, possibly reflecting the liver's earlier arrival at a functioning state, and the peak reached in the brain at the end of period II was not seen. Both chemically and functionally cerebral proteins comprise a very complex mixture and the course taken during development by some which can be characterized in enzymic terms is described separately below. Distinct from these is the proteolipid protein recognized as a myelin constituent (Chapter 12). This follows in development a distinct course which is more akin to that of cerebrosides in its increase during myelination (Folch, *Symposium*, 1959).

The cerebral content of any one protein species is to be seen as a balance between its synthesis and degradation, each a complex process susceptible to multiple controls. Approaches have been made to examining stages of the synthesis and breakdown during cerebral development. Protein synthetic rates are high at birth in many species and fall sharply soon afterwards: measured by amino acid incorporation to the brain of the mouse *in vivo*, incorporation per unit weight was at 15 days 0·1 of the neonatal value and remained at this lower level into adult life. To determine which aspects of protein metabolism had altered, aminoacyl RNA synthetase, RNA and transfer RNA binding capacity were measured but did not appear to be limiting in the adult animals (Johnson, 1969). A microsomal factor was concluded to have changed, resulting in a fall in incorporating activity per unit weight of ribosomal protein (A, Fig. 13.5); contributing also was a diminution in activity of the pH 5 enzymes with age.

Proteolytic enzymes reached their peak appreciably after birth, at 5–15 days of age in the rat. B, Fig. 13.5 shows this, and also that particular species of proteinase differ in their developmental course. The acidic proteinases are presumably lysosomal and subject to quite different control from those active at neutral pH, which reached their peak activity earlier (in period II rather than period III). After the first month of life the two categories of protease were

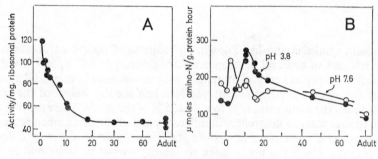

Age of animals, days

Fig. 13.5. Protein metabolism in the brain of young animals (Lerner & Johnson, 1970; Marks & Lajtha, 1970).
    A. Synthesis by ribosomal preparations from the brain of mice, measured as ^{3}H-phenylalanine incorporation in a cell-free system with ATP, GTP, a complete amino acid mixture, a standard amount of pH 5-enzyme, and added polyuridine.
    B. Hydrolysis at acid and at neutral pH by dispersions of rat brain, using a haemoglobin preparation as substrate.

numerically similar in their proteolytic activity, each corresponding to a protein turnover time of about 6 hr. if maximally active. Protein degradation has been indicated as contributing to metabolic regulation and adaptation in adult tissues as well as in development (Lajtha & Marks, 1969; Schimke, 1969; McIlwain, 1970b, 1971); in the brain, an additional role may be seen in relation to axoplasmic transport, when proteolysis can afford one route for the removal of material brought to the terminal regions of neurons.

The protein content or turnover in the brain has been measured in different situations of environmental stimulation or behavioural training, often parallelling the measurements of RNA described above (Weissman, 1967; Glassman, 1969). Sensory stimulation probably increases protein turnover as shown by amino acid incorporation, though protein quantity may be unchanged or diminished; incorporation also has been found to fall with electrical stimulation and in some instances with visual stimuli. Inhibitors of protein synthesis, acetoxycycloheximide and puromycin, administered in circumstances in which they allowed short-term retention of induced behavioural changes for periods up to about 30 min., prevented the long-term retention of the changes. Important in the interpretation of these phenomena are the instances of localized enzyme induction especially by neurohumoural agents, described in the following chapters. Induced changes of these categories can give a basis for cerebral development being influenced by sensory input (see McIlwain, 1970a, 1971b).

Cellular and Extracellular Phases, Electrolytes and Amino Acids

The proportion of water in the brain decreases during cerebral development, especially during the periods when myelination is active and the lipid content

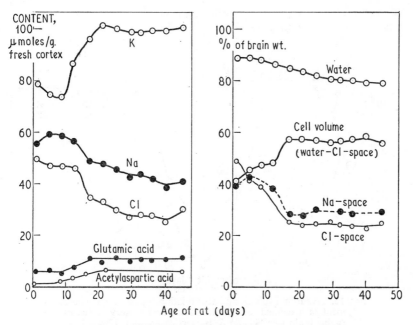

Fig. 13.6. Water and electrolytes of the cerebral cortex during development (Vernadakis & Woodbury, 1962). Rats of the ages quoted were exsanguinated and the blood plasma and cortex sampled. The "spaces" are those which would be occupied by the cerebral Na and Cl at the concentrations of the extracellular fluid. The data on N-acetylaspartic acid are from a separate investigation (Tallan, 1957).

of the tissue is increasing. Empirical equations giving average water contents of the human brain from males of 1 day to 98 years of age, have been derived by Rouser & Yamamoto (1969). It is during the earliest periods of growth, while cell division is dominant and many aspects of synthesis most active, that the tissues contain their highest proportion of water, some 90%, and of the 10% of solids a high proportion—about one-third—is water-soluble. Both the water and the water-soluble solids fall steadily during subsequent periods until the adult brain contains about 75% of water and only one-tenth of its solid constituents are water-soluble. Different parts of the cat and rabbit brain show some differences in time-course in arriving at their adult water-contents of 70–82% (Graves & Himwich, 1955; Agrawal *et al.*, 1967). The course of change in the cerebral cortex of the rat is shown in Fig. 13.6.

Cell Volume and Dendrite Development

Considerable changes take place also in the distribution of the fluid of the tissue between extracellular and intracellular phases. Estimating the extracellular phase from electrolyte distribution as outlined in Chapter 3, Flexner

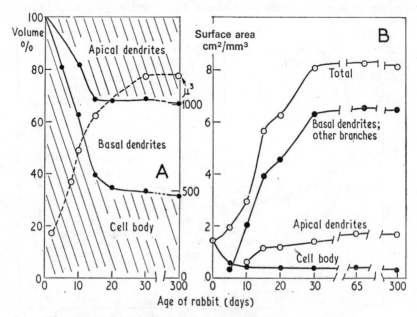

FIG. 13.7. Neuronal volume and area relationships during the development of a defined part of the motor and sensory cortex of the rabbit brain (see Schadé & Baxter, *Symposium* 1960). The data are calculated from linear measurements after rapid fixation of animals at the ages indicated.

A. Volume relationships. The left-hand scale and shaded portions give the percentage of the neuronal components of the cortex which are contributed by cell bodies, and by their apical and basal dendrites. The interrupted line and right-hand scale give average cell body volumes in μ^3.

B. Neuronal surface areas per cubic millimetre of cortex; the upper curve gives the total area (not including that of axons leaving the cortex), and the lower curves its distribution between the components named.

& Flexner (1949) found that in guinea pig cerebral cortex at the end of period I it accounted for 50% of the fluid, while in the adult, the proportion had fallen to 28%. A similar change in the rat, to be discussed more fully when the electrolytes themselves are considered below, is shown in Fig. 13.6. A histological counterpart of this phenomenon could be seen microscopically:

during periods II and III great growth in cell-processes took place, and the volume occupied by glia and by cell axons and dendrites was estimated to increase from 12 to 40% of the tissue; in the adult it was some 55%. Rapid increase in nerve-terminal numbers occurred in the rat brain at 14–24 days after birth; growth of horizontal cells and of their different types of synaptic contacts in the motor cortex of mice during the first few weeks of life has been quantitatively expressed (Aghajanian, 1967; Meller *et al.*, 1968).

Neuronal volumes and areas in the rabbit cortex during its first year of life are shown in Fig. 13.7. These were based on linear measurements made microscopically after rapid fixation, and refer specifically to neurons; the cell bodies are compared with their apical and basal dendrites, including their branches but without their more distant axons. The cell bodies increased four-fold in volume during the year, but their contribution per cu. mm. of cortex diminished. The cell processes, which occupied negligible space at birth, after a month had grown to occupy 70% of the neuronal volume. Because the cell processes were so elongated, their contribution to surface area in the cortex increased much more impressively, as shown in **B**, Fig. 13.7. The area of cell body per cu. mm of cortex diminished, for the cells were becoming sparser; but that of the processes increased until it was thirty times that of the cell bodies. Considering only the surfaces measured in this appraisal, it is seen that the area available for interchange between intracellular and extracellular phases has increased six-fold.

Inorganic Electrolytes

With diminution in water content, inorganic electrolytes, collectively, diminish in quantity in the developing brain; but several differential trends are evident and are of major significance in relation to the development of electrical activity in the brain (Fig. 13.6).

(i) Potassium content increases and sodium diminishes. Already at birth K is at a higher and Na at a lower concentration than in body fluids and these differences are accentuated after birth. This occurs especially during period III, in the rat between 10 and 20 days of age; and at this time the electroencephalograph develops, cerebral potentials occur in response to sound and changes in susceptibility to electroshock are observed (see Himwich, 1962). Thus the adult balance of active and passive Na and K movements described in Chapter 3 has presumably become established; the reciprocal change in Na and K shown in **A**, Fig. 13.6 is significant as the active process is one which exchanges Na and K.

(ii) Chloride content diminishes, especially during the same period, and to a proportional extent which is greater than the change in Na. This is to be seen in relation to concomitant changes: those above, (i), implying either a more negative membrane potential, or an increase in the cellular volume at a given negative potential. In either case, if chloride was or was nearly passively distributed between cellular and extracellular phases, its content in the brain as a whole would diminish. Further, this is a period when other cerebral anions increase. These anions are not distributed according to membrane potential and ion balance is thus maintained despite an increase in the sum of

Na and K. The anions which increase include especially those of the acidic lipids, and of amino acids, as is noted below.

(iii) The "chloride space" of the brain diminishes. In **B**, Fig. 13.6 this is expressed simply as the volume of fluid which would carry the cerebral Cl at the concentration of the extracellular fluid. A small proportion of this Cl is probably intracellular, assuming (Chapter 4) again passive distribution; this leaves 20–25 % of extracellular space in the adult brain.

Certain of the changes described occur in the white matter as well as in the grey matter of the guinea pig during corresponding periods; in addition, cerebral calcium diminished during period III (Flexner *et al.*, 1950; Wender & Hierowski, 1960). Tissue samples taken from the neocortex of rats and incubated in balanced glucose-salines *in vitro*, showed changes in water and electrolytes which were dependent on the age of the animal sampled (Frank, 1970; see Chapter 4). Tissues from 20-day-old animals showed little uptake of fluid *in vitro* under conditions in which 30-day samples absorbed some 11 % of fluid. This uptake was accompanied by Na and the K content of the tissues diminished. Much development of astrocytes occurred in rat cortex between 20 and 30 days and the changes are ascribed to a role of the astrocytes in regulating the ion environment of the mature neocortex.

Amino Acids

Considering first the amino acids which contribute appreciably to ion-balance: in the mammalian central nervous system glutamic acid preponderates, followed by *N*-acetylaspartic acid and aspartic acid. Fig. 13.6 shows that the first two of these increase two- to four-fold in cerebral concentration in the rat while the electrolyte changes just discussed are in progress. At this time, aspartic acid undergoes little sustained change; thus the change in all these amino acids, of about +15 μequiv./g., is to be compared with that in Cl⁻ of −20, in Na⁺ of −20 and K⁺, of +25 μequiv. By this appraisal the diffusible ions discussed remain at the same total but cations have increased by 5 μequiv./g. and anions diminished by 5. The conclusions of (ii) above thus remain after this more detailed consideration; see also Chapter 4. In kittens, cerebral glutamic acid doubled in concentration in the first 6 weeks of life and the distribution and metabolism of ^{14}C-glutamate applied to the surface of the brain also altered (Berl, 1965). Significant regional differences in glutamate metabolism were found on intracisternal administration of ^{14}C-glutamate to kittens, the hippocampus developing ahead of the brainstem and cerebellum (Berl & Purpura, 1966).

N-Acetylaspartic acid as noted above is diminished or absent in invertebrate species, certain of which contain much isethionic acid (Koechlin, 1955). The likely significance of the changes discussed in relation to ion balance is increased by the different course followed by glutamine, of which the level fluctuates but differs little at 32–40 days from its level at 5–12 days; this is true also of threonine (Tallan, 1957; Vernadakis & Woodbury, 1962).

γ-Aminobutyric acid in mouse, rat and rabbit increases relatively steadily from about 1–3 μmoles/g. in the first 30 days after birth, but a more remarkable increase occurs in the glutamate decarboxylase which forms it (Roberts, and

Baxter *et al.*, *Symposium*, 1960; Himwich, 1962). The enzyme increased about 30-fold in activity during this time. Enzyme mechanisms for removal of γ-aminobutyrate also show characteristic increases during development of the brain (Sims *et al.*, 1968). First to increase in rate of formation from 6 days of age in the rat, was succinic semialdehyde dehydrogenase. This was followed at 12 days of age by abrupt increase in the aminobutyrate:oxoglutarate aminotransferase which formed the aldehyde. The increases thus occur in periods II and III respectively, when dendrites and synaptic contacts are being formed. It has been noted that the arrival at adult EEG patterns in the rabbit coincides with the attainment of adult levels of γ-aminobutyrate (Baxter, 1970).

When free amino acids as a whole were surveyed in the rat brain during postnatal development to adults, the majority were found to undergo no great change in concentration (Agrawal *et al.*, 1966). This emphasizes the special roles of the compounds already discussed, which increased in concentration. Also, however, proline, valine, leucine, isoleucine, tyrosine and phenylalanine decreased in cerebral concentration, adult values being 10–50 % of those on the first day of life.

Energy Balance and Supply to the Developing Brain

The changes described in preceding sections imply increase in energy-consuming processes per unit weight of brain during periods II and III. For although synthesis of cell materials diminishes, greater ion gradients are now maintained over a much greater area of cell-interfaces; the electrical activity which is a manifestation of ion movements has increased. Several data are consistent with this view.

Respiration and Glycolysis

Considering first the cerebral uptake of oxygen itself, the determination of cerebral respiration in man by arteriovenous difference (Chapter 2) shows greatest rates in young children, falling to a relatively stable level in young adults. These periods are however relatively late in cerebral development. Studies with isolated cerebral tissues have given values at earlier ages and in different parts of the brain (Table 13.1; Fig. 13.8; Seiler, 1969). In the first few days after birth of the rat, respiratory rate of slices of their cerebral tissue in salt–glucose mixtures falls with age, but subsequently rises until at about 14 days of age the rate is close to its adult value which persists for 2 years. Mitochondrial numbers also increase (Kibler & Brody, 1942; Samson *et al.*, 1960). The rise in cerebral respiration takes place at a stage when the basal metabolic rate of the whole animal is still low, and it is therefore especially interesting to see that the period when the cerebral rate rises is that when electrical activity is first found at the cerebral cortex. Moreover, the cerebral respiration of the pig increases at a similar stage of development, which in this case is reached at about 100 days' gestation. L-Glutamate as oxidizable substrate for rabbit cerebral cortex supported respiratory rates which increased with the age of the animal yielding the tissue, between 1 and 16 days after birth

(Swaiman *et al.*, 1963); the increase closely paralleled that found when glucose itself was substrate. Thus increase is taking place in the major energy-yielding process of the tissue at the time when processes consuming metabolically-derived energy are also increasing.

Respiratory rates differ markedly in pieces of tissue taken from different parts of the adult central nervous system, the greatest differences being between samples of grey and of white matter. During development, while protein content is changing and myelination of some parts is proceeding, relative respiratory rates of different areas change. Thus during the first few

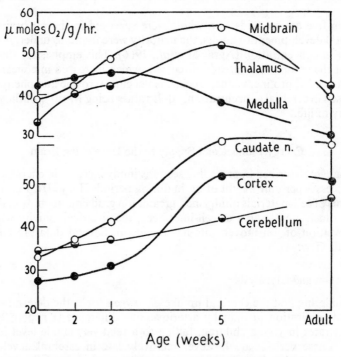

FIG. 13.8. Oxygen consumption *in vitro* of parts of the brain of dogs of different ages (Himwich, 1951).

weeks of life of the dog, the respiratory rate per unit weight of medulla falls, while it is undergoing myelination. At this time the respiration of the cortex and most other parts examined are increasing in parallel to their increase in dry weight.

Relationships between respiration and glycolysis change notably during development (Himwich, 1951; Seiler, 1969). The head of the chick embryo at its 4th to 6th day already contains energy-rich phosphates and shows both glycolysis and respiration (Needham & Nowinsky, 1937). Glycolysis appears however to play a more critical role as energy-yielding reaction in the early stages of mammalian development. After birth, respiration increases until its contribution greatly preponderates. The change to respiration as the most important energy-yielding process does not take place uniformly throughout the brain, but commences at the spinal cord and reaches last the cerebral cortex: there is thus to some extent an ontogenic recapitulation of this aspect of evolution in the central nervous system. The magnitude of cerebral respiratory rate at different ages and its relation to the concomitant glycolysis appears to condition the length of time for which animals of different ages can survive absence of oxygen. The effects of anoxia: excitement, then coma, suggest the central nervous system to be the limiting factor in survival under these conditions, and it is understandable that the higher respiratory rate and functional importance of the adult tissues should make them the more sensitive. This is seen in several species including man. Rats survived 50 min. in nitrogen on their day of birth, but only 3 or 4 min. from 11 days of age onwards. In nitrogen, iodoacetate (see below; Samson & Dahl, 1957) further shortened survival, which supports the view that glycolysis is then a critical factor.

Stimulating and Inhibitory Agents

Separated cerebral tissue as ordinarily examined *in vitro* respires more slowly than does the tissue *in vivo*, but values closer to those in the intact animal can be induced in the separated tissue by restoring to it an environment of fluctuating electrical potential gradients (see Chapter 4). The values quoted in Fig. 13.8 for adult animals are lower than those of the electrically excited tissue. However, this excitability has been found to change markedly during development (Table 13.1; Flexner; Greengard & McIlwain, *Symposium*, 1955). Electrical pulses brought about only a small increase in the respiratory rates of cerebral cortical tissues from newly-born rats or from guinea pigs at some 30–35 days' gestation; but during period III the respiratory rate was increased 70–110% by the applied pulses.

The change in excitability appeared to commence a little earlier only than the time at which electrical observations from the cortex of the living animal show continuous endogenous electrical activity. Of the many characteristics of the tissue which alter at about this time, those concerning electrolyte distribution are immediately relevant. Differential distribution, as noted above, becomes evident during period III, and implies that metabolic activities of the tissue are being employed in maintaining concentration gradients in Na^+ and K^+ salts. Regarding the electrical pulses as depolarizing tissue cells and briefly permitting ion exchange, the increased respiration associated with their application then represents the additional metabolic work necessary to restore the normal differential distribution.

High concentrations of potassium salts which also depolarize tissue cells, again increase the respiratory rate of adult cerebral tissues, but do not affect respiration at the early stages of development (Himwich 1951, 1962). The change again takes place during period III. It will be noted that the respiratory effects both of high concentrations of potassium salts and of electrical pulses imply not only the development at this time of systems utilizing metabolically-derived energy, but also of others which control energy-yielding processes.

With increase in respiratory rate, respiration of cerebral tissues has been found to become more sensitive to inhibitory agents. Malonate inhibition

(Chapter 6) increased in the first 10 postnatal days of the rat (Tyler, 1942) and inhibition by ethanol and pentobarbital (Himwich, 1951) was greater in adult than in infant rats. On the other hand, iodoacetate, which probably acts more immediately in glycolysis than in respiration, had greater effect on cerebral tissues from infant than adult rats.

Nucleotides and Phosphocreatine

Linking energy-yielding and energy-consuming processes are the nucleotides, especially adenosine and guanosine di- and triphosphates, and phosphocreatine (Chapter 6). It is remarkable that these collectively are at almost constant level in the brain during a major part of the development of the guinea pig and rat (Flexner *et al.*, 1953; Lolley *et al.*, 1961). In the guinea pig a change occurred in their distribution, for creatine phosphate increased in the later stages, after 40–50 days of gestation. This is the period at which electrical activity commences in the cortex and the increase in creatine phosphate is thus consistent with its representing a reserve of energy-rich substances available for sudden utilization during brief periods of activity. It would be especially interesting to know the histological distribution of the creatine phosphate.

In the rat, a calculation of the sum of $2(ATP + GTP) + ADP + GDP +$ phosphocreatine, at ages 1, 5, 10 and 21 days gave values of 9·4, 10·3, 9·6 and 8·8 μmoles/g. brain. Further evidence suggested, however, that these compounds were participating in regulation of energy-metabolism. For concentration ratios of ATP/ADP and of phosphocreatine/creatine, diminished during this period: the first from 15 to 5·4 and the second from 1 to 0·3. Taken together with the concomitant increase in respiration, these changes are consistent with respiratory and glycolytic systems retaining throughout development similar properties, in terms, e.g., of Michaelis constants, but being stimulated especially by ADP to operate at greater rates after the inception of greater functional activity in periods III and IV.

Column chromatographic methods have enabled some 15 nucleotides to be evaluated, so giving results in a detail which bears on questions of synthetic routes as well as on energy balance. The methods were applied to rapidly frozen samples from the brains of rats from 1 day of age to maturity (Mandel & Edel-Harth, 1966). The nucleotides collectively fell in concentration during this time but increased some 10-fold in amount per brain and three-fold per "cell" (DNA-P enumeration). Triphosphates collectively remained at 75–80% of the total free nucleotides during the development; adenine nucleotides increased at the expense of guanine-, uracil-, and especially of cytidine-nucleotides. The diminution was most notable in CMP, which fell from 111 to 3 nmoles/g. fresh weight; this was suggested as capable of limiting RNA synthesis in the adult. CDP-Choline ethanolamine, indicative of lipid synthesis, increased from 5 nmoles/g. on the first day of life to 93 on the second. Cerebral nucleotides were evaluated by similar methods in the brain of chick embryos from 6 days of incubation to hatching (Wegelin & Manzoli, 1967); during that time, they increased collectively 10-fold in quantity but diminished to a quarter of their initial concentration. Adenine nucleotides plus IMP, and guanine nucleotides, remained at relatively constant proportions of the whole, but cytidine nucleotides markedly diminished. This also was seen as support-ing a role for cytidine nucleotides in controlling RNA and hence protein synthesis.

Phosphatases

Observations on adenosine triphosphatases continue the theme of energy-utilization. Measured by brief incubation of ground cerebral cortex with adeno-sine triphosphate in the presence of different activating agents, adenosine

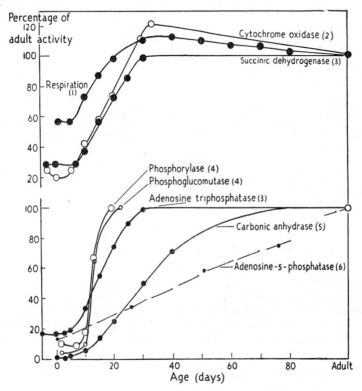

FIG. 13.9. Levels of enzyme activity in the brain of rats of different ages, expressed as percentages of the adult level. Data from (1) Tyler & van Harreveld, 1942; (2) Potter et al., 1945; (3) DuBois & Potter, 1943; (4) Shapiro & Wertheimer, 1943; (5) Ashby & Schuster, 1950; see also Giacobini, 1962; (6) Naidoo & Pratt, 1954.

triphosphatase of rat cerebral cortex and cerebellum increased especially between periods II and III. An appreciable proportion of this activity required added Na^+ and K^+ and was thus probably concerned with active cation move-ments (Jordan & March, *Symposium*, 1955; Samson *et al.*, 1964; Samson & Quinn, 1967; see also Fig. 13.9 and Chapter 12). The Na,K-ATPase in the brain of chick embryos increased sharply after 13 days incubation. It was microsomal and ouabain-sensitive; a Mg-ATPase, mitochondrial, was also in evidence. The Na,K-ATPase could be induced to appear rapidly by hydro-cortisone (Stastny, 1969). Development in the brain of the rat of adenosine 5′-monophosphatase is markedly different from that of the triphosphatase, being with carbonic anhydrase one of the most slowly-forming systems (Fig. 13.9); it is seen histochemically to be associated with myelination.

In ground cerebral tissues the level, per unit weight, of the systems liberating inorganic phosphate from glycerophosphate at pH 5 was found constant from the thirty-second day of gestation to birth. It then fell to half the foetal level, which is a greater fall than observed in other cerebral enzymes. Histo-chemically the enzyme has been detected in the cytoplasm and nuclei of neuro-blasts and neurons in guinea pigs at several stages of development (Flexner, *Symposium*, 1955), and in those of the adult rat (Naidoo & Pratt, 1951). Systems hydrolysing phenylphosphate at acid and alkaline pH have been found to undergo a small increase in rat brain during period II, followed by a decrease; in each case development in the hypothalamus preceded that in the cerebral cortex (Cohn & Richter, 1957). The behaviour of these systems contrasted markedly with that hydrolysing acetyl-β-methylcholine, which was investigated in parallel. In neural tissues from embryos of chick or man, alkaline phospha-tase was particularly high and diminished during development (Cohen, 1970). The acid phosphatase, probably lysosomal, was also at greatest activity at an early stage of development. The occurrence and activation of several lysosomal enzymes in the brain of the mouse have been measured during the first year of life (Verity *et al.*, 1968).

Respiratory and Glycolytic Enzymes

If the respiratory enzymes of cerebral cells all operated maximally or to some proportion of their maximal rate throughout development, there would be little to say in the present section; but this is not the case. Thus respiration of cerebral dispersions from the rat was essentially constant from birth to 2 years of age (Reiner, 1947), and the increase observed in the sliced tissue during period III was not in evidence. Systems which in the cell control respiratory rate are understandably altered in making the dispersion.

Succinic, Malic and Cytochrome Systems

These systems, all mitochondrial and involved in the oxidation of pyruvate through the tricarboxylic acid cycle, in general develop in parallel with cerebral respiration (Table 13.1; Fig. 13.9). Thus succinoxidase in guinea pig cerebral cortex doubled in activity about the time at which overt electrical signs appeared in the brain of the animals. Oxidation of succinate by guinea pig tissues during periods I and II was lower in cell-containing than in the cell-free systems from which the preceding data have been quoted. It is suggested that this may be due to the permeability changes occurring between periods II and III.

Succinic and malic dehydrogenases also underwent their most marked development in the rat between periods II and III. Malic dehydrogenase has been examined at different depths in the cerebral cortex, and the increase found to be localized at the outer cortical layers (Kuhlman & Lowry, 1956). Histochemical studies (Padykula, 1952) have shown succinic dehydrogenase to be markedly localized in the central nervous system of adult rats, being low in white matter, absent from nuclei, and present in grey matter especially in Purkinje cells. Its increase during development occurs after the nucleus has reached its adult size and to a large measure during the development of Nissl substance. Succinic dehydrogenase in the liver followed a markedly different course of development, being stable in level from the end of period I to the end of period III, and increasing in the guinea pig about the time of birth.

Systems reoxidizing reduced cytochrome c are throughout development at markedly higher levels than those of succinoxidase or of succinic dehydrogenase. It is understandable that this should be so, for succinic acid is only one of several substrates yielding hydrogen which passes through the cytochrome system. The adult rates of some 700 μmoles O_2/g. hr. in the guinea pig cerebral cortex, are approximately ten times those of succinoxidase; they are also about three times those of the cytochrome oxidase of the brain as a whole (Chapter 6). Again, increase between periods II and III is very evident.

Mitochondria in Development

It is to be noted that mitochondria themselves display characteristic developmental changes in the growing brain. Between 1-day-old and adult rats, the average cerebral mitochondrion increased 1·5-fold in protein, and four-fold in succinic dehydrogenase, cytochromes, and other components of the respiratory system (Gregson & Williams, 1969). Comparable changes did not occur in liver mitochondria from the same animals. Mitochondrial numbers/g. fresh brain were remarkably similar at the two ages, being 36×10^{10}, but the number per "cell" (DNA evaluation) doubled, to some 1,500 in the adult. Change during development in the amino acid utilization by cerebral mitochondria from rats and chicks is suggested by the data of Buniatian et al. (1969) and Simonian & Stepanian (1968).

Glucose- and Glycerol-phosphate Dehydrogenases

In contrast to the development of the enzymes just described, is that of *glucose-6-phosphate dehydrogenase*. This enzyme (Chapter 5) represents a route of glucose metabolism distinct from glycolysis plus the tricarboxylic acid cycle; its level was remarkably constant during periods II to IV in the development of the rat cerebral cortex. Its level during an earlier developmental period has been examined in chick brain and a high value observed after 3 days incubation. The glucose-6-phosphate dehydrogenase activity, indeed, was correlated with mitotic rate and RNA content (Burt & Wengler, 1961), and this could be considered to be associated with a need, at this period, for supply of metabolites from the pentose phosphate pathway. These metabolites include ribose as precursor of RNA, and NADPH which is involved in lipid synthesis.

It is also noteworthy that *glycerol phosphate dehydrogenase* develops quite slowly in the brain of the rat, with a peak at 40–50 days. The major increase does not occur until after period II and is thus associated with later stages of myelination (Laatsch, 1962). This is consistent with a role in supply of glycerol-3-phosphate for lipid synthesis. In particular, the enzyme differed in its development from *glyceraldehyde phosphate dehydrogenase* which in the same animals reached its maximum at 5–10 days, in period II. These two enzymes indeed compete for triose phosphates, and the changes described thus indicate glycolysis to be favoured at the earlier stages and at the later, a necessary preliminary to lipid synthesis. Such development can be recognized to be made feasible by the increase in respiratory enzymes in the immediately preceding period.

Glycogen and Glycolysis

Glycogen in the cerebral cortex of the dog or cat is at birth at only one-third or a quarter of its adult level (20, rising to 70 or 50 mg./100 g. fresh tissue). In the spinal cord or medulla, the change is as great or greater, but in the opposite sense (120–130, falling to 20–40 mg./100 g.). The quantity in other parts of the brain changes less and in, for example, the colliculi remains relatively constant (Chesler & Himwich, 1943). The general pattern of change is likely to have functional significance; the striking increase in the cerebral cortex is correlated with the inception of its functioning, and it has also been suggested that the additional glycogen is in a combined, more labile form (Palladin, *Symposium*, 1955). The decrease in glycogen content of the medulla appeared to be correlated with a fall in the activity of systems which degraded glycogen. For whereas in insulin hypoglycaemia the glycogen of the medulla or cord of new-born cats greatly decreased from its normal high level, the smaller quantity in the adult medulla or cord changed little if at all. The quantity in the cerebral cortex or hypothalamus fell by about the same proportion during hypoglycaemia in new-born or adult animals (Himwich, 1951). Studies of individual enzyme systems concerned in glycogen metabolism has given a partial understanding of certain of these changes. Preparations from rat brain (presumably all parts) showed an increase of some 70% in their ability to synthesize glycogen from glucose-1-phosphate during the first 3 weeks after birth. Systems degrading glycogen to glucose-6-phosphate increased to an even greater extent during the same period, and here the limiting factor was *phosphoglucomutase*, which in preparations from rats between 10 and 20 days of age increased about eight-fold (Shapiro & Wertheimer, 1943). Concomitant development of systems acting on glycogen occurred in muscle; embryonic tissues have previously been found to act much more slowly on glycogen than on glucose (Needham & Lehmann, 1937; Needham & Nowinski, 1937). In adult cerebral tissues glycogen breakdown to hexose phosphates was evenly distributed, grey and white matter showing similar activities.

Formation of lactic acid has been examined in tissues taken from the brain of rats of various ages. It is found, when examined anaerobically and with glucose as substrate, and expressed on a fresh weight basis, to increase after birth until 2–4 months of age and then possibly to decline (Himwich, 1951; Reiner, 1947). The increase is less than in respiratory rate, but otherwise the increase in glycolysis in different parts of the brain showed many similarities to those in respiration (Fig. 13.8). Medulla in the dog or cat again showed the higher rates at birth, but glycolysis in the caudate nucleus and cortex increased after birth so that in the young adult they possessed greater glycolytic activity than did other parts of the brain.

Of individual glycolytic enzymes, aldolase has been found at greater level in grey matter than in white, and to increase during development, as also does lactic dehydrogenase (Palladin, *Symposium*, 1955; Kuhlman & Lowry, 1956; Bennett *et al.*, 1959). Moreover, lactate dehydrogenase shows qualitative changes which appear to be of functional significance during development. The enzyme exists as tetramers of different subunits and the amounts and proportions of these change markedly in the first 50 days of the life of the rat (Bonavita *et al.*, 1964). In particular, isoenzyme 1 increased six-fold at the expense of isoenzyme 4. These two forms differed in susceptibility to inhibition by pyruvate, and this is suggested as related to the greater susceptibility of adult animals to anoxia. Aldolase also alters in isoenzyme components: towards form C, just before birth in the rat (Rensing *et al.*, 1967).

Non-Mammalian Neural Systems; Acetylcholine

Study of the nervous system in the chick embryo has contributed much to knowledge of development of the brain as of other organs, as is evident from preceding sections of this Chapter. Neurological and further biochemical data on the growth of the central nervous system of birds are given in Bernhardt & Schadé's (1967) account of developmental neurology and by Scarano & Augusti-Tocco (1967).

Notes on Comparative Neurochemistry

By far the greater part of the biochemical information available about the central nervous system has been obtained by investigating the brain of mammals. The preponderance is evident from the present book, and a relevant *Symposium* (1964), and is understandable in terms of human interests and the relatively large size of the brain in higher animals. However, aggregation of nerve cells to ganglia which can be regarded as the beginning of a central nervous system, are found in much more primitive animals. Thus in coelenterates neurons of different function from the individual sense organs appear in some cases to carry chemically different transmitting agents. Neural systems of snails and of insects have received some chemical study during development and regeneration (see Barondes, 1969; Kerkut, 1969). Neurosecretion has been recognized in the polychaete worm *Nereis virens*, which carries many bundles of some 2,000 neurons; and in annelids and leeches are neurons containing granules to which a transmitter or secretory function has been ascribed.

The giant fibres of crustaceae and squids have featured prominently in investigations of the ion movements fundamental to neural systems and described in Chapter 3. This is a reminder of how many important neural properties were established at this relatively early stage in development. Membrane potential, interestingly, is here also some 70–100 mv, and is thus to an appreciable extent independent of the ion composition of the nerve fibre: emphasizing, again, its relationship to properties of membrane constituents. Impressive also is the similarity in time-course of the nerve impulse in fibres of animals at different evolutionary stages and the quantities of Na and K exchanged per impulse. The similarities have however their limitations and the comparative neurophysiology of different excitable systems is an extensive subject (Grundfest, 1961; Eccles, 1964; *Symposia*, 1962, 1964; Horridge, 1968).

In insects the haemolymph is often high in potassium and a special role has been attributed to insect nerve sheaths in maintaining for the neural structures an extracellular fluid of normal Na and K content. A survey of nucleotides and organic phosphates in the cockroach central nervous system showed the presence of many compounds familiar from mammalian systems, but with enrichment of cytidine and uridine derivatives and with arginine phosphate as phosphagen. Concentrations of most amino acids high by mammalian standards are reported in the brain of the honey bee, and it and the housefly brain are rich in glutamic acid dehydrogenase and in γ-amino-butyric acid. Acetylcholine with potent synthesizing and degrading systems, is established in the brain of many insects; acetylcholine also occurs in non-neural sites, as in wasp venom. The neural cholinesterase has attracted attention as a point of action of potent insecticides; tetraethyl pyrophosphate causes accumulation of acetylcholine in the cockroach central nervous system (West & Hardy, 1961; Heslop & Ray, 1961; Treherne, 1962). Intriguingly specific are many of the insect attractants and repellants; and here it must be noted that in mammals also, neurochemical understanding of the chemical senses is limited.

Acetylcholine Metabolism

Neural tissues show relatively high cholinesterase activity from an early stage of development. The enzyme was determined in different minute parts of the embryo of the axolotl *Amblystoma punctatum* and at about the time when its neural fold was closing, the tissue of the fold increased its cholinesterase activity until it was five times that of normal ectoderm (Boell & Shen, 1944). Moreover, when secondary neural structures recognized as such histologically were induced by implantation the induced structures also were high in cholin-esterase. Choline acetylase in the guinea pig and rabbit increased prenatally in many parts of the brain, and postnatally in the cerebral cortex (McCaman & Aprison, 1964). At appropriate stages of the culture of cells from chick embryo brain, choline acetyltransferase and acetylcholinesterase could be greatly augmented by L-thyroxine or by cyclic adenosine monophosphate (Werner *et al.*, 1971).

The level, per unit weight of tissue, of systems hydrolysing acetylcholine increases about ten-fold during the development of the guinea pig brain (Table 13.1). It was determined in suspensions of ground cerebral cortex and throughout development hydrolysed acetyl-β-methylcholine but not benzoyl-choline and was thus similar to the acetylcholinesterase of most cerebral tissues or of red blood cells and distinct from that of blood serum. The greater part of the increase occurred nearly linearly with time between 35 and 55 days' gestation; and expressed as activity per cell the increase was centred round the period of 43–46 days' gestation when electrical stimulation of the cortex evokes motor responses and spontaneous electrical potential changes appear. The earlier time at which increase begins corresponds to the time when glial cells rather than neurones begin to differentiate, an observation to be compared with the finding (Koelle, 1950) that the enzyme in the adult rat is found at highest level histochemically in the glial cells.

In the new-born rat, true cholinesterase is at birth about equal to pseudo-cholinesterase in activity, but later the true enzyme preponderates (*Symposium*, 1955). After birth, the total cholinesterase of two areas of the cerebral cortex of the rat rose to a maximum at about 100 days, and later gradually fell; in subcortical structures the maximum was reached earlier. Differences were exhibited between different strains of rats; and also by using different substrates, several esterases hydrolysing α-naphthylacetate and homologues were shown to develop in the brain during the first 30 days of life of the rat (Bennett *et al.*, 1959; Himwich, 1962; Bernsohn *et al.*, 1963; Seiler, 1969).

Impeded or Modified Development of the Brain

The investigations of neural differentiation and proliferation described earlier in this Chapter offer instances in which cerebral development has been modified experimentally in order to understand its normal progress. Impeded cerebral development is also of practical concern in man and notes follow on its study in malnutrition and mental retardation.

Malnutrition

Dietary restriction in adults frequently has minimal immediate effects on the brain (Chapter 10). This relative protection of the brain extends to many consequences of general undernutrition in adults; the weight of the body may fall by 45 % with little or no change in that of the brain. At earlier ages, however, while the brain is still undergoing development, it is much more susceptible. Cerebral deficiencies can be induced during gestation of rats by restricting the mother's diet, and exhibited in the offspring, as in pyridoxine deficiency (Dakshinamurti & Stephens, 1969).

Deficiencies imposed postnatally can also have lasting effects, as in the protein–calorie undernutrition of kwashiorkor (q.v.). Inducing such undernutrition in the first 3 weeks of the life of rats, with normal diet subsequently, gave adult animals smaller in weight of body and brain than control animals (Davison & Dobbing, 1968). Even at a later stage, between 3 and 11 weeks of age, restriction of the quantity of otherwise adequate diet, gave subnormal adult animals. Significantly, cerebral DNA in the undernourished rats was 10 % lower than that of controls, suggesting a limitation of cell-division and emphasizing the continued postnatal proliferation of cells which normally occurs in the brain (Fig. 13.4). Cerebral cholesterol was also subnormal in the undernourished animals, and low contents of cerebral lipids have been reported in infants suffering malnutrition (Fishman *et al.*, 1969; and see Jervis, 1968).

In man, the corresponding period during which many cerebral constituents are accumulating at maximal rates and cerebral DNA also is still increasing, extends from the last few weeks of foetal life to about 1 year of age. It has been called a period of vulnerability or of growth spurt and corresponds approximately to periods II and III of Table 13.1, as shown by **A**, Fig. 13.3 and Fig. 13.4. Human infants which had suffered malnutrition in the first years of life, and possibly during gestation, were found below normal in cerebral lipid content.

The cerebral deficiencies in DNA and lipid content induced by dietary restriction, but persisting into adult life when nutrition is adequate, reflect the operation of factors similar to competence in embryonic induction. The possibility of a given development or response appears at a given stage and subsequently is lost. At this level the dietarily-conditioned subnormality is akin to subnormality caused by rearing animals with limited sensory input, or in isolation in an environment offering minimal scope for manipulation (see above, and Glassman, 1969).

Mental Retardation

Mental retardation in association with metabolic defect is a frequent consequence of genetic abnormality in man, as is evident from the accounts of amino acids and lipids in Chapters 8 and 11. Approaching 100 such abnormalities have been described (Eastham & Jancar, 1968; Chrome & Stern, 1967). Characterizing the conditions in terms of specified metabolites has frequently proved of great practical value; it is, however, part only of the linkage from a presumed change in DNA to modified protein make-up and changed mental functioning. It is to be noted that change in DNA has usually not been demonstrated chemically or cytologically in these abnormalities.

Investigation of Down's syndrome (mongolism) presents a converse situation in which the mental retardation is clearly associated with a chromosome abnormality. Trisomy in chromosome 21 or 22 has been observed and investigated by tissue culture techniques (*Study Groups*, 1967, 1971). Altered incorporation has been shown of ^{3}H-thymidine to DNA in lymphocytes from patients, and also increased incorporation of ^{14}C-orotic acid and -uridine to RNA of their leucocytes. However, investigation of numerous categories of circulating and urinary metabolites has shown only small, and not very characteristic, deviations from normality (Stern, in *Study Group*, 1971). Probably, therefore, the chromosomal abnormality expressed in the cells of the brain itself is responsible for the mental retardation.

The two preceding paragraphs are very relevant to the biochemical investigation of mental illness or defect in which inherited factors have been recognized genetically, but not yet specified either in chromosomal terms or by simpler metabolites. These two levels of specification are disparate. Between them lie the synthetic mechanisms of Chapter 9 and also the numerous controlling factors, rarely yet characterized in the brain, which condition genetic expression at the level of DNA or of the different categories of RNA and protein, and factors which govern the intracellular movements of these categories of substances. Such components of a normally developing brain, on disturbance would have primarily intracerebral effects and need involve minimal alteration in circulating or urinary metabolites.

A Note on Changes with Damage or Demyelination

In many parts of the nervous system, damage which is sufficient to cause loss of cells is followed by their regeneration, but this is limited in the mammalian central nervous system. In peripheral nerve and ganglia the sequence occurring after such damage: Wallerian degeneration and subsequent growth of new fibres: has received extensive chemical and enzymatic study (see *Symposium*, 1961; Klingman & Klingman, 1969). The loss of myelin and growth of scavenging cells during the degeneration, and subsequently the myelination of the newly grown fibres, involve large changes in most cell constituents: nucleic acids, proteins, lipids and enzyme systems. Neurons of the hypoglossal nucleus in the medulla of rats were examined after cutting or crushing the hypoglossal nerve (Watson, 1965). By quantitative microspectrography the nucleic acid content of both nucleolus and cell body were shown to increase, in the nucleolus from 2 to 3·2 and in the body from 140 to 300 pg./cell. The RNA changes in the nucleolus preceded those in the cell, and both began more promptly (1 day) after injuries which were close to the medullary nucleus, than after more distant injury (4 days). The increased RNA content lasted some 10–30 days and then returned to previous values. In the nucleus the increase coincided in time with an augmented incorporation of ^{3}H uridine, shown autoradiographically and susceptible to actinomycin D. The increased nucleolar production of RNA is pictured as involved in supply of ribosomes to the cell body. Observations of axoplasmic movement (q.v.) have shown supply of material from the cell body to distal regions and the experiments described suggest an augmented supply to the injured cells. Communication with distant parts of the cell to initiate such supply can evidently require some days; centripetal axonal movement and some release of normal DNA-inhibition, are presumably involved.

In amphibians, cutting the optic nerve is followed by comparable absorption and re-growth from the retina, giving vision adequate for coordinated movements, but this does not occur in mammals. The optic nerve in rabbits, or white matter tracts in the spinal cord of rats, after section, underwent changes akin to those of Wallerian degeneration, but quite slowly (McCaman & Robins, 1958; Karnovsky & Majno, *Symposium*, 1961). Thus several lipids were still diminishing at 100–200 days after section, e.g. cholesterol, then 32% of its original value and cerebroside-like compounds, then 17%. Marked but slow chemical changes were also observed in portions of the central nervous system when these are separated from the animal and kept at 37°C with their cell structure largely intact (Johnson *et al.*, 1949). When portions were taken from the brain of cats aseptically and incubated in a salt mixture anaerobically and without substrate, total phospholipid fell in a fortnight to 50% of its original value. Sphingomyelin and kephalin shared in this fall, but lecithin, cholesterol and cerebrosides did not change.

Demyelination is a feature of several diseases and intoxications (Thompson

& Cumings, 1964; Ansell & Hawthorne, 1964; Heath, 1961). Disseminated or multiple sclerosis is the commonest of these; of unknown origin but featuring patches of demyelination throughout the brain, in which nerve fibres remain but lose their myelin. Chemical examination of these areas shows diminution in almost all lipids, but the appearance of small amounts of cholesterol esters; this occurs also in Wallerian degeneration and is then pictured to be a stage in the disposal of cholesterol by scavenging cells. In multiple sclerosis and certain other demyelinating conditions, lipids of the cerebrospinal fluid are increased in quantity, being enriched in cerebral lipids and especially in kephalin components; this can be of diagnostic value (McArdle & Zilkha, 1962). The many conditions which can lead to demyelination include cyanide intoxication, severe hypoglycaemia, intoxication with tritolylphosphate and other organophosphorus compounds, some nutritional abnormalities (Chapter 10) including copper deficiency, and some allergic conditions induced experimentally or by disease. Immune and autoimmune responses have received much investigation in the nervous system; several cerebral lipids, notably cerebrosides and ganglioside preparations, act as haptens (Cumings & Kremer, 1968; Rapport, 1970). Allergic conditions may be involved in multiple sclerosis. They, together with the immunosympathectomy described at the beginning of this chapter, emphasize the little-understood chemical factors which are involved in cell-growth in the nervous system.

Comment

In a material sense much of the brain is made while its functioning is in progress. At birth in the rat or man, the brain contains only about a tenth of the solid matter of the adult organ. The temporal sequence of events in the brain becomes more significant with the knowledge that in other organs the time and order of the same chemical events is often different. Growth during functioning is common to the majority of organs of the body but is to be re-emphasized here as a very real phenomenon in the central nervous system. Electrical activity begins in the brain before the greater part of its substance has been assembled. From this point, material growth of the brain progresses while it is receiving impulses from the rest of the body and beyond. To take one example which has been considered from the point of view of information theory (*Symposium*, 1958): it is concluded that to specify particular neural connections between individual retinal elements and individual cortical cells would require more information than could be represented on all the chromosomes; consequently either the initial connnections must in part be random, or be dependent on signals received during development. It is thus understandable that some cerebral defects arising early in development are difficult or may be impossible to rectify later. The first few years of human life can be seen for chemical as for other reasons to be especially important in the making of the adult brain.

REFERENCES

AGHAJANIAN, G. K. (1967). *Brain Res.* **6**, 716.
AGRAWAL, H. C., BANIK, N. L., BONE, A. H., DAVISON, A. N., MITCHELL, R. F. & SPOHN, M. (1970). *Biochem. J.* **120**, 635.

AGRAWAL, H. C., DAVIS, J. M. & HIMWICH, W. A. (1966). *J. Neurochem.* **13**, 607.
AGRAWAL, H. C., DAVIS, J. M. & HIMWICH, W. A. (1967). *J. Neurochem.* **14**, 179.
ALTMAN, J. (1966). *Exper. Neurol.* **16**, 263.
ALTMAN, J. (1969). *Handbk. Neurochem.* **2**, 137.
ANSELL, G. B. & HAWTHORNE, J. N. (1964). Phospholipids: Chemistry, Metabolism and Function. Amsterdam: Elsevier.
ASHBY, W. & SCHUSTER, E. M. (1950). *J. biol. Chem.* **184**, 109.
BANIK, N. L. & DAVISON, A. N. (1969). *Biochem. J.* **115**, 1051.
BARONDES, S. H. (1969). (Ed.) *Sympos. Internat. Soc. Cell Biol.* **8**.
BAXTER, C. (1970). *Handbk. Neurochem.* **3**, 289.
BELLAMY, D. (1967). *Mem. Soc. Endocrinol.* **15**, 43.
BENNETT, E. L., KRETCH, D., ROSENZWEIG, M. R., KARLSSON, N., DYE, N. & OHLANDER, A. (1959). *J. Neurochem.* **3**, 144, 153.
BERL, S. (1965). *J. biol. Chem.* **240**, 2047.
BERL, S. & PURPURA, D. P. (1966). *J. Neurochem.* **13**, 293.
BERNHARDT, C. G. & SCHADÉ, J. P. (1967). *Progr. Brain Res.* **26**. Amsterdam: Elsevier.
BERNSOHN, J., BARRON, K. D., HESS, A. R. & HEDRICK, M. T. (1963). *J. Neurochem.* **10**, 783.
BOELL, E. J. & SHEN, S. C. (1944). *J. exp. Zool.* **97**, 21.
BOIVIN, A., VENDRELY, R. & VENDRELY, C. (1948). *C.R. Acad. Sci., Paris.* **226**, 1061.
BONAVITA, V., PONTE, F. & AMORE, G. (1964). *J. Neurochem.* **11**, 39.
BONDY, S. C. & ROBERTS, S. (1968). *Biochem. J.* **109**, 533.
BRACHET, J. (1960). The Biochemistry of Development. London: Pergamon.
BRANTE, G. (1949). *Acta physiol. scand.* **18**, suppl. 63.
BUNIATIAN, H. C., AFRIKIAN, G. V., SHAHINIAN, V. A. & NERCESSIAN, Z. M. (1969). Problems in Brain Biochemistry, Vol. 5, p. 35. Erevan: Armenian Acad. Sci.
BURT, A. M. & WENGLER, B. S. (1961). *Develop. Biol.* **3**, 84.
CHARGAFF, E. & DAVIDSON, J. B. (1955–60). The Nucleic Acids. New York: Academic Press.
CHESLER, A. & HIMWICH, H. E. (1943). *Arch. Biochem.* **2**, 175.
CHROME, L. C. & STERN, J. (1967). Pathology of Mental Retardation. London: Churchill.
COHEN, S. (1960). *Proc. Nat. Acad. Sci., U.S.* **46**, 302.
COHEN, S. R. (1970). *Handbk. Neurochem.* **3**, 87.
COHN, P. & RICHTER, D. (1957). *J. Neurochem.* **1**, 166.
CRAIN, S. M. (1963, 1964). *Science,* **141**, 427; *Exper. Neurol.* **10**, 425.
CRAIN, S. M., BORNSTEIN, M. B. & PETERSON, E. R. (1968). *Brain Res.* **8**, 363.
CROCKER, A. C. (1961). *J. Neurochem.* **7**, 69.
CUARÓN, A., GAMBLE, J., MYANT, N. B. & OSORIO, C. (1963). *J. Physiol.* **168**, 613.
CUMINGS, J. N. & KREMER, M. (1968). Biochemical Aspects of Neurological Disorders. Oxford: Blackwell.
DAKSHINAMURTI, K. & STEPHENS, M. C. (1969). *J. Neurochem.* **16**, 1515.
DAVISON, A. N. & DOBBING, J. (1968). Applied Neurochemistry, pp. 253, 287. Oxford: Blackwell.
DELLWEG, H., GERNER, R. & WACKER, A. (1968). *J. Neurochem.* **15**, 1109.
DEN, H., KAUFMAN, B. & ROSEMAN, S. (1970). *J. biol. Chem.* **245**, 6607.
DOBBING, J. & SANDS, J. (1970). *Nature, Lond.* **226**, 639.
DuBOIS, K. P. & POTTER, V. R. (1943). *J. biol. Chem.* **150**, 185.
EASTHAM, R. D. & JANCAR, J. (1968). Clinical Pathology of Mental Retardation. Bristol: Wright.
ECCLES, J. C. (1964). The Physiology of Synapses. Berlin: Springer.
FILOGAMO, G. (1969). *Sympos. Internat. Soc. Cell Biol.* **8**, 321.
FISHMAN, M. A., PRENSKY, A. L. & DODGE, P. R. (1969). *Nature, Lond.* **221**, 552.
FLEXNER, J. B. & FLEXNER, L. B. (1951). *J. cell. comp. Physiol.* **38**, 1.
FLEXNER, L. B., BELKNAP, E. L. & FLEXNER, J. B. (1953). *J. cell. comp. Physiol.* **42**, 151.
FLEXNER, L. B. & FLEXNER, J. B. (1949). *J. cell. comp. Physiol.* **34**, 115.
FLEXNER, L. B. & FLEXNER, J. B. (1950). *Anat. Rec.* **106**, 413.

15

FLEXNER, L. B., TYLER, D. B. & GALLANT, L. J. (1950). *J. Neurophysiol.* **13**, 427.

FRANK, G. (1970). Sur la composition ionique des tranches de cerveau de rat. Thesis: Université de Liège.

FUJITA, S. (1967). *J. Cell. Biol.* **32**, 277.

GARRIGAN, O. W. & CHARGAFF, E. (1963). *Biochim. Biophys. Acta,* **70**, 452.

GEIGER, R. S. (1963). *Internat. Rev. Neurobiol.* **5**, 1.

GIACOBINI, E. (1962). *J. Neurochem.* **9**, 169.

GLASSMAN, E. (1969). *Ann. Rev. Bioch.* **38**, 605.

GRAVES, J. & HIMWICH, H. E. (1955). *Amer. J. Physiol.* **180**, 205.

GREGSON, N. A. & WILLIAMS, P. L. (1969). *J. Neurochem.* **16**, 617.

GRUNDFEST, H. (1961). *Ann. N.Y. Acad. Sci.* **94**, 405.

HELLER, I. H. & ELLIOTT, K. A. C. (1954). *Canad. J. Biochem. Physiol.* **32**, 584.

HEATH, D. F. (1961). Organophosphorus Poisons. Oxford: Pergamon.

HESLOP, J. P. & RAY, J. W. (1961). *J. Insect. Physiol.* **7**, 127.

HILD, W. & TASAKI, I. (1962). *J. Neurophysiol.* **25**, 277.

HIMWICH, H. E. (1951). Brain Metabolism and Cerebral Disorders. Baltimore: Williams & Wilkins.

HIMWICH, W. A. (1962). *Internat. Rev. Neurobiol.* **4**, 117.

HORRIDGE, G. A. (1968). Interneurons. London: Freeman.

HUTTUNEN, M. O. (1969). Protein and RNA metabolism in rat brain cortex slices. Dissertation: Helsinki: Dept. of Medical Chemistry.

ITOH, T. & QUASTEL, J. H., (1969). *Science,* **164**, 79.

JERVIS, G. A. (1968). Expanding Concepts of Mental Retardation. Springfield: Thomas.

JOHNSON, A. C., MCNABB, A. R. & ROSSITER, R. J. (1949). *Biochem. J.* **45**, 500.

JOHNSON, T. C. (1969). *J. Neurochem.* **16**, 1125.

KANDEL, E. R. & SPENCER, W. A. (1968). *Physiol. Rev.* **48**, 66.

KERKUT, G. A. (1969). *Handbk. Neurochem.* **2**, 539.

KIBLER, H. H. & BRODY, S. (1942). *J. Nutrition,* **24**, 461.

KLINGMAN, G. I. & KLINGMAN, J. D. (1969). *J. Neurochem.* **16**, 261.

KOCH, W. & KOCH, M. L. (1913). *J. biol. Chem.* **15**, 423.

KOCH, W. & KOCH, M. L. (1917). *J. biol. Chem.* **31**, 395.

KOCH, W. & MANN, S. A. (1909). *Arch. Neurol. Psychiat., Lond.* **4**, 174.

KOECHLIN, B. A. (1955). *J. Biochem. Biophys. Cytol.* **1**, 511.

KOELLE, G. B. (1950). *J. Pharm. exp. Ther.* **100**, 158.

KUHLMAN, R. E. & LOWRY, O. H. (1956). *J. Neurochem.* **1**, 173.

LAATSCH, R. H. (1962). *J. Neurochem.* **9**, 487.

LAJTHA, A. & MARKS, N., (1969). *Dis. Nerv. System.* **30**, 36.

LANGMAN, J. & WELCH, G. W. (1967). *J. Comp. Neurol.* **131**, 15.

LAPHAM, L. W. (1968). *Science,* **159**, 310.

LENTZ, R. D. & LAPHAM, L. W. (1969). *J. Neurochem.* **16**, 379.

LERNER, M. P. & JOHNSON, T. C. (1970). *J. biol. Chem.* **245**, 1388.

LEVI-MONTALCINI, R. (1968). *Physiol. Rev.* **48**, 568.

LEVI-MONTALCINI, R. & ANGELETTI, P. V. (1961, 1962). *Proc. Internat. Neurochem. Sympos.* **4**, 362; *Ann. Rev. Physiol.* **24**, 11.

LOLLEY, R. N., BALFOUR, W. M. & SAMSON, F. E. (1961). *J. Neurochem.* **7**, 289.

LUMSDEN, C. E. (1968) In Structure & Function of Nervous Tissues. Ed. G. H. Bourne. New York: Academic Press.

MACARTHUR, C. G. & DOISY, E. A. (1918–19). *J. comp. Neurol.* **30**, 445.

MANDEL, P. & BIETH, R. (1952). *C.R. Soc. Biol., Paris,* **235**, 485.

MANDEL, P., REIN, H., HARTH-EDEL, S. & MARDELL, R. (1964). *Proc. Internat. Neurochem. Sympos.* **5**, 149.

MANDEL, P. & EDEL-HARTH, S. (1966). *J. Neurochem.* **13**, 591.

MARGOLIS, F. L. (1969). *J. Neurochem.* **16**, 447.

MARKS, N. & LAJTHA, A. (1970). Protein Metabolism of the Nervous System, p. 39. New York: Plenum.

MAY, R. M. (1945). La Formation du Système Nerveux. Paris: Gallimard.

MCARDLE, R. & ZILKHA, K. J. (1962). *Brain,* **85**, 389.

MCCAMAN, R. E. & ROBINS, E. (1958). *Neurology,* **8**, Suppl. 1, 86.

McCaman, R. E. & Aprison, M. H. (1964). *Prog. Brain Res.* **9**, 220.

McIlwain, H. (1970*a*). *Nature, Lond.* **226**, 803.

McIlwain, H. (1970*b*). In Wates Symposium on the Blood-Brain Barrier, p. 85. Ed. R. V. Coxon. Oxford: Physiol. Laboratory.

McIlwain, H. (1971*a*). In Defects in Cellular Organelles and Membranes in Relation to Mental Retardation. Ed. P. F. Benson. London: Churchill.

McIlwain, H. (1971*b*). *Essays in Biochemistry*, **7**, in press.

Meller, K., Breipohl, W. & Glees, P. (1968). *Z. Zellforsch.* **86**, 171.

Murthy, M. R. V. (1966). *Biochim. Biophys. Acta*, **119**, 599.

Naidoo, D. & Pratt, O. E. (1951). *J. Neurol. Neurosurg. Psychiat.* **14**, 287.

Naidoo, D. & Pratt, O. E. (1954). *Enzymologia*, **16**, 298.

Needham, J. (1942). Biochemistry and Morphogenesis. Cambridge: University Press.

Needham, J. & Lehmann, H. (1937). *Biochem. J.* **31**, 1210.

Needham, J. & Nowinski, W. W. (1937). *Biochem. J.* **31**, 1165.

Öhman, R. & Svennerholm, L. (1971). *J. Neurochem.* **18**, 79.

Padykula, H. A. (1952). *Amer. J. Anat.* **91**, 107.

Page, I. H. (1937). Chemistry of the Brain. Springfield, Illinois: Thomas.

Paoletti, R., Grossi-Paoletti, E. & Fumagalli, R. (1969). *Handbk. Neurochem.* **1**, 195.

Paul, J. & Gilman, R. S. (1968). *Sympos. Internat. Soc. Cell Biol.* **7**, 135.

Penn, N. W. & Suwalski, R. (1971). *Biochem. J.* **115**, 563.

Peters, V. B. & Flexner, L. B. (1950). *Amer. J. Anat.* **86**, 133.

Potter, V. R., Schneider, W. C. & Liebl, G. J. (1945). *Cancer Res.* **5**, 21.

Pritchard, E. T. (1966). *J. Neurochem.* **13**, 13.

Prives, C. & Quastel, J. H. (1969). *Biochim. Biophys. Acta*, **182**, 285.

Rapport, M. M. (1970). *Handbk. Neurochem.* **3**, 509.

Reiner, J. M. (1947). *J. Gerontol.* **2**, 315.

Rensing, U., Schmidt, A. & Leuthardt, F. (1967). *Hoppe Seyl. Z.* **348**, 921.

Rose, S. P. R. (1969). *FEBS Letters*, **5**, 305.

Rouser, G. & Yamamoto, A. (1969). *Handbk. Neurochem.* **1**, 121.

Samson, F. E., Balfour, W. M. & Jacobs, R. J. (1960). *Amer. J. Physiol.* **199**, 693.

Samson, F. E. & Dahl, N. A. (1957). *Amer. J. Physiol.* **188**, 277.

Samson, F. E., Dick, H. C. & Balfour, W. M. (1964). *Life Sciences*, **3**, 511.

Samson, F. E. & Quinn, D. J. (1967). *J. Neurochem.* **14**, 421.

Scarano, E. & Augusti-Tocco, G. (1967). Comprehensive Biochemistry. **28**, 55. Ed. Florkin, M. & Stotz, E. H. Elsevier.

Schimke, R. T. (1969). *Curr. Topics Cell Regul.* **1**, 77.

Seiler, N. (1969). *Handb. Neurochem.* **1**, 337.

Shapiro, B. & Wertheimer, E. (1943). *Biochem. J.* **37**, 397.

Shooter, E. M., Smith, A. P., Greene, L. & Varon, S. (1969). Second Internat. Neurochem. Meeting, p. 366. Milan: Tamburini.

Simonian, A. A. & Stepanian, R. A. (1968). Problems in Brain Biochemistry. Vol. 4, p. 123. Erevan: Armenian Acad Sci.

Sims, K. L., Witztum, J., Quick, C. & Pitts, F. N. (1968). *J. Neurochem.* **15**, 667.

Stastny, F. (1969). Second Internat. Neurochem. Meeting, p. 377. Milan: Tamburini.

Study Group (1967). Mongolism. Ed. G. E. W. Wolstenholme & R. Porter. London: Churchill.

Study Group (1971). Defects in Cellular Organelles and Membranes in Relation to Mental Retardation. Ed. P. F. Benson. London: Churchill.

Swaiman, K. F., Milstein, J. M. & Cohen, M. M. (1963). *J. Neurochem.* **10**, 635.

Symposium (1955). *Proc. Internat. Neurochem. Sympos.* **1**.

Symposium (1956). *Sympos. Soc. exp. Biol.* **10**, Cambridge: University Press.

Symposium (1958). Information Theory in Biology. Ed. Yockey. London: Pergamon.

Symposium (1959). The Biology of Myelin. Ed. Korey. London: Cassell.

Symposium (1960). Inhibition in the Nervous System and Gamma-aminobutyric Acid. Ed. E. Roberts. New York: Pergamon.

Symposia (1961, 1964). *Proc. Internat. Neurochem. Sympos.* **4, 5**. Oxford: Pergamon.

Symposium (1962). Properties of Membranes and Diseases of the Nervous System. Ed. M. D. Yahr. New York: Springer.

SZENTÁGOTAI, J. & HÁMORI, J. (1969). *Sympos. Internat. Soc. Cell Biol.* **8**, 301.

TALLAN, H. H. (1957). *J. biol. Chem.* **224**, 41.

THOMPSON, R. H. S. & CUMINGS, J. N. (1964). In Biochemical Disorders in Human Disease, p. 572. Ed. Thompson & King. London: Churchill.

THOMSON, D. A. (1942). On Growth and Form. Cambridge: University Press.

THOMSON, R. Y., HEAGY, F. C., HUTCHINSON, W. C. & DAVIDSON, J. N. (1953). *Biochem. J.* **53**, 460.

TIEDEMANN, H., BECKER, V. & TIEDEMANN, H. (1963). *Biochim. Biophys. Acta*, **74**, 557.

TOSCHI, G., DORE, E., ANGELETHI, P. U., LEVI-MONTALCINI, R. & DE HAËN, C. (1966). *J. Neurochem.* **13**, 539.

TREHERNE, J. E. (1962). *J. exper. Biol.* **39**, 193.

TYLER, D. B. (1942). *Proc. Soc. exp. Biol.* **49**, 537.

TYLER, D. B. & VAN HARREVELD, A. (1942). *Amer. J. Physiol.* **136**, 600.

UZMAN, L. L. & RUMLEY, M. K. (1959). *J. Neurochem.* **3**, 170.

VERITY, M. A., BROWN, W. J. & REITH, A. (1968). *J. Neurochem.* **15**, 69.

VERNADAKIS, A. & WOODBURY, D. M. (1962). *Amer. J. Physiol.* **203**, 748.

WATSON, W. E. (1968). *J. Physiol.* **196**, 655.

WEGELIN, I. & MANZOLI, F. A. (1967). *J. Neurochem.* **14**, 1161.

WEISS, P. (1968). *Sympos. Internat. Soc. Cell Biol.* **7**, ix.

WEISSMAN, A. (1967). *Internat. Rev. Neurobiol.* **10**, 167.

WELLS, M. A. & DITTMER, J. C. (1967). *Biochemistry*, **6**, 3169.

WENDER, M. & HIEROWSKI, M. (1960). *J. Neurochem.* **5**, 105.

WERNER, I., PETERSON, G. R. & SHUSTER, L. (1971). *J. Neurochem.* **18**, 141.

WEST, T. F. & HARDY, J. E. (1961). Chemical Control of Insects. London: Chapman & Hall.

WESTON, J. A. (1970). *Adv. in Morphogen.* **8**, 41.

WIGGLESWORTH, V. B. (1967). *Mem. Soc. Endocrinol.* **15**, 77.

YAMADA, T. (1967). *Comprehensive Biochemistry*, Vol. 28, p. 113. Ed. M. Florkin & E. H. Stotz. Amsterdam: Elsevier.

ZAMENHOF, S., BURSZTYN, H., RICH, K. & ZAMENHOF, P. J. (1964). *J. Neurochem.* **11**, 505.

ZOMZELY, C. E., ROBERTS, S., GRUBER, C. P. & BROWN, D. M. (1968). *J. biol. Chem.* **243**, 5396.

14 Chemical Factors in Neural Transmission

Cells in the central nervous system are distinct but clearly interact. A structural basis for this has been described in Chapter 12; much of the surface of a neuron may be occupied by a hundred or more terminal enlargements of processes from other cells, or a neuron may be enclosed by a basket-like ramification of dendrites from other cells. The mutual interaction involves chemical and electrical factors, which are often similar in peripheral and central neural systems, and in a wide range of animal species. Their investigation involves cytological, physiological and pharmacological as well as biochemical methods; for collected information, see Bourne (1969), Efron (1968), Akert & Waser (1969), Crossland (1967), Eccles (1964, 1966), de Robertis (1964) and the *Symposia*, (1964*a*, 1970).

The chemical and metabolic intricacy involved in cell interaction in the brain is adumbrated in Table 14.1. This lists several of the substances which are active in this regard, in the order in which they are discussed in this Chapter. Distinct stages have been recognized in the action of most of these compounds, and also in preparing them for action and in securing their release and subsequent dispersal. These processes have also been listed in Table 14.1: in broad outline, and with some probable additional complexities, they apply to each of the compounds listed. Some 50 chemically and physically distinct processes are thus implied by the table, granted some substrate-product relationships among the active compounds themselves. These processes are carried out in a variety of anatomically and histologically distinct sites; interactions based on serotonin release from junctions of the sparse, ramifying array of non-myelinated fibres in the neocortex, understandably differ from those based on the much more numerous myelinated fibres with acetylcholine-containing terminals.

Designation according to transmitter-substance is an important feature in understanding peripheral neural systems, and such designation is possible at cellular level in the brain. Also, multicellular aggregates and regions are often specialized in terms of one or a few transmitter-types. Thus a regional pattern is superposed on the chemical one, and histochemical methods have much application in the present subject, though they are described here in outline only.

Recognition of the twelve or so processes which may be involved in the action of a neurotransmitter has been greatly helped by blocking agents, many of which are therapeutically-useful drugs or are neurotoxic agents. Several such compounds receive comment below, and the scheme implied by Table 14.1 represents a biochemical framework for specifying psychopharmacological actions. The coordinated operation of many processes of Table 14.1 can be judged to involve numerous instances of metabolic regulation and adjustment, of which a minority are at present specified. Thus (i) there are quoted below processes of assimilation and synthesis of K_m appropriate to the concentration of active substance or precursor in surrounding fluids. (ii) Feedback inhibition in synthesizing enzymes also occurs and can be judged to maintain stability in

Table 14.1

Substances and processes involved in specialized cell interactions and in the central nervous system

1. Active substances	2. Processes involved in their action

Acetylcholine
Catecholamines:
  Dopamine
  Noradrenaline
  Adrenaline
Tryptamines:
  Serotonin
  Melatonin
Excitatory amino acids:
  Glutamic acid
Inhibitory amino acids:
  Glycine
  γ-Aminobutyric acid
Histamine
	Cellular uptake of:
	  Active substance itself
	  Precursors
	Intracellular changes:
	  Synthesis of active substance
	  Sequestering of active substance
	  Translocation of precursor, of substance or of
	    synthesizing enzyme
	Release
	Action on post-synaptic cell, modifying:
	  Membrane permeability and potentiating cell-firing
	  Intracellular effectors
	Dispersal of active substance:
	  Diffusion
	  Re-assimilation
	  Metabolism

Action of each of the substances in column (1) may involve the processes of column (2). The substances are described in this chapter in the order listed above.

the cell-content of active compounds. (iii) Induction and repression of synthesizing or degrading enzymes occurs and can modify the "set" of the homeostatic mechanisms implied by (ii).

Acetylcholine and the Brain *in situ*

Acetylcholine is the acetic acid ester of choline, the basic alcohol which is present in the brain and in most other parts of the body in relatively large quantities as the phosphatide, lecithin. The free choline of blood plasma is normally well maintained at about 10 μM and values of 115–150 nmoles/g. have been found for the free choline of mouse brain (Schuberth *et al.*, 1969). Acetylcholine itself has been isolated from extracts of ox brain and chemically identified; in many other species it has been shown to be present by a variety of pharmacological, enzymatic and chemical properties which differentiate it from chemically-related compounds (see Pepeu *et al.*, 1962; McLennan *et al.*, 1963; Whittaker, 1963; Hanin, 1969; Hebb & Morris, 1969). The quantity of acetylcholine demonstrated as present is consistently small, and varies with the state of an animal and the part of its brain which is examined. In several parts of the brain of man and of laboratory animals, 0·5–30 nmoles have been found per gram of fresh, excised tissue (a typical average value for the mouse: 13 nmoles/g.); similarly removed sympathetic nerves or ganglia may contain up to 200 nmoles/g. In the cerebral hemispheres and in the cord, grey matter contains much more acetylcholine than the white.

Cerebral Activity and Acetylcholine Content

Initial attempts at correlating the state of activity of the brain with its acetylcholine content were disappointing, relatively little change being found to be associated with strychnine convulsions, anoxia, or hypoglycaemia. However, it is probable that the effects of such conditions were overwhelmed by those of removing the unfixed tissue from the animals concerned. When, as has proved necessary in determining other labile cerebral constituents, the

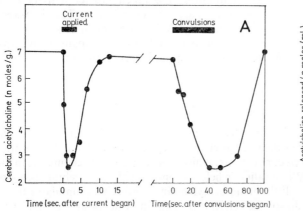 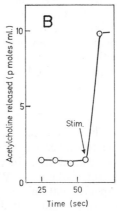

FIG. 14.1.A. Cerebral acetylcholine in young rats at different times before and after electro-shock (Richter & Crossland, 1949). Current was applied to electrodes on the head, from zero time for 3 sec. or until the animal was sacrificed when this was done before 3 sec. Convulsions began at periods 8–15 sec. after application of current. **B.** Release of acetylcholine from the surface of the rabbit occipital cortex to a small volume of saline, containing eserine and held in contact with the cortex by a small cup. Stimulation was by an electrode at the lateral geniculate body (Whittaker, 1969; see also Chakrin *et al.*, 1968).

brain has been fixed with liquid air, its acetylcholine content has been found to depend markedly on the condition of the animal at the time of fixation. To facilitate determinations in localized areas, such cooling has been halted just short of freezing, and the brain subsequently dissected at 0° (Takahashi & Aprison, 1964).

Adequate methods of analysis applied to young rats, in which the brain could be fixed by freezing within 1–4 sec. by dropping the animals into liquid air, were found to give an average cerebral acetylcholine of 7 nmoles/g. This was lower in animals in insulin hypoglycaemia, suggesting glucose metabolism to be needed for its maintenance (Crossland *et al.*, 1955). It rose to 8–10 nmoles/g. when normal animals were anaesthetized, and fell to 3–5 nmoles/g. with excitation and convulsions, as though the substance was consumed with increased cerebral activity. The change during electroconvulsions is especially interesting and is illustrated in Fig. 14.1. This shows an extremely rapid initial fall in acetylcholine such that the cerebral content was halved in animals put into liquid air 2 sec. after current was applied to the head. The change, occupying 3–6 sec., was thus proceeding at 0·6–1·2 nmoles/g. sec., or some 2–5 μmoles/g. hr. It began promptly, probably within a second of the application of current, but was rapidly followed by recovery when the current ceased. Only after the brain had recovered its initial acetylcholine content did the convulsions induced by the current commence; they ceased when, again, acetylcholine had fallen to about 40% of its normal value. The maximum rate of resynthesis of acetylcholine was about a quarter of its maximal rate of breakdown. Possibly, appreciable acetylcholine is needed not only for normal cerebral activity, but also for convulsive activity; and whereas in normal activity acetylcholine can be maintained, the much greater activity of a convulsion depletes it. The convulsions are thus intermittent. The time-scale of the breakdown and resynthesis of acetylcholine are similar to those of the changes in phosphocreatine which also precede or accompany convulsive activity: but the quantities of phosphocreatine involved are 500 times those of the acetylcholine.

Accumulation and Turnover; Administration

The cerebrospinal fluid normally contains no appreciable acetylcholine, but the substance has been detected there after epileptic attacks and also after experimentally-induced convulsions; it also can be caused to accumulate in the presence of eserine. When saline is held in contact with the cerebral cortex of experimental animals, little or no acetylcholine normally accumulates there, but can be caused to do so by electrical stimulation of the brain (**B**, Fig. 14.1). In small cups applied to the cortex of sheep or cats and containing salines with 0·4 mM-eserine, a normal output of acetylcholine corresponded to about 10 pmoles/cm^2 of cortex/min. during light anaesthesia. It was diminished by deeper anaesthesia and increased by a variety of forms of stimulation; convulsive activity caused by pentamethylene tetrazole (q.v.) yielded 25 pmoles/cm^2/min. (Mitchell, 1963; MacIntosh, 1963; Chakrin *et al.*, 1968; Schuberth *et al.*, 1969). During sensory stimulation of cats at moderate frequencies, greatest release of acetylcholine per stimulus from the somato-sensory cortex was obtained with 1 stimulus each 4 sec., and was of 0·5 pmoles/cm^2. If it is supposed that such a cup collects the acetylcholine released from a 1 mm. depth of cortex, the quantity released per stimulus is about 1/1000 of the acetylcholine available, and is yielded at a rate well within the synthetic abilities of the cortex. Presumably such stimulation brings into play only a proportion of the excitable elements of the cortex, in contrast to the general and abnormal stimulation which gave the much greater changes of **A**, Fig. 14.1.

Acetylcholine also appeared in eserinized salines which were caused to flow through the cerebral ventricles of cats (Bhattacharyya & Feldberg, 1958). The acetylcholine content of the perfusion fluid rose during the experiments and the output could continue for many hours at rates corresponding to 0·1 nmoles/min.

Thus the conditions of activity which are associated with loss of acetylcholine from the brain, permit it to diffuse and when it becomes diffusible, acetylcholine becomes more labile but can be protected by eserine. To understand these relationships it is necessary to turn to studies made with separated cerebral tissues. First, however, estimates of acetylcholine turnover may be given which have been based on administration of isotopically-labelled precursors. Using [Me-^{3}H]choline in mice, the normal turnover was estimated as 50 nmoles/g. min. diminishing to 10 with anaesthesia (Shuberth et al., 1969). The normal rate approximates to the rate of net change observed in vivo, e.g. in the experiments of A, Fig. 14.1.

The application of acetylcholine to the brain in quantities comparable in magnitude to those normally associated with the brain, can have considerable effects in whole animals. About 1 nmole injected to the carotid artery of cats greatly affects electrical activity of the brain, probably indirectly by action at the midbrain; at the cortex, amplitude, frequency and after-discharge may increase. Quantities of some 5 nmoles affect spinal cord activity. Larger doses intravenously or intracisternally produce generalized convulsions while local application to different parts of the central nervous system produces local discharges: the respiratory centre may be stimulated in this way, and also a variety of motor and behavioural effects have been produced (Feldberg, 1963). Impressively minute quantities of acetylcholine stimulate certain cells in the mammalian cerebral cortex when liberated in close proximity to them. This can be caused electrophoretically from micropipettes of tip-diameter 1 μ or less. Pyramidal cells deep in the cortex were found sensitive to acetylcholine and responded also to muscarine; atropine made acetylcholine ineffective in this respect (see Fig. 14.4; Krnjević & Phillis, 1963). A proportion of neurons in the visual cortex of cats responded by an increased rate of firing to acetylcholine similarly applied (Spehlmann, 1963); acetylcholine or prostigmine facilitated the discharge normally evoked in these cells by visual stimuli. Results of iontophoretic application of acetylcholine to various parts of the brain, with critical appraisal of the techniques, are given by Salmoiraghi & Stefanis (1967) and Bradley (1968). Liberation of acetylcholine probably contributes to the syndrome immediately following concussion; when reproduced in experimental animals, this is associated with electroencephalographic changes which are antagonized by atropine, and which may be simulated by intracisternal administration of acetylcholine.

Acetylcholine and Separated Cerebral Tissues

Though excision of parts of the brain may change their content of acetylcholine, the substance is unexpectedly stable in the separated tissue. Slices or suspensions in saline can retain some 10 nmoles of acetylcholine/g., but if acetylcholine in comparable amounts is added to such suspensions it is rapidly broken down. Thus much of the native acetylcholine of the brain is in bound forms: specifically, in the nerve terminals and vesicles described in Chapter 12. The acetylcholine-like material in such terminals has been examined in a number of ways, chemically and by biological assay, and concluded to be acetylcholine itself (Ryall *et al.*, 1964). Also, the subcellular distribution of acetylcholine has been investigated after its labelling by giving [Me-^{3}H]choline intracerebrally to anaesthetized cats, rabbits and guinea pigs (Chakrin & Whittaker, 1969; Takeno *et al.*, 1969). By fractionating tissue dispersions made in eserine-containing solutions, three forms of acetylcholine were recognized: the free compound, a labile-bound form present in the cytoplasm of nerve-terminals and a stable-bound form in synaptic vesicles. The labile-bound form

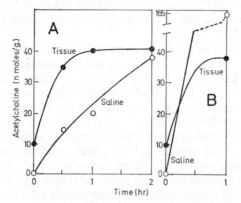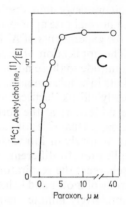

FIG. 14.2. Acetylcholine synthesis and uptake by sections of rat cerebral cortex incubated in glucose-salines (Mann *et al.*, 1939; Liang & Quastel, 1969).

A, B. Salines contained eserine, and potassium salts at the concentrations: A, 4 mM; B, 30 mM.

C. Salines with 5 mM-K$^+$, 40 μM added [^{14}C]-acetylcholine, and the concentrations of paroxon given by abscissae. The ordinate gives the ratio of labelled compound in a given quantity of tissue to that in the same quantity of saline.

was of highest specific activity and this contributed to the conclusion that, *in vivo*, most acetylcholine was synthesized cytoplasmically.

Acetylcholine not only is maintained, but also is synthesized in the separated tissue. For such synthesis, other reactions must be proceeding in the tissue, and again the acetylcholine formed must often be protected by a substance such as eserine to inhibit the cholinesterases which otherwise would break it down. Thus after sliced cerebral cortex from a guinea pig or rat has been respiring in an oxygenated salt mixture for an hour with glucose as substrate and with eserine, the initial 10 nmoles of acetylcholine/g. have been increased to about 59 (Fig. 14.2). Such synthesis does not take place in most other mammalian tissues; but in the rat brain, tissues of the striatum, which includes the caudate nucleus, were found especially potent in acetylcholine synthesis (Sattin, 1965). In media containing glucose, choline and other additions the tissue content of acetylcholine increased from 50 to 400 nmoles/g. in 30 min. Eserine was not needed and the acetylcholine synthesized was concluded to be in nerve-terminals, and partly within their synaptic vesicles.

The cerebral tissues produced acetylcholine while oxidizing either glucose, mannose, lactate, pyruvate or glutamate; but any synthesis with fructose, galactose or acetic, succinic, or α-oxoglutaric acids was small. The substrates which were effective are thus similar to, but not identical with, those maintaining creatine phosphate; presumably, under these conditions, supply of $\sim$P is one of the limiting factors. Studies using isotopically-labelled precursors show that in vitro, also, choline itself supplies the choline moiety. [U-^{14}C]Glucose and [2-^{14}C]pyruvate were equally effective in providing the acetyl moiety, which in double-labelling experiments using ^{3}H- and ^{14}C-glucose and rat cortex, carried isotopic ratios similar to those of the citrate formed concomitantly (Browning & Schulman, 1968; Sollenberg & Sorbo, 1969).

Acetylcholine added to or synthesized by incubated tissues, becomes distributed between extracellular and intracellular compartments. Determinations have been made of the compound in these two positions though the intracellular acetylcholine, as noted above, exists in more than one site or form. With suitable inhibition to prevent breakdown, acetylcholine itself accumulated in the free form in the fluid. The course of these changes is shown in Fig. 14.2. Here it is seen that although the synthesis is considerable, in the sense that the normal cerebral content of the material is observed to be formed in 10–15 min., production is very much slower than during the extremely rapid changes in vivo illustrated in Fig. 14.1. The ratio of tissue and fluid volumes in the experiments of A, Fig. 14.2 were such that acetylcholine remained at much higher concentration in the tissue than in the fluid. Adding [N-^{14}CH$_3$]acetylcholine to incubating fluids enabled the uptake of the compound to be studied. It was found to be inhibited by eserine but to be open to investigation in presence of an organophosphate anticholinesterase, diethyl-p-nitrophenylphosphate (Paroxon; Liang & Quastel, 1969; C, Fig. 14.2). To maintain the tissue/fluid ratios shown, glucose was required; in its presence, uptake of acetylcholine was inhibited by 2:4-dinitrophenol and by ouabain. These results were taken to suggest an uptake process which required $\sim$P and which was connected with the Na$^+$-pump of the tissue.

When acetylcholine has been synthesized by cerebral tissues it is stable anaerobically, and conditions affecting its release from the tissue can be studied. Thus the inclusion of 30 mM potassium salts in media in which sliced cerebral cortex was respiring, in place of the normal 4 mM, released acetylcholine. Addition of this concentration of potassium salts to tissue metabolizing aerobically with eserine, permitted a continuous and higher rate of formation of extracellular acetylcholine so that up to 250 nmoles/g. of fresh tissue was formed. This effect of potassium salts was seen primarily in cell-containing preparations, and not in finely minced tissue which could nevertheless synthesize acetylcholine. A similar change could also be brought about electrically in the cell-containing tissue. The electrical impulses which when applied to separated tissues respiring with glucose increased oxygen uptake and glycolysis, caused also a loss in cellular acetylcholine; and, with eserine, an increase in the extracellular form (Rowsell, 1954; Bowers, 1967). In cerebral tissues depleted of acetylcholine by impulses in absence of eserine, continued incubation with substrate restored the previous acetylcholine level. Incubation of neocortical tissues with ^{3}H-choline in presence of inhibitors of cholinesterase, yielded ^{3}H-acetylcholine and the specific activity and release of the compound was examined (Molenaar *et al.*, 1971; Richter & Marchbanks, 1971). With solutions 25 mM in K$^+$, about 0·12 of the acetylcholine content was released in 5–10 min., but this contained a disproportionately large amount of ^{3}H: preferential release of the newly-synthesized acetylcholine was thus indicated. Vesicles from the synaptosomes of tissues which had incorporated ^{3}H-choline to acetylcholine, yielded acetylcholine of lower specific activity than the cytoplasm. Release of acetylcholine from the tissues was diminished in media low in Ca^{2+}.

These and other findings contribute to a picture (Fig. 14.3) in which the level of acetylcholine is seen to result from the relative rates of its synthesis and breakdown, these two processes occurring by different routes. Synthesis of acetylcholine, its release from the tissue, and its breakdown can be judged by the preceding account to be intimately connected with functional activity in the intact central nervous system and in separated tissues. Increased potassium salts and applied electrical pulses *in vitro*, and neuronal activity *in vivo*, each involve depolarization of the cells of the tissue, as was noted in Chapter 4, and this, or associated phenomena (the entry of Na$^+$ or Ca^{2+}), can be judged to take an active part in the release of acetylcholine.

Acetylcholine and Convulsive Conditions

Occurrence of acetylcholine in the cerebrospinal fluid after convulsions, and initiation of convulsions by administered acetylcholine, have led to study of several aspects of acetylcholine metabolism in epilepsy. With human cerebral tissues removed during surgical treatment of epilepsy, acetylcholine metabolism has in some cases appeared abnormal. High cerebral content of acetylcholine has also been found in mice of a strain which was unusually susceptible to seizures (Tower, 1960; Pappius & Elliott, 1958; Kurokawa *et al.*, 1963). Convulsive tendency can also be induced in experimental animals by applying alumina cream to the surface of the cerebral cortex and also by feeding methionine sulphoximine (the toxic agent of "agenized" flour, that is flour treated with nitrogen trichloride). Study of tissues from such animals has shown their respiration and aerobic and anaerobic glycolysis to be normal. Abnormality has, however, been reported in their formation of acetylcholine and of glutamine (Stone, 1957; Folbergrova, 1963; Folbergrova *et al.*, 1969; see Chapter 8).

The defect reported in the human tissues lay specifically in a low retention in the tissue, of resynthesized acetylcholine. This was demonstrated by measurements in tissues before and after their respiration in glucose salines containing eserine, with either normal or high concentrations of potassium salts. The initial acetylcholine and also the acetylcholine which accumulated in the salines, were not abnormal in specimens from an epileptogenic focus. The cholinesterase of "focal" tissue was also somewhat higher than normal. In the animals treated with methionine sulphoximine, cerebral glutamine was diminished, and synthesis of glutamine by normal cerebral tissues *in vitro* was inhibited by 2 mM methionine sulphoximine. A link between the convulsive conditions induced by this agent and by lack of pyridoxine may thus lie in amino acid metabolism, with secondary effects on acetylcholine. These and other neurochemical mechanisms in epileptic conditions are appraised by Tower (1969).

Tissue from the alumina- or methionine sulphoximine-treated animals was also low in its retention of acetylcholine. A similar change could also be induced in slices of cerebral cortex from normal animals, *in vitro*, by partial anoxia; glutamine and asparagine then aided in restoring the acetylcholine.

Cell-free Systems

Synthesis of Acetylcholine

For detailed knowledge of the route of synthesis of acetylcholine, as of other substances, study of the component enzymes in cell-free systems has been necessary. The linkage between glucose metabolism and acetylcholine formation then proves to be indirect, the glucose acting as a source of energy-rich substances of which acetylcoenzyme A is, with choline, the immediate precursor of acetylcholine (Fig. 14.3).

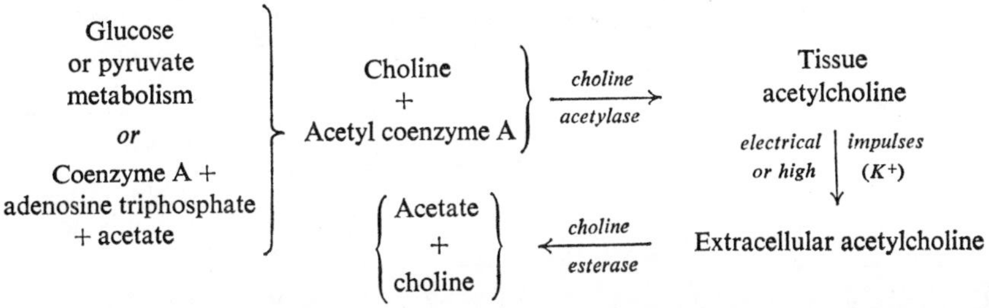

FIG. 14.3. Metabolism of acetylcholine.
Tissue acetylcholine is itself complex, existing free in nerve-terminals and also in synaptic vesicles. Choline acetylase is largely in solution cytoplasmically, while choline esterase is situated on the external surface of the outer cell membrane.

Acetylcoenzyme A with appropriate condensing enzymes will undergo a number of reactions in which an acetyl group is added to different molecules. Acetyl-CoA:choline O-acetyltransferase, or choline acetylase, which catalyses its condensation with choline, has been studied in a variety of extracts from cerebral tissues and from the head ganglion of the squid (Korkes *et al.*, 1952; Koelle, 1963). In a reaction mixture containing choline, potassium, magnesium, and phosphate ions, almost all of an 0·3 mM solution of acetylcoenzyme A underwent reaction with choline, forming acetylcholine which was determined chemically or by its pharmacological properties. An equivalent quantity of coenzyme A was formed concomitantly and determined by the appearance of its thiol group, the reaction being:

$$(CH_3)_3N^+.CH_2.CH_2OH + CoA.S.COCH_3 \rightleftharpoons (CH_3)_3N^+.CH_2.CH_2OCO.CH_3 + CoA.SH$$

Acetylcoenzyme A is normally present in cerebral and most other tissues in much smaller quantities than employed in this reaction mixture, and normally performs a role as carrier of acetyl groups. The coenzyme A formed in the reaction above may be reacetylated and then itself acetylate more choline. Reacetylation of coenzyme A may be brought about by several substances. A mixture of an acetate, adenosine triphosphate, and coenzyme A is effective (with the appropriate enzymes, which occur in cerebral tissues) in acetylating choline. In such reaction mixtures, eserine is usually added to prevent loss of acetylcholine, and fluoride to prevent breakdown of labile phosphates. When all other components of the acetylating systems are provided in excess, the rate

Table 14.2

Acetylcholine synthesis and hydrolysis in parts of the dog brain

Synthesis (Hebb & Silver, 1956; Hebb & Morris, 1969) was with acetone dried and extracted tissues; in calculation for the table it has been assumed that 1 g. of fresh tissue would yield 0·18 g. acetone powder. Reaction mixtures contained the extract, buffer, Mg salts, cysteine, choline, and an enzyme system yielding acetylcoenzyme A. Rates ascribed to the two cholinesterases were calculated from the rates of breakdown of acetylcholine, acetyl-β-methylcholine, and benzoylcholine; or with acetylthiocholine as substrate for the acetylcholinesterase, inhibiting the non-specific enzyme with ethopropazine HCl (Burgen & Chipman, 1951; Kasa & Silver, 1969). Sources of data for many other parts of the brain are quoted in the above papers; see also Foldes *et al.* (1962) for data from human brain.

Part	Rate of acetylcholine metabolism (µmoles/g. fresh tissue/hr.)		
	Synthesis	Hydrolysis	
		Acetyl cholinesterase	Non-specific cholinesterase
Cerebral cortex (different areas)	1·3–3·7	60–100	2–4
Cerebellar cortex	0·09	460	0·5
Corpus callosum	–	10–15	14
Caudate nucleus	13·0	1900	2
Thalamus	3·1	220–310	5
Hypothalamus	2·0	190	11

of formation of acetylcholine gives a measure of the activity of choline acetylase in the tissue, and several such assays have been made of the activity of different parts of the brain in acetylcholine formation.

Rates of synthesis of acetylcholine so determined are greatly dependent on the part of the brain examined. In general, they are such that the acetylcholine content of the brain could be synthesized in a few seconds, and so are in very satisfactory agreement with findings *in vivo* such as those of Fig. 14.1. Table 14.2 quotes values for different areas; at a typical rate of synthesis of 3 µmole/g. hr., the 8–12 nmoles/g. of cerebral tissues would require 10–15 sec. for its formation. Only a second or so would be required to produce the small quantities of acetylcholine which are observed to have marked effects when applied to the central nervous system. Synthesis is thus much more rapid in cell-free than has been observed in cell-containing systems. In general, areas high in choline acetylase, such as the caudate nucleus, are also high in acetylcholine content and in cholinesterases, though exceptions to this have been found.

Synthesis of acetylcholine in ground cerebral tissues may not need added coenzyme A, which already exists in the brain. That synthesis proceeds by the route outlined is however shown by effects of dialysis in removing the diffusible coenzyme A, when synthesis stops but can be initiated by coenzyme A preparations of known purity. Synthesis in the ground tissue is also susceptible to inhibition by agents such as iodoacetate which react with the thiol group of coenzyme A. The choline acetylating system shows considerable specificity with respect to the substances acetylated; ethanolamine and many of its derivatives did not act as substrates in place of choline; mono-, di- and triethyl analogues of choline were acetylated by a purified enzyme from bovine caudate nucleus (Hemsworth & Smith, 1970); the rates were below those for choline and diminished in the order named. With extracts from rat brain, only a few compounds of the general formula $HO.CH_2CH_2N^+(CH_3)_2.R$ were acetylated; R was required to be methyl, ethyl, n-propyl or n-butyl, the K_m rising in the order quoted. Limited substitution could be made in the acylating group, yielding the propionyl ester of choline. Higher homologues, e.g butyrate and palmitate, also gave choline esters in reaction mixtures containing aqueous extracts of acetone-treated mammalian or avian brain, but this activity was lost after ammonium sulphate purification of the choline acetylase (Dauterman & Mehrotra, 1963; Berry & Whittaker, 1959). For various choline esters of natural occurrence, see Koelle (1963) and Hebb & Morris (1969). Extremely rapid synthesis of acetylcholine is catalysed by the head of the blowfly, which can produce 70 μmole/g. hr. (Hebb, 1957).

Subcellular Localization of Acetylcholine Synthesis

The localization of choline acetylase in nerve terminal fractions from rat, guinea pig, rabbit and pigeon brain has been examined after disrupting the preparations by hypo-osmotic and other treatments (Whittaker, 1965; McCaman et al., 1965; Fonnum, 1967). Results suggested that under the osmotic conditions native to the tissue, the acetylase was free in the cytoplasm of the terminals; its behaviour in this respect resembled that of lactic dehydrogenase, also soluble. In particular, choline acetylase was not attached to the acetylcholine-containing vesicles. These vesicles, however, when examined in isolation, are capable of taking up acetylcholine from suspending fluids (Guth, 1969). Experiments in vivo which were discussed above suggested that the free cytoplasmic acetylcholine of nerve-terminals is the precursor of the stabler form which occurs in the vesicles, a finding consistent with the observed uptake. The terminals themselves in isolation, proved capable of assimilation of [^{14}C]choline and of its conversion to acetylcholine (Marchbanks, 1968, 1969). Uptake of acetylcholine by the vesicle suspensions was rapid, being largely complete in 30 sec. at 37°. Some 32–38 μl. of vesicles were calculated as present per gram of guinea pig brain.

Cholinesterases

As indicated above, acetylcholine can undergo rapid breakdown in cerebral tissues. The loss occurs by a simple hydrolysis to choline and acetic acid, and not by reversal of the reaction catalysed by choline acetylase; it is brought about by cholinesterases which require no coenzyme. Acetylcholine is also rapidly degraded by other tissues of the body (for reviews, see Koelle, 1963; Gerebetzoff, 1959; Augustinsson, 1960; Wilson, 1960). In demonstrating cerebral cholinesterase a chosen part of the brain is ground in a bicarbonate saline without substrate, and 1–10 mg. of tissue placed in apparatus, mano-metric or electrometric, arranged so that acetylcholine can be added and measurement made of the acid formed by the hydrolysis. In most parts of the brain, the enzyme so measured is largely the "true" cholinesterase, or acetyl-cholinesterase, which degrades acetylcholine itself more rapidly than other substrates. To demonstrate specifically the acetylcholinesterase, reaction is frequently carried out with related substrates broken down somewhat less rapidly but more specifically, such as acetyl-β-methyl choline; see Table 14.2. Other esterases also hydrolyse acetylcholine and have been termed non-specific, or pseudocholinesterases; they may be differentiated by their hydrolysis of benzoylcholine on which acetylcholinesterase has little action. The two classes of enzyme outlined (others acting on acetylcholine probably exist) can also be differentiated by their different susceptibility to inhibitory agents; etho-propazine, 2-diethylaminoethylphenothiazine HCl, in μM solutions inhibits preferentially the non-specific esterase. Much of the pseudocholinesterase of the brain appears by histochemical methods to be localized mainly at the walls of blood vessels, arterioles, venules, and capillaries; it is also at some glial cells. In the hypothalamus the true enzyme is at very high level in the cells of specific hypothalamic nuclei (Abrahams et al., 1957). Rodent cerebellar regions showed marked variation in acetylcholinesterase activity but activities were in parallel with those of choline acetylase (Kasa & Silver, 1969). This contributes to a picture of the enzyme functioning by limiting the spread of acetylcholine.

Values for the activity of cerebral cholinesterases given in Table 14.2, are seen to differ greatly in different parts of the brain. Average rates determined for the true acetylcholinesterase of the whole of the brain in different mam-malian species are between 200 and 500 μmoles acetylcholine hydrolysed/g.hr. Most other mammalian tissues: diaphragm, liver, stomach or lung, show less than a tenth of this activity. The true enzyme is, however, the predominating cholinesterase of erythrocytes, skeletal muscle and the electric organs possessed by certain fishes. On the other hand, heart muscle or intestinal mucosa may break down acetylcholine nearly as rapidly as mixed cerebral tissues, but by the non-specific enzyme in which the cerebral tissues are relatively much less potent. The cerebral acetylcholinesterase is firmly attached to membrane-structures (see Chapter 12 and below). A variety of procedures for solubilizing it for purification and further examination gave only limited success; but using an acetone-powder from the caudate nucleus, treatment with pancreatic lipase yielded a material which could be fractionated by salt precipitation, as also did a polyoxyethylene detergent (Lawler, 1963; Got & Polya, 1963). The acetylcholinesterase from the caudate nucleus of calf brain has been purified by extraction, column chromatography and zone electrophoresis, giving a 35-fold enrichment (Jackson & Aprison, 1966).

The rates attained by cerebral acetylcholinesterase show it to be among the more rapid cerebral processes. The mean rate is a quarter to a tenth that of several phosphokinases. To assess the significance of the speed of reaction of acetylcholinesterase, some properties of the system observed in material isolated from different parts of the brain including the nucleus caudatus, one of the most active centres, may be recounted (Nachmansohn, 1959; Koelle, 1963).

In these preparations, acetylcholine itself is degraded at greater speed than other substrates examined; propionylcholine, which also occurs naturally, reacting at about three-quarters of the rate and benzoylcholine or tributyrin not at all. 3,3-Dimethylbutyl acetate, in which a carbon atom replaces as nearly as possible the nitrogen atom of acetylcholine, is however hydrolysed by cerebral and other acetylcholinesterases. For optimum activity acetylcholine is required to be present at about 3 mM; higher concentrations inhibit the true but not the pseudo-enzyme, and this has contributed interestingly to the picture of how acetylcholine combines with the hydrolysing enzyme. More important to the action of the enzyme *in vivo* the rate also falls with decrease in substrate concentration below 3 mM; at 0·3 mM, the rate is some 5–10% of its maximal rate. The mean acetylcholine content of the whole brain is some 10 nmoles/g., corresponding to 10^{-5} M, and at this concentration the rate of acetylcholinesterase is probably not more than 1% of that determined at optimal substrate level. This in fact corresponds closely to the maximum rate of loss of acetylcholine observed in the whole brain, which at 2–5 μmoles/g. hr. is 1% of the 200–500 μmoles/g. hr. observed for the enzyme in the separated tissue at optimal acetylcholine concentration. More accurate comparison is made difficult by the uneven distribution of both enzyme and substrate in the tissue.

Acetylcholinesterase from the electric organ of the electric fish has been obtained in highly purified and crystalline form. The molecule contained aminosugar as well as amino acid residues, and consisted of 4 subunits of molecular weight approx. 64,000 (Leuzinger, 1969).

In the brain, both acetylcholine and acetylcholinesterase occur at higher level in grey than in white matter. In human cerebral cortex obtained at lobotomy, the true cholinesterase has been found to be of greatest activity in layers I, II and V, and at the II–IIIa junction, zones rich in fine arborizations (Pope *et al.*, 1952). Distribution is thus reminiscent of the occurrence of the enzyme at synaptic regions in the peripheral nervous system, and at the axonal surface rather than the axoplasm of the giant axon of the squid. The human specimens were derived from subjects with mental illness or intractable pain; small differences in enzyme level were found in certain groups of subjects and ascribed either to the illness or to previous therapeutic measures. Small deviations from normal level have also been found in the acetylcholinesterases of tissue from epileptogenic areas of human cerebral cortex (see above) and considerable deviations in cerebral tumours (Weber, 1952; Bulbring *et al.*, 1953).

Anticholinesterases

Much information on the importance of cholinesterases to the central nervous system has come from the study of substances which inhibit the enzymes. A wide variety of substances at relatively high concentrations will inhibit cholinesterases, as, for example, will methylene blue or strychnine. Several compounds rightly termed anticholinesterases inhibit the enzymes much more specifically and in concentrations between 10^{-9} and 10^{-6} M; the structures of some of these are compared with that of acetylcholine in Fig. 14.4. Prostigmine and physostigmine (eserine) show structural resemblances to acetylcholine which enable them to become attached to the cholinesterases at their active sites, apparently by forces similar to those involved in the normal

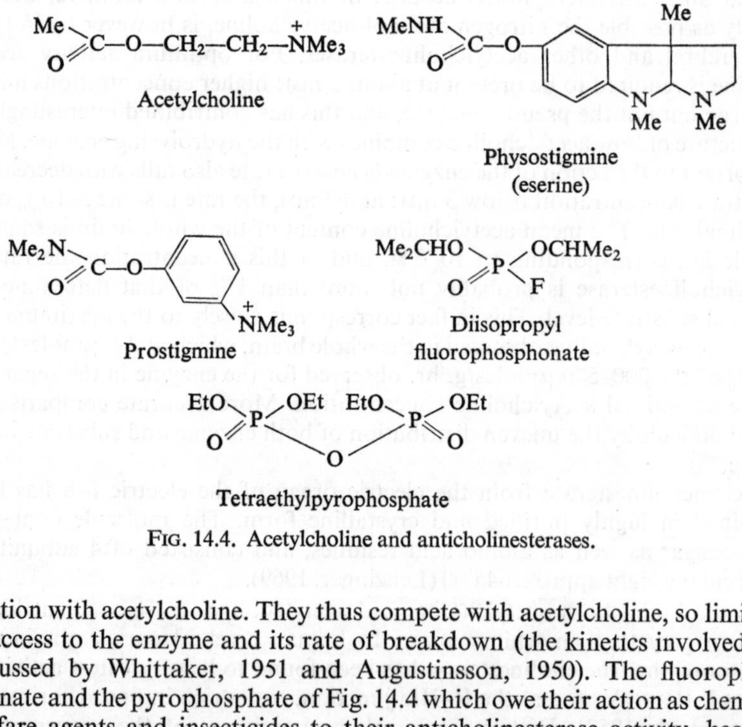

FIG. 14.4. Acetylcholine and anticholinesterases.

reaction with acetylcholine. They thus compete with acetylcholine, so limiting its access to the enzyme and its rate of breakdown (the kinetics involved are discussed by Whittaker, 1951 and Augustinsson, 1950). The fluorophosphonate and the pyrophosphate of Fig. 14.4 which owe their action as chemical warfare agents and insecticides to their anticholinesterase activity, become attached to that site on the enzyme which normally reacts with the ester link in acetylcholine, but then undergo further chemical reaction with the enzyme. Because of this further reaction, their effects are not easily, if at all, reversed by dilution or washing away the inhibitor, for example by the bloodstream; and they can inhibit at extremely low concentrations and in quantities of about one molecule of inhibitor for each molecule of enzyme. An effective antidote, pyridine-2-aldoxime methiodide, has, however, been designed on the basis of enzyme studies and applied therapeutically in poisoning by the agents (Wilson, in *Symposium*, 1962; see Heath, 1961 and Tower, 1969). Many thousands of cases of such poisoning have been associated with the industrial manufacture of organophosphorus compounds, and their use in agriculture.

Effects of anticholinesterases on the central nervous system can be seen most directly by their application to the cerebral cortex itself. Thus low concentrations of eserine, sufficient to inhibit acetylcholinesterase, potentiate the effects of locally applied acetylcholine and these effects are prevented by atropine. Epileptiform grand mal activity can be induced in the electroencephalogram of cats in this way by concentrations of acetylcholine which would not be effective alone. Applied to the hypothalamus, 8–59 μg. of eserine can produce sympathetic effects similar to certain of those elicited there electrically. Eserine intraperitoneally in rats also markedly affected the hypothalamus, inducing there a theta rhythm; with this came inhibition of the learning of a passive avoidance reaction (Bureš, *Symposium*, 1964). Tetraethylpyrophosphate given systemically to dogs led in the cerebral cortex to an accumulation of acetylcholine which was measured and correlated with electroencephalographic changes and convulsive activity (Stone, 1957; Tower, 1969).

When anticholinesterases are administered so that they reach the general circulation, not all of their effects are on the central nervous system. In particular, prostigmine is valuable for its peripheral action in myasthenia gravis and is excluded from the brain; but the use of di*iso*propylfluorophosphonate for the same purpose is limited by its central actions. These include electroencephalographic changes antagonized by atropine, and headache, emotional lability and insomnia. An insecticidal anticholinesterase, O,O-diethyl-S-ethyl-mercaptothiophosphate also has prominent central actions in man and had as its first detectable effect on rats an increase in errors in problem-solving; cerebral cholinesterase was then inhibited by 60% (Russell, *Symposium*, 1964; Heath, 1961). Much use has been made of anticholinesterases in investigating behavioural characteristics in laboratory animals and man; thus they affect arousal mechanisms, and they produce effects which mimic important aspects of psychotic illnesses (see Bradley & Fink, 1968; Efron, 1968).

Features in the Action of Acetylcholine

The conceptions of acetylcholine action developed in other systems, neural and neuromuscular, are likely to apply to its role in the brain, and they will not be appraised in detail here. The occurrence in nerve-terminal fractions of choline acetylase and of vesicles containing an appreciable proportion of the tissue's acetylcholine have been described above and in Chapter 12, together with the likely release of vesicle contents to the synaptic cleft on stimulation. Evidence suggests, however, that not all cerebral release of acetylcholine on stimulation occurs from a "stable-bound" vesicular pool (Whittaker, 1969). Following its release, it is then pictured that acetylcholine increases the permeability of the postsynaptic membrane to Na^+, so diminishing membrane potential and contributing to cell-discharge. In this sequence, which is terminated by removal of the acetylcholine by diffusion and by cholinesterase, the following points may be noted regarding the enzyme velocities which have been observed in the mammalian brain.

Speed of Acetylcholine Synthesis

The formation of acetylcholine consumes energy-rich substances: the necessary acetylcoenzyme A can be formed by the expenditure of 1 mole of adenosine triphosphate per mole of acetylcholine synthesized. By comparing the maximum rate of cerebral choline acetylase with the respiratory rate of the brain, an impression may be gained of the proportion of metabolically-derived energy which could be expended in the acetylcholine system. The proportion is small. Thus acetylcholine is formed in preparations from mammalian brain at about 3 μmoles/g. of mixed tissue/hr. (Table 14.2). The formation of energy-rich phosphate, at an efficiency of 2–3 moles/atom of oxygen with a respiratory rate of 60–150 μmoles O_2/g. hr., can occur at 240–900 μmoles/g. hr. Thus even if choline acetylase is working at the maximal observed rate, continually, only 0·3 to 1 % of metabolically-derived energy can be utilized in acetylcholine metabolism by known routes. For such an assessment the rate of hydrolysis of acetylcholine is irrelevant. Cholinesterases could catalyse the hydrolysis of acetylcholine at 100 times the rate of synthesis, but it is the synthesis which conditions the rate of expenditure of energy through acetylcholine.

Nevertheless, small quantities of acetylcholine comparable to those synthesized in brief periods by choline acetylase, can cause convulsive activity with its large increase in energy-yielding and energy-consuming reactions. Thus in the central as in the peripheral nervous system acetylcholine is acting as a trigger and the major energy-consuming reactions which it initiates are considered to be those of the active ion movements needed after cell discharge (Chapter 3).

Diffusion and Breakdown of Acetylcholine

In assessing the functioning of acetylcholine in transmission its rate of release from the tissue, and the rate of breakdown of the liberated compound, become very important. The rates of release and breakdown would be expected to condition the onset of transmission and the rate of recovery before a second impulse could be fired. The rate of release has been little studied in isolated systems, but must be high. It may be supposed that under resting conditions in a nerve-terminal, transient contacts constantly occur between vesicle and outer membrane by Brownian movement, and that these become effective in liberating transmitter when the membrane is sufficiently depolarized. Possibly the depolarization diminishes repulsive forces exerted on a vesicle which has acidic groups at its outer surface, or exposes new groups at the inside of the membrane and encourages the fusion illustrated in Fig. 12.2. Acetylcholine is calculated to exist at 110 mM in the vesicles of some neuromuscular junctions, and thus on liberation a large concentration gradient transitorily exists across the 300 Å of the synaptic cleft; μsec. may suffice for its arrival in adequate concentration at the postsynaptic side and less than a msec. for a large proportion to have been removed by diffusion to a distance of a few μ (Ogston, 1955; Eccles, 1964; De Robertis, 1964). Synaptic vesicles from the mammalian cerebral cortex have also been computed to contain an approximately isotonic solution of acetylcholine or some 300–3000 molecules/vesicle; $3·8 \times 10^{12}$ vesicles, not necessarily all from cholinergic endings, are estimated/g. tissue

(Whittaker & Sheridan, 1965). Calcium ions may be involved in the release of acetylcholine, which in a non-cerebral preparation had as counter-ion a small polyacidic protein; in cerebral systems, see Matsuda *et al.* (1971).

Cholinesterase present at the synaptic region and beyond acts during and after this time. The rate of breakdown of acetylcholine has been noted above to average 200–500 μmoles/g. tissue/hr. but to reach this rate acetylcholine is required at about 3 mM. Though this is 300 times its mean concentration in the brain *in vivo*, the localization of acetylcholine means that suitably localized cholinesterase could be working at maximal capacity shortly after liberation of the substrate. If in such a localized area 1 % of the cerebral acetylcholine was released: that is, 0·07 nmoles/g. tissue, its hydrolysis at 350 μmoles/g. hr. would require 0·7 msec. Thus quantitative aspects of diffusion and breakdown of acetylcholine appear consistent with the highest rates of cell firing found in the brain, of some 1,000/sec.

The means by which acetylcholine causes the change in membrane permeability which is involved in its acting as a transmitting agent is uncertain but may be related to its effect in dissociating lipo-protein complexes or penetrating surface films of lipids. This can be brought about by 10^{-6} M acetylcholine and and if such actions took place at the cell surface at the synapse, release of acetylcholine could be understood to alter the polarization of cells by making their outer membranes more permeable at this point. Deductions have been made about molecular configurations at acetylcholine receptor sites, from structures of pharmacological agents which act in relation to acetylcholine (Chothia, 1970; Beers & Reich, 1970). A proteolipid which may be present at the cholinergic receptor site has been isolated from nerve terminal fractions on the basis of its combination with ^{14}C-dimethyltubocurarine and the binding of acetylcholine to lipoprotein and other components extracted from synaptic membranes had been examined (De Robertis, 1969; Hauser *et al.*, 1970). Electroplax tissues yielded a proteolipid of high affinity for acetylcholine; in a lipid membrane, reaction of the proteolipid with acetylcholine caused increased conductance (De Robertis, 1971).

Catecholamines

Noradrenaline, 3-hydroxytyramine (or dopamine) and adrenaline have their chief cerebral occurrence in the lower parts of the brain (Table 14.3). Their concentrations there are quite small but not remote from those found in the sympathetic nervous system where their functional importance is undoubted. Much of the characterization and measurement of these compounds, the components of cerebral sympathin, has therefore depended upon chromatography, biological assay and fluorometric measurements; but by these means the compounds can be differentially determined and a variety of their properties demonstrated. For collective information on the catecholamines in neural systems generally, see Himwich & Himwich (1964), Iversen (1967), Efron (1968), Akert & Waser (1969), Fuxe *et al.* (1970) and Snyder *et al.* (1970).

Occurrence in the Brain; Turnover and Release

Catecholamine-containing structures of the brain, as of other organs, have been visualized microscopically by the fluorescence of their condensation

Table 14.3

Cerebral catecholamines, serotonin and related enzymes

	Content[1], human brain (nmoles/g.)			Enzyme activity (μmoles/g. hr.)		
	Noradrenaline	Dopamine	Serotonin	Dopa decarboxylase[2]	Catechol O-methyl transferase[3,5]	Mono-amine oxidase[4,5]
Cerebral cortex	0·3 (2·3)	0·5	0·2 (3·5)	(0·1)	0·45	4·2
White matter	0·05	0·3	–	–	0·55	2·4
Caudate nucleus	0·45 (0·2)	24 (26)	1·8 (8·2)	3 (2·2)	0·58	4·8
Thalamus	0·65 (0·8)	1·6	1·3 (2·2)	2·1 (0·4)	–	5·0
Hypothalamus	6·0 (14)	4·8	2·6 (13)	3·4 (1·5)	0·50	8·4
Medulla oblongata	0·8	0·1	2·1	2·6	0·50	6·0

For further data, including values for other mammalian species, see Robson & Stacey (1962), McCaman *et al.* (1965) and Kindwall & Weiner (1966).

[1] Bertler *et al.* (1960); Sano *et al.* (1960) and Hornykiewicz (1964, 1966). Values in parentheses are for the cat (Bertler *et al.*, 1960; Kuntzman *et al.*, 1961).
[2] Holtz & Westermann (1956), in ox brain; Kuntzman *et al.* (1961), in cat brain, in parentheses.
[3] Axelrod *et al.* (1960), in monkey brain.
[4] Bogdanski *et al.* (1957), in dog brain.
[5] Similar values were obtained in samples of human brain (Vogel & Orfei, 1967).

products with formaldehyde, and are found to correspond to complex neuronal systems (see Dahlström, 1969; Iversen, 1967; Lichtensteiger & Langemann, 1966). Fine nerve fibres with catecholamine-containing terminals or varicosities occur in many regions from the spinal cord to the neocortex, and originate from cell bodies, especially the brain stem and substantia nigra, which also contain catecholamines.

Of the three catecholamines, (Fig. 14.5) adrenaline preponderates in the amphibian brain but in mammals it forms only some 4–12% of the cerebral catecholamines (Carlsson, *Symposium*, 1959; Montagu, 1963). Of the other two compounds, dopamine preponderates in the corpus striatum, including both the caudate nucleus and the putamen of the lentiform nucleus, but noradrenaline preponderates elsewhere; in the brain as a whole the two are present in similar concentrations in a number of mammalian species including man. The cortical grey matter contained only some 0·5 nmoles of the catecholamine/g., and white matter, down to one-tenth of that level. Some contribution to the very low values may come from sympathetic nerves supplying the blood vessels. The richest areas, however, are akin functionally in being the parts of the brain connected with the activity of the sympathetic nervous system. On stimulation they have among their effects the peripheral release of adrenaline, with consequential glycosuria and increase in blood pressure and heart rate. This occurs notably by stimulation of parts of the hypothalamus and of the floor of the fourth ventricle.

Moreover, stimulation of specific areas has led to measured release of cerebral catecholamines or their metabolites. This occurred from the putamen of cats, which liberated dopamine on excitation from the substantia nigra; similar stimulation led to increased homovanillic acid, a major metabolite of dopamine, in the lateral ventricle (McLennan, 1965; Portig & Vogt, 1969). Perfusion of of the third ventricle of cats with solutions containing first [^{14}C]noradrenaline

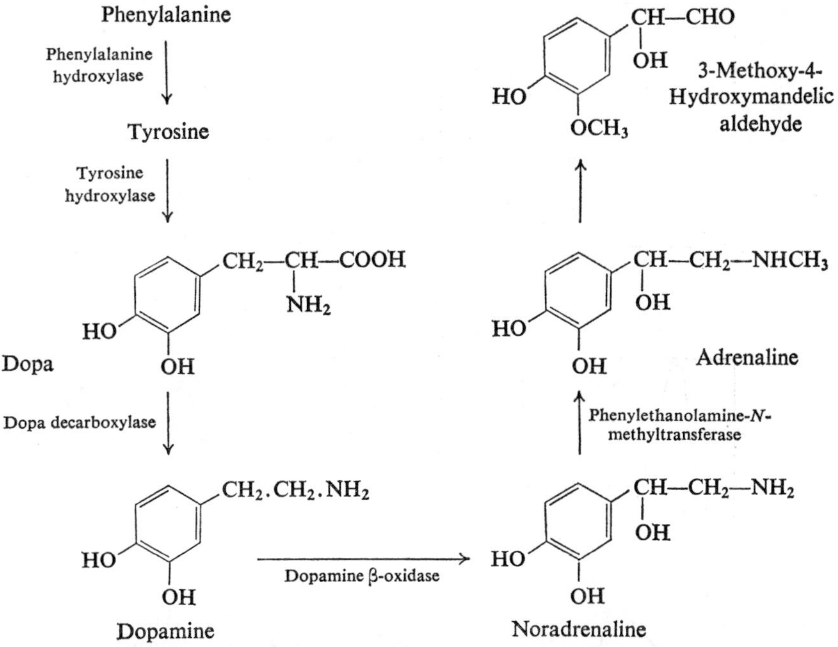

Phenylalanine

Phenylalanine hydroxylase

Tyrosine

Tyrosine hydroxylase

CH_2—CH—$COOH$
       |
      NH_2

HO

Dopa   OH

Dopa decarboxylase

$CH_2.CH_2.NH_2$

HO

OH

Dopamine

$\xrightarrow{\text{Dopamine } \beta\text{-oxidase}}$

CH—CHO
  |
  OH   3-Methoxy-4-
HO   Hydroxymandelic
    OCH_3 aldehyde

CH—CH_2—$NHCH_3$
  |
  OH
HO
    OH   Adrenaline

Phenylethanolamine-N-methyltransferase

CH—CH_2—NH_2
  |
  OH
HO
    OH

Noradrenaline

FIG. 14.5. Formation of the catecholamines, and an intermediate in their breakdown. Phenylalanine, its hydroxylation, and tyrosine are described in Chapter 8. Dopa is an established abbreviation given in the 1920s to "*dioxyphenylalanine*" for which the systematic name is now 3:4-dihydroxyphenylalanine or 3-hydroxytyrosine. Adrenaline and noradrenaline are synonymous with epinephrine and norepinephrine.
3-Methoxy-4-hydroxymandelic aldehyde is an intermediate in the breakdown of the catecholamines, and can lead either to acidic metabolites terminating in homovanillic acid: see Axelrod (1965), Rutledge & Jonason (1968) and Calne & Sandler (1970); or to neutral metabolites, e.g. 4-hydroxy-3-methoxyphenylethyleneglycol (Taylor & Laverty, 1969).

and subsequently nialamide as inhibitor of its degradation, allowed observation of release of noradrenaline from the hypothalamus. Release was increased by electrical stimulation of hypothalamic nuclei, and also by addition of acetylcholine to the perfusion fluids (Philippa *et al.*, 1970); significantly, the release by acetylcholine required the concomitant presence of calcium ions.

Turnover of cerebral catecholamines *in vivo* has been measured after intraventricular administration of [^{3}H]noradrenaline or dopamine; a half-life

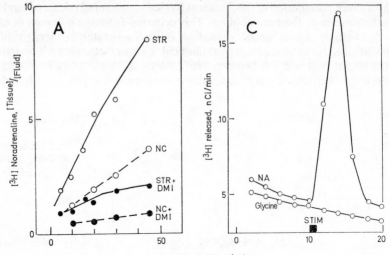

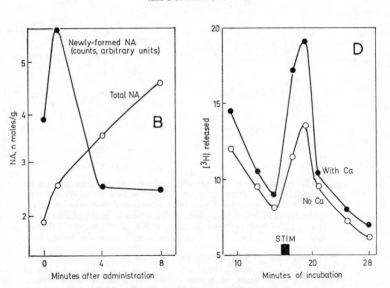

Fig. 14.6. Accumulation, synthesis and release of noradrenaline by cerebral tissues (Baldessarini & Kopin, 1967; Spector, 1968; Snyder *et al.*, 1968; McIlwain & Snyder, 1970).

A. Uptake. Tissues from the striatum (STR) or neocortex (NC) of rats were incubated in a few ml. glucose bicarbonate salines which contained [^{3}H]noradrenaline, and some of which also contained desmethylimipramine (DMI).

B. Synthesis of noradrenaline (NA) from administered [^{3}H]L-dihydroxyphenylalanine by guinea pigs; monoamine oxidase was inhibited by N-methyl-N-2-propynylbenzylamine HCl (pargyline), and the diminution of incorporation of precursor after 1 hr. is attributed to feedback inhibition by NA.

C. Tissues from the piriform cortex of guinea pigs were incubated in salines containing either [^{3}H]glycine, or [^{3}H]noradrenaline with of between 2 and 4 hr. was found in several regions of rat brain. These values agreed with data obtained by determining the net change in the amines after inhibiting their endogenous synthesis and represent a more rapid turnover than occurs in the catecholamines of other tissues studied, e.g. of spleen, adrenal or heart (Glowinski *et al.*, 1965; Iversen, 1967).

Catecholamines in Separated Tissues

The endogenous catecholamines of isolated cerebral tissues are relatively stable and on incubating the tissues in fluid media, undergo exchange with added catecholamines. Uptake of [³H]noradrenaline in such systems has been measured as indicated in **A**, Fig. 14.6; initial uptake proceeded at about 15 nmoles/g. hr. with 0·1 μM-noradrenaline. By examining uptake from noradrenaline solutions of different concentrations, apparent K_m values were obtained, and these ranged from 0·4 to 2 μM with tissues from different regions of rat brain. Uptake was inhibited by drugs, notably by desmethylimipramine (Dengler *et al.*, 1961; Snyder *et al.*, 1968). It was inhibited also by reagents disturbing energy-metabolism, by ouabain, and was diminished when reserpine had been administered to the cats which yielded the tissue.

After its uptake by the isolated tissue, noradrenaline was gradually released from the tissue and circumstances conditioning its release can be studied. Electrical stimulation, notably, caused prompt release of noradrenaline. Such stimulation causes depolarization of cells of the tissue and changes in major metabolites, but release of labelled compounds is nevertheless selective: from cortical samples, [³H]glycine was not released by stimuli which released noradrenaline (Fig. 14.5). Bromides, lithium salts or tetrodotoxin depressed the release of noradrenaline caused by electrical stimulation (Katz & Kopin, 1969; Goodwin *et al.*, 1969), which was, moreover, depressed also by omission of Ca^{2+} salts from incubating media. Each of these four agents affects other responses which cerebral tissues give to stimulation presumably through modifying at cell-membrane level, the cation movements of neural excitation. Release of the amines on stimulating isolated tissues thus appears to give a valid means of examining processes normal to their release in the brain.

Dopamine synthesis and release has also received study in isolated tissues from the brain (Baldessarini & Kopin, 1966; Besson *et al.*, 1969). The striatum of rats incubated in oxygenated salines was initially exposed to [³H]tyrosine, and subsequently superfused. [³H]Dopamine, identified by column chromatography was formed in the tissue (see below) and appeared in the outflow from

---

FIG. 14.6.—*cont.*
ascorbic acid and nialamide. A flow of glucose bicarbonate saline was then started (apparatus: Fig. 4.1), and the effluent saline collected at 2-min. intervals for determination of noradrenaline. Electrical stimulation was applied to both tissues as indicated.

D. Coronal sections of rat brain, including parts of the hypothalamus and thalamus, were incubated in substrate-Ringer solutions with or without Ca^{2+}, and with [³H]noradrenaline; electrical stimulation was applied as indicated.

superfusion at a rate implying a half-life of about 1 hr. for the compound. Release of the ^{3}H of dopamine but not of other substances examined was accelerated by D-amphetamine and by acetylcholine.

Subcellular Occurrence of Catecholamines

Noradrenaline was noted in Chapter 12 to be associated with nerve-terminals when the fraction containing the terminals was separated centrifugally from the brain as a whole. Further, comparable behaviour has been found in specifically the hypothalamus and caudate nuclei of cats or rabbits, after dispersion in sucrose and density-gradient or differential centrifugation: 70% of the nor-adrenaline in such sites was deposited not at 5000 g. min., but at 3×10^6 g. min. and between similar speeds, some 30% of the dopamine was deposited (Bertler et al., 1960; Chrusciel, Symposium, 1960; see also Maynert et al., 1964). Further separation showed the noradrenaline to be associated with particles resembling nerve-terminals. These may presumably derive from the varicosities described above as well as from terminal regions; the term synaptosome is used with this in mind. From such synaptosomal fractions, brief exposure to hypo-osmotic conditions enabled a vesicle fraction to be separated which was enriched in the catecholamine (de Robertis, 1964).

The brain stem of rats, sampled 17 hr. after intraventricular injection of [^{3}H]noradrenaline to the animals, also yielded by differential and density gradient centrifugation a synaptosomal fraction carrying much of the nor-adrenaline of the tissue (Bogdanski et al., 1968). For maintenance of the noradrenaline content of the terminals, Na$^+$ at about 140 mM was needed in suspending fluids; the half-life of the noradrenaline was then about 3·5 hr., which approximated to in vivo values. Moreover, Na$^+$ was needed for uptake of further noradrenaline to the synaptosomal fraction in vitro.

Dopamine of the rat hypothalamus also occurred in particles with synapto-somal properties; by in vitro uptake of the ^{3}H-labelled amines, particles carry-ing dopamine were found to be separable centrifugally from those carrying noradrenaline (Iversen & Snyder, 1968). In the dopamine-containing nigro-neostriatal system of the rat, nerve-cell bodies contained about 2 pg. of dopamine each and the 5×10^5 varicosities in the terminal arborizations (some decimetres in total length) from the average neuron collectively carried about 125 pg. (Dahlström, 1969). The amine-carrying varicosities in the brain generally, are credited with a content of biologically-active bases equivalent to about 50 mM (Glowinski, 1970). The nature of the acidic counter-ion is thus important; in the adrenal it is adenosine triphosphate, which is liberated together with adrenaline but undergoes degradation to adenosine 5'-phosphate and this compound is secreted together with adrenaline when the gland is stimulated. In preparations from the brain, adenosine itself is liberated by stimulation, together with catecholamines and serotonin, and conceivably a similar storage mechanism is operating (Sattin & Rall, 1970; McIlwain, 1971).

It is thus evident that the occurrence and release of catecholamines in cerebral systems have several features in common with those of catecholamines of other tissues of the body, including the adrenal and peripheral nerve (Iversen, 1967; Banks et al., 1969; Blaschko & Smith, 1970). Further resemblances will be found in the account which follows and which concerns processes of synthesis and degradation of the catecholamines.

Synthesis; Tyrosine Hydroxylase and Dihydroxyphenylalanine

A route for the synthesis of the catecholamines from tyrosine has been established in cerebral and other tissues and is outlined in Fig. 14.5; alternative routes have been explored but are not prominent in neural systems under normal conditions (Axelrod, *Symposium*, 1963*a*; Lipton & Udenfriend, 1968). The initial stage, catalysed by tyrosine hydroxylase, was demonstrated with dispersions incubated aerobically with 10 mM-tyrosine enriched in [^{3}H]- or [1-^{14}C]tyrosine (Nagatsu *et al.*, 1964). This yielded 3:4-dihydroxyphenyl-alanine (dopa) which was separated on an alumina column and shown to be formed by a dispersion of guinea pig brain at about 8 nmoles/g. hr. Activity was markedly greater in the brain stem, which gave 12, than in the cerebellum or cortex which gave 0·9–2·3 nmoles/g. hr. The whole of this activity was deposited at 0·3 × 10^6 g. min. The brain from other mammalian species showed comparable activity; an adrenal dispersion yielded 16, but heart, liver and spleen gave only 0·1–0·6 nmoles/g. hr.

Tyrosine hydroxylase of the caudate nucleus of bovine brain was also particulate, and deposited in synaptosomal fractions (McGeer *et al.*, 1967; Fahn *et al.*, 1969). From these, vesicle-containing fractions prepared by hypoosmotic treatment were enriched in the enzyme. This is likely to be of much significance in the control of catecholamine synthesis, for the hydroxylase was inhibited by noradrenaline: about 50% at 1 mM. The mean tissue concentration of noradrenaline is much below this value, which could however be reached in the synaptosomes or vesicles. As tyrosine hydroxylase is the rate-limiting step in the sequence yielding noradrenaline, it is thus susceptible to feedback inhibition and this process can control noradrenaline level. In the experiment of **B**, Fig. 14.6, noradrenaline was caused to accumulate through inhibition of monoamine oxidase (q.v.) and after a small elevation of noradrenaline from its normal level, synthesis from [^{3}H]dopa greatly diminished.

Much of the hydroxylase from the adrenal, unlike that from the brain, was in the soluble portion of the dispersions. After purification, it was shown to require a tetrahydropteridine for activity, and to be stimulated by ferrous salts. The formation of tyrosine itself from phenylalanine (Chapter 8) will be recalled as an analogous reaction which also required reduced pteridines. The cerebral tyrosine hydroxylase was inhibited 80–90% by 0·1–1 mM-L-phenyl-alanine, and thus the accumulation of phenylalanine in phenylketonuria may well disturb catecholamine metabolism in the phenylketonurics. Much tyrosine is of dietary origin and tyrosine levels in the body as a whole are controlled by processes which include hepatic *tyrosine transaminase*, EC 2.6.1.5. The activity of this enzyme in rat liver proves to be under control from the brain (Black *et al.*, 1971). Transection of the spinal cord was followed by an increase in activity of the hepatic enzyme which was counteracted by subcutaneous noradrenaline. Lesions in the lateral hypothalamus of rats also augmented the tyrosine transaminase and abolished a natural daily rhythm in its activity. Noradrenaline appeared to have its effect on the transaminase through combination with its pyridoxal coenzyme (q.v.); in addition, the transaminase could be increased in activity by stimulation of the vagus and by cholinergic agents (Black & Reis, 1971). This increase was suppressed by cycloheximide, and proved to involve net increase in hepatic tyrosine transaminase, which is of rapid turnover (half-life approx. 1·5 hr.).

Dopa Decarboxylase

In the synthetic route of Fig. 14.5, the first catecholamine synthesized is 3-hydroxytyramine or dopamine, yielded by decarboxylation. This reaction occurs in the brain itself (Table 14.3) and has been measured by incubating 20–100 mg. cerebral samples anaerobically, dispersed in buffered dopa solutions containing added pyridoxal phosphate; the dopamine was then extracted and determined fluorometrically. The decarboxylase is a pyridoxal phosphate-requiring enzyme found in many organs of the body and depleted in pyridoxine deficiency. It is not uniformly distributed in the brain but has been found at markedly greater activity in the hypothalamus, caudate nucleus, and medulla than in the cerebral cortex. Examination of about forty areas led to the conclusion (Kuntzman et al., 1961) that the enzyme was localized in regions which coordinated behavioural and autonomic activities: in the reticular formation, hypothalamus, and certain parts of the thalamus and rhinencephalon. These were usually but not always regions highest also in noradrenaline. The decarboxylase is important again in relation to serotonin, as described below. An interesting account is given by Blaschko (*Symposium*, 1964a) of how the properties of L-dopa decarboxylase condition the choice of metabolic routes among the catecholamines. The non-natural amino acid, α-methyl-m-tyrosine, and also certain hydrazides are effective inhibitors of the decarboxylase, showing action *in vivo* and *in vitro*, including the depletion of cerebral dopamine and noradrenaline (Fig. 14.11; Jepson; Pletscher, *Symposium*, 1963a; Costa & Brodie, *Symposium*, 1964a; Sourkes et al., 1961; Efron, 1968).

β-Hydroxylation; Adrenaline

Continuing the synthetic route (Fig. 14.5), the formation of noradrenaline now requires a side-chain hydroxylation and again parts of the brain have been shown to possess the enzymes concerned. Using [1-^{14}C]dopamine in reaction mixtures with cerebral dispersions and a number of cofactors, aerobic incubation followed by chromatographic separation yielded ^{14}C-noradrenaline (Udenfriend & Creveling, 1959). Rat brain gave about 0·3 nmoles of noradrenaline/g. tissue/hr. but, examining parts of the brain of the ox or dog, much greater *dopamine-β-hydroxylase* activity was found in the caudate nucleus and hypothalamus: these yielded 2·5–3·5 nmoles/g. hr., with little or no activity in the cerebral cortex. The adrenal medulla also yielded about 3 nmoles/g. hr.; the purified enzyme from this source required ascorbic acid and oxygen, and could hydroxylate tyramine and certain cognate substances, so providing alternative routes to the catecholamines. The cerebral enzyme was inhibited by p-hydroxybenzyloxamine, which is isosteric with tyramine (Creveling et al., 1962; Costa & Brodie, *Symposium*, 1964a). It is copper-containing and inhibited by disulphiram (q.v.). Adrenal dopamine increased, and noradrenaline decreased, after administering disulphiram.

The final stage in the adrenaline synthesis of Fig. 14·5 is catalysed by a phenylethanolamine-N-methyltransferase. This catalyses reaction between S-adenosylmethionine and a number of phenylethanolamines and has been purified from the adrenal. In the rabbit, activity was detected in the midbrain, but was small (Axelrod, 1962), a result compatible with the small quantity of cerebral adrenaline.

Administration of Catecholamines and Dopa; Parkinsonism

Noradrenaline can, in limited fashion, arrive at the brain from the blood-stream as well as by synthesis. After administering minute quantities of ^{3}H-noradrenaline intravenously to cats, parts of the brain were extracted and the bases separated and purified by chromatography on alumina (Weil-Malherbe et al., 1961). Entry was slow and sparse; only in a few areas was the noradrenaline appreciably assimilated, and in these uptake was still increasing 2 hr. after the injection: in the pituitary, which reached a level fifteen times that of blood plasma and in the hypothalamus, which approached blood level. Little or no ^{3}H was found in the cortex; these experiments did not involve appreciable net uptake of noradrenaline, for the maximum quantity measured in the hypothalamus was only 0·2% of its normal noradrenaline content. The limitation to uptake of noradrenaline by the cerebral cortex appears to be largely at the blood-brain barrier, for, as noted above, the compound is assimilated after intraventricular administration, or by cerebral tissues in vitro. This ability, indeed, appears to come into operation in vivo in reassimilating a significant amount of noradrenaline after its release on stimulation. It is not however, entirely specific to noradrenaline and analogues can become assimilated as "false adrenergic transmitters".

Adrenaline, also, is found by similar techniques to have only limited access to the brain (Axelrod et al., 1959), and it is thus to be concluded that the cerebral catecholamines generally originate endogenously from amino acids and not by uptake as amines produced elsewhere in the body. Dopa itself, however, penetrates to the brain much more readily than do the amines and after injecting [2-^{14}C]dopa to rats, part of the ^{14}C was found as amines: half of this portion being dopamine and the remainder, noradrenaline and 3-methoxytyramine (B, Fig. 14.6; Gey & Pletscher, 1964; Symposium, 1964a). Although the amino acid reached most parts of the brain which were examined, the amines were found at higher levels in the caudate nucleus, mesencephalon, diencephalon and medulla oblongata, than in the cerebral hemispheres or cerebellum: thus reflecting the distribution of the decarboxylase recorded in Table 14.3.

In the brain of sufferers from Parkinsonism, those parts normally rich in catecholamines were found to be of unusually low dopamine content, and administration of L-dopa ameliorated the condition, as also did inhibitors of amine oxidase (q.v.; Hornykiewicz, 1964; Sourkes, Symposium, 1964a). The central effects of administering dopa to normal animals include increased spontaneous movements. Also, animals sedated with reserpine (q.v.) can be restored to almost normal behaviour by dopa. Parkinsonism, a disorder with disabling tremor and rigidity of the limbs developing slowly in old age, is associated with visible lesions in the basal ganglia. The lesions are especially in the substantia nigra and corpus striatum and may have a variety of origins, including virus infections and chemical intoxications. Experimental lesions in the brain stem also cause depletion of noradrenaline in the striatum, presumably by interrupting axonal flow. L-Dopa can be judged by data appraised above to be a feasible manner of increasing cerebral catecholamines. It is however degraded on administration, and the relatively large doses involved in treatment (some 8 g./day) frequently produced nausea; thus their use was necessarily approached with caution, but is now realized as likely to be successful in ameliorating the disease in about half the instances treated (see Calne & Sandler, 1970; Goldstein et al., 1969). The large doses of L-dopa have several cerebral effects apart from increase in dopamine content; serotonin was decreased and 5-hydroxyindole acetic acid increased. Using isolated synaptosomal preparations treated with suitable precursors in vitro 10 μM-dopa caused partial release of labelled noradrenaline, dopamine and serotonin; these actions were prevented by an inhibitor of dopamine decarboxylase and were attributed to displacement by newly-formed dopamine (Ng et al., 1971).

Catecholamine Actions and Further Metabolism

The parts played by noradrenaline and by other catecholamines in the central nervous system constitute major physiological and pharmacological subjects which can only be adumbrated here. Catecholamines come under consideration in investigating mechanisms of attention, sleep, learning, of cognitive tests and of elevation and depression of mood (Carlsson, and Costa & Brodie, Symposium, 1964a; De Robertis, 1964; Iverson, 1967; Efron, 1968).

Noradrenaline or adrenaline applied close to the brain itself, intraventricularly or intracisternally, has effects similar in some respects only to those of its general administration; the route necessarily selects the systems which can be affected. Blood glucose rises, but anaesthesia or analgesia and sleep may result, and blood pressure and heart rate do not increase; the electroencephalogram is affected. The anaesthesia and sleep were induced in the cat by 0·1–0·5 μmole of either substance, intracisternally; and in man by 11 μmoles of adrenaline (Leimdorfer, 1950; Feldberg, 1963). Changes produced in body temperature (Fig. 14.10) are described below and other actions in Chapter 15. That major effects are produced on intraventricular administration emphasizes the localization of several of the cerebral systems concerned with the catecholamines; administration by this route has proved valuable also in metabolic studies described elsewhere in this chapter. Noradrenaline sensitivity has also been shown in individual cerebral neurons by micropipette techniques. Some 20 examples are quoted by Bloom (1968). Of subsequent instances: applied electrophoretically in the region of spontaneously firing cells of the cat neocortex, firing rate was frequently increased by noradrenaline and the increase found susceptible to adrenergic antagonists; neurons of the brain stem were increased or decreased in firing rate by noradrenaline (Johnson et al., 1969; Bradley, 1968).

Actions of catecholamines in certain other systems are mediated by the cyclic adenosine-3′,5′-phosphoric acid (cyclic AMP) described in Chapter 9. This compound exists in the brain and was shown to be formed by cerebral extracts, but at a rate independent of catecholamines; in parallel experiments, a catecholamine was required for its formation by preparations from mammalian muscles (Rall & Sutherland, 1958; see Robson & Stacey, 1962). The glycogen level of the brain of the rabbit is unaffected by adrenaline in a variety of dosage levels and by different routes (Kerr et al., 1937). This is in contrast to liver and muscle glycogen of the same animals which was lost with the typical increase in blood glucose and lactate. Examination of cell-containing systems has however shown major influence of neurotransmitters on cerebral cyclic AMP (Kakiuchi & Rall, 1968; Kakiuchi, Rall & McIlwain, 1969). These include increase up to eight-fold in the cyclic AMP of rabbit cerebellar preparations following the addition of 4–100 μM noradrenaline, and about a two-fold increase in the cerebral cortex. Neocortical tissues however increased greatly in cyclic AMP following electrical stimulation, as described in Chapter 9. General discussion on systems concerned with cyclic AMP as representing catecholamine receptors is given by Costa & Weiss (1968) and Greengard & Costa (1970).

Catechol-O-methyl Transferase

^{14}C-Noradrenaline injected to the lateral ventricle of cats gave as the main ^{14}C-products in the brain 3 hr. later, 3-O-methyl noradrenaline, 4-hydroxy-3-methoxymandelic acid and 4-hydroxy-3-methoxyphenyl glycol (Mannarino et al., 1962); the latter two compounds are no longer catecholamines and do not have the pharmacological properties of the noradrenaline. This and other evidence (see below) suggested for the inactivation of the cerebral catecholamines a route already established in other organs, namely: noradrenaline → the 3-O-methyl derivative → 4-hydroxy-3-methoxymandelic aldehyde (see Fig. 14.5) → the mandelic acid and the glycol. Similar results have been obtained with rats (Glowinski et al., 1965) and the noradrenaline initially taken up, found in nerve terminal fractions. For consideration of different metabolites from dopamine and noradrenaline, administered intraventricularly and intravenously to dogs and other species, see Chase et al. (1971).

The first two reactions are catalysed respectively by catechol-O-methyl transferase and by monoamine oxidase. These enzymes have moderately wide specificity and can act also on adrenaline and dopamine; in particular species and situations, they may not always act in the sequence quoted. The catechol-O-methyltransferase operates at moderate speed in most parts of the brain (Table 14.3: Axelrod et al., 1960; McCaman, 1965). It has been measured by incubating KCl-extracts from the different tissues with β-^{3}H-adrenaline and S-adenosylmethionine in buffered Mg^{2+} solutions, mixtures then being extracted at pH 10 to determine the methylated products. The liver and a few other organs displayed activities two to ten times those of the brain; the highest cerebral activity was in the neurohypophysis which formed 1 μmole 3-O-methyladrenaline/g. tissue/hr. It has also been demonstrated that cerebral tissues can produce the S-adenosylmethionine from methionine and adenosine triphosphate.

Cerebral noradrenaline can be increased three-fold by administration of pyrogallol to the lateral ventricles of cats (Masami *et al.*, 1962). This action was concluded to be due to inhibition of the transferase, and to show the role of the enzyme in inactivation of noradrenaline; for behavioural and other effects of related inhibitors, see White & Nash (1963), the *Symposium* (1964*a*) and Iversen (1967). 4-Tropolone acetamide was employed as an inhibitor of catechol-O-methyltransferase in experiments with rabbit cerebral tissues *in vitro*, and found to lead to increase in 3:4-dihydroxyphenylacetic acid as terminal product rather than homovanillic acid (Rutledge & Jonason, 1968). The acidic metabolites collectively have been regarded as characteristic products from the cerebral removal of exogenous catecholamines, rather than from the smaller amounts of endogenous catecholamines released locally in normal functioning: these latter circumstances yielding, rather, 3-hydroxy-4-methoxyphenylethylene glycol and other neutral derivatives (Taylor & Laverty, 1969).

Monoamine Oxidase; Speed of Metabolism

Removal of the amino group from the various catecholamines is catalysed in cerebral and in many other tissues by monoamine oxidases (EC1.4.3.4.). As examined in cerebral dispersions the enzymes react with many substrates, but are distinct from diamine oxidase and amino-acid oxidases; they will oxidise a number of primary amines, and also secondary amines provided the substituent R' is a methyl group:

$$R.CH_2.N^+H_2R' + O_2 \rightarrow R.CHO + {}^+NH_3R' + H_2O_2$$

the aldehydes produced can be substrates of a distinct *aldehyde oxidase* (q.v.). The monoamine oxidase reaction was initially measured by O_2 uptake and showed, e.g., with mixed cerebral tissues from the mouse acting on tyramine, 32; serotonin, 21; tryptamine, 10 and *iso*amylamine, 8 μmoles O_2/g./hr. (Table 14.3; Blaschko, 1963; Hope & Smith, 1960). That the enzyme acts on tryptamine as well as on tyramine derivatives is noteworthy, and led to some confusion in interpreting actions of inhibitors. Subsequent methods have depended on spectrophotometric measurement of the aldehydes produced. By such means, monoamine oxidase activity has been extensively investigated in relation to cerebral development, localization, the action of drugs and behavioural characteristics (Hoijer, 1969).

The cerebral amine oxidase activity has been shown by several criteria to be largely mitochondrial. Moreover, it is complex: at least four forms exist in the brain of the rat and of man (Youdim *et al.*, 1969; Collins *et al.*, 1970). These have been separated after treating mitochondria with detergent in the presence of benzylamine as protective substrate, by ammonium sulphate fractionation, column chromatography and gel electrophoresis. Fractions so obtained differed markedly in substrate velocity and affinity, and in susceptibility to inhibitors (Table 14.4). Thus from rat, reaction rates/mg. protein decreased in the order *1–4* with tyramine as substrate, whereas fraction *4* was the most rapidly reacting with tryptamine. The two inhibitors quoted acted on the four fractions differently: pargyline most depressed *1* and *3*; *2* was inhibited most by · harmaline.

Prior to separation of mitochondrial amine oxidases from human brain, measurement of activity in the presence of increasing concentrations of inhibitor gave a triphasic concentration/inhibition curve, suggesting three components differing in K_i. Thus the fractions obtained by separation were not engendered by the fractionation procedures, but pre-existed. The occurrence of the four amine oxidases in different regions of the human brain was not uniform; the brain stem gave greatest specific activity, with fraction *4* and dopamine as substrate, but in the cerebral cortex greatest activities were with

Table 14.4

Properties of monoamine oxidases from rat brain

Characteristic measured	Monoamine oxidase fraction			
	1	2	3	4
Electrophoretic migration, to:	cathode	cathode	cathode	anode
	nmoles deamination/hr. mg. protein			
Velocity with substrate:				
Tyramine	360	185	111	0·6
Tryptamine	46	29	7	47
Benzylamine	20	10	1·2	0
Kynuramine	19	40	24	25
Michaelis constant* $M \times 10^5$	2·4	3·8	8·3	4·5
Inhibitory constants* K_i:				
Pargyline, $M \times 10^8$	1·4	5·9	2·6	5·8
Harmaline, $M \times 10^5$	12	1·5	17	14

The fractions separated as bands on polyacrylamide gel at pH 9·1 in 1–2 hr.
* Measured with kynuramine as substrate. Youdim *et al.*, 1969.

fraction *1* and tyramine as substrate. Thus the suggestion that the same enzyme oxidizes catecholamines and indolealkylamines does not appear to be true when examined in specific regions and at isoenzyme level.

Aldehyde Dehydrogenase: Speed of Catecholamine Oxidation

The aldehydes formed by amine oxidases are substrates for *aldehyde dehydrogenase* (EC 1.2.1.3; Erwin & Deitrich, 1966) which yields the corresponding acids and is also in the brain a mitochondrial enzyme, with small activity remaining in a supernatant fraction. From mitochondria of bovine brain, material carrying the dehydrogenase was extracted by sonication and purified by ammonium sulphate fractionation. It required NAD^+ and assays measured the NADH formed. Column chromatography separated the dehydrogenase from succinic aldehyde dehydrogenase. A less pure preparation oxidized a wide variety of aldehydes, including 3,4-dihydroxyphenylacetaldehyde at about 1 μmole/g. brain/hr. and 5-hydroxyindoleacetaldehyde at 0·5

16

μmoles/g. hr.; K_m values for these substrates were 10 and 2 μM. The products, phenylacetic acids and indoleacetic acids, are inactive pharmacologically.

Calculating values for aldehyde dehydrogenation on a whole-brain basis, they are thus ample in rate for participation in oxidation of the cerebral catecholamines and indolamines, which occur in quantities of nmoles/g. and have half-lives of 0·5 to a few hr. Also, as the monoamine oxidases which form the aldehydes are also mitochondrial enzymes, accessibility to and concentration of substrate would not be expected to limit dehydrogenase action. The *in situ* functioning of this inactivation system may therefore be appraised in terms of the monoamine oxidases. These are relatively rapid (Table 14.3: 2–10 μmoles/g. hr.) when acting on substrates at a few mM; for these rates, action must be supposed to be in volumes about 1/1,000 of the tissue, and rates would then be such as to cause inactivation of the cerebral amine content in 0·5–20 sec. The values in relation to catecholamine-O-methyltransferase do not require as high a degree of localization, but reaction would need some 5–200 sec. These are markedly slower rates than were computed in relation to acetyl-choline (q.v.). It is noteworthy that catecholamine action can be terminated not only by metabolic change but also by reassimilation (see above).

Inhibitors of amine oxidases, some of which are useful drugs (see Fig. 14.11), have proved valuable in indicating the role of the enzyme and its substrates in the brain. After systemic administration of iproniazid to rabbits or mice, it rapidly reached the brain and inhibited the monoamine oxidase. Cerebral noradrenaline increased, as also did dopamine and serotonin; similar results followed nialamide, pheniprazine or harmine (Spector *et al.*, 1960; Carlsson *et al.*, *Symposium*, 1960; Brill, 1967; Efron, 1968). The increase was in several instances accompanied by excitement of the animals. The rate of increase of the catecholamines approximated to 1 nmole/g. tissue/hr., which is compatible with properties noted above in the synthesizing enzymes; serotonin increased at about 3 nmoles/g. hr.

Serotonin

Serotonin or 5-hydroxytryptamine (Fig. 14.7; Page, 1954, 1969; *Symposia*, 1957, 1958, 1964*a*) was first characterized and isolated from animal tissues as a vasoconstrictor: to the resultant increase in blood pressure it owes its name. It acts as vasoconstrictor in concentrations of 0·5 μM, and acts at some sensory nerve endings at a tenth of this level. In the brain, pharmacological and fluoro-metric methods applied to tissue removed without the rapid freezing methods found necessary in determining acetylcholine, have shown an average level of about 3 nmoles/g. It is, however, highly localized, the cerebral cortex containing about 1 and the amygdala and hypothalamus, about 10 nmoles/g.; the limbic cortex contained much more than the neocortex (Table 14.3; Paasonen *et al.*, 1957; Bogdanski *et al.*, 1957). The pineal gland is particularly rich in serotonin and related systems, as is described more fully below. Other investigations have connected cerebral serotonin with temperature-regulation, reactions to light and to pain and the control of sleep (see Bloom, 1969).

Aspects of the comparative biology of serotonin are described by Welsh (1968); for pharmacological, behavioural and clinical studies see Garattini & Shore (1968).

Manner of Occurrence and Formation in the Brain

Serotonin in freeze-dried cerebral sections can be visualized admirably by treating them with formaldehyde vapour and examining by fluorescence-microscopy; serotonin yields a 6-hydroxy-3,4-dihydrocarboline of strong yellow fluorescence (Fuxe *et al.*, 1968). The cell bodies so characterized are mainly in the raphe nuclei of the lower brain stem. The fluorescence is accentuated when tissues are taken from animals which have been treated with inhibitors of monoamine oxidase (q.v.), as nialamide, some hours previously. Fluorescence then extends to processes from these cells which are unmyelinated and analogous to C fibres and is seen in varicosities at their terminal ramifications, e.g. in certain nuclei of the pons and medulla. Techniques of subcellular fractionation have shown the serotonin in the brain of guinea pig and rat to occur in particulate fractions distinct from those which carry acetylcholine (Michaelson & Whittaker, 1962, 1963; Pellegrino de Iraldi *et al.*, 1968). These serotonin-enriched particles presumably correspond to the varicosities seen microscopically; by hypotonic and ultrasonic disruption, serotonin-containing vesicles have been obtained from them.

The localization and course and also some indication of a function of the nerve fibres concerned with serotonin has been given by nerve section. The serotonin content of rat brain fell after certain lesions, especially after section of the medial forebrain bundle (Heller & Moore, 1968; Lints & Harvey, 1969). This lesion increased the sensitivity of the animals to painful stimuli, but normal sensitivity was restored by administration of 5-hydroxytryptophan.

The route of formation of serotonin in the brain commences with the dietarily essential amino acid, tryptophan (Fig. 14.7). Formation of serotonin from [2-^{14}C]tryptophan was demonstrated by injecting the compound intracerebrally to pigeons (Gal & Marshall, *Symposium*, 1964a); acid extracts of the brain were chromatographed and ^{14}C-serotonin identified and measured. That the synthesis occurred in the brain itself was shown by absence of ^{14}C-serotonin in the extracts when much larger quantities of ^{14}C-tryptophan were administered intraperitoneally. An inhibitor of amine oxidase (q.v.), β-phenyliso-propylhydrazine, administered systemically before the tryptophan was given intracerebrally, increased the yield of serotonin which could then rise within 10 min. to 1 % of the administered ^{14}C; see also Eccleston *et al.* (1965).

Accumulation of serotonin in the brain of rats commences within a few minutes of the administration of pargyline, a relatively irreversible inhibitor of monoamine oxidase. It proceeded almost linearly at 1·7–2·5 nmoles/g. hr. for about 2 hr., and comparable rates of metabolism have been obtained by independent methods applied to unanaesthetized rats (Neff *et al.*, 1969). After inhibition of monoamine oxidase with pargyline, the formation of hydroxyindole acetic acid from serotonin declined at 2·1–4·3 nmoles/g. hr. in different cerebral areas, in each of which a half-life of 1·2 hr. was implied. Turnover at similar rates was found by measuring the incorporation to cerebral serotonin of ^{14}C from ^{14}C-tryptophan given intravenously at a small, steady rate of about 250 nmoles/hr. The data so obtained suggested also that the tryptophan of the cells concerned, equilibrated within about 30 min. with that administered; and that the neuronal store of 5-hydroxytryptophan, inter-

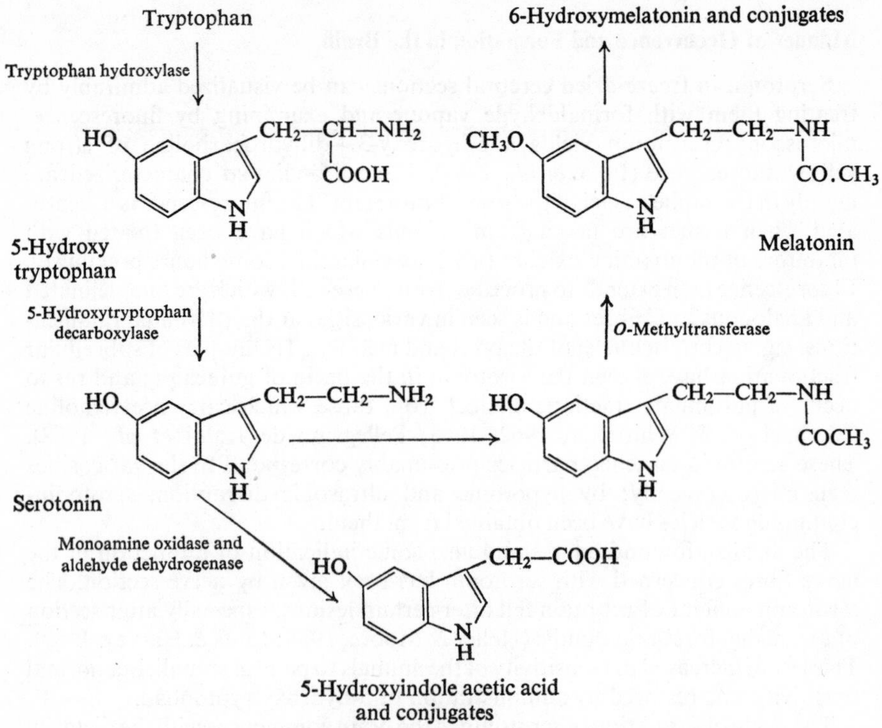

Tryptophan   6-Hydroxymelatonin and conjugates

Tryptophan hydroxylase

$CH_2—CH—NH_2$
$COOH$

$CH_2—CH_2—NH$
$CO.CH_3$

5-Hydroxy
tryptophan

Melatonin

5-Hydroxytryptophan
decarboxylase

O-Methyltransferase

$CH_2—CH_2—NH_2$

$CH_2—CH_2—NH$
$COCH_3$

Serotonin

Monoamine oxidase and
aldehyde dehydrogenase

$CH_2—COOH$

5-Hydroxyindole acetic acid
and conjugates

FIG. 14.7. Indolealkylamine metabolism in the brain. Formation of
serotonin from tryptophan, and its subsequent inactivation and
excretion. Formation of melatonin, as it takes place in the pineal,
and its subsequent inactivation.

mediary in serotonin formation (Fig. 14.7) was relatively small. Accumulation
of serotonin under these conditions can be largely prevented by p-chlorophenyl-
alanine, an inhibitor of the hydroxylase now to be described (Diaz *et al.*, 1968).

Tryptophan 5-Hydroxylase

Of the enzymes involved in the synthesis of serotonin (Fig. 14.7) the first,
tryptophan hydroxylase, yields 5-hydroxytryptophan which readily gives
serotonin in the brain itself and in cerebral preparations. Administration of 5-
hydroxytryptophan to animals is followed by marked central actions, including
catatonia and apparent fear or rage, which are accompanied by an increase in
the serotonin of the brain. To produce central effects by serotonin itself, it
must be given by intraventricular or comparable routes, or intravenously at high
dosage, for it passes with difficulty from the blood to the brain. Giving
5-hydroxytryptophan intramuscularly to pigeons, followed by removal of the
brain and its dissection and extraction, showed a net increase to be caused in
the cerebral serotonin. The increase was small in the cerebellum but in the
pons, medulla and telencephalon values increased from about 5 to 20 nmoles/g.,
returning to normal about 2 hr. later. During this period the animals were

abnormal in behaviour, being depressed in a specific fashion (Aprison et al., 1962).

Tryptophan hydroxylase has been purified from the brain stem of the rabbit, and also demonstrated to be present in a number of tissues and animal species (Grahame-Smith, 1967; Ichiyama et al., 1968; Lovenberg et al., 1968). The cerebral enzyme was of monooxygenase type, atmospheric O_2 yielding $1H_2O$ and $1[O]$ to L-tryptophan. It required a reduced pteridine coenzyme, but not NADPH or ascorbic acid. Half-maximal velocity was given with tryptophan at 20 μM. On dispersing brainstem in isotonic sucrose, little of the hydroxylase was found in the soluble, the nuclear, or the microsomal fractions but almost all in the crude mitochondrial fraction, and this on further separation showed the hydroxylase to be associated with nerve teminals. From lyophilized preparations, activity could be extracted with phosphate buffer, stabilized by mercaptoethanol, and purified by ammonium sulphate fractionation.

Tryptophan hydroxylase under optimal assay conditions, yielded some 6 nmoles product/g. hr. from the rat or rabbit brain stem. The cerebral cortex showed about 2% of this activity, while the pineal (q.v.) was much more active. In several cerebral regions the subsequent step needed for serotonin synthesis, namely 5-hydroxytryptophan decarboxylase, proceeded at 30–300 times the rate of the hydroxylase: thus the hydroxylase is clearly the rate-limiting step in serotonin synthesis, as is shown also by effects of inhibitors of the two reactions. Tryptophan-5-hydroxylase was inhibited by phenylalanine (K_i, 0·1–1 mM) and also by several related compounds, of which p-chlorophenylalanine has received extensive pharmacological study (see Garattini & Shore, 1968). With tryptophan hydroxylase in vitro, 0·5 mM p-chlorophenylalanine gave about 60% inhibition and this was reversible by dialysis; in vivo interactions were more complex. Appraisal has been given of tryptophan assimilation and hydroxylation as processes controlling the cerebral synthesis of serotonin (Grahame-Smith & Parfitt, 1970; Macon et al., 1971).

5-Hydroxytryptophan Decarboxylation; Tissue Serotonin

Decarboxylation of 5-hydroxytryptophan to serotonin, the second stage in its synthesis, is catalysed by an enzyme which is probably identical with the decarboxylase which forms noradrenaline and which is termed aromatic L-amino acid decarboxylase. Cerebral dispersions incubated anaerobically with added pyridoxal phosphate, were noted above to catalyse the liberation of CO_2 from dopa and from 5-hydroxytryptophan at similar rates, and an almost constant ratio between the two activities persisted in some twenty parts of the brain (Kuntzman et al., 1961). The decarboxylation of 5-hydroxytryptophan was depressed in pyridoxine-deficient rats (Eberle & Eiduson, 1968); production of apoenzyme was little affected during the first two weeks of life, but was found to be only 12% saturated with coenzyme in the cerebral cortex of animals raised on a B_6-deficient diet in contrast to 63% saturation in normal animals.

It is important to the synthetic route for serotonin that the cerebral decarboxylase has much greater affinity for 5-hydroxytryptophan than for tryptophan, the K_m values being respectively 50 μM and 3 mM (Ichiyama et al., 1968).

Thus with substrates at 40 μM, 5-hydroxytryptophan was decarboxylated at 700 times the rate of tryptophan.

Both the decarboxylase and serotonin are in part localized in a particular subcellular fraction, as shown by dispersing rat brain in isotonic sucrose and centrifuging (De Robertis; Whittaker, *Symposium*, 1964*a* and Chapter 12). The fraction contained nerve terminals; on treatment with hypotonic solutions the enzyme became soluble and was concluded to occur normally in the cytoplasm within the terminals, but not otherwise bound. Serotonin presented as such to cerebral tissues can be assimilated, and exogenous ^{3}H serotonin administered intraventricularly in small amounts appears to localize preferentially in serotonergic neurons (Synder *et al.* 1970; McIlwain & Synder, 1970; Kuhar *et al.*, 1971). At higher concentrations of serotonin, accumulation has been found to take place also in neurons which normally carried catecholamines. Uptake of 50 nM ^{3}H-serotonin to sections from the hypothalamus and midbrain of several species gave preparations from which synaptosomes could be derived; on gradient centrifugation, ^{3}H and endogenous serotonin were found in the same subfractions. This gives valuable control data for some of the experiments of subsequent sections. Among other tissues in which serotonin is enriched, blood platelets are of interest through their accessibility for diagnosis and research; in platelets, serotonin is associated with adenosine triphosphate and both components were found to be lowered in specimens from children suffering a form of Down's syndrome (mongolism; q.v.) (Boullin & O'Brien, 1971).

Serotonin and Cell-Firing

Much evidence for judging the status of serotonin as a neurotransmitter came first with invertebrate systems (Gerschenfeld & Stefani, 1968). Mammalian preparations also have now been shown electrophysiologically to respond to serotonin, *in vivo* and *in vitro*; and, moreover, these preparations release serotonin on excitation.

In lightly anaesthetized rats, electrical stimulation of different regions of the mesencephalon showed that excitation of the mid-brain raphe diminished the serotonin of the animal's forebrain (Sheard & Aghajanian, 1968; Aghajanian *et al.*, 1969). The raphe was noted above to contain the cell bodies of serotonin-rich neurons; stimulation at an optimal frequency of 10/sec. caused a small decrease in the forebrain serotonin, and an 80% increase in 5-hydroxyindole acetic acid, its major metabolite (Fig. 14.7).

Micropipette application of serotonin has been made to many parts of the mammalian central nervous system (Weight & Salmoiraghi, 1968; Bloom, 1968). A proportion of cells sensitive to serotonin was found in the spinal cord and in various parts of the brain stem, diencephalon and telencephalon. Depression of firing rate was more often found than acceleration, though the two were about equally frequent in the medulla and pons. The onset of responses to serotonin was relatively slow, as is consistent with unmyelinated fibres with dispersed terminals. In exploring the brain stem of rats with microelectrodes (Aghajanian *et al.*, 1969) about 60% of the neurons whose firing was observed, stopped firing after the animals had received 25–50 μg./kg lysergic acid diethylamide, a dose at which behavioural effects of the drug were becoming evident. These susceptible neurons were all situated in the midbrain raphe.

Serotonin and Excitation in Isolated Tissues

Tissues from the mammalian brain display a number of metabolic and electrophysiological aspects of indolealkylamine functioning. This is the case with sections of the brain stem and also with piriform cortex and neocortex

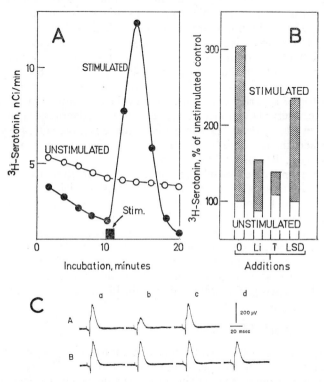

FIG. 14.8. Serotonin and the excitation of isolated tissues from the brain.

A. Time-course of serotonin release from guinea pig piriform cortex, with and without electrical stimulation. Tissues were preincubated with ^{3}H-serotonin and nialamide, superfused to remove excess reagents and the outflow collected at the times indicated, during 1 min. of which some tissues were stimulated at 100 pulses/sec.

B. Inhibition of serotonin output in experiments similar to those of A, but with striatal tissues from coronal sections of rat brain. Reagents present during incubation: LiCl, 2–4 mM; T, tetrodotoxin, 1 μM; LSD, lysergic acid diethylamide, 2 μM.

C. Potentials evoked in the superior colliculus in bicarbonate salines with additions: A.a, none; A.b, 2 μM serotonin; A.c, washed free; B.a, 1 μM lysergic acid diethylamide; B.b, 2 μM serotonin; B.c, washed free; B.d, 2 μM serotonin.

Data from Katz & Kopin (1969); Kawai & Yamamoto (1968) and McIlwain & Snyder (1970).

despite their much smaller content of these compounds. The tissues' native serotonin is largely maintained on incubation in oxygenated glucose-salines, and isotopically-labelled serotonin added with an inhibitor of amine oxidase reaches with cortical sections an intracellular/extracellular ratio of about 10/1. This ratio, based on total cell volume, implies a much higher ratio in the sparsely-distributed regions which are specifically concerned with the compounds. Electrical stimulation of cortical or striatal tissues now caused the release of serotonin, characterized chromatographically, to superfusing salines (Katz & Kopin, 1969; McIlwain & Snyder, 1970). The release was subject to modification by the agents indicated in Fig. 14.8, being diminished by lithium salts and by lysergic acid diethylamide, but not by certain LSD analogues which did not share its pharmacological actions. Inhibition of release by tetrodotoxin indicates an association with neural excitation.

The ability of serotonin to depress neuronal response has been reproduced in portions taken from the brain of the guinea pig (Fig. 14.8), maintained in glucose salines as described in Chapter 4. Stimulation of an optic nerve, still attached to the superior colliculus, gave evoked potentials in the colliculus which were observed by surface electrodes. Serotonin depressed such responses, in a fashion readily reversible by washing with saline. On adding lysergic acid diethylamide, the response to excitation was unaffected but serotonin was no longer active in depressing the response.

Serotonin undergoes metabolic conversion in cerebral tissues during *in vitro* incubation; striatal and cerebellar preparations yielded [^{3}H]-5-hydroxy-indoleacetic acid from [^{3}H]-5-hydroxytryptophan (Chase *et al.*, 1969). Addition of serotonin to incubating tissue has further metabolic consequences: the cyclic 3′.5′-adenosine monophosphate content of rabbit cerebellar preparations could be increased three-fold in 6 min. by 0·1 mM serotonin—though this increase is much less than that which can be caused by electrical stimulation, it may nevertheless be correspondingly large in the cell-elements which are concerned with serotonin (Kakiuchi & Rall, 1968; Kakiuchi *et al.*, 1969).

Metabolic Disposal of Serotonin

The several references already made to monoamine oxidase give ample evidence for a role of the oxidase in degrading serotonin. The reaction presumably proceeds through the relatively unstable aldehyde which may be trapped as a hydrazide but normally yields mainly 5-hydroxyindole acetic acid. Under some conditions the alcohol, 5-hydroxytryptophol, may be given; these two compounds are without the pharmacological actions of serotonin (Keglevic *et al.*, 1968).

The brain carries also an enzyme catalysing the transfer of sulphate from 3′-phosphoadenosine 5′-phosphosulphate to serotonin (Hidaka *et al.*, 1969). This *PAPS:serotonin sulphotransferase* was found mainly in the soluble fraction of cerebral dispersions and acted at rates of 0·1–1 μmoles/g. hr. in four mammalian species. The enzyme was partly purified from rabbit brain and was not inhibited by amine oxidase inhibitors including isonicotinic acid 2-isopropylhydrazine.

The brain stem of the rabbit showed two to three times more activity than the cerebral cortex. Again, the product, serotonin-*O*-sulphate, was without physiological activity.

Pineal Indolealkylamines

In Gladstone & Wakeley's (1940) monograph on the pineal is quoted one of the opinions of Tristram Shandy, that the soul could not be where DesCartes had fixed it upon the pineal gland, which formed a cushion no larger than a pea.

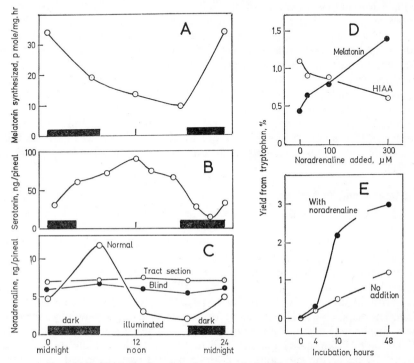

FIG. 14.9. Control of melatonin synthesis by illumination and by noradrenaline. (Wurtman *et al.*, 1968; Axelrod *et al.*, 1969).

A–C. Diurnal variation in pineal melatonin, serotonin and noradrenaline.

D, E. Pineals from adult rats were examined under tissue-culture conditions in media containing 0·1 mM-^{14}C-tryptophan and the noradrenaline additions stated.

Metabolically, the pineal is distinguished by a metabolic route proceeding through serotonin to melatonin, and by knowledge of how this route is controlled by sensory perception and enzyme induction.

The serotonin content of the brain in several lower vertebrates is markedly greater than in mammals, being for example 45 nmoles/g. in the toad, or twenty times that of the rat (Brodie *et al.*, 1964). Examination of several parts of the brain showed that a given part from different species was fairly constant in serotonin content per unit weight, and that the species variation depended on the proportional contribution by different parts. In particular, in species which included many reptiles, the olfactory bulb and cerebellum were lowest in serotonin and the pineal was unusually high (Quay & Wilhoft, 1964; Quay, *Symposium*, 1964a).

In the pineal of animals including man and the rat, serotonin is the most plentiful of a group of indole compounds (Fig. 14.7), but its concentration is variable: it depended on the time of the day at which the pineal was sampled. With circadean alternation of light and darkness, a marked rhythmic change in serotonin was found and is shown in Fig. 14.9. This is reminiscent of the conclusion that the mammalian pineal is derived from a visual sense organ of more primitive animals (see Wurtman, Axelrod & Kelly, 1968), and that it may be a gland of internal secretion. Exposure of animals to prolonged illumination indeed modified the size, cytological structure, and other chemical and enzymic constituents of the pineal. The serotonin of the hypothalamus, sampled in the same investigation, did not show such changes. Altering the daily period of illumination altered the rise or fall in pineal serotonin. The pineal is rich also in catecholamines and histamine. It has characteristic pinealocytes as a major cellular component, a neural input, and nerve terminals containing vesicles. The nerve terminals are close to perivascular spaces and are thus concluded to represent the secreting unit (De Robertis, 1964; *Symposium*, 1971).

Melatonin and its Actions

The specialized relationships of the pineal to serotonin derivatives include its content of melatonin, N-acetyl-5-methoxytryptamine (Fig. 14.7). The substance was identified in investigating the means by which frogs, and other lower vertebrates, adapt to the light and colour of their environment. The adaptation is effected by aggregation or dispersion of black or coloured granules about the nucleus of specialized cells in the skin, and these processes are brought about by a combination of visual reflexes and a humoural mechanism. The dispersion has been known for some time to be promoted by a melanocyte-dispersing hormone of the pituitary (q.v.). The aggregation, and hence the lightening of skin-colour, was found to be caused by minute quantities of naturally occurring substances, of which neutral tissues formed an effective source. Of all materials examined, aqueous extracts of the pineal were the most potent and the agent responsible was termed melatonin. Countercurrent distribution of an extract from many kg. of ox pineal in ethylacetate–heptane–water, followed by silicic acid chromatography, concentrated the material to a stage when biological activity was recognized as associated with an indole derivative. Of the indoles from the gland, 5-hydroxyindole-3-acetic acid and its O-methylated derivative were first identified and occurred at about 2 μg./g. fresh pineal. The melanocyte aggregation was associated with an indole present in only about one-tenth of this concentration. It was characterized and identified by comparison with synthetic compounds and shown to be N-acetyl-5-methoxytryptamine (Fig. 14.7). This was done while the quantities available were only about 0·1 mg., by making much use of fluorescence and adsorption characteristics as well as biological activity (Lerner *et al.*, 1960).

The pineal in man is rich in melatonin activity, which is found also in urine. Melatonin is active at 4 pM in aggregating the melanocyte granules and in opposing the action of the pituitary melanocyte-dispersing hormone. This hormone also is present in the pituitary of mammals including man, and acts in concentrations as minute as does melatonin. Conceivably here as in the control of the circadean rhythm, the continued elaboration of the substances in higher vertebrates represents the persistence of some aspect of their previous function, in this case one of adaptation to environment. Such persistence or transfer of function is made more likely with melatonin and the melanocyte-dispersing agent as they constitute a pair of opposing hormones, each still elaborated at commensurate activity in a situation irrelevant to the actions by which they were first characterized.

Melatonin indeed functions in mammals, in several cases in mediating biological responses of a diurnal or seasonal character. Administered, it can produce sleep in cats, and delay the onset of sexual maturity in rats. This includes delaying and depressing the growth of the ovaries in the female and diminishing the weight of seminal vesicles in the male. It also depressed the contractility of certain smooth muscles, spontaneous or induced by serotonin, and diminished the wheel-running activity of rats (Wurtman & Axelrod, 1968; Wong & Whiteside, 1968; Reiter, 1967). To understand the control of these actions in a biological setting, details of the synthesis of melatonin are needed.

Synthetic Route to Melatonin

The pineal is active in tryptophan hydroxylase and in hydroxytryptophan decarboxylase, with the hydroxylase as rate limiting step: thus the production of serotonin is by the route already described. Acetylation of serotonin can occur in a number of tissues and in the pineal was demonstrated by incubating serotonin, an acetyl-CoA generating system (coenzyme A, acetylphosphate and the phosphotransferase) and a soluble pineal extract: this yielded N-acetyl-serotonin (Weissbach et al., 1960). The methylating system is much more specifically localized: examining a number of tissues of the monkey for the methylating system (Axelrod et al., Symposium, 1961), only the pineal of about thirty sites showed appreciable activity, with the habenula at much lower potency and others without detected action. A pineal extract formed melatonin at 6 μmoles/g. tissue/hr. from acetylserotonin and S-adenosylmethionine. A few related indoles were methylated also, but more slowly than acetylserotonin. Intravenously administered melatonin, ^{3}H-labelled in the acetyl group, was taken up by many organs including the brain and excreted after hydroxylation in the 6-position and conjugation with sulphate or glucuronate (Kopin et al., 1961; Wurtman et al., 1968).

Control of Melatonin Synthesis

Illumination controls a daily rhythm in the pineal content of melatonin as well as of serotonin (A, Fig. 14.9). Moreover, both actions appear due to the level of the rate-limiting enzyme of melatonin synthesis, hydroxyindole O-methyltransferase, which is most active when the animals are in darkness. Light affected the rat through its eyes: melatonin production no longer responded with the eyes obscured or the optic tract severed. Further nerve-section displayed an unusual route for the fibres concerned, for they proceeded by the accessory optic tract to the spinal cord, through a sympathetic ganglion and re-entered the skull to terminate in the pineal (Wurtman *et al.*, 1968).

The sympathetic neurotransmitter, noradrenaline, was accordingly examined in rat pineal and found also to display a light-dependent fluctuation which was eliminated when the animals were blind or when the optic tract was severed (C, Fig. 14.9). It would appear, therefore, that nerve impulses from the retina released noradrenaline at the pineal nerve terminals and so diminished the noradrenaline content of the pineal. Actions were therefore sought of noradrenaline on pineal metabolism, and found as indicated in D, E, Fig. 14.9. In pineal glands from adult rats incubated under tissue-culture conditions in fluids with ^{14}C-tryptophan, the production of melatonin proceeded steadily for 48 hr. Addition of 0·1–0·3 mM noradrenaline accelerated this synthesis, the effect becoming evident at 4 hr. and large at 10 hr. Concomitantly, the production of 5-hydroxyindole acetic acid, a metabolite of serotonin but not of melatonin, diminished.

The action of noradrenaline was by enzyme induction. Thus the acceleration by noradrenaline in E, Fig. 14.9 was blocked by cycloheximide. Moreover, the 5-hydroxyindole O-methyltransferase itself was assayed in the pineals of rats which had received different sequences in light and darkness. When animals which had been in the light were transferred to darkness, the pineal transferase increased up to three-fold. This increase could be stopped by administering puromycin at 10 mg./kg. body weight (Axelrod *et al.*, 1965). The mode of action of noradrenaline as an enzyme-inducing agent, and the examination of pineal metabolism in various biological settings, remain intriguing subjects (Wurtman *et al.*, 1968; Zweig & Axelrod, 1969; *Symposium*, 1971).

Actions Involving Both Tryptamines and the Catecholamines

Several metabolic similarities and interactions between the catecholamines and serotonin have already received comment. Their functional interconnection extends further, as will now be indicated.

Regulation of Body Temperature

Applied close to the hypothalamus, serotonin and the catecholamines have opposing actions on the body temperature of mammals (Feldberg & Myers, 1964; Feldberg *et al.*, 1967; Giarman *et al.*, 1968). Effects on intraventricular injection are shown in Fig. 14.10: the small quantities indicated of adrenaline or noradrenaline depressed the cat's temperature for 2–3 hr. Comparable additions of serotonin by the same route raised the temperature, which could then be depressed towards normal by either catecholamine. Observation of the animals showed that the changes in body temperature were brought about by a number of factors: vasodilatation or vasoconstriction, alteration in muscle tone, shivering, and possibly by other means: that is, the amines caused a coordinated adjustment of heat loss and heat production which altered temperature within appropriate limits. On microinjection in the hypothalamus, quantities of 5–10 nmoles of the amines acted: amounts commensurate with the hypothalamic content of the amines. It is thus pictured that body temperature is normally adjusted by processes which include the release of the native hypothalamic serotonin and noradrenaline, at centres which coordinate many bodily activities which can affect an animal's heat production or heat loss. Extremes of heat or cold lowered the serotonin content of the brain of rats; in other organs the serotonin was unaffected, and that of the brain also was unaffected by other stresses examined (Toh, 1960). Results of intraventricular administration of catecholamines and serotonin are species-specific: the dog and rhesus monkey responded similarly to the cat, while the rabbit showed altered relationships. Also, procedures which changed the cerebral content of the amines altered the response to them, to pyrogens and to other drugs (see Bligh *et al.*, 1971).

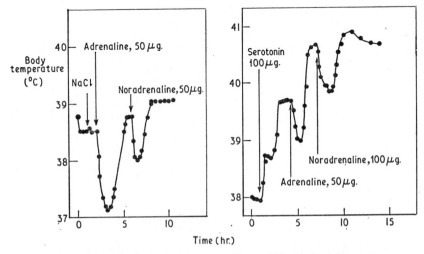

FIG. 14.10. The body temperature of cats which received catecholamines or serotonin intraventricularly (Feldberg & Myers, 1964). Implanted cannulae led to the lateral cerebral ventricles and the additions noted were made in 0·1 ml. of solution. Rectal temperatures were measured; room temperature was 20–30°.

Synthetic drugs and natural products which are pyretic or antipyretic on systemic administration have been studied since the 1880s and many concluded to act on two interconnected centres, in the hypothalamus, which control body temperature and which are of marked chemical specificity (see McIlwain, 1957). There is much in common between these and the systems responding to serotonin and catecholamines, for some of the agents examined earlier are β-phenylethylamines and others interact with the catecholamines and serotonin: bacterial pyrogens in minute quantities intraventricularly gave prolonged increase in body temperature, again lowered by adrenaline or noradrenaline as well as by acetylsalicyclic acid and by chlorpromazine (q.v.). Catecholamines can in specific situations share the analgesic properties of acetylsalicylic acid; antipyretic actions in chlorpromazine contributed to its selection as a centrally-acting drug. Intriguingly, it appears that capsaicin, a substance giving pungency to red pepper, is capable on intraperitoneal injection

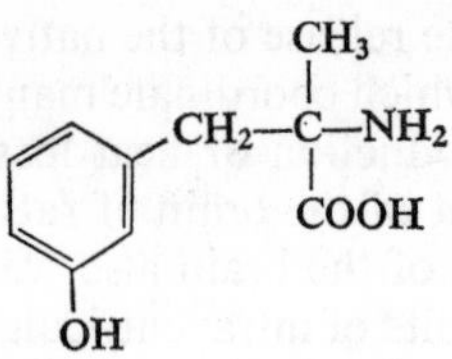

I

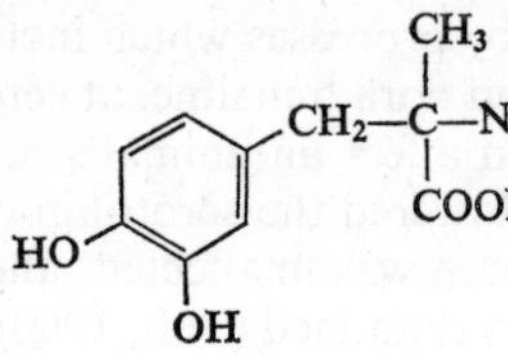

II

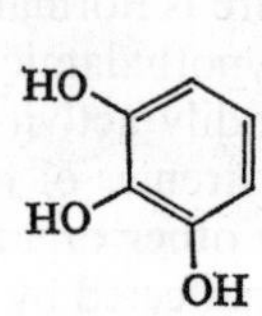

III

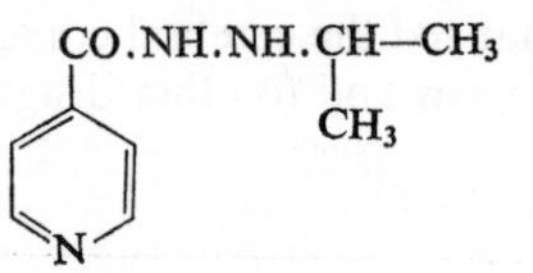

IV

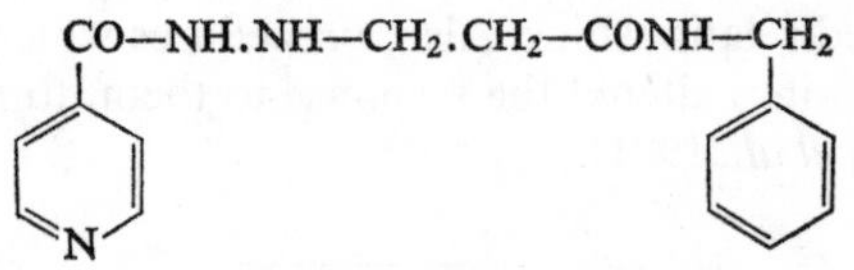

V

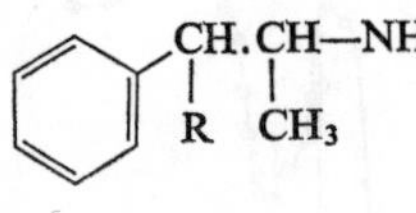

VI

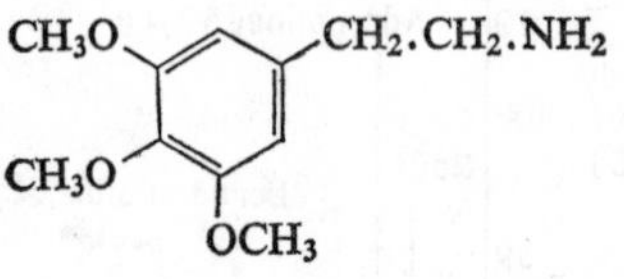

VII

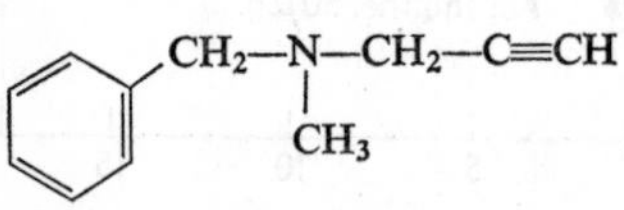

VIII

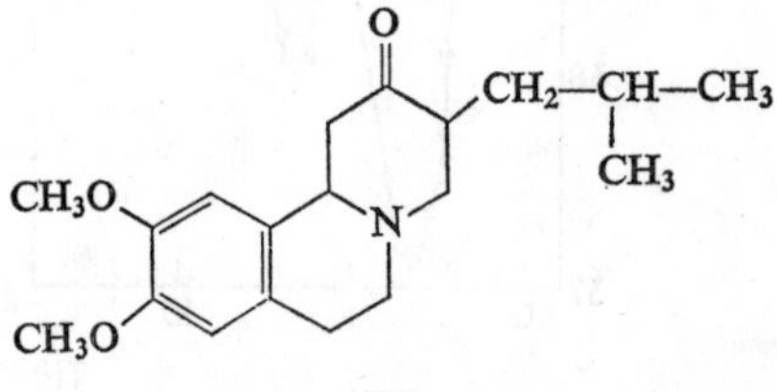

IX

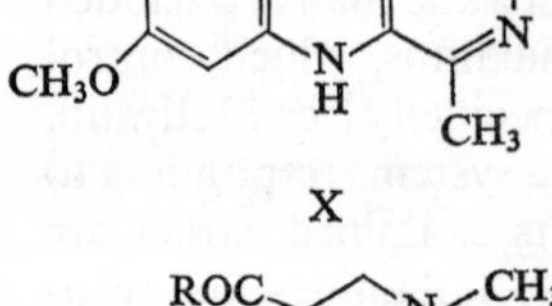

X

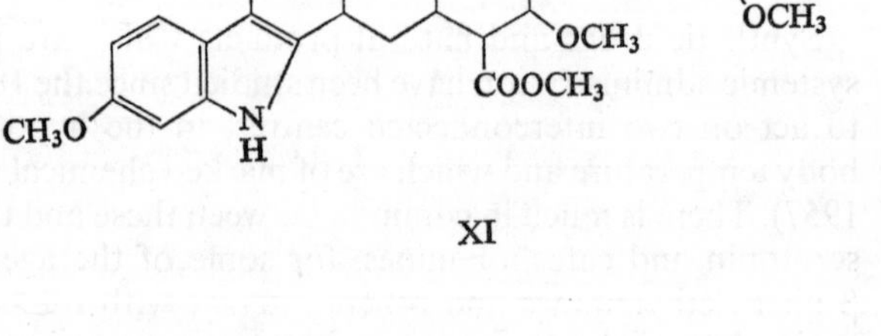

XI

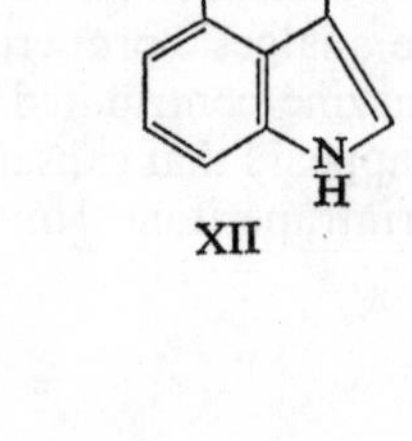

XII

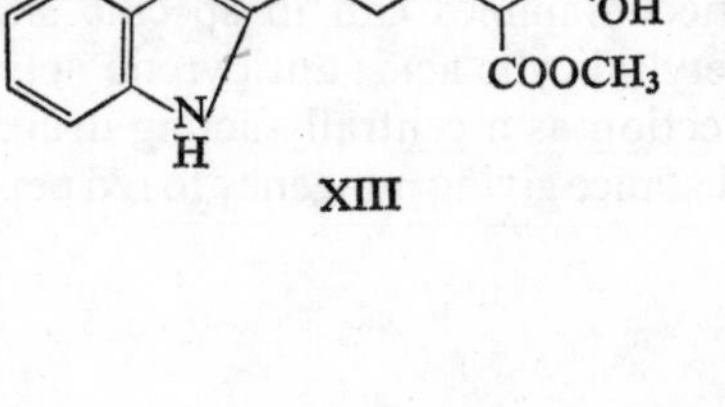

XIII

to rats of first stimulating and subsequently inactivating the hypothalamic warmth-detectors (Jancsó-Gábor *et al.*, 1970).

Reserpine and the Bound Catecholamines and Serotonin

The existence in cerebral dispersions of bound forms of serotonin and noradrenaline, which could be deposited by centrifuging, has been recounted above in describing the nerve terminals and vesicles in which the two amines occur. Before this was established, investigation of reserpine (Fig. 14.11) had shown the two amines to be bound in the brain *in vivo*, for reserpine caused a remarkable release of both compounds. Reserpine acted specifically at the intracellular or vesicular storage sites, and not at the outer cell membrane. Thus loss of stainable material concluded to be aromatic amines, from small terminal vesicles was observed in reserpine-treated animals (Tranzer *et al.*, 1969; Carlsson, 1969). Fig. 14.12 shows the action of reserpine on the amines of the brain-stem; depletion is caused also at other sites in the body, though the cerebral action is that most relevant to the sedative or tranquillizing effect of the drug. In this regard both amines are important; thus it is possible by administering reserpine to rats kept at 4° to deplete cerebral catecholamines without action on serotonin. Such animals were not sedated but became so on regaining room temperature, when cerebral serotonin fell. In certain reserpine analogues, sedative action was better correlated with fall in noradrenaline than in serotonin; and also, 3:4-dihydroxyphenylalanine aroused from reserpine sedation (Carlsson; Vogt: *Symposium*, 1960; see Lucas, 1963). The neural systems involved in a process as complex as the maintenance of behaviour normally associated with consciousness, are understandably manifold. At adrenergic neuromuscular junctions, more defined effects follow reserpine, analogous to those after partial denervation (see Eccles, 1964).

Reserpine not only caused loss of catecholamines from the brain, but modified cerebral (and other) tissues so that they were less capable of assimilating added amines (Brodie *et al.*, 1960; Weil-Malherbe, *Symposium*, 1960). Administering ^{3}H-adrenaline to cats, the pituitary normally reached ^{3}H contents three to five times those of the blood plasma, but after reserpine the ratios were 0·7–1. Tissues taken from the pituitary, pineal, cerebral cortex and hypothalamus of the animals and incubated in bicarbonate–blood serum

---

Fig. 14.11. Compounds related to the catecholamines and serotonin.
I and II. α-Methyl-*m*-tyrosine and an analogous hydrazide, inhibitors of dopa decarboxylase.
III. Pyrogallol, inhibitor of catechol-O-methyltransferase.
IV and V. Iproniazid and nialamide, inhibitors of amine oxidase.
VI. R = R′ = H, amphetamine; R = H, R′ = CH$_3$, methamphetamine; R = OH, R′ = CH$_3$, ephedrine; R = H, R′ = NH$_2$, pheniprazine.
VII. Mescaline.
VIII. Pargyline, an antidepressant drug.
IX. Tetrabenazine, a tranquillizer.
X. Harmine.
XI. Reserpine.
XII. R = NEt$_2$, lysergic acid diethylamide.
XIII. Yohimbine.

mixtures, normally reached noradrenaline contents four times those of the media, but this also was diminished in tissues from reserpinized cats, to ratios of about 1·5. Dopa also yielded little noradrenaline in the brain of the rabbit even 3 days after reserpine administration; this was attributed to a lack of ability to retain the dopamine formed and synthesis was increased towards normal by β-phenylisopropylhydrazine, an amine-oxidase inhibitor. Recovery from reserpine sedation has been observed to occur at the time when the vesicular storage mechanism begins to recover, and before the cerebral content of amines has returned to normal.

Sedation without anaesthesia is induced not only by reserpine and structur-ally analogous compounds, but also by some substituted aralkylamines,

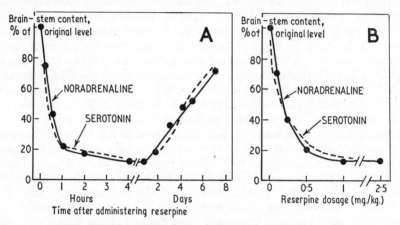

FIG. 14.12. Reserpine action in depleting the brain stem of rabbits in noradrenaline and serotonin.
  A. Loss and slow recovery after 5 mg. reserpine/kg.; initial nor-adrenaline, about 3 nmoles/g. and serotonin, 2·5 nmoles/g. (Shore & Brodie, 1957).
  B. Loss 4 hr. after reserpine at the dose-levels indicated.

including bis(3,4-dichlorophenylethyl)amine, and by benzoquinolizines as tetrabenazine (Fig. 14.11). Though of varied structural types, these compounds were all found to impair the cerebral storage of indolealkylamines and catechol-amines. Monoamine oxidase inhibitors antagonized the autonomic and behavioural effects of each group of drugs; metabolic and pharmacological rationale in their actions has been appraised by Sulzer & Bass (1968).

In the pineal of rats, structures have been identified electron-microscopically which are lost or changed after administration of reserpine (De Robertis, 1964). The pineal nerve-endings noted above contained vesicles staining lightly with osmium tetroxide, and others which stained deeply. After reserpine administra-tion, the dark-staining vesicles or granules diminished rapidly in number, following a time-course almost exactly that of Fig. 14.12. The vesicles are thus pictured to owe their dark staining to the abilities of the catecholamines and serotonin to reduce OsO_4, and reserpine to cause these vesicles to discharge their contents. Rats treated with the amine oxidase inhibitor iproniazid, yielded pineals enriched in dark-staining nerve-ending granules.

Central Effects of Related Substances

Chemically or metabolically related to the catecholamines or serotonin are many compounds which have characteristic actions on the central nervous system; for an indication of the extensive chemical and pharmacological investigation of such compounds, see Gordon (1967) and Efron (1968). Reference to Fig. 14.11 shows several compounds whose actions have already received comment, and others which will now be noted briefly. In each case the biochemical action indicated may be one property only among several which are relevant to a compound's pharmacological effect.

Thus *amphetamine* and methedrine (VI, Fig. 14.11) are both sympatho-mimetic amines and inhibitors of amine-oxidase (Hope & Smith, 1960). Amine-oxidase in cerebral and other tissues does not oxidize amines in which the amino group is placed in the middle rather than at the end of a carbon chain. Certain such bases, however, retain affinity for the enzyme and block its action. Notable in this respect is the group of β-amino-*n*-propylbenzenes (VI, Fig. 14.11) which include the naturally occurring ephedrine and the widely used amphetamine and methedrine. These compounds cause restlessness and insomnia; oppose the action of depressants and rouse in narcolepsy. Effects can depend on the personality and mood of the subject to whom the agents are given, but include increased attention, alertness, initiative and feeling of well-being, possibly associated with dizziness and succeeded by fear and fatigue; in addicts, their effects may simulate schizophrenia (Connell, 1958; McConnell, 1963). Amphetamine and methamphetamine have been administered for the purpose of relieving the symptoms of mild depressive illnesses; and also in order to maintain wakefulness and alertness in normal people when, after fatigue, sleep would otherwise result. The metabolism of amphetamine, and metabolic and behavioural consequences of its administration, are described in the following chapter.

Hallucinations and delusions, especially in vision, but also in touch and in smell, are major effects of *mescaline* (Fig. 14.11), a naturally-occurring β-phenylethylamine. Disturbances of the sympathetic system also follow the administration of 0·3–0·6 g. in man (Guttmann, 1936; *Symposia*, 1957); and comparable levels of 0·3 mM prevent the metabolic response to electrical pulses in separated cerebral tissues (Lewis & McIlwain, 1954). Synthetic drugs related in structure to amphetamine, being mainly derivatives of β-phenyl-ethylamine, have been the subject of several assays designed to select those with maximal effect on the central nervous system. The assays have measured the effects of the compounds on the movement and behaviour of experimental animals, as well as on their body temperature and the duration of sleep after giving depressant drugs. Such assays have confirmed the considerable central activity of amphetamine and methamphetamine, and also shown potency in other compounds including pipradrol, α-2-piperidylbenzhydrol, which has received clinical trial in depressive states.

Several of the complex effects of the ergot alkaloids can be related to the sympathetic nervous system or to adrenaline (see Barger, 1938; Rothlin, 1947; *Symposium*, 1960). Thus prior subcutaneous injection of 0·2 μmole/kg. of ergotamine or ergotoxine to the rabbit prevents the three-fold increase in blood glucose which normally follows 0·5 μmole/kg. of adrenaline. Ergotamine and dihydroergotamine affect circulation and body temperature by routes which in part involve the central nervous system; ergotamine is applied in treatment of *migraine* possibly through its effect on the cerebral blood vessels, but it may also produce vomiting, excitement and confusion. Tyramine-containing foods cause migraine episodes in about 30% of patients suffering migraine, and in a group of susceptible patients a defect in conjugation of tyramine was detected (Youdim *et al.*, 1971).

Central effects are the most prominent features of the action of *lysergic acid diethylamide* (Fig. 14.11), which is produced synthetically from lysergic acid, the polycyclic substance common to the ergot alkaloids. The diethylamide can induce hallucinations and marked changes of mood when 1 μg./kg. (3 nmoles/kg.) is taken orally or by other routes. Many of its effects have been described as schizophrenia-like and the substance has been widely studied (*Symposia*, 1957; Garattini & Shore, 1968); it antagonizes serotonin in several systems and a major basis for this has been described above. Small doses of lysergic acid diethylamide have been administered to mentally ill subjects and have caused a variety of changes of mood, usually temporarily only. The physiological and mental changes induced by lysergic acid diethylamide in men and dogs have been concluded to be similar to those following infusion of tryptamine, suggesting an action of the diethylamide at tryptamine receptors (Martin & Sloan, 1970).

The impressively low dosage in which lysergic acid diethylamide acts as a hallucinogen is adequate also to affect the cerebral heat-regulating centres in the rabbit and is also a feature in the action of other of the ergot alkaloids; some affect isolated organs at 4 nM (2 μg./l.). The β-phenylethylamine structure of adrenaline is discernible not only in mescaline, methedrine and the ergot alkaloids, but also in bulbocapnine, which has central effects which include the production of catatonia. Structural features common to lysergic acid diethylamide and the phenylethylamine and other hallucinogenic agents are discussed by Snyder & Richelson (1968). Substances without such structure, but whose action is related to adrenergic mechanisms, include dibenamine, $Cl.CH_2.CH_2.N(CH_2.C_6H_5)_2$, which has a variety of central effects.

Glutamic Acid and Related Cerebral Excitants

Investigation of tissue extracts for action on neural systems showed the mammalian brain to be a source of both excitant and depressant compounds. The excitant materials include glutamic acid, which on application to regions of the brain and spinal cord can greatly increase the rate of cell-firing. An example is shown in Fig. 14.13; the threshold concentrations required for such effects are about 0·15 mM. This is a significantly low value when it is recalled that the average cerebral content of glutamic acid is about 8 mM, and that the acid can be rapidly formed and degraded. Indeed the major metabolic roles played by glutamic acid (Chapter 8) are always to be borne in mind in appraising the properties of the acid as a cerebral excitant.

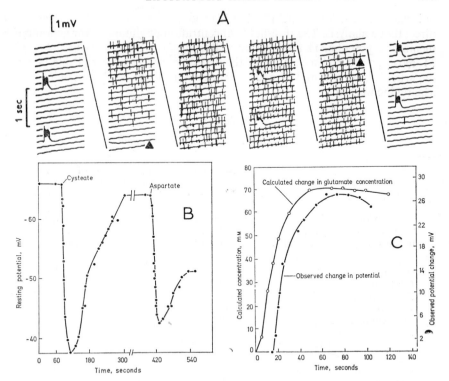

FIG. 14.13. Cell-firing and depolarization induced by acidic amino acids.

A. Extracellular records from a cell of the spinal cord of a cat, firing in response to the iontophoretic application of glutamate between the two signs ▲. The time base of an oscilloscope proceeds from left to right and bottom to top, as indicated (Curtis *et al.*, 1960).

B, C. Intracellular records from cells of the guinea pig neocortex, in tissues maintained *in vitro*, following the application of glutamate, cysteate and aspartate by micropipette. In C the time-course of the change in potential (displaced by an addition of about 8 sec. in the Fig.) is compared with that of the change in glutamate concentration in the region of the cell (Bradford & McIlwain, 1966).

Specificity and Ionic Bases for Action

Structural specificity among glutamate congeners gives important data in differentiating between their metabolic and cell-firing properties. In particular, homocysteic acid which is a sulphonic acid analogue of glutamic acid, is as potent an excitant as is glutamic acid (Table 14.5), but does not undergo comparable metabolic changes. The excitant amino acids all carry two acidic groupings and include aspartate and certain substituted aspartates. The ω-amino acids, which are depressant, receive comment below.

The basis for cell-firing by glutamate proves to have factors in common with cell-firing by other excitants. Glutamates depolarize: within some milliseconds of their application in the region of spinal or cortical neurons, the intracellularly measured cell membrane potential diminishes, later spontaneously recovering (Krnjević & Schwartz, 1967; Curtis, 1969). This action has been reproduced in isolated neocortical tissues (Fig. 14.13) and its ionic basis demonstrated by direct tissue analysis. The threshold concentration of glutamate for action on membrane potential *in vitro*, as on cell-firing *in vivo*, was about 0·2 mM. Moreover, structural specificity for the two actions were similar (Table 14.5); in particular, aspartic and homocysteic acids were active, while glutamine and asparagine were not.

Table 14.5

Amino acids and cell-firing in the brain and spinal cord

Compound (of stereoisomerides, L, unless otherwise specified)	System examined and degree of action (increasing from 0–3)		
	Neocortex *in vitro*: depolarization[1]	Spinal neurons: increased firing[2]	Pericruciate cortex: cell-firing[2]
Aspartate	3*	3	1
Glutamate	3*	3	1
Asparagine, glutamine	0	0	0
Glutaric	0	0	–
DL-αAminoadipic	2*	–	–
N-Acetylaspartate	0	0	–
N-Methyl-D-aspartate	1	2	3
N-Propyl-DL-aspartate	0	–	–
N-Methyl-DL-glutamate	0	0	–
Cysteate	3*	3	–
DL-Homocysteate	3*	–	3
Glycine	0	–2	–
β-Alanine	0	–3	–
γ-Amino-n-butyrate	0	–3	–3
ω-Amino-caprylate	–	0	0
α-Amino-n-butyrate	–	0	–

Degree of action is represented by an arbitrary scale from –3 (maximum inhibition) to 3 (maximum action).
Cats and guinea pigs were examined in systems similar to those of Fig. 14.13.
[1] Hillman & McIlwain, 1961; Gibson & McIlwain, 1965; Bradford & McIlwain, 1966. The compounds asterisked also increased intracellular Na, and diminished phosphocreatine.
[2] Curtis & Watkins, 1960; Crawford & Curtis, 1964. A negative sign means diminution in firing.
Valine, leucine, serine were among some 20 compounds which showed no activity.

Tissues sampled in the first few minutes or so after glutamate addition had increased in Na^+ content (Fig. 14.14; Bradford & McIlwain, 1966; McIlwain *et al.*, 1969). Thus a simple explanation for the diminution of potential across cell-membranes could be by entry of Na^+ to the cell interior, normally negatively charged in relation to extracellular fluids. Calculation from the likely area and capacity of neuronal membranes in neocortical samples gave an ion equivalence of 10–50 n equiv./g. tissue for a 10 mv change in potential (Harvey & McIlwain, 1968). The initial net rate of entry of Na^+ caused by glutamate corresponded to 160 nequiv./g. sec.; supposing a 10 mv change to be sufficient to initiate cell firing, this could be reached in 60–300 msec.: a time consistent with the observed actions of added glutamate.

The marked effect of glutamate on Na movements was also shown isotopically, using $^{22}Na^+$ with isolated neocortical tissues (McIlwain *et al.*, 1969). Glutamate increased Na^+ influx from 400 to 1,200 μequiv./g. tissue/hr. and this increase was inhibited by tetrodotoxin, which inhibited also the net entry of Na^+ (Fig. 14. 14). Structural relationships between glutamates, tetrodotoxin and membrane phospholipids have led to suggestions regarding the membrane reorganization which appears to be involved in neural excitation (Chapter 12; McIlwain *et al.*, 1969).

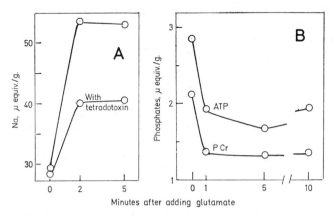

FIG. 14.14. Changes in tissue composition induced by sodium
  L-glutamate.
    A. Increase in the Na of the non-inulin compartment of guinea pig neocortical tissue, on adding 5 mM glutamate to glucose bicarbonate salines bathing the tissue. The solutions indicated were 60 nM in tetrodotoxin (McIlwain, Harvey & Rodriguez, 1969).
    B. Diminution in adenosine triphosphate and phosphocreatine in the tissues following a similar addition of glutamate. The changes following cysteate and homocysteate were similar (Bradford & McIlwain, 1966).

The sodium entry initiated by glutamate and its congeners has, understandably, a number of other consequences: in particular, the ATP and phosphocreatine of the tissues fall (Fig. 14.14), presumably through activation of the Na,K-activated adenosine triphosphatase. Again, it is the excitatory amino acids of Table 14.5 which bring about this change, while glutamine and alanine were without action; the fall in ~P caused by glutamate or homocysteate was nearly complete within 1 min. after which ATP remained at a lower, relatively stable level with increased ADP and P_i. These latter changes presumably cause the increased glucose utilization, respiration and lactic acid formation which characteristically follow the addition of glutamates to cerebral tissues in glucose salines (Chapters 4 and 8; for a description of these and subsequent changes see Tower, 1960; Bradford & McIlwain, 1966). Many of these changes are caused by a toxic excitatory amino acid of natural occurrence, β-N-oxalyl-L-α,β-diaminopropionic acid (Cheema *et al.*, 1970). This acid contributes to causing lathyrism, a nutritional disorder with convulsive episodes. Such episodes occur in young rats within 5 min. of their receiving 5 mg. of the acid intraperitoneally.

Release of Glutamates on Excitation

The free amino acids of cerebral tissues exchange to varying degrees with fluids surrounding the tissue, and this exchange is altered selectively when the tissue is electrically stimulated (Chapter 8). Evidence suggested that the release of glutamate from striatal tissues was increased on stimulation (Katz et al., 1969), and that this occurred also from synaptosomal preparations from the rat cerebral cortex (Bradford, 1970), as well as from invertebrate systems (Kerkut, 1969).

Glutamate thus has several of the characteristics of an excitatory neuro-transmitting agent, and some aspects of its differential localization in the spinal cord have been interpreted as supporting such a role (Graham & Aprison, 1969). Localized liberation of small quantities of glutamic acid at points in the hypothalamus of adult unanaesthetized rats evoked quite complex behavioural responses which were similar to those given by electrical stimulation of the same sites (Brody et al., 1969). Caution in accepting a neuro-transmitter role for glutamates has been expressed on the basis of electrophysiological measurements, which give a reversal potential for depolarization of mammalian motoneuron membranes by glutamate at a more polarized level than is characteristic of neural excitation (Curtis & Watkins, 1965); some corresponding data in a lower vertebrate has however been interpreted in favour of a transmitter role for the acid (Martin et al., 1970). Release of glutamate has been implicated in the process of spreading depression in retinal preparations, and may play a similar role in the cortex (van Harreveld & Fifkova, 1971).

Study of the mechanism and site of glutamate release at subcellular level can be seen to be important to further understanding of its role. Neural excitation in other situations has involved Ca^{2+}; glutamates at neocortical tissues caused a prompt, small increase in intracellular Ca (Ramsay & McIlwain, 1970; Pull et al., 1970). With $^{45}Ca^{2+}$, this was shown to be due to glutamate accelerating the influx of Ca and diminishing its efflux. The Ca entry stimulated by glutamate was inhibited by tetrodotoxin, which confirms a relationship with neural excitation for this is also inhibited by tetrodotoxin.

Inhibitory Amino Acids

Two major inhibitory amino acids, distinct in their central occurrence and action, are described below (see also Table 14.5): glycine and γ-aminobutyric acid.

γ-Aminobutyric Acid

γ-Aminobutyric acid occurs in the brain at 2–4 μmoles/g. and is formed in the tissues themselves from glutamic acid, as has been described already in

Chapters 7 and 8, where its metabolic role in the mammalian brain is appraised. The role of γ-aminobutyrate in inhibiting nerve-impulse generation was first realized through study of the stretch-receptor neurons of the crayfish. The impulse-generation was found to be inhibited by extracts of natural materials of which the mammalian brain proved a very active source. Chemical fractionation suggested the cerebral constituent responsible to be γ-aminobutyric acid with a lesser contribution from glutamic acid. In this situation, 20 nM-γ-aminobutyric acid, natural or synthetic, inhibited impulse generation. Of related compounds, racemic β-hydroxy-γ-aminobutyric acid showed half this potency while β-alanine or δ-aminovaleric acid were effective only in much greater concentrations (Elliott & Florey, 1956; Bazemore et al., 1957).

Moreover, γ-AB was found to have inhibitory effects in the brain itself. These were exhibited in experiments of the type illustrated in Fig. 14.13, as is noted in Table 14.5; cell-firing by single neurons of the pericruciate cortex of anaesthetized cats was depressed by γ-AB. The sulphonic analogue, 3-amino-1-propane sulphonic acid was among structurally related compounds which were also inhibitory: thus, as with glutamate (q.v.) the structural specificity of γ-AB is such as to dissociate its metabolic properties from its properties in relation to cell-firing. The effect of γ-AB was a sharp and easily reversible blocking action; the development of this picture of cortical inhibition is described by Krnjević et al. (1966). Similarity between properties of γ-AB and of the native inhibitory transmitter extended to observations with intracellular electrodes, and the central inhibitory properties of γ-AB are applicable to man: the compound showed effective anticonvulsant properties in a proportion of epileptic conditions (Tower, in Roberts, 1960).

Metabolic appraisal of γ-AB in Chapter 8 indicated that part of the cerebral content of γ-AB was attached to subcellular particles. Using ^{14}C-γ-AB, preferential attachment was found to nerve-terminal fragments, and to vesicles from nerve-terminal fractions (Varon et al., 1965; Kuriyama et al., 1968). Such fractions were enriched in glutamate decarboxylase which formed γ-AB (De Robertis, 1964); by contrast, the transaminase (q.v.) which removed γ-AB was largely a mitochondrial enzyme.

γ-Aminobutyrate Release

Release of γ-AB from the brain to surrounding fluids has been demonstrated both in vitro (Table 8.5) and in vivo. It was released on local superfusion of the monkey brain (DeFeudis et al., 1969) to fluids in contact with the neocortex of cats (Mitchell & Srinivasan, 1969) and also to those of the fourth ventricle (Obata & Takeda, 1969). In the latter situation, release of γ-AB (in the presence of an inhibitor of its transamination, amino-oxyacetic acid) was increased three-fold by stimulation of the cerebellum, then reaching about 1·5 nmoles γ-AB/min. It was reasoned that the γ-AB had originated as an inhibitory transmitter liberated from the axon terminals of Purkinje cells, which end at cerebellar subcortical nuclei in the region of the fourth ventricle. From the visual cortex of the cat, γ-AB was released at 30 pmoles/cm^2.min. in absence of stimulation, and this rate was increased 3–6 fold by stimulation of the cortex or of the lateral geniculate nucleus (Iversen et al., 1971). Analysis of effluent samples showed γ-aminobutyrate to be the only amino acid responding in this way to such stimulation.

From the cat cortex, release of γ-AB in presence of amino-oxyacetic acid was doubled by a rapid succession of stimuli which inhibited cortical cell-firing, and which was suggested to act by nerve-terminal release of γ-AB. Basis for the inhibitory action of γ-AB appears to lie in its causing hyperpolarization of the postsynaptic cell. The reversal potential for this action has the same value as that for the hyperpolarization induced by stimulation of inhibitory tracts: evidence favouring a neurotransmitter role for γ-AB. Pharmacological evidence for this has also been obtained: the action of γ-AB in depressing the firing of cerebellar Purkinje cells was blocked by bicuculline, an isoquinoline alkaloid, at concentrations commensurate with those at which bicuculline was convulsant (Curtis, 1969; Curtis et al., 1970).

Glycine as Spinal Inhibitor

Investigation of numerous amino acids for effect on cell-firing in several neural systems revealed inhibitory properties in the simplest of α-amino acids, glycine, especially in preparations of the spinal cord (Table 14.5; Purpura et al., 1959; Curtis & Watkins, 1960; Curtis et al., 1968). Cell-firing by neural routes in the dorsal horn of the cat cord was found in the majority of instances to be more depressed by glycine than by γ-AB, though in other situations this order of activity could be reversed.

Special properties in the spinal actions of glycine were emphasized by their susceptibility to strychnine. Strychnine opposed inhibition of cell-firing caused by glycine, but not that caused by γ-aminobutyrate. This clearly bears on the action of strychnine as a convulsant agent, when it acts preferentially in removing inhibitory actions normally operating in the spinal cord. Markedly higher concentrations are required of strychnine for cerebral effects, so supporting γ-aminobutyrate as the main cerebral inhibitory agent. Strychnine enabled the inhibitory effects of amino acids on cell-firing to be classified to glycine-like and γ-aminobutyrate-like; the glycine-like, susceptible to strychnine, were given also by α-alanine and serine, which were, however, less potent than glycine.

The grey matter of the spinal cord was found to be enriched in glycine in comparison with spinal white matter; the grey matter also showed a relatively high activity of D-amino acid oxidase, which converts glycine to glyoxylate. Glyoxalate had little or no action on cell-firing in the spinal cord; the oxidase activity was over 2 μequiv./g. hr. in spinal grey matter, 0·4–0·8 in spinal white matter and 0·1–0·6 μequiv./g. hr. in neocortex (de Marchi & Johnston, 1969). The oxidase was inhibited by p-chloromercuribenzoate; use of this compound in electrophysiological experiments was not straightforward but gave results suggesting that it prolonged the action of an inhibitory transmatter (Curtis et al., 1968).

Glycine was among the amino acids liberated in vivo on superfusion of parts of the monkey brain (De Feudis et al., 1970). Fig. 14.6 gives an instance in which stimulation of cerebral cortical tissue did not affect the release of glycine, but a normal, slow output of ^{14}C from preparations of rat spinal cord pretreated with ^{14}C-glycine, was doubled promptly in response to electrical excitation (Hopkin & Neal, 1970). The ^{14}C released was shown chromatographically to consist of glycine. Cerebral glycine can originate from the bloodstream, from cerebral proteins, and by synthesis through serine from glucose. The latter route appeared to preponderate in the brain of the rat (Shank & Aprison, 1970).

Histamine and Other Substances

Described first below is histamine, which, interestingly, repeats the pattern of a pharmacologically-active agent produced by decarboxylation from an amino acid. A few other substances then receive comment. A survey of amines of cerebral occurrence independently of their pharmacological properties, showed the presence of many simple bases including β-hydroxypropylamine and n-butylamine (Perry et al., 1965).

In rat and guinea pig brain histamine has been found at 0·5–2 nmoles/g. and has been examined in a number of experimental and pathological conditions (Michaelson & Dowe, 1963; Green, 1964; Adam, Symposium, 1961). Histidine (q.v.) is present at much higher level and cerebral tissues are capable of decarboxylating it to yield histamine (see below). The most notable occurrence of histamine in the mammalian brain is in the pituitary, especially in the stalk and the posterior lobe. In samples from the pituitary, centrifugation suggests the histamine to occur in entities akin to mast cells. This is not, however, the case with the smaller quantity of histamine in the hypothalamus, which appears to be attached to smaller particles. Most mast cells were also found in the pituitary: an association of histamine with mast cells has been found elsewhere in the body. Release of histamine may contribute to vasodilatation; the pituitary stalk carries some unusual blood vessels (see Chapter 16). A methyltransferase which acts on histamine has been found in the brain, but diamine oxidase, which oxidizes histamine and other diamines, has extremely small if any activity in mammalian brain (Burkard et al., 1963; Snyder & Hendley, 1968). Antihistamine drugs have notable central effects, not however rigidly specified as directly related to histamine.

Histamine undergoes quite rapid turnover in the brain, but does not readily enter the brain from the bloodstream (Schayer & Reilley, 1970). ^{14}C-Histidine gave ^{14}C-histamine in the brain of mice, at maximal level within 10 min. of its intraperitoneal administration. Following intracerebral administration of ^{14}C-histamine, methylhistamines rapidly appeared; methylation appears to be the route of inactivation of histamine in some species although histamine is oxidized in others. The histidine decarboxylase, EC 4.1.1.22, which forms histamine has been characterized in preparations from the brain of the rat (Schwartz et al., 1970). It showed K_m of 0·4 mM for histidine, acted specifically on the L-isomeride, and was inhibited by 0·1 mM-hydrazino-histidine but not by α-methyldihydroxyphenylalanine. These properties differentiate it from the aromatic L-amino acid decarboxylase. In nine regions examined in rats, histidine decarboxylase was at greatest potency in the hypothalamus which produced 6 nmoles/g.hr.; this was also the region of greatest histamine content.

Histamine increased the cyclic AMP of neocortical tissues incubated *in vitro*, from about 1 to 8 nmoles/g. tissue; still greater increase was found, to some 40–80 nmoles/g. when adenosine was added or the tissue was electrically stimulated in the presence of histamine (Kakiuchi *et al.*, 1969; Sattin & Rall, 1970). These proportionally large increases were in part antagonized by antihistamine drugs and the effects of electrical stimulation on cyclic-AMP were augmented by theophylline in a fashion which may contribute to explaining its central actions.

Substance P, a polypeptide which also is a vasodilator, is present in the mammalian brain, especially in areas with little acetylcholine. Certain parts of the midbrain and medulla showed greatest activity and a variety of different assays have established its individuality (Amin *et al.*, 1954; Gaddum, 1960; Cleugh *et al.*, 1964). The prostaglandins, C_{20}-hydroxylated and cyclic fatty acids, include members which occur in the brain and others which produce catatonia on intraventricular injection (Horton & Main, 1965; see also Chapter 11). Liberation of adenosine on stimulating isolated cerebral tissues was noted in the preceding description of catecholamines. It will be recalled from Chapter 9 that adenosine increases the tissue's content of cyclic adenosine monophosphate; in doing so, it acts synergistically with catecholamines and certain other bases. As the cyclic monophosphate (q.v.) can act as an inducing agent in altering cellular enzymic content, the liberation of adenosine may contribute to long-lasting effects of cerebral excitation (McIlwain, 1971).

Comment

It is a general biological observation that cells produce and evolve to surrounding media, substances which affect the actions of other cells and organisms. Both carbon dioxide and ammonia feature in symbiosis in unicellular organisms as well as affecting the excitability of the central nervous system. Neurotoxins or antibiotics can be recognized as specialized for such interactions, and chemical factors in neural transmission give a further example of this phenomenon. Their close relation to general metabolites is thus understandable; the precursors of those described here: choline, aromatic amino acids, histidine and glutamic acid often require no more than one or two enzymic steps to yield their active products. Possibly the compounds discussed above represent varying degrees of specialization in cell interaction: acetylcholine forming part of systems highly adapted for such a role while those concerned with glutamic acid remain less specialized. In a search for pharmacologically active substances from the brain, the effects of cerebral extracts were examined using intestinal muscles from different species as test-system (Toh, 1963, 1964). A number of substances present in the extracts caused contraction or relaxation; these included known compounds, as adenosine triphosphate, and also unidentified nucleotide-like materials, unsaturated fatty acids and a phosphopeptide.

Cerebral tissues thus contain a number of substances which can act on neural and on other types of cells. Search for such substances using cerebral systems has not been intensive, possibly because means of testing their effects specifically on the brain are not so well developed as are those for judging the response of several other organs. The cerebellum of decerebrate rabbits has been developed as a test system and tissue extracts, especially from the cerebellum, shown to be excitatory (Crossland, 1960). At present the hypothalamus and neighbouring regions display the greatest variety of substances known to act upon other cells. These parts also include regions highly sensitive to circulating hormones, and in this way also can form part of regulating systems.

Neural structures of a variety of functions are closely packed in the brain. Localization of the action of given cells is largely determined anatomically, but where such elements are closest, chemical specificity becomes more important. Thus inhibitory and excitatory impulses from different fibres are postulated as acting on a single motor cell of the spinal cord by liberating different substances from the two types of fibre-terminals. Acetylcholine and now glycine can be conceived in these two roles, lowering and raising membrane potential, but much is probably still to be learned of the carefully-engineered synapses which form an extremely important unit of neural structure and action. Scope for further specific consequences of neurotransmitter action in the brain is also considerable, and receives comment in the two chapters which follow.

REFERENCES

ABRAHAMS, V. C., KOELLE, G. B. & SMART, P. (1957). *J. Physiol.* **139**, 137.
AKERT, K. & WASER, P. G. (1969). *Progr. Brain Res.* **31**. Amsterdam: Elsevier.
AGHAJANIAN, G. K., FOOTE, W. E. & SHEARD, M. H. (1968). *Science,* **161**, 706.
AMIN, A. H., CRAWFORD, B. B. & GADDUM, J. H. (1954). *J. Physiol.* **126**, 596.
APRISON, M. H., WOLF, M. A., POULOS, G. L. & FOLKERTH, T. L. (1962). *J. Neurochem.* **9**, 575.
AUGUSTINSSON, K-B. (1950). The Enzymes, Vol. 1, p. 443. Ed. Summer & Myrbäck. New York: Academic Press.
AUGUSTINSSON, K-B. (1960). The Enzymes, Vol 4, p. 521. Ed. Boyer. New York: Academic Press.
AXELROD, J. (1962). *J. biol. Chem.* **237**, 1657.
AXELROD, J. (1965). *Rec. Progr. Horm. Res.* **21**, 597.
AXELROD, J., ALBERS, W. & CLEMENTE, C. D. (1960). *J. Neurochem.* **5**, 68.
AXELROD, J., SHEIN, H. M. & WURTMAN, R. J. (1969). *Proc. nat. Acad. Sci.* **62**, 544.
AXELROD, J., WEIL-MALHERBE, H. & TOMCHICK, R. (1959). *J. Pharmacol.* **127**, 251.
AXELROD, J., WURTMAN, R. J. & SNYDER, S. H. (1965). *J. biol. Chem.* **240**, 949.
BALDESSARINI, R. J. & KOPIN, I. J. (1966). *Science,* **152**, 1630.
BALDESSARINI, R. J. & KOPIN, I. J. (1967). *J. Pharmacol.* **156**, 31.
BANKS, P., BIGGINS, R., BISHOP, R., CHRISTIAN, B. & CURRIE, N. (1969). *J. Physiol.* **200**, 797.
BARGER, G. (1938). *Handbuch exp. Pharmakol.* **6**, 85. Berlin: Springer.
BAZEMORE, A. W., ELLIOTT, K. A. C. & FLOREY, E. (1957). *J. Neurochem.* **1**, 334.
BEERS, W. H. & REICH, E. (1970). *Nature, Lond.,* **228**, 917.
BERRY, J. F. & WHITTAKER, V. P. (1959). *Biochem. J.* **73**, 447.
BERTLER, Å., HILLARP, N-Ä. & ROSENGREN, E. (1960). *Acta Physiol. Scand.* **50**, 113.
BESSON, M. J., CHARAMY, A., FELTZ, P. & GLOWINSKI, J. (1969). *Proc. Nat. Acad. Sci. N.Y.* **62**, 741.
BHATTACHARYYA, B. K. & FELDBERG, W. (1958). *Brit. J. Pharmacol.* **13**, 156, 163.
BLACK, I. B., AXELROD, J. & REIS, D. J. (1971). *Nature new Biol.* **230**, 185.
BLACK, I. B. & REIS, D. J. (1971). *J. Physiol.* **23**, 421.
BLASCHKO, H. (1963). The Enzymes, Vol. 8, p. 337. Ed. Boyer, New York: Academic Press.
BLASCHKO, H. K. F. & SMITH, A. D. (1970). Discussion Meeting, Roy Soc. (to be published).

BLIGH, J., COTTLE, W. H. & MASKREY, M. (1971). *J. Physiol.* **212**, 377.

BLOOM, F. E. (1968). In Efron (1968), p. 355.

BLOOM, F. E. (1969). *Adv. Biochem. Pharmacol.* **1**, 27.

BOGDANSKI, D. F., TISSARI, A. & BRODIE, B. B. (1968). In Efron (1968) p. 17.

BOGDANSKI, D. F., WEISSBACH, H. & UDENFRIEND, S. (1957). *J. Neurochem.* **1**, 272.

BOULLIN, D. J. & O'BRIEN, R. A. (1971). *J. Physiol.* **212**, 287.

BOURNE, G. H. (1969). (Ed.). The Structure and Function of Nervous Tissue. New York: Academic Press.

BOWERS, M. B. (1967). *Internat. J. Neuropharmacol.* **6**, 399.

BRADFORD, H. F. (1970). *Brain Res.* **19**, 239.

BRADFORD, H. F. & McILWAIN, H. (1966). *J. Neurochem.* **13**, 1163.

BRADLEY, P. B. (1968). *Internat. Rev. Neurobiol.* **11**, 12.

BRADLEY, P. B. & FINK, M. (1968). (Ed.). *Progr. Brain. Res.* **28**.

BRILL, H. (1967). Neuropsychopharmacology. Amsterdam: Excerpta Medica.

BRODIE, B. B., BOGDANSKI, D. F. & BONOMI, L. (1964). *Proc. Internat. Neurochem. Sympos.* **5**, 367.

BRODIE, B. B., CHO, A. K., STEFANO, F. J. E. & GESSA, G. L. (1969). *Adv. Biochem. Psychopharm.* **1**, 219.

BRODIE, B. B., DENGLER, H. J., TITUS, E. & WILSON, C. W. M. (1960). *J. Physiol.* **154**, 37P.

BRODY, J. F., DeFEUDIS, P. A. & DeFEUDIS, F. V. (1969). *Nature*, **224**, 1330.

BROWNING, E. T. & SCHULMAN, M. P. (1968). *J. Neurochem.* **15**, 1391.

BULBRING, E., PHILPOT, F. J., & BOSANQUET, F. D., (1953) *Lancet*, **i**, 865.

BURGEN, A. S. V. & CHIPMAN, L. M. (1951). *J. Physiol.* **114**, 296.

BURKARD, W. P., GEY, K. F. & PLETSCHER, A. (1963). *J. Neurochem.* **10**, 183.

CALNE, D. B. & SANDLER, M. (1970). *Nature, Lond.* **226**, 21.

CARLSSON, A. (1969). *Progr. Brain Res.* **31**, 53.

CHAKRIN, L. W., SHIDEMAN, F. E. & MARRAZZI, A. S. (1968). *Internat. J. Neuropharm.* **7**, 351.

CHAKRIN, L. W. & WHITTAKER, V. P. (1969). *Biochem. J.* **113**, 97.

CHASE, T. N., BREESE, G. R., GORDON, E. K. & KOPIN, I. J. (1971). *J. Neurochem.* **18**, 135.

CHASE, T. N., KATZ, R. I. & KOPIN, I. J. (1969). *J. Neurochem.* **16**, 607.

CHEEMA, P. S., PADMANABAN, G. & SARMA, P. S. (1970). *J. Neurochem.* **17**, 1295.

CHOTHIA, C. (1970). *Nature, Lond.* **225**, 36.

CLEUGH, J., GADDUM, J. H., MITCHELL, A. A., SMITH, M. W. & WHITTAKER, V. P. (1964). *J. Physiol.* **170**, 69.

COLLINS, G. C. S., SANDLER, M., WILLIAMS, E. D. & YOUDIM, M. B. H. (1970). *Nature, Lond.* **225**, 817.

CONNELL, P. H. (1958). Amphetamine Psychosis. Maudsley Monograph, **5**. London: Chapman & Hall.

COSTA, E. & WEISS, B. (1968). In Efron (1968), p. 39.

CRAWFORD, J. M. & CURTIS, D. R. (1964). *Brit. J. Pharmacol.* **23**, 313.

CREVELING, C. R., VAN DER SCHOOT, J. B. & UDENFRIEND, S. (1962). *Biochem. Biophys. Res. Comm.* **8**, 215.

CROSSLAND, J. (1960). *J. Pharm. Pharmacol.* **12**, 1.

CROSSLAND, J. (1967). *Progr. med. Chem.* **5**, 251.

CROSSLAND, J., PAPPIUS, H. M. & ELLIOTT, K. A. C. (1955). *Amer. J. Physiol.* **183**, 27, 32.

CURTIS, D. R. (1969). In Basic Mechanisms of the Epilepsies, p. 105. Ed. Jasper, Pope & Ward. Boston: Little, Brown.

CURTIS, D. R., DUGGAN, A. W., FELIX, D. & JOHNSTON, G. A. (1970). *Nature, Lond.* **226**, 1222; **228**, 676.

CURTIS, D. R., PHILLIS, J. W. & WATKINS, J. C. (1960). *J. Physiol.* **150**, 656.

CURTIS, D. R. & WATKINS, J. C. (1965). *Pharm. Rev.* **17**, 347.

CURTIS, D. R., HOSLI, L. & JOHNSTON, G. A. R. (1968). *Exper. Brain Res.* **6**, 1.

DAHLSTRÖM, A. (1969). In Basic Mechanisms of the Epilepsies, p. 212. Ed. Jasper, Pope & Ward. Boston: Little, Brown.

DAUTERMAN, W. C. & MEHROTRA, K. N. (1963). *J. Neurochem.* **10**, 113.

DENGLER, H. J., SPEIGEL, H. E. & TITUS, E. O. (1961). *Science,* **133,** 1072.
DEFEUDIS, F. V., DELGADO, J. M. R. & ROTH, R. H. (1970). *Brain Res.* **18,** 15.
DE MARCHI, W. J. & JOHNSTON, G. A. R. (1969). *J. Neurochem.* **16,** 355.
DE ROBERTIS, E. (1964). Histophysiology of Synapses and Neurosecretion. Oxford: Pergamon.
DE ROBERTIS, E. (1969). *Sympos. Internat. Soc. Cell Biol.* **8,** 191.
DE ROBERTIS, E. (1971). *Science,* **171,** 936; **172,** 56.
DIAZ, P., NGAI, S. H. & COSTA, E. (1968). *Adv. Pharmacol.* **6B,** 73.
ECCLESTON, D., ASHCROFT, G. W. & CRAWFORD, T. B. B. (1965). *J. Neurochem.* **12,** 493.
EBERLE, E. D. & EIDUSON, S. (1968). *J. Neurochem.* **15,** 1071.
ECCLES, J. C. (1964). The Physiology of Synapses. Berlin: Springer.
ECCLES, J. C. (1966). (Ed.). Brain & Conscious Experience. Berlin: Springer.
EFRON, D. H. (1968). (Ed.). Psychopharmacology. Washington: U.S. Govt. Printing Office.
ELLIOTT, K. A. C. & FLOREY, E. (1956). *J. Neurochem.* **1,** 181.
ERWIN, V. G. & DEITRICH, R. A. (1966). *J. biol. Chem.* **241,** 3533.
FAHN, S., RODMAN, J. S. & COTE, L. F. (1969). *J. Neurochem.* **16,** 1293.
FELDBERG, W. (1963). A Pharmacological Approach to the Brain from its Inner and Outer Surfaces. London: Arnold.
FELDBERG, W., HELLRON, R. F. & LOTTI, V. J. (1967). *J. Physiol.* **191,** 501.
FELDBERG, W. & MYERS, R. D. (1964). *J. Physiol.* **173,** 226.
FOLBERGROVA, J. (1963). *J. Neurochem.* **10,** 775.
FOLBERGROVA, J., PASSONNEAU, J. V., LOWRY, O. H. & SCHULZ, D. W. (1969). *J. Neurochem.* **16,** 191.
FOLDES, F. F., ZSIGMOND, E. K., FOLDES, V. M. & ERDOS, E. G. (1962). *J. Neurochem.* **9,** 559.
FONNUM, F. (1967). *Biochem. J.* **103,** 262.
FUXE, K., HÖKFELT, T. & UNGERSTEDT, U. (1968). *Adv. Pharmacol.* **6A,** 235.
FUXE, K., HÖKFELT, T. & UNGERSTEDT, U. (1970). *Internat. Rev. Neurobiol.* **13,** 93.
GADDUM, J. H. (1960). In Polypeptides which Affect Smooth Muscle and Blood Vessels. Ed. M. Schachter. London: Pergamon.
GIARMAN, N. J., TANAKA, C., MOONEY, J. & ATKINS, E. (1968). *Adv. Pharmacol.* **6A,** 307.
GARATTINI, S. & SHORE, P. A. (1968). *Adv. Pharmacol.* **6,** A, B.
GEREBETZOFF, M. A. (1959). Cholinesterases. London: Pergamon.
GERSCHENFELD, H. M. & STEFANI, E. (1968). *Adv. Pharmacol.* **6A,** 369.
GEY, K. F. & PLETSCHER, A. (1964). *Biochem. J.* **92,** 300.
GIBSON, I. M. & MCILWAIN, H. (1965). *J. Physiol.* **176,** 261.
GLADSTONE, R. J. & WAKELEY, C. P. G. (1940). The Pineal Organ. London: Baillière, Tindall & Cox.
GLOWINSKI, J. (1970). *Handbook Neorochem.* **4,** 91. New York: Plenum.
GLOWINSKI, J., KOPIN, I. J. & AXELROD, J. (1965). *J. Neurochem.* **12,** 25.
GOLDSTEIN, M., ANAGUOSTE, B., BATTISTA, A. F., OWEN, W. S. & NAKATANI, S. (1969). *J. Neurochem.* **16,** 645.
GOODWIN, J. S., KATZ, R. I. & KOPIN, I. J. (1969). *Nature,* **221,** 556.
GORDON, M. (1967). Psychopharmacological Agents. New York: Academic Press.
GRAHAME-SMITH, D. G. (1967). *Biochem. J.* **105,** 351.
GRAHAME-SMITH, D G. & PARFITT, A. G. (1970). *J. Neurochem.* **17,** 1339.
GRAHAM, L. T. & APRISON, M. H. (1969). *J. Neurophysiol.* **16,** 559.
GOT, K. & POLYA, J. B. (1963). *Nature, Lond.* **198,** 884.
GREEN, J. P. (1964). *Fed. Proc.* **23,** 1095.
GREENGARD, P. & COSTA, E. (1970). Edit.: *Advanc. Biochem. Psychopharmacol.* **3.**
GUTH, P. S. (1969). *Nature, Lond.* **224,** 384.
GUTTMANN, E. (1936). *J. ment. Sci.* **82,** 203.
HANIN, I. (1969). *Advances in Biochem. Pharmacol.* **1,** 111.
HARVEY, J. A. & MCILWAIN, H. (1968). *Biochem. J.* **208,** 269.
HAUSER, H., PHILLIPS, M. C. & MARCHBANKS, R. M. (1970). *Biochem. J.* **120,** 329.

HEATH, D. F. (1961). Organophosphorus Poisons. Oxford: Pergamon.
HEBB, C. O. (1957). *Physiol. Rev.* **37**, 196.
HEBB, C. & MORRIS, D. (1969). In Structure & Function of Nervous Tissue, Vol. 3. Ed. G. H. Bourne. New York: Academic Press.
HEBB, C. O. & SILVER, A. (1956). *J. Physiol.* **134**, 718.
HELLER, A. & MOORE, R. Y. (1968). *Adv. Pharmacol.* **6A**, 191.
HEMSWORTH, B. A. & SMITH, J. C. (1970). *J. Neurochem.* **17**, 171.
HIDAKA, H., NAGATSU, T. & YAGI, K. (1969). *J. Neurochem.* **16**, 783.
HILLMAN, H. H. & MCILWAIN, H. (1961). *J. Physiol.* **157**, 263.
HIMWICH, H. E. & HIMWICH, W. A. (1964). (Ed.). *Progr. Brain Res.* **8**.
HOIJER, D. J. (1969). A Bibliographic Guide to Neuroenzyme Literature. New York: Plenum.
HOLTZ, P. & WESTERMAN, E. (1956). *Arch. exp. Pathol. Pharmakol.* **227**, 538.
HOPE, D. B. & SMITH, A. D. (1960). *Biochem. J.* **74**, 101.
HOPKIN, J. M. & NEAL, M. J. (1970). *Brit. J. Pharmac. Chemother.* 136P.
HORNYKIEWICZ, O. (1964). *Proc. Internat. Neurochem. Sympos.* **5**, 379.
HORNYKIEWICZ, O. (1966). *Pharmacol. Rev.* **18**, 925.
HORTON, E. W. & MAIN, I. H. M. (1965). *Int. J. Neuropharmacol.* **4**, 65.
ICHIYAMA, A., NAKAMURA, S., NISHIZUKA, Y. & HAYASHI, O. (1968). *Adv. Pharmacol.* **6A**, 5.
IVERSEN, L. L. (1967). Uptake and Storage of Noradrenaline in Sympathetic Nerves. Cambridge Univ. Press.
IVERSEN, L. L., MITCHELL, J. F. & SRINIVASAN, V. (1971). *J. Physiol.* **212**, 519.
IVERSEN, L. L. & SNYDER, S. H. (1968). *Nature, Lond.* **220**, 796.
JACKSON, R. L. & APRISON, M. H. (1966). *J. Neurochem.* **13**, 1351, 1367.
JANCSÓ-GÁBOR, A., SZOLCZÁNYI, J. & JANCSÓ, N. (1970). *J. Physiol.* **206**, 495.
JOHNSON, E. S., ROBERTS, M. H. T., SOBIESZEK, A. & STRAUGHAN, D. W. (1969). *Internat. J. Neuropharm.* **8**, 549.
KAKIUCHI, S. & RALL, T. W. (1968). *Mol. Pharmacol.* **4**, 367, 379.
KAKIUCHI, S., RALL, T. W. & MCILWAIN, H. (1969). *J. Neurochem.* **16**, 485.
KASA, P. & SILVER, A. (1969). *J. Neurochem.* **16**, 389.
KATZ, R. I. & KOPIN, I. J. (1969). *Biochem. Pharmacol.* **18**, 1935; *Pharmacol. Res. Commun.* **1**, 54.
KATZ, R. I., CHASE, T. N. & KOPIN, I. J. (1969). *J. Neurochem.* **16**, 961.
KAWAI, N. & YAMAMOTO, C. (1968). *Brain Res.* **7**, 325.
KEGLEVIĆ, D., KVEDER, S. & ISKRIŤ, S. (1968). *Adv. Pharmacol.* **6A**, 79.
KERKUT, G. A. (1969). *Endeavour*, **28**, 22.
KERR, S. E., HAMPEL, C. W. & GHANTUS, M. (1937). *J. biol. Chem.* **119**, 405.
KINDWALL, E. P. & WEINER, N. (1966). *J. Neurochem.* **13**, 1523.
KOELLE, G. B. (1963). (Ed.). *Handbuch d. exper. Pharmacol.* **15**. Cholinesterases and Anticholinesterase Agents. Berlin: Springer.
KOPIN, I. J., PARE, C. M. B., AXELROD, J. & WEISSBACH, H. (1961). *J. biol. Chem.* **236**, 3072.
KORKES, S., CAMPILLO, A. DEL, KOREY, S. R., STERN, J. R., NACHMANSOHN, D. & OCHOA, S. (1952). *J. biol. Chem.* **198**, 215.
KRNJEVIĆ, K. & PHILLIS, J. W. (1963). *J. Physiol.* **166**, 296, 328.
KRNJEVIĆ, K., RANDIĆ, M. & STRAUGHAN, D. W. (1966). *J. Physiol.* **184**, 78.
KRNJEVIĆ, K. & SCHWARTZ, S. (1967). *Exper. Brain Res.* **3**, 306, 320.
KUHAR, M. J., SHASKAN, E. G. & SYNDER, S. H. (1971). *J. Neurochem.* **18**, 333.
KUNTZMAN, R., SHORE, P. A., BOGDANSKI, D. & BRODIE, B. B. (1961). *J. Neurochem.*, **6**, 226.
KURIYAMA, K., ROBERTS, E. & KAKEFUDA, T. (1968). *Brain Res.* **8**, 132.
KUROKAWA, M., MACHIYAMA, Y. & KATO, M. (1963). *J. Neurochem.* **10**, 341.
LAWLER, H. C. (1963). *Biochim. Biophys. Acta*, **81**, 280.
LEIMDORFER, A. (1950). *J. Pharmacol.* **98**, 62.
LERNER, A. B., CASE, J. D. & TAKAHASHI, Y. (1960). *J. biol. Chem.* **235**, 1992.
LEUZINGER, W. (1969). *Progr. Brain Res.* **31**, 241.
LEWIS, J. L. & MCILWAIN, H. (1954). *Biochem. J.* **57**, 680.
LIANG, C. C. & QUASTEL, J. H. (1969). *Biochem. Pharmacol.* **18**, 1169.

LICHTENSTEIGER, W. & LANGEMANN, H. (1966). *J. Pharmacol.* **151**, 400.

LINTS, C. E. & HARVEY, J. A. (1969). *Physiol. Behaviour*, **4**, 29; *J. comp. Physiol. Psychol.* **67**, 23.

LIPTON, M. A. & UDENFRIEND, S. (1968). In Efron (1968), p. 7.

LOVENBERG, W., JEQUIER, E. & SJERDSMA, A. (1968). *Adv. Pharmacol.* **6B**, 21.

LUCAS, R. A. (1963). *Progr. med. Chem.* **3**, 146.

MACINTOSH, F. C. (1963). *Canad. J. Biochem. Physiol.* **41**, 2555.

MACON, J. B., SOKOLOFF, L. & GLOWINSKI, J. (1971). *J. Neurochem.* **18**, 323.

MANN, P. J. G., TENNENBAUM, M. & QUASTEL, J. H. (1939). *Biochem. J.* **33**, 822.

MANNARINO, E., KIRSHNER, N. & NASHOLD, B. S. (1962). *Fed. Proc.* **21**, 182.

MARCHBANKS, R. M. (1966). *J. Neurochem.* **13**, 1481.

MARCHBANKS, R. M. (1968). *Biochem. J.* **110**, 533.

MARCHBANKS, R. M. (1969). *Biochem. Pharmacol.* **18**, 1763; *Sympos. Intern. Soc. Cell Biol.* **8**, 115.

MARTIN, A. R., WICKELGREN, W. O. & BERANEK, R. (1970). *J. Physiol.* **207**, 653.

MARTIN, W. R. & SLOAN, J. W. (1970). *Psychopharmacologia*, **18**, 231.

MASAMI, M., HIROSHI, Y. & REIJI, I. (1962). *Biochem. Pharmacol.* **11**, 1109.

MATSUDA, T., SAITO, K., KATSUKI, S., HATA, F. & YOSHIDA, H. (1971). *J. Neurochem.* **18**, 713.

MAYNERT, E. W., LEVI, R. & DE LORENZO, A. J. D. (1964). *J. Pharmacol.* **144**, 385.

MCCAMAN, R. E. (1965). *Life Sci.* **4**, 2353.

MCCAMAN, R. E., MCCAMAN, M. W., HUNT, J. M. & SMITH, M. S. (1965). *J. Neurochem.* **12**, 15.

MCCAMAN, R. E., ARNAIZ, G. R. DE L. & DE ROBERTIS, E. (1965). *J. Neurochem.* **12**, 927.

MCCONNELL, W. B. (1963). *Brit. J. Psychiat.* **109**, 218.

MCGEER, E. G., GILSON, S., WADA, J. A. & MCGEER, P. L. (1967). *Canad. J. Biochem.* **45**, 1943.

MCILWAIN, H. (1957). Chemotherapy and the Central Nervous System. London: Churchill.

MCILWAIN, H. (1971). In *Effects of Drugs on Cellular Control Mechanisms*. Ed. Rabin & Freedman. London: Macmillan.

MCILWAIN, H., HARVEY, J. A. & RODRIGUEZ, R. (1969). *J. Neurochem.* **16**, 363.

MCILWAIN, H. & SNYDER, S. H. (1970). *J. Neurochem.* **17**, 521.

MCLENNAN, H. (1965). *Experentia*, **21**, 725.

MCLENNAN, H., CURRY, L. & WALKER, R. (1963). *Biochem. J.* **89**, 163.

MICHAELSON, I. A. & DOWE, G. (1963). *Biochem. Pharm.* **12**, 949.

MICHAELSON, I. A. & WHITTAKER, V. P. (1962–3). *Biochem. Pharmacol.* **11**, 505; **12**, 203.

MITCHELL, J. F. (1963). *J. Physiol.* **165**, 98.

MITCHELL, J. F. & SRINIVASAN, V. (1969). *Nature*, **224**, 663.

MOLENAAR, P. C., NICKOLSON, V. J. & POLAK, R. L. (1971). *J. Physiol.* **213**, 64P.

MONTAGU, K. (1963). *Biochem. J.* **86**, 9.

NEFF, N. H., LIN, R. C., NGAI, S. H. & COSTA, E. (1969). *Adv. Biochem. Psychopharm.* **1**, 91.

NG, K. Y., COLBURN, R. W. & KOPIN, I. J. (1971). *Nature, Lond.* **230**, 331.

OBATA, K. & TAKEDA, K. (1969). *J. Neurochem.* **16**, 1043.

OGSTON, A. G. (1955). *J. Physiol.* **128**, 222.

NACHMANSOHN, D. (1959). Chemical and Molecular Basis of Nerve Activity. New York: Academic Press.

NAGATSU, T., LEVITT, M. & UDENFRIEND, S. (1964). *J. biol. Chem.* **239**, 2910.

PAASONEN, M. K., MACLEAN, P. D. & GIARMAN, N. J. (1957). *J. Neurochem.* **1**, 326.

PAGE, I. H. (1954). *Physiol. Rev.* **34**, 563.

PAGE, I. H. (1969). In Bourne (1969), p. 289.

PAPPIUS, H. M. & ELLIOTT, K. A. C. (1958). *J. Appl. Physiol.* **12**, 319.

PELLEGRINO DE IRALDI, A., ZIEHER, L. M. & ETCHEVERRY, G. J. (1968). *Adv. Pharmacol.* **6A**, 257.

PEPEU, G., SCHMIDT, N. F. & GIARMAN, N. J. (1962). *Biochem. Pharmacol.* **12**, 385.

PERRY, T. L., HANSEN, S., FOULKS, J. G. & LING, G. M. (1965). *J. Neurochem.* **12**, 397.

PHILIPPA, A., HEYD, G. & BURGER, A. (1970). *Europ. J. Pharmacol.* **9**, 52.
POPE, A., CAVENESS, W. & LIVINGSTONE, K. E. (1952). *Arch. Neurol. Psychiat.* **68**, 425.
PORTIG, P. J. & VOGT, M. (1969). *J. Physiol.* **204**, 687.
PULL, I., MCILWAIN, H. & RAMSAY, R. L. (1970). *Biochem. J.* **116**, 181.
PURPURA, D. P., GIVADO, M., SMITH, T. G., CALLAN, D. A. & GRUNDFEST, H. (1959). *J. Neurochem.* **3**, 238.
QUAY, W. B. & WILHOFT, D. C. (1964). *J. Neurochem.* **11**, 805.
RALL, T. W. & SUTHERLAND, E. W. (1958). *J. biol. Chem.* **232**, 1065.
RAMSAY, R. L. & MCILWAIN, H. (1970). *J. Neurochem.* **17**, 781.
REITER, R. J. (1967). *Neuroendocrinol.* **2**, 138.
RICHTER, D. & CROSSLAND, J. (1949). *Amer. J. Physiol.* **159**, 247.
RICHTER, J. A. & MARCHBANKS, R. M. (1971). J. *Neurochem.* **18** (in press).
ROBERTS, E. (1960) (Ed.). Inhibition in the Nervous System and γ-Aminobutyric acid. Oxford: Pergamon.
ROBSON, J. M. & STACEY, R. S. (1962). Recent Advances in Pharmacology. London: Churchill.
ROTHLIN, E. (1947). *Bull. Acad. suisse Sci. med.* **2**, 1.
ROWSELL, E. V. (1954). *Biochem. J.* **57**, 666.
RUTLEDGE, C. O. & JONASON, J. (1968). *Europ. J. Pharmacol.* **4**, 264.
RYALL, R. W., STONE, N. & WATKINS, J. C. (1964). *J. Neurochem.* **11**, 634.
SALMOIRAGHI, G. C. & STEFANIS, C. N. (1967). *Int. Rev. Neurobiol.* **10**, 1.
SANO, I., TANIGUCHI, K., GAMO, T., TAKESADA, M. & KAKIMOTO, Y. (1960). *Klin. Wochschr.* **38**, 5.
SATTIN, A. (1965). *Biochem J.* **96**, 48P.
SATTIN, A. & RALL, T. W. (1970). *Mol. Pharmacol.* **6**, 13.
SCHAYER, R. W. & REILLY, M. (1970). *J. Neurochem.* **17**, 1649.
SCHUBERTH, J., SPARF, B. & SUNDWALL, A. (1969). *J. Neurochem.* **16**, 965.
SCHWARTZ, J. C., LAMPERT, C. & ROSE, C. (1970). *J. Neurochem.* **17**, 1527.
SHANK, R. P. & APRISON, M. H. (1970). *J. Neurochem.* **17**, 1461.
SHEARD, M. H. & AGHAJANIAN, G. K. (1968). *J. Pharmacol.* **163**, 425.
SHORE, P. A. & BRODIE, B. B. (1957). In Psychotropic Drugs. Ed. Garattini. Amsterdam: Elsevier.
SNYDER, S. H., GREEN, A. I. & HENDLEY, E. D. (1968). *J. Pharmacol.* **164**, 90.
SNYDER, S. H. & HENDLEY, E. D. (1968). *J. Pharmacol.* **163**, 386.
SNYDER, S. H., KUHAR, M. J., GREEN, A. I., COYLE, J. T. & SHASKAN, E. G. (1970). *Internat. Rev. Neurobiol.* **13**, 127.
SNYDER, S. H. & RICHELSON, E. (1968) *Proc. nat. Acad. Sci. U.S.A.* **60**, 206.
SOLLENBERG, J. & SORBO, B. (1969). *J. Neurochem.* **17**, 201.
SOURKES, T. L., MURPHY, G. F., CHAVEZ, B. & ZIELINSKA, M. (1961). *J. Neurochem.* **8**, 109.
SPECTOR, S. (1968). In Efron (1968), p. 13.
SPECTOR, S., SHORE, P. A. & BRODIE, B. B. (1960). *J. Pharmacol.* **128**, 15.
SPEHLMANN, R. (1963). *J. Neurophysiol.* **26**, 127.
STONE, W. E. (1957). *Amer. J. Phys. Med.* **36**, 222.
SULZER, F. & BASS, A. D. (1968). In Efron (1968), p. 1065.
Symposium (1957a). *Ann. N.Y. Acad. Sci.* **66**, 417.
Symposium (1957b). *Proc. Internat. Sympos. Psychotropic Drugs.* Amsterdam: Elsevier.
Symposium (1958). 5-Hydroxytryptamine. Ed. Lewis. London: Pergamon.
Symposium (1959). *Pharmacol. Rev.* **11**, 232.
Symposium (1960). Adrenergic Mechanisms. Ed. Vane, Wolstenholme & O'Connor. Ciba Foundation. London: Churchill.
Symposium (1961). *Proc. Internat. Neurochem. Sympos.* **4**.
Symposium (1962). Enzymes and Drug Action. Ed. Mongar & De Reuck. Ciba Foundation. London: Churchill.
Symposium (1963). The Clinical Chemistry of Monoamines. Ed. Varley & Gowenlock. Amsterdam: Elsevier.
Symposium (1964). Animal Behaviour and Drug Action. Ed. Steinberg, De Reuck & Knight. Ciba Foundation. London: Churchill.

Symposium (1964*a*). Biogenic Amines. Ed. Himwich & Himwich. Amsterdam: Elsevier.
Symposium (1970). V. Internat. Symp. on Neurosecretion. Ed. Bargmann, W. & Scharrer, B. Berlin: Springer.
Symposium (1971). *The Pineal Gland.* Edit. Wolstenholme, G. E. W. & Knight, J. London: Churchill Livingstone.
TAKAHASHI, R. & APRISON, M. H. (1964). *J. Neurochem.* **11**, 887.
TAKENO, K., NISHIŌ, A. & YANAGIYA, I. (1969). *J. Neurochem.* **16**, 47.
TAYLOR, K. M. & LAVERTY, P. (1969). *J. Neurochem.* **16**, 1367.
TOH, C. C. (1960). *J. Physiol.* **151**, 410.
TOH, C. C. (1963, 1964). *J. Physiol.* **165**, 47; **173**, 420.
TOWER, D. B. (1960). Neurochemistry of Epilepsy. Springfield: Thomas.
TOWER, D. B. (1969). In Basic Mechanisms of the Epilepsies, p. 611. Ed. H. H. Jasper, A. A. Ward and A. Pope. Boston: Little, Brown.
TRANZER, J. P., THOLMEN, H., SNIPES, R. L. & RICHARDS, J. G. (1969). *Progr. Brain Res.* **31**, 33.
UDENFRIEND, S. & CREVELING, C. R. (1959). *J. Neurochem.* **4**, 350.
VAN HARREVELD, A. & FIFKOVÁ, E. (1971). *J. Neurobiol.* **2**, 13.
VARON, S., WEINSTEIN, H., KAKEFUDA, T. & ROBERTS, E. (1965). *Biochem. Pharmacol.* **14**, 1213.
VOGEL, W. H. & ORFEI, V. (1967). *Fed. Proc.* **26**, 615.
WEBER, G. (1952). *Bull. schweiz. Akad. med. Wiss.* **8**, 263.
WEIGHT, F. F. & SALMOIRAGHI, C. C. (1968). *Adv. Pharmacol.* **6A**, 395.
WEIL-MALHERBE, H., WHITBY, L. G. & AXELROD, J. (1961). *J. Neurochem.* **8**, 55.
WEISSBACH, H., REDFIELD, B. G. & AXELROD, J. (1960). *Biochim. biophys. Acta.* **43**, 352.
WELSH, J. H. (1968). *Adv. Pharmacol.* **6A**, 171.
WHITE, R. P. & NASH, C. B. (1963). *Internat. J. Neuropharmacol.* **2**, 249.
WHITTAKER, V. P. (1951). *Physiol. Rev.* **31**, 312.
WHITTAKER, V. P. (1963). *Handb. d. exper. Pharmakol.* **15**, 1.
WHITTAKER, V. P. (1965). *Progr. Biophys. mol. Biol.* **15**, 41.
WHITTAKER, V. P. (1969). *Progr. Brain Res.* **31**, 1.
WHITTAKER, V. P. & SHERIDAN, M. N. (1965). *J. Neurochem.* **12**, 363.
WILSON, I. (1960). The Enzymes, 4, 501. Ed. Boyer. New York: Academic Press.
WONG, R. & WHITESIDE, C. B. C. (1968). *J. Endocrinol.* **40**, 383.
WURTMAN, R. J., AXELROD, J. & KELLY, D. E. (1968). The Pineal. New York: Academic Press.
WURTMAN, R. J. & AXELROD, J. (1968). *Adv. Pharmacol.* **6A**, 141.
YOUDIM, M. B. H., CARTER, S. B., SANDLER, M., HANINGTON, E. &. WILKINSON, M. (1971). *Nature,* **230**, 127.
YOUDIM, M. B. H., COLLINS, G. G. S. & SANDLER, M. (1969). *Nature, Lond.* **223**, 626.
ZWEIG, M. & AXELROD, J. (1969). *J. Neurobiol.* **1**, 87.

17

15 Drugs Acting on the Central Nervous System

Drug action displays the extreme susceptibility of the brain to alteration in its chemical environment. The traditional materia medica which selected naturally-occurring substances for medicinally-useful actions included many materials which acted centrally, either by deliberate choice or as undesirable side-effects to action elsewhere in the body. The same themes persist in currently produced synthetic drugs: probably every cerebral function can be modified by administered substances, but it remains a major problem to devise compounds with specified, therapeutically-useful properties.

Biochemical factors are involved with centrally-acting drugs at numerous points: (1) in their design; (2) in determining at what parts of the brain they arrive, and in what form: this is a specialized aspect of the bodily distribution and metabolism of the drug; (3) in understanding their immediate action at cellular level; and (4) in observing how the brain adapts to the drug: this is especially important in drugs of addiction but features also in, for example, the action of anticonvulsants

The drugs described below display the biochemical factors just enumerated. More chemical aspects of recently-devised centrally-acting agents are given by Gordon (1967); pharmacological aspects by Brill et al (1967), Efron (1968) and Burger (1968); animal behavioural aspects by Steinberg et al. (1964, 1969).

General Depressants

The first success in synthesizing chemical substances to control cerebral activities was achieved with the anaesthetics used surgically. Several of the substances introduced over 100 years ago are still in use: nitrous oxide, ether and chloroform. Recently-developed anaesthetics as halothane, $CF_3 . CHClBr$, have much the same action but a minimum of undesirable side-effects or incidental properties. The loss of sensation caused by these substances is accompanied by loss of consciousness and their effects considered collectively are not clearly distinguishable except in degree from those of the class of depressants used more frequently as hypnotics, for example the barbiturates. Their common effect of depression of the central nervous system is, curiously, usually preceded by a stage of excitement which varies in prominence with the different depressants and also in different individuals, and which receives comment

506

below (see Table 15.4). Consciousness and control of bodily activities are modified in various ways before finally being lost, and during this progression of events both the electrical and metabolic activities of the brain are observed to undergo change.

Metabolic Effects *in vivo*

Two main techniques have given information on chemical changes in the brain during anaesthesia. Respiration has been measured by determining the arteriovenous difference in oxygen and the rate of blood flow in experimental animals and in man, and labile cerebral constituents have been determined after rapidly fixing the brain of anaesthetized experimental animals.

During early stages of the action of depressants, when frequency and potential seen in the electroencephalogram may increase, little or no change in overall cerebral respiration has been found. It falls, however, by some 30% when, with sleep or light surgical anaesthesia induced by pentobarbitone, "spindles" are seen in the EEG, and by some 45% with deep anaesthesia when the frequency and potential of all components of the EEG have fallen. Thus the major energy-yielding reaction of the brain is very considerably depressed. Comparable depression of cerebral respiration can be brought about in other ways (Chapter 2) but is always associated with major changes in cerebral functioning. Barbiturates have also been shown to lower the respiration of the perfused brain. The partly-isolated brain remains susceptible to depressants: in the *cerveau isolé* of the cat, halothane, pentobarbitone, diallylbarbituric acid and a thiobarbiturate diminished the frequency of cell-firing. This occurred with concentrations of the barbiturates used as hypnotics, when the cell-firing was spontaneous and when it was induced by acetylcholine (Crawford, 1970).

Analysis of the brain itself during anaesthesia gives information on the linkage between the depression of activity and that in respiration. The cerebral tissues of normal and of anaesthetized animals are found to differ in their content of important metabolites and these differences are given in Chapter 3. They include, firstly, another change which can be taken as indicating a decrease in energy-yielding reactions of the tissue: the cerebral content of lactic acid is low in animals anaesthetized with pentobarbitone or allobarbitone. Nevertheless, in spite of this decrease and of that in cerebral respiration, the content of energy-rich substances in the brain of the anaesthetized animals is high. Cerebral glycogen can be increased three-fold by barbiturates in mice or rats; phosphocreatine is a third above its normal level, adenosine triphosphate is slightly increased and the inorganic phosphate formed when they break down in supporting cerebral activities, is low (Lowry *et al.*, 1964; Nelson *et al.*, 1968).

Thus, of the changes in respiration and of functioning in the anaesthetized animals, it would appear that the depression in functioning was the preponderating action and that this led to a lesser utilization of substances including glycogen and phosphocreatine. Their accumulation is thus understandable, as also is the lower level of their products, lactate, inorganic phosphate and phosphate acceptors; and this is known from previous consideration (Chapter 7) to lead to lowered respiration and glycolysis in cerebral tissues.

Respiration of cerebral tissues may also, as will be indicated shortly, be lowered directly by the depressants but must be predominantly affected by the route just described. For if the preponderating effect had been to inhibit respiration, then cerebral levels of glycogen and phosphocreatine would have been expected to be low and of lactic acid to be high, as is the case in anoxia or in cyanide intoxication: circumstances which also lower cerebral activities but in a fashion very different from general anaesthesia. Also, interestingly, it would appear that the toxic effects of general depressants themselves, effects which are clearly distinguishable from their effects as depressants, are due in large measure to direct inhibition of cerebral respiration. In an instance in which analyses were carried out in animals with a toxic dose of pentobarbital, cerebral energy-rich phosphates were low and their products, and lactic acid, were high (LePage, 1946).

Metabolic and Electrical Effects *in vitro*

The pattern of biochemical changes induced in the brain during anaesthesia is not brought about when depressants are added to separated cerebral tissues respiring under normal conditions *in vitro*. The differences are listed in Table 15.1: with sufficient depressant, respiration of the tissue may be lowered, but

Table 15.1

Pattern of chemical change during the action of depressant and convulsive agents

	Changes caused by depressants				
	In the brain *in vivo*		In cerebral tissues *in vitro*		Changes caused by convulsants
Property measured	During anaesthesia	At toxic levels	Under ordinary conditions	With electrical stimulation	
Respiration	−	−	−	−	+
Lactic acid accumulation	−	+	+	−	+
Phosphocreatine level	+	−	−	+	−
Inorganic phosphate level	−	+	+	−	+

Increase: +; decrease: −, caused by concentrations of the agents just sufficient to bring about the changes noted in respiration, and when compared with tissues lacking the agent but otherwise under identical conditions. Changes *in vivo*: see Chapters 2 and 3. Changes *in vitro*: Quastel, Colloquium, 1951; Anguiano & McIlwain, 1951; Buchel & McIlwain, 1950; McIlwain, 1953 and *Symposium*, 1962; Cohen & Heald, 1960.

this lowering is accompanied by decrease in phosphocreatine and by increase in lactic acid. These changes are the reverse of those occurring during anaesthesia and are akin rather to the toxic effects of the depressants; indeed, the concentrations of depressants needed for these effects correspond to the toxic rather than to the anaesthetic levels of the drugs.

This phenomenon is understandable when it is recalled that *in vivo* measurements indicate that the depressants affect first the functioning of the brain, and only in consequence or in higher concentrations, its respiration. Thus they might act *in vitro* in converting a higher to a lower level of activity, and this can be tested by examining their effects on the electrically stimulated tissue described in Chapter 4. It is then found, as shown in Fig. 15.1 that a concentration of phenobarbitone which has little or no action on the respiration of the tissue in absence of applied electrical pulses, in their presence inhibits respiration by some 40%. Butobarbitone and chloral behaved similarly. Inhibition is also increased when respiration is stimulated by other means, and the effect of depressants on the stimulated tissue, as *in vivo*, is not a permanent one, but is

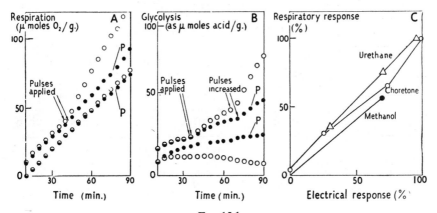

FIG. 15.1.

A and B. Selective effect of depressants on the metabolism of electrically stimulated respiration A and glycolysis B of separated guinea pig cerebral cortex. Data obtained manometrically with the vessels of B, Fig. 4.2 (McIlwain, 1953). Tissues were unstimulated during the first 40 minutes, after which electrical pulses were applied to the two indicated. P: containing 0·7 or 1·7 mM-phenobarbitone; the others contained no depressant but were otherwise similar. Some ordinates displaced for clarity.

C. Parallelism in the effect of three depressants on electrical and respiratory responses to stimulation of the stellate ganglion of the cat (Larrabee & Bronk, 1952; Edwards & Larrabee, 1955). Respiratory response was measured potentiometrically in the apparatus of A, Fig. 4.2. The electrical response measured was the height of the postganglionic action potential. Different points with a given depressant represent the effects of different concentrations of the substance.

lost when the depressant is removed. Moreover, glycolysis in the separated electrically stimulated tissue is depressed and the breakdown of phosphocreatine which normally follows electrical pulses is diminished, again in parallel with events *in vivo* during anaesthesia (Table 15.1).

These findings have been explored further by electrical observations of conduction and cell discharge in isolated cerebral tissues (Yamamoto & McIlwain, 1966; Campbell, 1967; McIlwain, 1968b). A non-toxic level of phenobarbitone is shown by Fig. 4.10 to permit conduction in a sensory tract in the brain, but to prevent the normal cortical response to such conducted impulses. The normal postsynaptic responses reappeared when the barbiturate was washed away from the tissue. Ether displayed a similar reversible inhibition.

Synaptic transmission at certain ganglia is affected also by depressants at concentrations equal to or often only a little greater than those giving anaesthesia (Table 15.2). On stimulating a suitable isolated ganglion such as the stellate ganglion of the cat several phenomena can be observed simultaneously: transmission by a direct, non-synaptic route; transmission by a synapse within the ganglion, and also the respiratory change associated with the induced activity. Depressants are found to act on these processes as shown in Table 15.2 and Fig. 15.1. Synaptic transmission proves much more sensitive to most

Table 15.2

Concentrations and activities of depressants

Depressant	Concentration needed for surgical anaesthesia (mM)	Concentration blocking ganglion			
		Synaptic transmission		Axonal conduction	
		(mM)	Activity[1]	(mM)	Activity[1]
Ethanol	76	478	0·032	240	0·02
Ethyl ether	18	34	0·042	96	0·12
Chloroform	2·7	4·4	0·063	13·2	0·19
Pentobarbitone	0·2	0·2[2]	–	1·8	–
n-Octanol	–	0·12	0·027	0·55	0·12

Data from Posternak & Larrabee (*Colloquium*, 1951), Larrabee & Posternak (1952) and sources quoted by those authors. Concentrations needed for surgical anaesthesia are mainly from observations in man; the ganglion studied was the stellate ganglion of the cat. For application of similar considerations to anaesthesia in other systems, see Larsen, Van Dyke & Chenoweth, in Burger (1968); and Mullins, (1971).

[1] Thermodynamic activity measured by: the partial pressure of the substance concerned in the vapour phase in equilibrium with its solution of the strength quoted, as a fraction of the vapour pressure of the pure substance.

[2] 0·2 or less in the cat; 0·14 in the cervical ganglia of the rat and 0·35 in those of the rabbit.

depressants than is axonal conduction by the non-synaptic route; and there is remarkably close parallelism between the lowering of the postsynaptic action potential and depression of the respiration of the ganglion.

Action of the depressants both in ganglia and in isolated cerebral tissues, involves both the raising of the threshold for response, and diminution of the response obtained. This is shown in cerebral tissues by the respiratory data plotted in Fig. 15.3.

General and Physical Properties of the Depressants

Substances causing anaesthesia in man or experimental animals include some which are chemically almost inert, as argon, krypton or xenon, and also nitrogen gas (Haldane, *Colloquium*, 1951; Featherstone & Muehlbaecher, 1963). These substances as well as the anaesthetics or hypnotics already discussed have depressant effects on a wide range of living organisms including those without distinct nervous systems, though concentrations greater than those needed for anaesthesia are commonly needed in the other circumstances. Effects then include inhibition of cell-division, of motility, photosynthesis and bioluminescence.

Curiously, if a series of depressants is placed in an order of effectiveness depending on the concentration required to cause one such effect, the order is often the same as that of the order of effectiveness in a quite distinct system. Further, these relationships can be expressed quantitatively: the ratio of effective concentrations of two depressants may be closely similar for action on weevils and on mice. These relatively simple relationships hold especially for the more chemically inert depressants, and not for substances actively metabolized *in vivo*.

Moreover, it has been found possible to correlate the concentrations of different depressants which are effective in a given biological system, with several of their purely physical properties. The first such correlations noted were with lipid solubility and adsorption: when depressants were shaken in oil–water or in charcoal–water mixtures, until the composition of the different phases was constant, the substances whose distribution was most in favour of the oil or the charcoal were the more active biologically. Adsorption and liquid–liquid distribution are two properties which can be expressed simply in terms of the chemical potential or thermodynamic activity of a substance, as also can its vapour pressure or solubility. Expressed in this way, substances very diverse in structure can bring about a similar degree of depression at comparable thermodynamic activities (Ferguson, 1939). Thus the concentrations needed of the five substances of Table 15.2, in order to block synaptic transmission through the stellate ganglion of the cat, vary over a 4,000-fold range: but their thermodynamic activities differ by little more than two-fold.

The purely physical effects of depressants make understandable several features in their action and although they do not themselves localize this they limit the types of action possible. Two types of action remain feasible, despite the limited reactivity of the inert gases. (i) The depressants may act by their mere presence, as diluents or forming a barrier or displacing components at some structure or interface. This leads to ideas of solution in or association with lipids of cell membranes, so diminishing membrane permeability. Conclusions regarding the actions of local anaesthetics are relevant here: examination of a series of compounds including alcohols and cocaine (Skou, 1961), suggested that penetration to lipid monolayers, with resultant effects on the entry of Na^+ during the nerve impulse, were involved in their action. (ii) The depressants may interact with water in a fashion which occurs even with xenon and leads to clathyrate compounds or labile micro-crystalline associations between the water molecules around the xenon (Pauling, 1961; Miller, 1961). It is pictured that the polar groups of proteins take part in such associations and so become less available for their normal functioning (Featherstone & Muehlbaecher, 1963). Association of xenon with cerebral proteins was made likely by finding that the solubility of the gas in preparations from the brain was greater than the amount which would dissolve in the water and the lipids which the preparations contained (Kwan & Trevor, 1969).

Balance of Inhibition during Anaesthesia

The correlations noted above suggest a mechanism devised in relation to the inert gases to apply also to other general depressants. Results which include those of Table 15.2 then suggest the structures most sensitive to depressants to be associated with synaptic transmission. Possibly it is the multiplicity of membrane structures in the fine dendrites and nerve endings of the cerebral cortex which constitute surfaces making it the most sensitive part of higher animals to the action of the depressants.

The level of activity of the cerebral cortex has, further, been shown electro-physiologically to be susceptible to increase or decrease from lower parts of the brain (see below; Table 15.4). It is probably important that a general depressant includes in its action the brain-stem activating system and that this contributes to inducing sleep by a relatively normal route. Cerebral blood flow in most grey-matter areas of the brain of cats was diminished in light thiopentone (pentothal) anaesthesia; action at the sensory cortex (-50%) was especially prominent, and a small diminution (-17%) was observed at the reticular formation of the brain stem (Kety, *Symposium*, 1963). The main occasion for the use of general depressants in surgical anaesthesia, involves depression of cerebral activities to a much greater degree than does sleep, but nevertheless this is done reversibly and in many aspects of cerebral functioning.

Knowing the actions of depressants in a wide range of biological systems, enables their effects in different cerebral preparations to be seen in adequate perspective. Thus parallelism is found in a series of depressants between the order of their effectiveness as anaesthetics, and in inhibiting respiration during ordinary, unstimulated metabolism of the separated tissue. Such parallelism is however a feature of depressant action in very diverse systems and does not imply that the respiratory inhibition is the basis for anaesthesia. The depressants also inhibit respiration and phosphorylation in cerebral and other mitochondria (Bain, 1957; Aldridge, McIlwain: *Symposium*, 1962). Physical association between components of the respiratory chain is important to their action and it is presumably such structural relations which are affected by the depressants. But, especially in view of the results of Table 15.1, it appears unlikely that mitochondrial structures should be those most sensitive to depressants in the brain *in vivo*, and indeed there is clear evidence from phosphocreatine levels that during anaesthesia energy-yielding processes are not depressed as much as are the processes utilizing the phosphates produced.

It is probable, however, that during the action of a successful anaesthetic some degree of balance is necessary between inhibition of energy-yielding and of energy-consuming processes. Inhibition of one or the other of these does not produce anaesthesia. The effects of anoxia or hypoglycaemia on the one hand, or of a blocking agent such as atropine on the other, are very different from anaesthesia. It can hardly be coincidence that the successful anaesthetics have widespread effects in a multiplicity of biological systems. Probably to depress successfully the action of so complex an organization as that of the brain, inhibition is necessary of a variety of very different pro-cesses including some outside the brain. A greater or lesser imbalance in such inhibition (for example, of energy-yielding and energy-consuming processes) may contribute to certain barbiturates being convulsant, and to the transient phase of excitation in the action of most depressants.

Anticonvulsants and Epilepsy

Chemical involvement in the initiation of convulsive seizures has been described in discussing anoxia, galactose, glutamic acid, cerebral cations, acetylcholine, electrical excitation and pyridoxine (q.v.). The multiplicity of initiating factors contributes to the viewpoint that such seizures represent a very general reaction-type to which the brain is susceptible. The initiating factors have been taken as neurochemical models in understanding epilepsy or in devising anticonvulsants (Tower, 1960, and in Jasper et al., 1969).

Chemical initiating factors which produce chronic epileptic foci include metallic powders, especially cobalt, and hydrated alumina. These when placed on the cerebral cortex cause spontaneous convulsive episodes, starting from the site of application and recurring over a period of months or years (Ward, in Jasper et al., 1969). In this they are analogous to the many instances of epilepsy which follow local injury to the brain. An important model in suggesting causation in these instances is that afforded by denervation hypersensitivity. Also, the local escape of endogenous substances may be involved. Seizures, once initiated by these various agents may be pictured to extend beyond the initial foci by neural connections and by processes analogous to those of spreading depression (q.v.); they then involve the large expenditure of metabolically-derived energy described below in discussing convulsive agents.

Anticonvulsant Drugs

An initial seizure tendency can be chemically augmented by convulsants or depressed by anticonvulsants. Anticonvulsants proper are not general depressants, although some compounds including phenobarbitone show both properties. Anticonvulsants are clearly required to depress particular types of cerebral activities: those associated with the epilepsies or with convulsions which can be caused experimentally to originate in the central nervous system. Their success in clinical use depends on doing this with minimal action as general depressants. The two or three main types of epilepsy are antagonized most effectively by different drugs several of which exhibit intriguing structural relationships (Fig. 15.2): trimethadione and ethosuccimide are of most value in petit mal, diphenylhydantoin in grand mal, and primidone in grand mal and psychomotor epilepsy. These agents, in concentrations used as anticonvulsants, have little or no effect on the electroencephalogram or on other indications of cerebral activity observed in normal subjects, but specifically depress the sudden bursts at high frequency and high voltage which occur in the brain in epilepsy, and at the same time minimize the seizures which are associated with the electrical changes. Several anticonvulsants are, however, not closely related in structure to those named; for instance, certain propanediols. For accounts for the development of anticonvulsants, see McIlwain (1957) and Spinks & Waring (1963).

The anticonvulsants have general metabolic effects in so far as they antagon- ize the normal metabolic sequelae to convulsive activity. More specific effects in the animal body as a whole have not been found to be of general occurrence among anticonvulsants, though many factors which affect bodily physiology affect the frequency of seizures in epileptic subjects. Pyridoxine and glutamic acid have already been discussed in this connection (Chapters 8 and 10). The factors include also salt and water balance, and either for this reason, or because steroids have direct effects on cerebral excitability, the level of adrenal

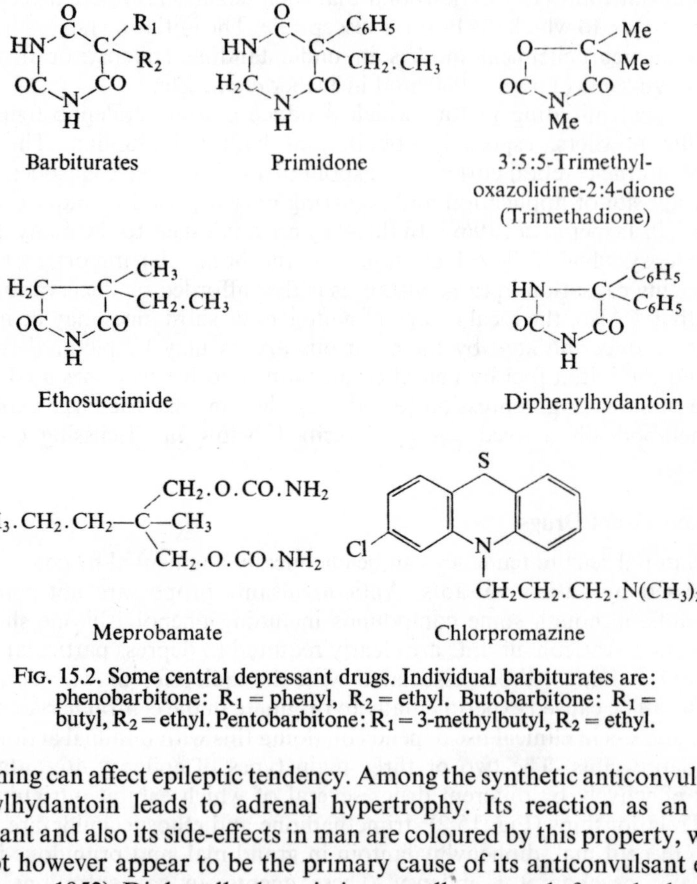

Barbiturates   Primidone   3:5:5-Trimethyl-
oxazolidine-2:4-dione
(Trimethadione)

Ethosuccimide   Diphenylhydantoin

Meprobamate   Chlorpromazine

FIG. 15.2. Some central depressant drugs. Individual barbiturates are: phenobarbitone: R_1 = phenyl, R_2 = ethyl. Butobarbitone: R_1 = butyl, R_2 = ethyl. Pentobarbitone: R_1 = 3-methylbutyl, R_2 = ethyl.

functioning can affect epileptic tendency. Among the synthetic anticonvulsants diphenylhydantoin leads to adrenal hypertrophy. Its reaction as an anti- convulsant and also its side-effects in man are coloured by this property, which does not however appear to be the primary cause of its anticonvulsant effect (Woodbury, 1952). Diphenylhydantoin is normally excreted after p-hydroxyla- tion; individuals genetically lacking this reaction are unusually susceptible to toxic side-effects of the drug, which include nystagmus, drowsiness and ataxia (Kutt et al., 1964).

Cerebral Metabolic Effects

Diphenylhydantoin and certain other anticonvulsants alter electrolyte concentrations in the brain itself, and also the excitability of isolated cerebral tissues (Koch & Woodbury, 1960; Greengard & McIlwain, 1955; Woodbury, and McIlwain, in Jasper *et al.*, 1969). After giving rats four doses of diphenyl-hydantoin, of 40 mg./kg. at 6-hr. intervals, their cerebral Na decreased when expressed as a concentration in a (theoretical: see Chapter 4) non-chloride space; a fall of 35% occurred. Administration of a ^{22}Na salt now showed a more rapid entry of ^{22}Na to the brain of the treated than of control animals, suggesting therefore that ^{22}Na extrusion had been made more effective by the drug. A compound of different type which has anticonvulsant properties, acetazolamide, also diminished cerebral Na but by a distinct mechanism.

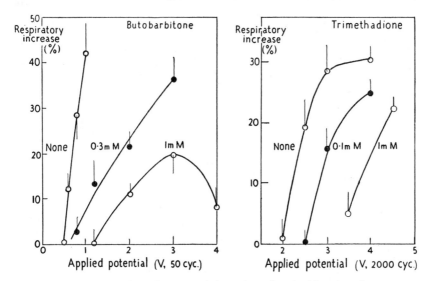

FIG. 15.3. Action of a general depressant (butobarbitone) and an anticonvulsant (trimethadione) on the respiratory response of isolated cerebral tissues to sine-wave alternating currents of the different characteristics noted. Points give mean values and lines extend from them for a distance equal to the standard error of the mean; 0·1 mM-diphenylhydantoin and 0·35 mM-phenobarbitone behaved similarly to trimethadione (Greengard & McIlwain, 1955).

Acetazolamide, 5-acetamide-1,3,4-thiadiazole-2-sulphonamide, is an in-hibitor of carbonic anhydrase and in this case entry of ^{22}Na to the brain of the treated animals was diminished. The lowered cerebral Na content could thus be obtained without effect on Na extrusion. Other circumstances affecting cerebral excitability also affect cerebral sodium. In rats exposed to cold, Na accumulated, the ratio of extracellular to intracellular Na diminished, and excitability increased. Overbreathing, or alteration in the CO_2 concentration of the air breathed, could also increase cerebral excitability and was associated in the latter case with decreased membrane potential (Petschek & Timiras, 1963; Krnjević *et al.*, 1965).

Effects on tissue excitability were observed when electrical pulses were applied to sections of mammalian cerebral cortex while these were respiring in glucose-saline solutions (see Chapter 4). The respiration of such tissues can be increased to similar degrees by pulses of a variety of electrical character-istics, for example by sine-wave alternating currents of different frequencies and voltages, and by brief condenser pulses of different potential, duration and frequency. Anticonvulsants were found to antagonize the respiratory response specifically to pulses at high frequency (Fig. 15.3). In this their effects differed from those of the general depressants, which antagonized the increase in respiration brought about by all types of pulses examined. In this and in certain other experimental arrangements, the anticonvulsants display proper-ties akin to those applied therapeutically, when they depress the excessively frequent or rapid cerebral discharge while allowing normal activity. Possibly

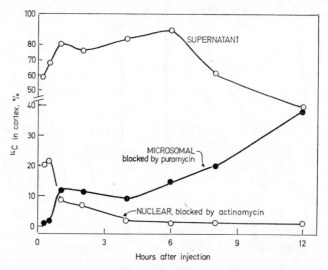

FIG. 15.4. The subcellular distribution of diphenylhydantoin in cerebral dispersions from rats which received the ^{14}C-labelled drug by in-jection. Free ^{14}C-diphenylhydantoin was yielded from the fractions by alkali. The ordinate gives the proportion of the drug in each fraction as a percentage of the total brain content at the intervals quoted; the mitochondrial content was between 3% and 8% of the total (Kemp & Woodbury, 1969).

this is mediated by lengthening the refractory period between successive im-pulses; hindrance of ion movements could in general terms be understood to have such an effect.

Diphenylhydantoin shows other metabolic properties which may be the basis for its actions on cerebral membrane phenomena and electrolytes. It is assimilated preferentially to the brain where its concentration rises to 10 times that in blood plasma. In the brain of experimental animals ^{14}C-diphenyl-hydantoin was initially found to be attached to nuclear fractions (Fig. 15.4) but gradually during 12 hr. the peak radioactivity transferred to the micro-somal fraction. Here it was attached to proteins, but hydrolysis yielded again ^{14}C-diphenylhydantoin. Its initial nuclear accumulation was inhibited by actinomycin D while the subsequent association with the microsomes was blocked by puromycin (Fig. 15.4). Moreover, diphenylhydantoin proved to augment the incorporation of orotic acid to the nucleic acids of nuclei but to inhibit its incorporation to microsomes (Kemp & Woodbury, 1969). It thus appears that aspects of protein synthesis, possibly connected with axoplasmic flow, are being affected by the drug; this brings its action into the category of phenomena related to denervation hypersensitivity which received comment above.

Before development of the specific anticonvulsants mentioned above, administration of paraldehyde or bromides were among the measures adopted in epilepsy. Paraldehyde has the characteristics of a general depressant. The bromide ion has a more specific action, possibly connected with the role of chloride ions in the central nervous system. In concentrations not very different from those causing depression, it leads to mental confusion and disorientation which has been studied as an experimentally-induced psychosis. Several steroids also affect electroshock threshold and certain of the earlier measures adopted to alleviate epilepsy may have included changed balance of steroid hormones or of electrolytes in their mode of action. The actions of diphenylhydantoin on protein synthesis and on Na movements show similarities to actions of aldosterone.

Reserpine and Chlorpromazine

These two substances receive comment as examples of the tranquillizing agents more fully described elsewhere (*Symposium*, 1957, 1962; *Conference*, 1962; Root & Hofmann, 1963). Although both compounds produce a type of sedation without loss of consciousness they are very distinct in biochemical action and in chemical structure. Reserpine as described in Chapter 14 acts potently in releasing several biologically active amines from their sites of storage in the body. Thus a daily dose in man is often 1–5 mg., and comparable dose-levels act in many mammalian species in causing loss of serotonin from the gut, the blood platelets and the brain; lower animals are however more resistant to the drug (Brodie *et al.*, *Symposium*, 1964). Confirmation that these chemical effects on the brain are close to the action of the drug is given by the arousal from reserpine sedation which is caused by 3:4 dihydroxyphenylalanine (see above). Reserpine itself is found in most parts of the brain after its administration and its action thus appears to proceed by release of the catecholamines and serotonin from their sites of storage, including vesicles of the particular nerve endings in the brain which are concerned with the amines. The specific type of sedation following reserpine then reflects the normal activities of the parts of the brain which carry these amines and of which the usual functioning is disturbed.

Chloropromazine does not cause comparable release of catecholamines or serotonin from the brain or elsewhere in the body. It was at one time believed to act by inhibiting uptake of those amines to their cerebral depots, but this has proved to be secondary to the hypothermia caused by chlorpromazine: uptake was normal in sedated animals when their body temperature was maintained. This is a reminder of the marked control of body temperature exerted from the brain (Fig. 14.10); of the pronounced metabolic sequelae to a lowering of body temperature by some 10°C: cerebral protein synthesis is inhibited by 75% (Pletscher et al., Symposium, 1964a; Shuster & Hannam, 1964); and also of how chlorpromazine was selected as a central depressant drug partly on the basis of its hypothermic effect. Chlorpromazine undergoes extensive metabolic alteration in the body, in particular to demethylated compounds and to sulphoxides which, however, are less active pharmacologically than is chlorpromazine itself (see Efron, 1968).

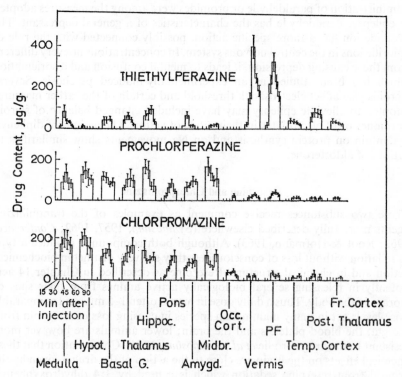

Fig. 15.5. Distribution of phenothiazines in the brain after their systemic administration to dogs (Jaramillo & Guth, 1963). Specimens were obtained from 14 areas at each of the intervals indicated, from 15 to 90 min. after injection of the drugs. Cortical areas: Fr., frontal; Occ., occipital. Cerebellar parts: PF., paraflocculus; and vermis.

The analogy between the sedation caused by chlorpromazine and that caused by reserpine appears rather to lie in the function of the parts of the brain on which they act. The parts overlap but are not identical; major areas affected by chlorpromazine include the hypothalamus and reticular formation (Table 15.4). Distribution of phenothiazines within the brain is very relevant to the type of central actions which they exhibit. In Fig. 15.5 chlorpromazine and prochlorperazine which is also a tranquilliser are seen to be at highest levels in the medulla, hypothalamus, hippocampus and midbrain with little in the cerebellum or neocortex. By contrast, triethylperazine was at highest level in the cerebellum and thalamus: this compound has anti-vertigo, antiemetic and antinauseant properties.

The action of chlorpromazine on the neural systems which it affects can be described generally as one of causing diminished excitability. A primary metabolic site for chlorpromazine action has not been determined; an appraisal (McIlwain, *Symposium*, 1962; 1969) of actions reported on respiration, tissue phosphates and phosphorylation has indicated that these are unlikely to constitute points of action sensitive to the low concentrations of chlorpromazine which have therapeutically useful effects. These metabolic processes in isolated cerebral tissues are not affected by 5–10 μM chlorpromazine until the tissues are electrically stimulated, when normal responses to excitation are inhibited. Chlorpromazine can also diminish the changes normally caused by excitation in the tissues' Na, K and membrane potential, and an action at systems involved in nerve-impulse generation or transmission thus appears likely as primary effect. Membrane permeability features as a likely point of action for phenothiazines in the assessment of Gabay (1971).

Ethanol and Alcoholism

Some centuries of scientific and other writing have described effects of alcoholic drinks on mental and social phenomena (see Lucia, 1963), and ethanol remains the substance manufactured on the largest scale for its central effects. The mixture of excitation and depression in outward behaviour which it produces has also long attracted attention and has contributed to ideas on the heterogeneity and evolutionary organization of the brain. Hughlings Jackson in 1873 and on several subsequent occasions writes or quotes that with "... alcohol, the nervous system appears to be paralysed in inverse order of its development, the highest centres going first, next the middle, and then the lowest". This is a sequence seen in the action of several general depressants but among them, alcohol occupies an unusual position; it is in a real though limited sense, both food and drug and any at all complete account of its effects on cerebral processes needs to invoke many scientific disciplines, from the physicochemical to the psychosocial (see Trémolières, 1970).

Ethanol and the Brain

Small quantities of material determined as ethanol by methods including gas chromatography are normally present in animals; blood levels in man are equivalent to about 0·03 mM ethanol (Lester, 1962). In the brain of the rat, an average value of 0·37 μmoles/g. was found; other organs carried 0·1–1 μmoles/g. and ^{14}C-ethanol was formed from [2-^{14}C]pyruvate by tissue preparations from the liver and the heart (McManus *et al.*, 1966). A reconstructed system containing pyruvate dehydrogenase, pyruvate, NADH, thiamine pyrophosphate and magnesium salts yielded ethanol; probably free acetaldehyde acted as intermediary. Ethanol is thus a normal metabolite of the mammalian body, independently of its dietary intake.

After administration of ethanol, it quickly becomes generally distributed in all the body water and converted largely to CO_2 within a few hours; a small proportion of [1-^{14}C]ethanol remained in the brain, as in other tissues (Fig. 15.6). When consumed or administered intravenously in quantities producing facial vasodilatation and mild inebriation, no changes were observed in cerebral blood flow or respiration. At higher levels, about 20 mM when behavioural effects are evident, there were little or no indications of lowered cerebral blood flow and respiration, but these become clearly evident with the severe intoxication associated with levels of 70 mM (Hine *et al.*, 1952; Sutherland *et al.*, 1960). No inhibition in respiration of separated cerebral

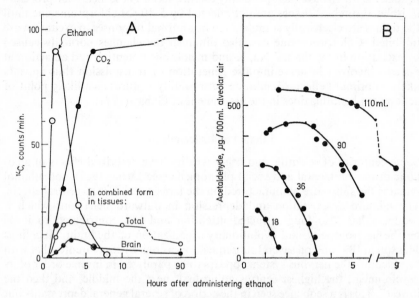

Hours after administering ethanol

FIG. 15.6. Metabolism of ethanol.
A. Blood constituents and tissue constituents of mice which received ^{14}C from [1-^{14}C]ethanol with an ethanol dose of 3·75 g/kg. (Casier, 1967).
B. Acetaldehyde as intermediary in oxidation of ethanol in man; the exhaled compound was determined by specific gas-chromatographic methods after a person had received the amounts of ethanol quoted (Freund, 1967).

tissues is caused by ethanol until very high concentrations—some 800 mM—are reached. Nor is ethanol oxidized in the brain at a rate sufficient to replace glucose in supporting normal cerebral functions, when administered to hypoglycaemic subjects.

Administered ^{14}C-ethanol nevertheless takes part in a number of metabolic interchanges in the brain and the scheme of Fig. 15.7, which as is indicated below summarizes general metabolic routes from ethanol, can be regarded as applying also to the brain. The demonstrated stages include *alcohol dehydrogenase*, identified as the nicotinamide-adenine dinucleotide oxidoreductase EC 1.1.1.1 (Raskin & Sokoloff, 1968) and found, when derived from the brain, to have properties similar to those of the enzyme from the liver described below. Its rate is, however, relatively small: some 2·4 μmoles/g. brain/hr.

contrasting with 9 mmoles/g. liver/hr. in the same animals. The acetaldehyde produced by the dehydrogenase in the brain, as well as that arriving from the bloodstream, undergoes further cerebral metabolism. An *aldehyde dehydrogenase* has been identified in various parts of the brain in a number of mammalian species (Erwin & Deitrich, 1966). It produced acetate from acetaldehyde at about 1–2 μmoles/g. tissue/hr., was largely a mitochondrial enzyme and oxidized also, several other aldehydes. On partial purification, however, succinic semialdehyde was not oxidized; nicotinamide adenine dinucleotide was required.

On administering ^{14}C-ethanol, a small proportion of the ^{14}C is found as non-volatile compounds in the brain. Fig. 15.6 shows this, and indicates that 15–40% of the ^{14}C "fixed" from ethanol in such experiments, is found in the brain; the greater part of the ethanol is, however, oxidized to CO_2 and exhaled. The amount "fixed" does not necessarily imply a large net conversion, as much mixing of ^{14}C-compounds with metabolic pools of the corresponding

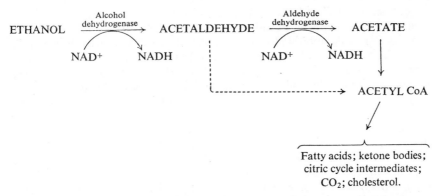

FIG. 15.7. Routes of ethanol metabolism.

endogenous ^{12}C-compounds inevitably occurs. The persistence of a proportion of the "fixed" ^{14}C (Fig. 15.6) is also understandable in these terms, supposing acetate or acetyl-CoA to be involved as suggested in Fig. 15.7 and to include such products as cholesterol.

Ethanol causes a small increase in the respiration of isolated cerebral tissues, as do other general depressants in moderate concentrations (Sutherland *et al.*, 1956; Wallgren & Kulonen, 1960; McIlwain, *Symposium*, 1962). The respiratory response of cerebral tissues to electrical stimulation is, however, progressively inhibited by concentrations above some 60 mM ethanol; depression was 9% at 87mM and 12% at 130 mM. The rapid fall in phosphocreatine which normally occurs when isolated cerebral tissues are electrically stimulated, was markedly depressed by ethanol; 87 mM permitted only 50% of the normal rate. Four other simple aliphatic alcohols used at concentrations which gave similar thermodynamic activities (see Table 15.2), inhibited the electrically stimulated tissue to similar degrees (Lindbohm & Wallgren, 1962; Wallgren, 1963, 1971). In these respects, therefore, ethanol appears to be acting as a general depressant; high concentrations impede Na^+ and K^+ movements

(Kalant & Israel, 1967). Isolated, electrically stimulated cerebral tissues also reproduce changes in the amino acids of the brain which occur during alcoholic intoxication (Häkkinen *et al.*, 1961, 1963).

Ethanol: General Bodily Metabolism

Reactions to ethanol are however conditioned not only by its properties as a general depressant but also by its bodily metabolism summarized in Fig. 15.7 and by a variety of metabolic and social adaptations prompted by its frequent consumption. These can receive only brief comment here; in man, up to 400 ml. of ethanol can be oxidized per day and so contribute largely to overall energy supply. Much metabolic reorganization is involved in this (see, for example, Williamson *et al.*, 1969). When this large quantity was first taken in frequent small doses by volunteers under controlled conditions and with adequate dietary supplements, it produced gross intoxication and blood levels of 4–10 mM-ethanol. However, after 10–14 days of this regimen blood alcohol fell to "nearly zero" and intoxication diminished (Wikler, 1964); some adjustment could also be made to still greater intake, while blood levels of ethanol were 30–50 mM. Adaptation to the ethanol was thus made both by its increased metabolism, described below, and by modification of the nervous system to function in its presence. Withdrawal of ethanol then produced hallucinations, tremors and other physical and mental disturbance; tranquillizing drugs have been used to control such withdrawal symptoms in alcoholics (*Symposium*, 1957; Popham & Schmidt, 1962).

Administration of ethanol to rats at about 0·6 g./kg. led to increase of a number of simple substances in their blood, especially acetaldehyde, acetates and acetoacetates (Forsander & Räihä, 1960; Russell & Van Bruggen, 1964). Within 1 hr. of giving 1- or 2-^{14}C-ethanol these compounds, with ethanol and CO_2, contained much of the ^{14}C of the blood and so were produced from ethanol itself rather than by diversion of other intermediary metabolites. In several tissues, also, cholesterol became isotopically labelled from ^{14}C-ethanol as rapidly as from ^{14}C-acetate; ^{14}C-acetylsulphanilamide was also formed from the ^{14}C-ethanol. Metabolism of ethanol thus appeared to proceed through acetaldehyde and acetylcoenzyme A (Fig. 15.7). The liver was demonstrated as a major site of formation of acetate and acetoacetate by perfusing isolated rat liver with ethanol. Also, blood levels of ethanol remained higher in eviscerated animals and by perfusing the liver was shown to account for at least 60–80% of the alcohol metabolized in the whole animal (Hine *et al.*, 1952; Jacobsen, 1952; Mardones, 1963). For comment on other metabolic routes, see Kalant (1962) and Maickel (1967).

The alcohol dehydrogenase of mammalian liver which yields acetaldehyde from ethanol is an active and interesting enzyme (McKinley-McKee & Donninger, 1963). The liver carries also the aldehyde dehydrogenase which yields acetic acid from acetaldehyde, but as indicated some acetaldehyde reaches the blood after ingestion of ethanol; it rose for example to 0·1–0·2 mM when blood ethanol was about 20 mM, during the first hour after giving 1 g./kg. ethanol to men (institutionalized; Sutherland *et al.*, 1960). Acetaldehyde serves as cerebral substrate when it is caused to accumulate in the body. Its level in the cerebral venous blood is markedly lower than in arterial blood, and when added to cerebral dispersions acetaldehyde is rapidly lost, to a considerable extent in formation of acetoin, a reaction promoted by thiamine pyrophosphate and by pyruvate (Stotz et al., 1944). By this route acetaldehyde accelerates pyruvate removal; the formation of acetoin can amount to 80% of that expected stoichiometrically.

Adaptive Changes to Ethanol: Acetaldehyde

The level of alcohol dehydrogenase, especially in the liver, can be rate-limiting in ethanol metabolism; the subsequent stage, aldehyde dehydrogenase (Fig. 15.7) can proceed at much greater rate. Animals have been found to react to administration of ethanol by an adaptive increase in alcohol dehydrogenase. The activity of the enzyme per unit weight of tissue could double, and increase also in the stomach and small intestine. Moreover, such changes were associated with self-administered ethanol; a strain of rats which drank dilute ethanol in preference to water showed over twice the hepatic alcohol dehydrogenase of a strain without this preference; aldehyde dehydrogenase increased to an even greater extent. Alcohol dehydrogenase in the gastro-intestinal tract and liver of rats increased in 4–10 hr. after a single dose of ethanol and the increase was prevented by actinomycin-D or cycloheximide. Thus adaptation by new protein synthesis was demonstrated (Mistilis & Birchall, 1969; Sheppard et al., 1968; Wilson, 1967).

In the body as a whole acetaldehyde is ordinarily metabolized rapidly for it serves as substrate for several enzymes in different tissues (see Hunter & Lowry, 1956; Kiessling, 1963), but when blood levels of some 50–200 μmoles/l. are maintained by infusion, breathing and pulse rates are increased, the face flushes and a nausea akin to alcoholic hangover is experienced. Acetaldehyde, indeed, plays a large part in the unpleasant and toxic effects of ethanol. After ingestion of ethanol, acetaldehyde can be caused to accumulate in the blood to levels comparable with those produced by infusion, when further oxidation of acetaldehyde is inhibited. Several substances have this inhibitory property including cyanamide, which was noticed by workers handling it to cause an intolerance to alcohol. This intolerance can be deliberately induced as an aid to the treatment of alcoholism, and for this purpose is used disulphiram, bis(di-ethylthiocarbamyl)disulphide: $Et_2N.CS.S.S.CS.NEt_2$. Acetaldehyde can be further metabolized in the liver and in mixtures containing liver preparations, by dismutations which require nicotinamide coenzymes (Lundquist et al., 1959) and by oxidative routes. At least one of these routes is highly sensitive to inhibition by disulphiram, which itself is capable of inducing psychotic episodes. A flavoprotein-containing aldehyde oxidase from rabbit liver was inhibited by 0·3 μM disulphiram while 0·6 mM-disulphiram markedly inhibited the oxidation of acetaldehyde by xanthine oxidase prepared from rat liver (Kjeldgaard, 1949; Westerfeld et al., 1959; Palmer, 1962; Rajagopalan et al., 1962).

Several endocrinological changes also follow the consumption of ethanol (see Kalant, 1962; Maickel, 1967). Thus diuresis occurs after alcohol ingestion in part through diminution in the release of pituitary antidiuretic hormone, and the excretion of several physiologically active compounds is modified, including tryptamine, catecholamines and their metabolites. Although the major immediate effects of ethanol are those of a general depressant the associated metabolic events, as can be judged by the properties of acetaldehyde, appreciably colour its actions in man. Ethanol also acts as depressant in a wide variety of other organisms (*Colloquium*, 1951). For a description of general and hepatic pathology associated with high ethanol intake or with alcoholism, see Maickel (1967); and of psychological social factors involved in alcoholism, see Steinberg (1969) and Lucia (1963).

Morphine and Related Drugs

Opium, or the morphine alkaloids prepared from it (Fig. 15.8), has been for over 1,000 years a major means of controlling central reactions to pain, and of inducing euphoria in those accustomed to its use. The analgesia can

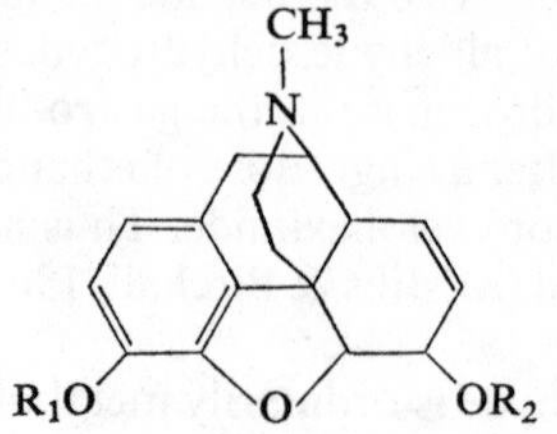

Morphine: I, $R_1 = R_2 = H$.
Codeine: I, $R_1 = CH_3$; $R_2 = H$.
Heroine: I, $R_1 = R_2 = COCH_3$.
Nalorphine: I, $R_1 = R_2 = H$, with
$-CH_2-CH=CH_2$ replacing $-CH_3$.

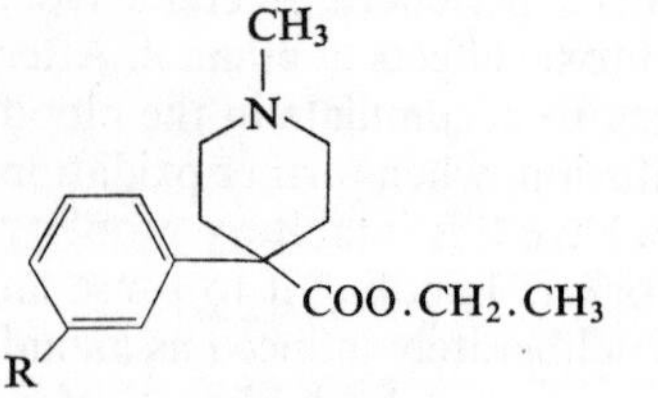

Meperidine (pethidine)

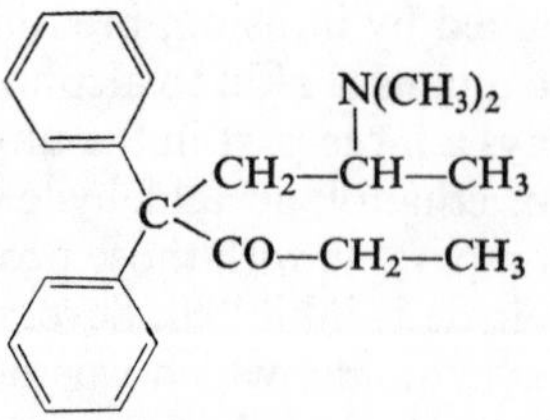

Methadone (amidone)

FIG. 15.8. Morphine and synthetic analgesics.

be reproduced in experimental animals, as can also the acquisition of tolerance to the drug on repeated administration in the increased dosage necessary to maintain analgesia. The increased dosage can, in suitable circumstances, be self-selected by experimental animals. When administration of morphine is stopped, the ensuing withdrawal syndrome includes disturbances of many aspects of homeostasis normally controlled from the brain (see Clouet, 1968; Steinberg, 1969; Wikler, 1968). Chemical and metabolic studies of the action of morphine have been very numerous and varied, and the present account selects those which seem most closely connected with the complex of actions just described.

Metabolic Reactions to Morphine

Pharmacological specification of the action of morphine in several parts of the body including the gastro-intestinal tract and the brain, connects its action with neurotransmitters, especially acetylcholine (Paton, 1969; Clouet, 1968; Hano et al., 1964; Wikler, 1968). Morphine diminished the release of acetylcholine normally caused by stimulation of the superior cervical ganglion; it diminished the acetylcholine released to an intraventricular superfusion fluid; in mice, it caused an accumulation of cerebral acetylcholine. Moreover, the acetylcholine so accumulating diminished when, with repeated administration of morphine, the animals became tolerant to it; but after the repeated administration was stopped, the accumulation increased to its former level in about 15 days (Hano et al., 1964). Chemical correlates to the development of tolerance and withdrawal were thus observed. Possibly, morphine blocks the release of acetylcholine in the parts of the brain in which it acts, and some receptor component in those parts proliferates in response to the block; this is one only of the wide range of responses to the drug (see for example Clouet 1971). Topical application of morphine, and intravenous morphine, both diminished the rate of release of acetylcholine from a number of cortical areas of the cat (Jhamandas et al., 1970). Morphine antagonists, as naloxone, prevented this action.

Study of isolated cerebral tissues has yielded cognate information. Morphine competes with acetylcholine for uptake to sections of mouse brain in vitro (K_i, 3×10^{-5} M; Schuberth & Sundwall, 1967). When animals become tolerant to morphine, it is not because less of the drug is taken up by the brain (Table 15.3); but the tissues have changed in the respiratory response which they afford to the addition of KCl. This response is no longer susceptible to inhibition by morphine but morphine sensitivity is restored when withdrawal effects are induced by nalorphine, the morphine antagonist (Fig. 15.8). Moreover, a phenomenon akin to cross-tolerance is exhibited by the isolated tissues: the sensitivity of the respiratory response to inhibition by methadone and by meperidine is diminished, as well as that to morphine; after nalorphine, response increases in its sensitivity to all three analgesics.

In seeking further specification of how the tissues had altered, the incorporation of ^{32}P from inorganic phosphate into phospholipids was examined during incubation in vitro. Such incorporation was itself sensitive to morphine: cerebral samples from guinea pigs which had received a single dose of morphine showed increased incorporation of ^{32}P to most of the eight phospholipid fractions which were examined. In animals made morphine-tolerant or morphine-abstinent, incorporation to some phospholipids, as diphosphoinositide, changed relatively little while to phosphatidylcholine or to the triphosphoinositide it altered considerably (Table 15.3). Sensitivity to morphine was also shown to the incorporation of glycerol and inositol. The phospholipids are membrane-localized but do not specify a membrane type. Of cerebral enzymes associated with microsomal membrane-structures, an adenosine triphosphatase diminished in activity with chronic morphine administration, apparently through alteration in its relationship to Mg^{2+} (Ghosh & Ghosh, 1968). Examination of the subcellular localization of

³H-morphine administered to guinea pigs showed a small proportion of the cerebral ³H to be in a microsomal fraction; most was present in the post-microsomal supernatant (Mulé, 1969).

Table 15.3

Tolerance to morphine: induction and loss in rats and guinea pigs

Groups of animals	1 Normal	2 Tolerant	3 Withdrawal or antagonism
Treatment (guinea pigs or rats*)	Saline injections controlling Group 2; morphine, 40 mg./kg. given 1 hr. before sampling	Morphine, 5 mg./ kg. each 8 hr., increased until stabilized on 40 mg./kg.	After treatment as Group 2, morphine withdrawn or nalorphine* administered
Condition just after morphine	Sedated	Active	–
Morphine in cerebral:			
Grey matter	1·31	1·70	0
White matter	0·71	1·11	0
Respiratory response* to KCl (% of control)	53	97	53
Incorporation of ³²P, (% of control) to:			
Phosphatidyl-choline	60	5	4
Diphosphoinosi-tide	15	−1	−15
Triphosphoinosi-tide	63	38	126

Rats* (Takemori, 1962) were injected with saline or morphine (15 mg./kg.) twice daily for 7–10 days, and when indicated with nalorphine, 10 mg./kg., 30 min. before sampling. Guinea pigs (Mulé, 1967) in Group 3 did not receive nalorphine, but morphine was withdrawn 24 hr. before sampling.

The respiratory response was measured in the presence of 1 mM morphine; quantitative data were determined also in the presence of other analgesics. The incorporation of ³²P was measured in the presence of 0·1 mM morphine and animals including the non-tolerant but not those used to control the ³²P incorporation, received morphine before sampling. Data were obtained for six other phospholipid fractions, and at other intervals after morphine administration.

Inhibiting the Development of Morphine Tolerance

Demonstration of changes in cerebral metabolism when animals become morphine-tolerant, indicates that processes of metabolic adaptation are occurring, and prompts corresponding investigation of the process of development of tolerance.

Tolerance in many experiments has required several days for its induction, but this is most typically the case when the administration of morphine is intermittent. When morphine was administered to rats by intravenous infusion, so that blood and tissue levels were more constant and defined, tolerance developed in about 4 hr. Fig. 15.9 shows that by such infusions analgesia required about an hour to reach its maximum value, which was maintained for 2 hr. but was already diminishing at the third hour. When actinomycin D was added with morphine to the infusion fluid, establishment of analgesia was not affected but its subsequent loss was delayed: that is, the development of tolerance was inhibited. Actinomycin D did not itself affect the animals' response to pain, as indicated by the lower lines of Fig. 15.9. In a similar group of experiments in which analgesia was established by intravenous infusion of morphine plus actinomycin D, omission of the actinomycin without alteration

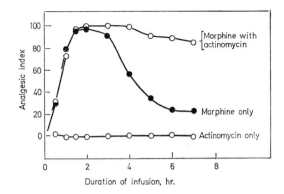

FIG. 15.9. Acute tolerance to intravenous morphine.
Rats received intravenous infusions of saline containing morphine, actinomycin, or both. Analgesia was measured by the pressure required to be applied to the tail to elicit a specified response from the animal.
Dose-levels in mg./kg./hr.: morphine, 7·5 and actinomycin, 0·01. Ordinate scale: 100 represents maximum analgesia (Cox, Ginsburg & Osman, 1968).

in the level of morphine allowed tolerance to begin to develop in about an hour. However, when tolerance had developed it was not overcome by actinomycin D.

The known point of action of actinomycin D is on DNA-directed RNA synthesis (see Chapter 9), and the time-course outlined for actinomycin action above is consistent with the fashion in which it would be expected to modify metabolic characteristics such as those of Table 15.3. This would be pictured to occur after the RNA had taken part in protein synthesis, and this has been confirmed by examination of a wider range of compounds which interfere with synthesis of either RNA or protein (Cox & Osman, 1970; Loh, Shen & Way, 1969). Cycloheximide, also, prevented the development of tolerance to morphine in both mice and rats and was shown during the same experiments to have much greater effect on cerebral synthesis of protein than of RNA. Interestingly, the toxicity of morphine is increased when it is administered together with cycloheximide, suggesting that the reaction to morphine by modification of synthetic processes, is indeed protective to the animal.

Synthesis of a wide range of protein types is inhibited by the blocking agents. The associated studies may suggest connection with phospholipid metabolism, with acetylcholine or with serotonin; several possible mechanisms are discussed by Cox & Ginsburg (1969) and by Loh *et al.* (1969); see also Wikler (1968).

Comments on Depressants and Excitants of the Central Nervous System

The agents described above are preponderantly depressant and those which follow, preponderantly excitant; normal cerebral functioning is itself a

Table 15.4

Specificity in the action of depressants of the central nervous system

Part of the CNS	Barbiturates	Meprobamate	Morphine	Chlorpromazine
Cerebral cortex	⬇R↓	O ↓	O ⬇↑	O ⬇⇡(broken)
Thalamus: specific relay nuclei	⬇R↓	⇣(broken)↓	O ↓	O ⬇↑
diffuse projections	⬇R↓	⇣(broken)↓	⬇R↑(broken)	⬇R↓
Hypothalamus	⬇↓	⇣(broken)↓	⬇↓	⬇↓
Limbic system	⬇↓	⇣(broken)↓	O ↓	O ⇡(broken)
Brain-stem reticular formation	⬇↓	O ↓	⇣(broken)↓	⇣(broken)⬇↑
Spinal cord	⬇↓	⬇↓	⬇↑	O O

The scheme, adapted from Domino (1962) can give approximate indications only of the actions of the drugs. Downward-pointing arrows mean depression of activities, judged electrophysiologically or by overt effects; upward-pointing, stimulation. Bold arrows give their major effects, seen soon after administration or with small doses only. The thin arrows which follow give the effect of larger doses; R indicates that the depression of the reticular formation appears to be causing a stimulation in these parts of the brain at some stages in their action. Broken arrows indicate that the effects are slight or partial.

balance of excitant and depressant actions. Much interpretation and differentiation in central depressant actions are necessarily through electrophysiology and the behavioural sciences. Some of the differences which have been demonstrated among central depressants by electrophysiological and pharmacological methods, are indicated in Table 15.4. This emphasizes that even barbiturates and meprobamate, which are fairly general in their depressant action, have specific features. In the barbiturates some stimulant action can appear in the cortex through inhibition elsewhere. With meprobamate (Fig. 15.2) which is a mild tranquillizing agent but developed from muscle-relaxant drugs, a proportionally greater effect is retained on the spinal cord. Markedly differential effects appear with more complex agents exemplified by morphine and chlorpromazine. The theme of metabolic adaptation by the brain to many agents which alter its level of functioning, will be found to continue in the cerebral excitants now to be described.

Convulsants

Agents causing widespread cerebral excitation may first be considered, with subsequent comment on more specific agents. Administration of a convulsive agent such as pentamethylene tetrazole (Fig. 15.10), or the application of

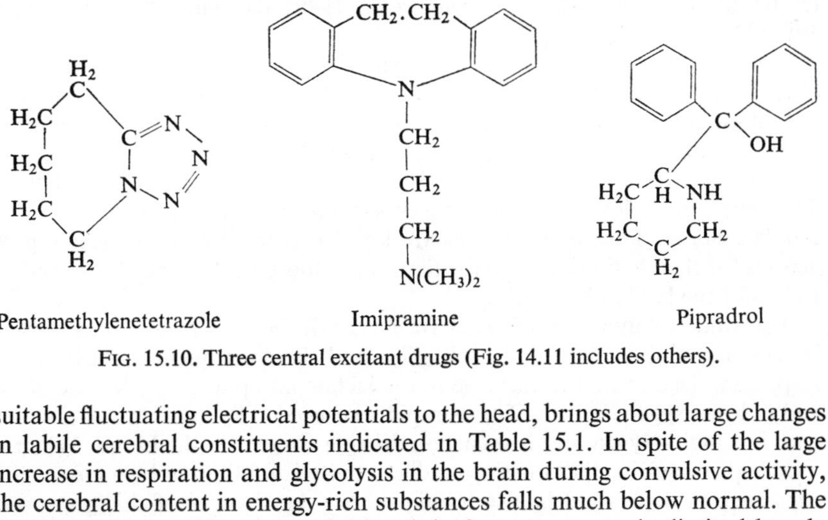

Pentamethylenetetrazole   Imipramine   Pipradrol

FIG. 15.10. Three central excitant drugs (Fig. 14.11 includes others).

suitable fluctuating electrical potentials to the head, brings about large changes in labile cerebral constituents indicated in Table 15.1. In spite of the large increase in respiration and glycolysis in the brain during convulsive activity, the cerebral content in energy-rich substances falls much below normal. The duration of convulsions, once initiated, in fact appears to be limited largely by metabolic factors, for when additional oxygen or glucose is provided, convulsions are prolonged (Ruf, 1951).

The metabolic events following convulsions *in vivo* include several which can readily be measured in separated mammalian cerebral tissues. Addition of convulsive drugs to such tissues respiring in the ordinary way in balanced salt mixtures with glucose or other substrates in most cases does not alter their respiration, glycolysis, or phosphate content. One convulsive agent is, however, fully effective in bringing about *in vitro* all the metabolic changes induced *in vivo*. This is the application of electrical pulses whose effects have been described in Chapter 4. Thus the separated tissue is fully capable of responding in a fashion similar in this respect to the whole brain (Anguiano & McIlwain, 1951; McIlwain & Greengard, 1957).

In intact animals, a number of convulsive agents greatly increase the frequency of discharge from the pyramidal cells of the motor area of the cerebral cortex (Adrian & Moruzzi, 1939). Such cells normally give impulses at 5–50/sec., without limb movements but strychnine, picrotoxin, pentamethylenetetrazole and thujone caused bursts of impulses at up to 1,000/sec. for brief periods. This, with other characteristics of their action, was interpreted to mean that a convulsive agent inhibited processes normally operating to end a period of activity. Description of this in terms of strychnine preventing the inhibitory action of glycine was given in Chapter 14.

General Metabolic Changes after Convulsions

The convulsive agents described act primarily at the central nervous system but their action there has metabolic among other consequences in the body as a whole. Many of the consequences are common to convulsive activity induced either by drugs or electrically and they have been studied not only in experimental animals but also in man through the use of convulsive agents in treatment of mental disease (*Symposium*, 1949; Russell, 1960; Holmberg, 1963; Dobkin, 1970).

Firstly, exchange between the brain and the blood or cerebrospinal fluid is altered. Apart from the initially increased uptake of oxygen and glucose and output of their products, inorganic phosphate and potassium salts are increased in the cerebral venous blood; acetylcholine as well as phosphates and possibly nucleotides and protein also increase in the cerebrospinal fluid. This represents a loss from the brain of substances which normally are intracellular. Some of these substances are known to require energy-yielding reactions for their assimilation to the tissue and thus their loss may be secondary to loss of the labile phosphates.

A second and much more extensive group of changes result from muscular activity of the convulsion itself. This and the consequent disturbance of respiration lead at first to increase in the lactate and phosphates of the blood and to low oxygen content. This is rapidly succeeded by hyperventilation and with it a high oxygen and low carbon dioxide content in the blood. When in modified convulsive therapies muscular activity is minimized by a curare-like substance (a depressant is also administered) the changes of this group are much smaller.

A further group of changes reflects the stimulation of the autonomic nervous system during seizures. Catecholamines increase in blood and urine, and release of serotonin also occurs. Blood glucose begins to rise within a minute of the convulsion and reaches some 10–20 min. later, its peak of perhaps 7 mM from a resting level of 4·5 mM. Mediation of the changes has been studied in experimental animals. In vagotomized rats the increase in glucose is greater than normal while in adrenalectomized animals the glucose level falls following electrically-induced convulsions. It is unaffected by electroshock in animals with both operations. Other signs of adrenal stimulation are an increase in blood pressure, and the respiratory changes described above.

Secretion not only from the adrenal medulla but also from the adrenal cortex is increased following convulsions. This may occur through release of adrenocorticotrophic hormone from the pituitary as a result of events purely within the brain itself, or as a result of changes in the rest of the body; the changes have many but not all characteristics in common with those following administration of adrenocorticotrophic hormone. Thus they include increase in urinary 17-oxosteroids and cortins. Excretion of phosphates, uric acid and potassium salts also increase; fluid and sodium balance is altered. The volume of blood plasma decreases, the level of lymphocytes in the blood falls as also does that of eosinophils. Possibly related are changes in glucose and insulin tolerance.

After electrically inducing convulsions in mentally ill subjects on several occasions over some weeks and with therapeutic intent, the changes described tend to persist for weeks or months after the convulsions, and to an extent which has been reported to be greatest in subjects showing most clinical improvement, though such correlation does not always occur. Electro-convulsive therapy is concluded to be of greatest value in depressive states.

Repeated electroshock in experimental animals and in man has been found to raise the threshold necessary to induce electroshock on subsequent days (Essig et al., 1963). The threshold in cats rose during 3 weeks from 6 to 16 mamp. and on cessation of periodic electroshock, returned to its previous value in 10 days. Elevation of threshold occurred also in response to repeated electroshock of adrenalectomized animals, which increased the likelihood that the elevation depended on changes in the brain rather than elsewhere in the body. Thus numerous changes in amino acids and neurotransmitters take place in the brain with electroshock (Engel et al., 1968; Dobkin, 1970): for example, increased release and turnover of catecholamines.

Amphetamine

Amphetamine (2-amino-1-phenylpropane: Fig. 14.11) was noted in the preceding chapter as a centrally-acting excitant, a sympathomimetic agent and inhibitor of monoamine oxidase. It is now considered in more detail, because its actions after administration to animals or man are markedly dependent on the concomitant level of sensory stimulation or other environmental factors, and also because amphetamine and amphetamine–barbiturate mixtures can be drugs of addiction. The term "amphetamine(s)" will be used to include D, L and DL isomerides, and also methamphetamine, N-methylamphetamine, unless specifically differentiated.

On their systemic administration to mice or cats, amphetamines arrive promptly at the brain and remain at appreciable level there for 2 hr. or more (A, Fig. 15.10; Young & Gordon, 1962). They are also widely distributed in the body but are gradually converted to mixtures of metabolites (Dring et al., 1970; Hewick & Fouts, 1970), with benzoic acid preponderating in six species including man, though this is replaced by conjugates of 4-hydroxyamphetamine in the rat. Nevertheless, in man and in two other species, about 30% of a pharmacologically active dose was excreted unchanged and excretion continued for about 3 days after the administration, which is valuable in diagnosis of suspected amphetamine addiction or psychoses (see Connell, 1958; Kalant, 1966; Phillipson, 1970). Some alterations have been noted in the rate of disposal of amphetamine in rats under changed physiological conditions. Hexobarbitone or diphenylhydantoin administered with amphetamine had little effect on its metabolism (Groppetti & Costa, 1969), but chlorpromazine and imipramine increased the concentration and persistence of amphetamine in the brain; desmethylimipramine inhibited the hydroxylation of amphetamine (Sulser & Sanders-Bush, 1970; Consolo et al., 1967; Valzelli, 1969). The rate of excretion of amphetamine fluctuated with urinary pH, and in man could increase from 1 to 6 μg./min. when pH fell from 8 to 5 (Beckett, 1969).

Amphetamine Action and Cerebral Constituents

The structure and properties of amphetamine led to examining tissue catecholamines in interpreting its action and as is shown in **B**, Fig. 15.11, the cerebral noradrenaline of mice was depleted by doses of amphetamine which caused excitement and running. Moreover, amphetamine was found to release cerebral dopamine and noradrenaline in a specific fashion (Carlsson, 1969; Gunne & Lewander, 1968). In doses which had relatively little action on levels of the catecholamines in normal animals, amphetamine lowered cerebral catecholamines in reserpinized animals treated with dihydroxyphenylalanine. This treatment led to the cytoplasmic accumulation of catecholamines, the vesicular accumulation having been blocked by reserpine (q.v.). The O-methylated metabolites of the catecholamines increased following amphetamine administration, this presumably resulting from the release of noradrenaline and also from inhibition of monoamine oxidase which constitutes an alternative pathway for their metabolism and inactivation (q.v., Iversen, 1967). Inhibition by amphetamine of the re-uptake of catecholamines following their release, has been proposed also in interpretation of the yield of methylated metabolites.

As a sympathomimetic agent, the action of amphetamine appears to be indirect and mediated by noradrenaline, for it no longer occurred after administration of α-methyltyrosine which by inhibiting tyrosine hydroxylase (q.v.) blocked noradrenaline formation. Thus in presence of α-methyltyrosine, amphetamine no longer increased the spontaneous or psychomotor activity of rats (Sulser & Sanders-Bush, 1970). L-Dihydroxyphenylalanine (q.v.), however, restored this action of amphetamine to animals treated with α-methyltyrosine. Electrophysiological observations have also displayed situations in which amphetamine acts by releasing endogenous catecholamines. Amphetamine applied iontophoretically to the brain stem of the rat or cat mimicked the changes in cell-firing caused by noradrenaline, similarly applied. After treatment of the animals with reserpine, noradrenaline retained its action but the action of amphetamine was lost (Boakes et al. 1971). In the substantia nigra of rats, lesions which depleted the endogenous catecholamines (preponderantly dopamine) also diminished behavioural responses to amphetamine (Simpson & Iversen, 1971).

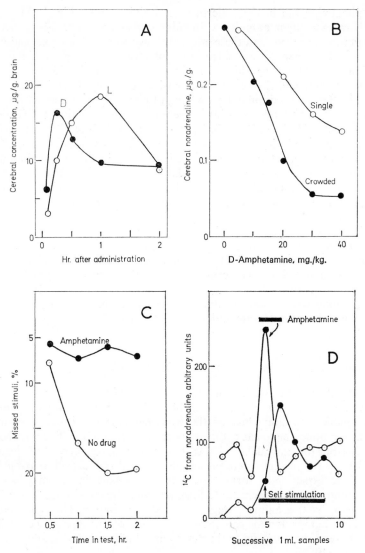

FIG. 15.11. Amphetamine: arrival at, and actions in, the brain.

A. Cerebral concentrations of amphetamine isomerides after their intraperitoneal injection at 15 mg./kg. to mice (Benakis & Thomasset: *Symposium*, 1969).

B. Depletion of cerebral noradrenaline by D-amphetamine in mice which were kept for 4 hr. either singly, or crowded (four in a small cage). L-Amphetamine was also studied (Moore, 1963).

C. Increase in errors in signal-detection by radar operators, on continuing a test beyond 30 min.; amphetamine (10 mg., orally 1 hr. before testing) prevented the increase (Mackworth, 1950; Weiss, 1969).

D. Release of ^{14}C administered to rats as ^{14}C noradrenaline, to saline solutions perfusing the region of the amygdala of rats, at approx. 0·1 ml./min. D-Amphetamine: 3 mg./kg., intraperitoneally; self-stimulation, by electrodes in the medial forebrain bundle (Stein & Wise, 1969).

Amphetamine can increase alertness and vigilance (**C**, Fig. 15.11) and is used therapeutically in narcolepsy. In animals also, restlessness, hyperactivity and agitation are seen, and these effects in mice were accentuated and could result in death when the animals were kept several in a cage rather than in isolation. In interpreting this phenomenon the determinations of **B**, Fig. 15.11 were made and showed more extensive depletion of cerebral catecholamines in the crowded animals; lowering of cerebral glycogen also occurred and was intensified by crowding; cerebral phosphocreatine fell (Estler & Ammon, 1967; Clark *et al.*, 1967). By examining animals at different environmental temperatures, it was concluded that an increase in body temperature resulting from amphetamine contributed to death in the crowded animals; so also did a fall in blood glucose. In isolated animals, blood glucose rose after amphetamine administration, as would be expected from a sympathomimetic agent; but in association with the crowding and hyperthermia, blood glucose fell.

Action of amphetamine in raising body temperature has been associated with its *anorexic* effect, which has been one reason for its therapeutic administration. Contributing to both these actions is the ability of amphetamine to release noradrenaline at nerve terminals in the fatty tissues of the body, which induces the formation of free fatty acids from the fat depots (see Brodie *et al.*, 1969). Administered noradrenaline could itself increase the circulating free fatty acids, body temperature and anorexia.

Regional, Behavioural and Persistent Effects of Amphetamine

Release of cerebral catecholamines by amphetamine shows some selectivity when examined in different parts of the brain. In rats with indwelling cannulae which enabled the amygdala or the hypothalamus to be perfused, intraperitoneal amphetamine caused the appearance of noradrenaline metabolites in fluids from the amygdala only (**D**, Fig. 15.11). Specific types of electrical stimuli from the medial forebrain bundle released noradrenaline from both sites. These experiments formed part of an investigation from which the forebrain bundle was concluded to form part of a "reward system" (see Olds, 1962; Stein, 1968) as animals sought to cause its excitation. That systemically-administered amphetamine can activate a system of this type may contribute to the abuse of the drug and to the development of amphetamine-dependence (see Collier, 1969).

Amphetamine and amphetamine–barbiturate mixtures have some clinical use in mild depressive states (see Efron, 1967) and are discussed as drugs of addiction in the symposia edited by Sjöqvist & Tottie (1969) and Phillipson (1970). Counterparts to some of the effects in man of amphetamine and of amphetamine–barbiturate mixtures, especially the 1:6·5 mixture of amphetamine–amylobarbitone which constitutes "purple hearts", have been found in experimental animals. The mixture is remarkable for its interacting with environmental influences and in inducing long-lasting behavioural changes in rats and mice; these changes appear to be metabolically-conditioned and have been described as extending the impression of novelty in a limited environment

(Steinberg *et al.*, 1961; Dickins *et al.*, 1965; Rushton *et al.*, 1968; McIlwain, 1968; Cooper *et al.*, 1969).

Persistent changes at metabolic level also have been observed on administering amphetamines. Thus tyrosine hydroxylase of chicken adrenal gland increased three-fold following 2 days' administration of methedrine; similar changes occurred in the brain, were accompanied by increased turnover of noradrenaline, and were inhibited by cycloheximide (Mandell & Morgan, 1970). The hydroxylase, which is the rate-limiting enzyme in noradrenaline synthesis (q.v.), was induced also on treating animals with reserpine, which though quite different in most of its actions as a drug, also modified cerebral noradrenaline. Thus the level of tyrosine hydroxylase appears to be controlled by the β-phenylethylamines present at particular subcellular sites; as these can be modified also by sensory input, basis is given for interaction of environmental factors and amphetamine.

Long-term administration of amphetamines produces very persistent cerebral changes, some of which can again be related to cerebral catecholamine precursors. On administering methamphetamine for 20–70 days to guinea pigs, their cerebral monoamine oxidase measured with tyramine as substrate was depressed by some 30%; but after administration had been stopped for a few days the oxidase levels became some 30% higher than those of control animals (Utena *et al.*, 1959). Increased monoamine oxidase persisted for some weeks and during this time the glycolysis of cerebral tissues also was increased. Conceivably the glycolytic changes are related to those in tyramine metabolism, which may be greater in the cerebral regions or isoenzymic components most affected by methamphetamine.

Experimental Psychoses; Antidepressant Drugs

The mental disturbances caused by amphetamine have been appraised in detail in comparison with those of mental illnesses; they resemble features of schizophrenic episodes sufficiently for amphetamine-takers to have been diagnosed repeatedly as suffering schizophrenia, as is described on p. 489. Persistent changes in behaviour follow the administration of methamphetamine to rodents, cats and monkeys as well as to man. (Utena, 1966; Machiyama *et al.*, 1970). After daily administration of methamphetamine for about a month, animals not then receiving the drug showed diminution of motor activity, loss of responsiveness to defined stimuli, and other changes which were considered to be analogues of schizophrenia in man. Some of the persistent effects were ameliorated by administering chlorpromazine. Among cerebral constituents which were examined for correlation with behavioural activity in cats, serotonin was found to increase in several parts of the brain while methamphetamine was exhibiting its long-term action, and to be transitorily diminished by the chlorpromazine administration.

A valuable appraisal of amphetamine and of other model psychoses is given by Lipton (1970). Methoxyamphetamines termed DOM, DOET and STP show several of the features of amphetamine and mescaline and have been examined as psychotropic agents in man (Snyder *et al.*, 1970) with appraisal of the structural and metabolic features involved. Substances related to sero-

tonin, as well as to catecholamines, induce experimental psychoses, as will be
be evident from the properties of lysergic acid diethylamide (q.v.); alkyl-
tryptamines including bufotenin, 5-hydroxy-N-N-dimethyltryptamine, investigated as psychotomimetic agents showed, as well as immediate mental
disturbances, some persistent effects which were attributed to enzyme induction
(Szara, 1970).

As antidepressant drugs in addition to amphetamines, are employed two
other groups of substances. These comprise inhibitors of monoamine oxidases: hydrazine derivatives, phenylcyclopropylamine and pargyline (q.v.);
and tricyclic antidepressants. Imipramine (Fig. 15.10) the parent substance of
the tricyclic group, probably acts largely after conversion to desmethylimipramine and among its effects interacts with adrenergic systems; it potenti-
ates amphetamine and inhibits cellular uptake of noradrenaline at cerebral
tissues.

Comment

Examples only have been given in this chapter of how the study of centrally-
acting drugs has been the occasion for enlarging biochemical knowledge of the
working of the brain. In devising or using such drugs intentions have usually
been therapeutic, the correcting of identified ills; but extending or improving
some aspect of normal performance has also been an objective, as in the use of
amphetamine to increase vigilance. The subject of psychopharmacology is now
very large and has specialized texts and journals concerned with both the use
and abuse of centrally-acting drugs: a duality which has been a recurrent
theme in the study of such drugs, as ethanol and morphine exemplify. A
psychopharmacologist (see Brill *et al.*, 1967) can view himself in oracular position at the crossroads of biological and moral sciences; but so, possibly, could
many investigators of the brain. Cerebral changes induced by drugs are seen
in the following chapter as one of several aspects of the biology of the brain
in which chemical mediation is prominent.

REFERENCES

ADRIAN, E. D. & MORUZZI, G. (1939). *J. Physiol.* **97**, 153.
ANGUIANO, G. & MCILWAIN, H. (1951). *Brit. J. Pharmacol.* **6**, 448.
BAIN, J. A. (1957). *Progr. Neurobiol.* **2**, 139.
BECKETT, A. H. (1969). In Steinberg, H. (1969).
BOAKES, R. J., BRADLEY, P. B. & CANDY, J. M. (1971). *Nature, Lond.* **229**, 496.
BRILL, H., COLE, J. O., DENIKER, P., HIPPIUS, H. & BRADLEY, P. B. (1967). Neuro-
    psychopharmacology. Amsterdam: Excerpta Medica.
BRODIE, B. B., CHO, A. K., STEFANO, F. J. E. & GESSA, G. L. (1969). *Adv. Bioch.
    Psychopharm.* **1**, 219.
BUCHEL, L. & MCILWAIN, H. (1950). *Brit. J. Pharmacol.* **5**, 465.
COHEN, M. & HEALD, P. J. (1960). *J. Pharmacol.* **129**, 361.
BURGER, A. (1968). (Ed.). Drugs Affecting the Central Nervous System. London:
    Arnold.
CAMPBELL, W. J. (1967). *J. Neurochem.* **14**, 937.
CARLSSON, A. (1969). In Symposium (1969), pp. 305, 353.
CASIER, H. (1967). In Maickel (1967), p. 73.
CLARK, W. C., BLACKMAN, H. J. & PRESTON, J. E. (1967). *Arch. internat. Pharm. Ther.*
    170, 350.
COLLIER, H. O. J. (1969). In Steinberg (1969), p. 49.

CLOUET, D. (1968). *Internat. Rev. Neurobiol.* **11**, 100.
CLOUET, D. H. (1971). *Handb. Neurochem.* **6**, 479.
Colloquium (1951). Méchanisme de la Narcose. Paris: Centre National de la Recherche Scientifique.
Conference (1962). *Psychopharm. Service Centre Bull.* **2**, 29.
CONNELL, P. H. (1958). Amphetamine Psychosis. London: Institute of Psychiatry.
CONSOLO, S., DOLFINI, E., GARATTINI, S. & VALZELLI, L. (1967). *J. Pharm. Pharmacol.* **19**, 253.
COOPER, S. J., JOYCE, D. & SUMMERFIELD, A. (1969). *Proc. Brit. Pharmacol. Soc.* 25.
COX, B. M., GINSBURG, M. & OSMAN, O. H. (1968). *Brit. J. Pharmacol. Chemother.* **33**, 245.
COX, B. M. & GINSBURG, M. (1969). In Steinberg (1969), p. 97.
COX, B. M. & OSMAN, O. H. (1970). *Brit. J. Pharmacol.* **38**, 157.
CRAWFORD, J. M. (1970). *Neuropharmacology*, **9**, 31.
DICKINS, D. W., LADER, M. H. & STEINBERG, H. (1965). *Brit. J. Pharmacol. Chemother.* **24**, 14.
DOBKIN, J. (1970). *J. Neurochem.* **17**, 237.
DOMINO, E. F. (1962). *Ann. Rev. Pharmacol.* **2**, 215.
DRING, L. G., SMITH, R. L. & WILLIAMS, R. T. (1970). *Biochem. J.* **116**, 425.
EDWARDS, C. & LARRABEE, M. G. (1955). *J. Physiol.* **130**, 456.
EFRON, D. H. (1968) (Ed.). Psychopharmacology: A Review of Progress. Washington, D.C.: U.S. Govt. Printing Office.
EFRON, D. H. (1970) (Ed.). Psychotomimetic Drugs. New York: Raven Press.
ENGEL, J., HANSON, L. C. F., ROOS, B-E. & STROMBERGSSON, L-E. (1968). *Psychopharmacologia*, **13**, 140.
ERWIN, V. G. & DEITRICH, R. A. (1966). *J. biol. Chem.* **241**, 3533.
ESSIG, C. F., GRACE, M. E. & WILLIAMSON, E. L. (1963). *Science*, **140**, 828.
ESTLER, C. J. & AMMON, H. P. T. (1967). *J. Neurochem.* **14**, 799.
FEATHERSTONE, R. M. & MUEHLBAECHER, C. A. (1963). *Pharm. Rev.* **15**, 97.
FERGUSON, J. (1939). *Proc. roy. Soc. B.* **127**, 387.
FORSANDER, O. A. & RÄIHÄ, N. C. R. (1960). *J. biol. Chem.* **235**, 34.
FREUND, G. (1967). In Maickel (1967), p. 89.
GABAY, S. (1971). *Handb. Neurochem.* **6**, 325.
GHOSH, S. K. & GHOSH, J. J. (1968). *J. Neurochem.* **15**, 1375.
GORDON, M. (1967) (Ed.). Psychopharmacological Agents. New York: Academic Press.
GREENGARD, O. & MCILWAIN, H. (1955). *Biochem. J.* **61**, 61.
GROPPETTI, A. & COSTA, E. (1969). *Internat. J. Neuropharmacol.* **8**, 209.
GUNNE, L-M. & LEWANDER, T. (1968). *Proc. Assoc. Res. nerv. ment. Dis.* **46**, 106.
HÄKKINEN, H-M. & KULONEN, E. (1961). *Biochem. J.* **78**, 588.
HÄKKINEN, H-M., KULONEN, E. & WALLGREN, H. (1963). *Biochem. J.* **88**, 488.
HANO, K., KANETO, H., KAKUNAGA, T. & MORIBAYASHI, N. (1964). *Biochem. Pharmacol.* **13**, 441.
HEWICK, D. S. & FOUTS, J. R. (1970). *Biochem. J.* **117**, 833.
HINE, C. H., SHICK, A. F., MARGOLIS, L., BURBRIDGE, T. N. & SIMON, A. (1952). *J. Pharmacol.* **106**, 253.
HOLMBERG, G. (1963). *Internat. Rev. Neurobiol.* **5**, 389.
HUNTER, F. E. & LOWRY, O. H. (1956). *Pharm. Rev.* **8**, 89.
IVERSEN, L. L. (1967). Uptake and Storage of Noradrenaline in Sympathetic Nerves. Cambridge: University Press.
JACOBSEN, E. (1952). *Nature, Lond.* **169**, 645; *Pharm. Rev.* **4**, 107.
JARAMILLO, G. A. V. & GUTH, P. S. (1963). *Biochem. Pharmacol.* **12**, 525.
JASPER, H. H., WARD, A. A. & POPE, A. (1969). Basic Mechanisms of the Epilepsies. Boston: Little, Brown.
JHAMANDAS, K., PINSKY, C. & PHILLIS, J. W. (1970). *Nature, Lond.* **228**, 176.
KALANT, H. (1962). *Quart. J. Stud. Alcohol.* **23**, 52.
KALANT, H. & ISRAEL, Y. (1967). In Maickel (1967), p. 25.
KALANT, O. J. (1966). The Amphetamines: Toxicity and Addiction. Toronto: University Press.

18

KEMP, J. W. & WOODBURY, D. M. (1969). In Jasper *et al.* (1969), p. 666.
KIESSLING, K-H. (1963). *Exper. Cell. Res.* **30**, 569.
KJELDGAARD, N. O. (1949). *Acta pharmacol. toxicol.* **5**, 397.
KOCH, A. & WOODBURY, D. M. (1960). *Amer. J. Physiol.* **198**, 434.
KRNJEVIĆ, K., RANDIĆ, M. & SIESJÖ, B. K. (1965). *J. Physiol.* **176**, 105.
KWAN, E. & TREVOR, A. (1969). *Mol. Pharmacol.* **5**, 236.
KUTT, H., WINTERS, W., KOKENGE, R. & MCDOWELL, F. (1964). *Arch. Neurol.* **11**, 642.
LARRABEE, M. G. & BRONK, D. W. (1952). *Cold Spr. Harb. Sym. quant. Biol.* **17**, 245.
LARRABEE, M. G. & POSTERNAK, J. M. (1952). *J. Neurophysiol.* **15**, 91.
LEPAGE, G. A. (1946). *Amer. J. Physiol.* **146**, 267.
LESTER, D. (1962). *Quart. J. Stud. Alcohol.* **23**, 17.
LINDBOHM, R. & WALLGREN, H. (1962). *Acta Pharm. Toxicol.* **19**, 53.
LIPTON, M. A. (1970). In Efron (1970), p. 231.
LOH, H. H., SHEN, F-H. & WAY, E. L. (1969). *Biochem. Pharmacol.* **18**, 2711.
LOWRY, O. H., PASSONNEAU, J. V., HASSELBERGER, F. X. & SCHULZ, D. W. (1964). *J. biol. Chem.* **239**, 18.
LUCIA, S. P. (1963) (Ed.). Alcohol and Civilization. New York: McGraw-Hill.
LUNDQUIST, F., FUGMANN, U., KLANING, E. & RASMUSSEN, H. (1959). *Biochem. J.* **72**, 409.
MACHIYAMA, Y., UTENA, H. & KIKUCHI, M. (1970). *Proc. Jap. Acad.* **46**, 738.
MACKWORTH, N. H. (1950). Researches on the Measurement of Human Performance. London: H.M.S.O.
MAICKEL, R. P. (1967) (Ed.). Biochemical Factors in Alcoholism. Oxford: Pergamon.
MANDELL, A. J. & MORGAN, M. (1970). *Nature, Lond.* **227**, 75.
MARDONES, J. (1963). See Root & Hofmann, p. 99.
MCILWAIN, H. (1953). *Biochem. J.* **53**, 403.
MCILWAIN, H. (1957). Chemotherapy and the Central Nervous System. London: Churchill.
MCILWAIN, H. (1968*a*). *Nature, Lond.* **220**, 889, 1364.
MCILWAIN, H. (1968*b*). *Brit. med. Bull.* **24**, 174.
MCILWAIN, H. (1969). In Experimental Approaches to the Study of Drug Dependence. Ed. H. Kalant & R. D. Hawkins. Toronto: University Press.
MCILWAIN, H. & GREENGARD, O. (1957). *J. Neurochem.* **1**, 348.
MCKINLEY-MCKEE, J. S. & DONNINGER, C. (1963). *Biochem. J.* **85**, 23P.
MCMANUS, I. R., CONTAG, H. O. & OLSON, R. E. (1966). *J. biol. Chem.* **241**, 349.
MILLER, S. L. (1961). *Proc. Nat. Acad. Sci.* **47**, 1515.
MISTILIS, S. P. & BIRCHALL, A. (1969). *Nature, Lond.* **223**, 199.
MOORE, K. E. (1963). *J. Pharmacol.* **142**, 8.
MULÉ, S. J. (1967). *J. Pharmacol.* **156**, 92.
MULÉ, S. J. (1969). In Steinberg (1969), p. 97.
MULLINS, L. J. (1971). *Handb. Neurochem.* **6**, 395.
NELSON, S. R., SCHULZ, D. W., PASSONNEAU, J. V. & LOWRY, O. H. (1968). *J. Neurochem.* **15**, 1271.
OLDS, J. (1962). *Physiol. Rev.* **43**, 554.
PALMER, G. (1962). *Biochim. Biophys. Acta*, **56**, 444.
PATON, W. D. M. (1969). In Steinberg (1969), p. 31.
PAULING, L. (1961). *Science*, **134**, 15.
PETSCHEK, R. & TIMIRAS, P. S. (1963). *Amer. J. Physiol.* **205**, 1163.
PHILLIPSON, R. V. (1970). Modern Trends in Drug Dependence and Alcoholism. London: Butterworths.
POPHAM, R. E. & SCHMIDT, W. (1962). A Decade of Alcoholism Research. Toronto: University Press.
RAJAGOPALAN, K. V., FRIDOVICH, I. & HANDLER, P. (1962). *J. biol. Chem.* **237**, 992.
RASKIN, N. H. & SOKOLOFF, L. (1968). *Science*, **162**, 131.
ROOT, W. S. & HOFMANN, F. G. (1963) (Ed.). Physiological Pharmacology. New York: Academic Press.
RUF, H. (1951). *Arkiv. f. Psychiat. u. Z. Neurol.* **187**, 97.
RUSHTON, R., STEINBERG, H. & TOMKIEWICZ, M. (1968). *Nature, Lond.* **220**, 885.

RUSSELL, G. F. M. (1960). *Clin. Sci.* **19**, 327.
RUSSELL, P. T. & VAN BRUGGEN, J. T. (1964). *J. biol. Chem.* **239**, 719.
SCHUBERTH, J. & SUNDWALL, A. (1967). *J. Neurochem.* **14**, 807.
SHEPPARD, J. R., ALBERSHEIM, P. & MCCLEARN, G. E. (1968). *Biochem. Genetics*, **2**, 205.
SHUSTER, L. & HANNAM, R. V. (1964). *J. biol. Chem.* **239**, 3401.
SIMPSON, B. A. & IVERSEN, S. D. (1971). *Nature New Biol.* **230**, 31.
SJÖQVIST, F. & TOTTIE, M. (1969) (Ed.). Abuse of Central Stimulants. Stockholm: Almqvist & Wiksell.
SKOU, J. C. (1961). *J. Pharm. Pharmacol.* **13**, 204.
SNYDER, S. H., WEINGARTNER, H. & FAILLACE, L. A. (1970). In Efron (1970), p. 247.
SPINKS, A. & WARING, W. S. (1963). *Progr. Med. Chem.* **3**, 261.
STEIN, L. (1968). In Efron (1968), p. 105.
STEIN, L. & WISE, D. C. (1969). *J. comp. Physiol. Psychol.* **67**, 189.
STEINBERG, H. (1969). (Ed.). Scientific Basis of Drug Dependence. London: Churchill.
STEINBERG, H., RUSHTON, R. & TINSON, C. (1961). *Nature, Lond.* **192**, 533.
STEINBERG, H., DE REUCK, A. V. S. & KNIGHT, J. (1964). Animal Behaviour and Drug Action. London: Churchill.
SULSER, F. & SANDERS-BUSH, E. (1970). In Efron (1970) p. 83.
STOTZ, E., WESTERFELD, W. W. & BERG, R. L. (1944). *J. biol. Chem.* **152**, 41.
SUTHERLAND, V. C., HINE, C. H. & BURBRIDGE, T. N. (1956). *J. Pharmacol.* **116**, 469.
SUTHERLAND, V. C., BURBRIDGE, R. N., ADAMS, J. E. & SIMON, A. (1960). *Appl. Physiol.* **15**, 189.
Symposium (1949). *Proc. R. Soc. Med.* **42**, Supplement, 1.
Symposium (1957). *Ann. N.Y. Acad. Sci.* **66**, 417.
Symposium (1962). Enzymes and Drug Action. Ed. Mongar & de Reuck. Ciba Foundation. London: Churchill.
Symposium (1963). Selective Vulnerability of the Brain in Hypoxaemia. Ed. Schade & McMenemey. Oxford: Blackwell.
Symposium (1964). *Proc. Internat. Neurochem. Sympos.* **5**.
Symposium (1964a). Biogenic Amines. Ed. Himwich & Himwich. Amsterdam: Elsevier.
Symposium (1969). Abuse of Central Stimulants. Ed. A. Sjöqvist & M. Tottie. Stockholm: Almqvist & Wiksell.
SZARA, S. (1970). In Efron (1970), p. 275.
TAKEMORI, A. E. (1962). *J. Pharmacol.* **135**, 89.
TOWER, D. B. (1960). Neurochemistry of Epilepsy. Springfield: Thomas.
TRÉMOLIÈRES, J. (1970). (Edit.) *Internat. Encyclop. Pharmacol. Therap. Sect.* 20, vol. I, II. Oxford: Pergamon.
UTENA, H. (1966). *Progr. Brain Res.* **21B**, 192.
UTENA, H., EZOE, T., KATO, N. & HADA, H. (1959). *J. Neurochem.* **4**, 161.
VALZELLI, L. (1969). *Proc. Coll. Internat. Neuropsychopharm.* **6**, 355.
WALLGREN, H. (1963). *J. Neurochem.* **10**, 349.
WALLGREN, H. (1971). *Handb. Neurochem.* **6**, 509.
WALLGREN, H. & KULONEN, E. (1960). *Biochem. J.* **75**, 150.
WEISS, B. (1969). In Sjöqvist & Tottie (1969), p. 31.
WESTERFELD, W. W., RICHERT, D. A. & BLOOM, R. J. (1959). *J. biol. Chem.* **234**, 1889.
WESTERFELD, W. W., RICHERT, D. A. & HIGGINS, E. S. (1959). *J. biol. Chem.* **234**, 1897.
WIKLER, A. (1964). Proc. 26th Internat. Congr. Alcohol Alcoholism. Stockholm: Eklunds & Vaastryck.
WIKLER, A. (1968) (Ed.). The addictive States. *Proc. Assoc. Res. nerv. ment. Dis.* **46**.
WILLIAMSON, J. R., SCHOLZ, R., BROWNING, E. T., THURMAN, R. G. & FUKAMI, M. H. (1969). *J. biol. Chem.* **244**, 5044.
WILSON, E. C. (1967). In Maickel, R. P. (1967), p. 115.
WOODBURY, D. (1952). *J. Pharmacol.* **105**, 46.
YAMAMOTO, C. & MCILWAIN, H. (1966). *J. Neurochem.* **13**, 1333.
YOUNG, R. L. & GORDON, M. W. (1962). *J. Neurochem.* **9**, 161.

16 The Brain and the Body as a Whole

The central nervous system, like many other parts of the body, is to be under-stood in two ways: in itself, and in its relationship to the rest of the body. In this final chapter these two ways of viewing the brain will be exemplified. First is described a little of the intricate chemical control of the body from the hypothalamus and pituitary, which are linked not only anatomically by intriguingly specialized blood-vessels and nerve fibres, but also functionally. The purpose of such description is not to summarize this aspect of endocrin-ology but to emphasize the chemical versatility of the central nervous system. Second is discussed the speed of chemical change in the brain, in a way which enables it to be regarded as one metabolic unit, despite its obvious diversity and complexity.

The Pituitary and Pituitary Hormones

Removal of the pituitary gland or damage to it in the living animal has effects so drastic and bearing on so many clinical problems that its study has been deservedly widespread. Its key position in the hormonal regulation of the body as a whole is well documented from endocrinological, chemical, pathological and pharmacological studies (Harris & Donovan, 1966; Levine, 1966; Berde, 1968; Reiss, 1970; Sachs, 1970). Chemically, the pituitary is remarkable in its content of biologically active peptides and proteins (Table 16.1) organized in elaborate neurosecretory systems. Many of its more general biochemical properties are nevertheless similar to those of other parts of the nervous system, in spite of the origin of the anterior pituitary or adenohypophysis from non-nervous tissue.

Metabolism of the Pituitary

The pituitary, in a bony cavity at the base of the brain, is difficultly placed for metabolic studies *in situ*. As a separated gland it is, however, readily available, because techniques for its removal in small experimental animals have been developed in producing hypophysectomized animals for assay of the pituitary hormones. In the rat the pituitary weighs typically 10 mg. or less, and in man, 500–600 mg.; aspects of its metabolism can thus be studied by incubating the whole gland or slices from it, in oxygenated salines. Under these conditions, whole pituitaries from the rat respired at rates between 35 and 60 μmoles

540

O_2/g. fresh tissue/hr. and in short experiments these rates were not greatly increased by added glucose. Anterior and posterior pituitary each respired at 55–60 μmoles O_2/g. hr. in one set of experiments, in which lactic acid was formed from glucose at 10 μmoles/g. hr. by the anterior and about 15 μmoles/g. hr. by the posterior pituitary (Roberts & Keller, 1955). Slices of beef anterior pituitary formed $^{14}CO_2$ from 1-^{14}C-glucose, and the reaction was found to be stimulated by β-phenylethylamine and several of its derivatives; these were concluded to act by virtue of the aldehydes yielded by monoamine oxidase (Barondes, 1962). In the ground tissue, relations rather similar to those of A, Fig. 6.1, were displayed: pyruvate was oxidized at rates greatly increased by fumarate and adenine nucleotides. Succinate and oxoglutarate also served as oxidizable substrates, but not glycine, alanine nor glutamate. Transamination between glutamate and oxaloacetate could however proceed at 360 μmoles/g. hr.

Tissues from the pituitary, maintained under good metabolic conditions in oxygenated glucose salines have been employed in studies of the release of pituitary hormones; instances are given subsequently (see Fig. 16.3). Also, rat anterior pituitary so incubated established defined levels of cyclic adenosine 3',5'-phosphate of about 6 nmoles/g. which were augmented about 10-fold by hypothalamic extracts, concomitantly with eight-fold release of luteinizing hormone (q.v.; Zor et al., 1970). Adrenaline did not cause such release, although it released other of the anterior pituitary hormones under similar circumstances

After grinding pituitary tissues in sucrose and centrifuging, fractions rich in nuclei and smaller subcellular entities can be obtained by the techniques developed for other tissues (Chapter 12 and see below). Again, the denser nuclear fraction was rich in deoxyribonucleic acid and poor in systems oxidizing succinate. Fractions less easily sedimented had properties akin to mitochondria and microsomes. In particular the "large granules" stained with Janus green and were rich in succinoxidase. A specific feature, which can give pituitary fractions a characteristic visual appearance during preparation, is their content of secretory granules; lysosomes are also in evidence (McDonald et al., 1968 and see below). Cholinesterase, however, was not concentrated in microsomal fractions (q.v.) to the extent found in the cerebral cortex, but in both lobes of beef pituitary was found also in mitochondrial and supernatant fractions (Parmar et al., 1961). It had, moreover, a greater admixture of non-specific cholinesterase.

Proteinases, Peptidases and Amidases of the Pituitary

These enzymes of the pituitary draw much importance from the protein and peptide nature of the hormones secreted by both lobes of the gland. The pituitary carries an active protease of pepsin-like properties which can in-activate certain of the pituitary hormones and is itself inhibited by constituents of blood plasma (Melchior & Hilker, 1955; Ellis, 1960; Lewis, 1963). Three arylamidases have been characterized in the pituitary; these act on model substrates which have short peptide chains attached to β-naphthylamine (Ellis & Perry, 1966; McDonald et al., 1968a, b). When purified these three differ in their cofactor requirements, pH optima and substrate specificity.

A dipeptidyl arylamidase II from rat or ox anterior pituitary was relatively specific in its action on lysylalanyl-β-naphthylamine among analogous compounds examined. To the lysylalanyl derivative it showed K_m 10 μM, and an optimum activity at pH 5·5 which was inhibited competitively by a number of cations including Na^+ (K_i, 5 mM) and by puromycin (K_i, 20 μM). Also it acted on simple peptides and here among 9 greatest activity was on trialanine and was maximal at pH 4·5 with K_m 2·5 mM. From aqueous extracts of ox anterior pituitary it was purified 1,000-fold by ammonium sulphate, DEAE-cellulose and gel electrophoresis; the arylamidase and peptidase activities throughout purification were 2·5-fold greater with trialanine than with the arylamine peptide as substrate, and rose to 2·64 moles/hr. g. protein. Dipeptides and tetrapeptides were not attacked.

When this peptidase was examined in tissue dispersions made in isotonic sucrose, it separated in a fraction which was distinct from nuclei, mitochondria and secretory granules and which was shown electron-microscopically to be enriched in lysosomes. This fraction contained the peak acid phosphatase activity, and the peak also of a distinct seryltyrosyl arylamidase I. The arylamidase I and II activities in this fraction were largely latent, showing prior to activation with a surface-active agent, only 5–10% of their maximal activity. By contrast, an arginylarginyl arylamidase III was not particulate-bound and was active at pH 9. Arylamidases I and II were separable by ammonium sulphate.

Forms of Occurrence of the Pituitary Hormones

Histological studies of the intact pituitary associated several of its secretions (Table 16.1) with the presence of granules, 0·1–0·3 μ across, in both anterior and posterior lobes.

After dispersing parts of the gland in isotonic sucrose and centrifuging, the granules are still recognizable in particulate fractions. From the *posterior pituitary* of the dog, dispersion in buffered sucrose and differential centrifuging deposited a nuclear fraction; the supernatant at higher speed yielded a pellet containing 50% of the vasopressin of the gland. Density gradient centrifuging now separated the fraction containing vasopressin from mitochondria; the vasopressin remained in granules, relatively inactive biologically but released by a detergent or by hot dilute acetic acid. Electron-microscopically the granules displayed stainable material within a distinct outer membrane (Pardoe & Weatherall, 1955; Weinstein *et al.*, 1961; Barer *et al.*, 1963). Greatest enrichment of vasopressin in dispersions of the hypothalamus (q.v.) has also been found in a granule-fraction.

Neurosecretory granules from the neural lobes of bovine pituitaries were found to contain the vasopressin and oxytocin in association with larger molecules: proteins, termed *neurophysins* (La Bella *et al.*, 1967; Dean & Hope, 1968). After separating the granules in quantity by centrifuging in sucrose gradients, they were observed by electron microscopic control to be freed from other subcellular particles. Lysis in 0·1 N-HCl gave in solution the neurohypophysial hormones and the neurophysins. Some 16% of the protein of the granules was insoluble, while 62% of the soluble protein consisted of neurophysins I and II in equal amounts. The neurophysins were separable by electrophoresis and prepared on larger scale by direct acid extraction of acetone-dried posterior pituitaries (Hollenberg & Hope, 1968; Wuu & Safran, 1969; Uttenthal & Hope, 1970). Two major components were obtainable in this way from bovine tissues: I, apparent molecular weight 19,000 and II, 21,000. They were of similar amino acid composition but I lacked histidine present in II; they differed also in methionine content. Each neurophysin formed complexes with both oxytocin and vasopressin and several of the complexes were obtained in crystalline form. By chemical modification of neurophysin II the molecular unit was found to be of molecular weight about 10,000 (Furth & Hope, 1970); this neurophysin II was concluded to be associated in the pituitary mainly with vasopressin, by non-covalent forces at a defined binding site. Neurophysin preparations from pig pituitaries have also been fractionated to two major components and characterized by amino acid analyses and by their combination with oxytocin and vasopressin. In this case the main components were of molecular weight about 9,000 and 14,000 and firm combination took place between 1 g-mole of lysine vasopressin (the porcine hormone: see Fig. 16.2) and some 13,000 g. of the latter component (Ginsburg & Thomas, 1969). Neurophysin did not form complexes with histamine, catecholamines, substance P nor with a number of other compounds. A third neurophysin has been prepared and characterized from bovine posterior pituitaries (Rauch et al. 1969).

Dispersions of the *anterior pituitary* from rats, made in sucrose and polyvinylpyrrolidone, have been fractionated by filtration to remove larger particles, followed by gradient-density and differential centrifugation. This gave fractions shown electron-microscopically to contain granules of different sizes. Those of 0·3–0·45 μ across were akin to "A granules" seen in acidophilic cells of the intact pituitary. Smaller particles of 0·1–0·2 μ across were similar to "B granules" from basophilic cells. Neither of these fractions contained appreciable cytochrome oxidase, succinic dehydrogenase or ribonucleic acid and thus were distinct from mitochondria and ribosomes. Moreover, assay for the pituitary hormones showed them to be distinctively distributed among the fractions: the A granules, containing only 5% of the protein of the dispersion, carried the greater part of the lactogenic and growth hormones. The B granules with 8% of the original protein were enriched in thyroid-stimulating hormone and gonadotrophins. Adrenocorticotrophic hormone was found in a distinct fraction, which also contained microsomes (Hymer & McShan, 1963; see Ziegler & Melchior, 1956).

Biosynthesis of Pituitary Hormones

Protein synthesis in several cerebral systems has been described in Chapters 9 and 13; synthesis of *adrenocorticotrophic hormone* in the pituitary is noteworthy as an example of synthesis of a specific protein species by the brain and by a cerebral preparation *in vitro*. Considering first the formation *in vivo*, the synthesis was demonstrated to occur in the pituitary itself by administering 1-14C-serine to rats 12 min. before they were killed and their anterior and posterior pituitaries and hypothalamus separately extracted and fractionated. By

chromatographic separation and biological assay, newly-incorporated serine
was shown to be present in adrenocorticotrophic hormone in the extracts.
Animals now subjected to a stress known to cause release of adrenocorticotrophic hormone, showed increased incorporation of 1-^{14}C-serine to the
hormone from specifically the anterior pituitary (Jacobowitz *et al.*, 1963).

In vitro incorporation of amino acids to proteins generally, in isolated
pituitaries from the rat has been demonstrated using ^{35}S-methionine (Ziegler &
Melchior, 1956). With the intact or sliced gland incubated for 0·5–2 hr. in

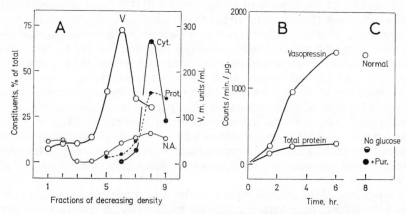

FIG. 16.1. Vasopressin: occurrence and synthesis in tissues from the
hypothalamus plus median eminence of dogs (Sachs, 1963, 1970).
    A. Occurrence: dispersions of the tissue after differential centrifuga-
tion were centrifuged in a sucrose gradient, continuous between 1·5 and
2 M. Vasopressin-containing granules, *V*, are largely separated from
mitochondria indicated by cytochrome oxidase, *cyt.*, and from much of
the protein and nucleic acid-containing particles, *NA*.
    B. Incorporation of ^{35}S-cysteine to vasopressin on incubating
tissue from the hypothalamus plus posterior pituitary of guinea pigs,
in glucose bicarbonate–Ringer solutions. After a period in a diluted
tissue-culture medium, tissues were incubated in the bicarbonate plus
cysteine, nucleotides and an antibiotic for the periods indicated. They
were then extracted with trichloroacetic acid for determination of
vasopressin, total protein and the ^{35}S in each.
    C. In a similar experiment some tissues were incubated without
glucose and others with glucose plus 0·5 mM puromycin; all data quoted
refer to vasopressin; incorporation to protein was similarly depressed.

salines containing the methionine, and succinate as oxidizable substrate, rates
of incorporation up to 0·1 μmoles methionine/g. fresh pituitary/hr. were found.
During these experiments net protein synthesis was not observed, but protein
diffused from the tissue to the medium. The rates of incorporation observed
were several times those for incorporation of methionine to liver proteins in
parallel experiments, though the status of succinate as an energy-yielding
substrate for pituitary tissue does not appear to have been appraised. Thus with
cerebral cortex, succinate supports respiration but not labile phosphates
(Chapter 4). On grinding pituitary tissue, the rate of methionine incorporation
decreased but the phenomenon could be reproduced, at diminished rates, by
mixtures containing the large-granule fraction. Synthesis of adrenocortico-

trophic hormone was demonstrated by again incubating rat pituitaries, specifically the anterior lobe, in salines containing ^{14}C-phenylalanine (Wool *et al.*, 1961). After adding carrier corticotrophin, the tissues were extracted with hot dilute acetic acid; adsorption, elution and chromatography gave material containing no free phenylalanine but retaining ^{14}C. The incorporation proceeded almost linearly for 4 hr., and the product was characterized in several fashions as adrenocorticotrophin. Moreover, prior adrenalectomy of the animals yielding the tissue increased incorporation to adrenocorticotrophin-like material but not to other fractions.

When maintained *in vitro* under tissue-culture conditions for some days, anterior pituitary samples can synthesize certain of their constituent hormones. The rat gland during 3 days' incubation liberated lactogenic hormone to a surrounding fluid in quantities up to ten times the amount initially present in the explant (Gala & Reece, 1963). Further studies with isolated pituitary preparations are quoted subsequently in describing releasing factors for the pituitary hormones (Fig. 16.3).

Synthesis of *vasopressin*, which occurs largely if not entirely in the hypothalamus, is described below. The further metabolism and inactivation of the pituitary hormones are often linked with their actions on target organs outside the brain, which are not described in detail here (see Smith & Sachs, 1961; Rudman *et al.*, 1964; Harris & Donovan, 1966).

Active Pituitary Constituents

Before the localization and synthesis of pituitary hormones were understood in the detail just described, extraction and fractionation of the whole gland had yielded many pure substances which could restore particular bodily functions which were disturbed when the gland was removed. This very impressive display of chemical control from the pituitary is summarized in Table 16.1 in the order in which comment is given below. It is to be emphasized that this information covers only a very small part of the complex end-results on metabolism and behaviour, which are effected by materials from the gland. It is not entirely certain that materials extracted from the gland are the hormones as they are normally released to the bloodstream, but accepting a common usage the term hormone is applied to them. All are peptides or proteins; in general, no small prosthetic groups have been recognized as carrying their activity. The source of the purified compounds has usually been the pituitaries of pig, sheep or ox removed at slaughter. Their activities are not markedly species-specific, but instances are noted of given hormones from different species differing in chemical structure. Material from human pituitaries has also received systematic fractionation (Wilhelmi; Li: *Colloquium*, 1960; see Harris & Donovan, 1966 and Sachs, 1970). The pituitary hormones have been compared with other proteins secreted by vertebrates, and common chemical features noted (Adelson, 1971).

Anterior Lobe (Adenohypophysis)

The large molecule of the *growth hormone* has been prepared from several animal species in forms homogeneous by physical criteria, and found to consist

Table 16.1

Active materials from pituitary extracts

Substance (synonyms)	Brief indication of actions and assay	Chemical nature
Anterior pituitary		
1. Growth hormone (somatotrophin)	Accelerates growth of body as a whole; assays measure body weight or the width of a cartilage of the tibia	From human pituitary, a protein with 188 amino acid residues, mol. wt. 21,500
2. Adrenocortico-trophic hormone (ACTH; cortico-trophin)	Stimulates adrenal cortex as measured by increase in adrenal weight, depletion of ascorbic acid, or release of steroid hormones	From sheep or pig, a polypeptide of thirty-nine residues (Fig. 16.2); mol. wt. about 3,500
3. Thyrotrophic hormone (thyrotrophin)	Stimulates thyroid gland; assays measure the size of the gland or discharge of isotopic iodine compounds from it	From ox, a glycoprotein; mol. wt. about 10,000
4. Lactogenic hormone (prolactin; luteotrophin)	Maintains corpus luteum and elicits milk secretion; stimulates crop gland in immature pigeons	From ox or sheep, a protein; mol. wt. about 26,500
5. Follicle-stimulating (gameto-trophic) hormone	Promotes maturation of ovarian follicles and spermatozoa; an assay measures ovarian size	A glycoprotein; mol. wt. about 17,000
6. Interstitial cell stimulating (luteinizing) hormone	Promotes ovulation; stimulates the corpus luteum and interstitial cells of ovary and testis	A glycoprotein; mol. wt. about 23,000
Posterior pituitary		
1. Vasopressin (pressor-anti-diuretic hormone)	Raises blood pressure of anaesthetized or spinal animals; assays are by intravenous injection to dog, cat or rat. Delays flow of urine when water and then hormone are given to rats or mice	Peptide of nine amino-acid residues (Fig. 16.2); mol. wt. 1,056 or 1,084
2. Oxytocin	Contracts uterine muscle. Assays use isolated guinea-pig or rat uteri in saline. Also causes diuresis and milk-ejection	Peptide of nine amino acid residues (Fig. 16.2); mol. wt. 1,007

entirely of known amino acids. Their sequence has been determined in several instances, including the human hormone (Li *et al.*, 1966; Niall, 1971). The bovine hormone, on treatment with carboxypeptidase releases two molecules of phenylalanine from a terminal position, and other amino acids, without marked change in activity. Some degradation beyond this is also compatible with activity, but potency is lost while the residue is still a large molecule. In this molecule certain substitutions may be made, for example by iodine and guanidine groups, while retaining activity. Ox anterior pituitaries yield 3·5 g./kg. of nearly pure hormone, of which 20 µg./day restores normal growth to hypophysectomized rats according to the criteria of a quantitative assay. Plasma assays of growth hormone showed its prompt release in association with hypoglycaemia, block of glucose utilization by 2-deoxyglucose, or by exercise and certain stressful situations; the release could be suppressed by increased blood glucose. In the action of the hormone on growth many metabolic adjustments occur in the body as a whole, and certain of these have been observed in separated tissues: for example in the metabolism of isolated diaphragm suspended in glucose salines and on the incorporation of precursors to ribonucleic acids and proteins of liver slices, which was accelerated by

(I) Ser-Tyr-Ser-Met-Glu-His-Phe-Arg-Try-Gly-Lys-Pro-Val-Gly-Lys-Lys-Arg-Arg-Pro-Val-
1   10   20

-Lys-Val-Tyr-Pro-Ala-Gly-Glu-Asp-Asp-Glu-Ala-Ser-Glu(NH$_2$)-
30

-Ala-Phe-Pro-Leu-Glu-Phe
39

(II) Cys-Tyr-Ileu-Glu(NH$_2$)-Asp(NH$_2$)-Cys-Pro-Leu-Gly(NH$_2$)

FIG. 16.2. (I) Sequence of amino-acids in α-corticotrophin from sheep anterior pituitary (Li, 1956, Lee et al., 1961). Corticotrophin-A from the pig contains .leu.ala. in positions 31 and 32 and differs also at positions 25–28. Human corticotrophin differs between positions 26 and 33. (II) Oxytocin of ox or pig. Vasopressin is also a peptide of nine amino acid residues, but with phenylalanine in place of the isoleucine and arginine in place of the leucine of oxytocin (in material from the ox; from the pig lysine replaces leucine: du Vigneaud, 1955; see Symposium, 1962; Acher, 1966 and Sachs, 1970).

bovine growth hormone at 10 ng./ml. Moreover, effects in microsomal protein-synthesizing systems suggest a primary point of action for the hormone to be in the formation of ribonucleic acids (Korner, 1964; Clemens & Korner, 1969; Ganong & Martini, 1969).

The *adrenocorticotrophic hormone* is chemically the smallest and most completely understood of the anterior pituitary hormones. As extracted by acid organic solvents it proved to be a polypeptide of which the structure in several species is now completely known (Fig. 16.2; Evans et al., 1966). An active hormone has been synthesized, and also peptides approaching the structures and activities of the natural hormones; thus much data on structure and corticotrophic activity relationships are available. Small differences in composition occur in the materials from sheep and from pig pituitaries. From the polypeptide of thirty-nine amino acid residues, at least eleven residues may be removed from one end of the chain without much loss of activity. Biological assay of the hormone is sufficiently sensitive for it to be determined in different parts of the body. The activity of mammalian pituitaries has been found relatively uniform, corresponding to 1–3 mg. corticotrophin/g. from the rat to man or the whale. Levels from zero to 2 μg./100 ml. have been found in blood plasma or serum from man; in the rat it has been reported as not normally detectable but to rise to 2 μg./100 ml. on adrenalectomy. When the bovine hormone is injected intravenously to the rat it rapidly passes to the tissues, where it loses its activity. Endogenous corticotrophin in the rat is also estimated to have a half-life of only 1 min. Incubated *in vitro*, corticotrophin is quickly inactivated by several tissues but not by blood plasma.

The adrenocorticotrophic hormone stimulates both synthesis and release of the active steroids from the adrenal, and acts promptly: rates of secretion are increased within 2 min. in the dog. It also will act on the perfused adrenal, and on slices of the adrenal of the rat, incubated *in vitro*. In this way one action of the pituitary hormone has been shown to be on a particular stage in synthesis of the corticosteroids: on the conversion of cholesterol to pregnenolone. Action of ACTH on the adrenal appears to be mediated by cyclic adenosine 3',5'-phosphate, as is also its action on adipose tissue (Skosey, 1970). Dosage with corticotrophin over a period of days or weeks results in growth in size of the adrenal, and changes in the pattern of the steroids synthesized and excreted by it. The daily dose necessary to bring about nearly maximal adrenal growth in hypophysectomized rats, is 4–8 μg. It has been suspected that different pituitary fractions have some degree of selective action on different aspects of adrenal functioning, measured by adrenal weight or by the depletion in its content of ascorbic acid which is associated with hormone synthesis. Chemical treatment of pure corticotrophin has also yielded materials more active in one respect than another.

The β-*melanocyte-stimulating* hormone from pig pituitary is also a small peptide of high activity (see Chapter 14); of its eighteen amino acid residues, many are in a sequence found also in adrenocorticotrophic hormone (Harris, 1959). Structures of the hormone in other species have been determined and have a large sequence in common; the human β-melanocyte-stimulating hormone has twenty-two residues (Harris, Lee *et al.*: *Symposium*, 1962). Dodecapeptides of melanocyte-stimulating activity have been characterized from the dogfish pituitary, and evolution of the larger, more active peptides considered (Lowry & Chadwick, 1970).

The *gonadotrophic hormones* (4, 5 and 6 of Table 16.1) may be considered together. The large molecule of the *lactogenic hormone* has been obtained in a yield of about 2 g./kg. sheep pituitary and acts at a total dose of less than 1 mg. in inducing milk secretion in suitably prepared rabbits or guinea pigs. It appears to have a direct action on metabolic systems in mammary tissue. The follicle-stimulating, luteinizing and also the thyrotrophic hormones on purification proved to be glycoproteins and from histological studies appear to be associated with particular basophilic cells of the pituitary. The *follicle-stimulating* hormone was found to be the most soluble in ammonium sulphate and the most resistant to tryptic digestion among the anterior pituitary hormones. It has been highly purified (Duraiswami *et al.*, 1964) and contained fucose, mannose, galactose, a hexosamine and sialic acid residues; of a preparation obtained at about 1 g./kg. sheep pituitary, a total dose of 50 μg. over 3 days was effective in rats. The *luteinizing hormone* proved active in hypophysectomized rats in a dose of some 1–5 μg. The characterized and homogeneous hormone has been dissociated to subunits, their content of 17 amino acids, fucose, mannose, glucosamine and galactosamine residues reported, and considerable reassociation to the active hormone demonstrated by bioassay and immunological techniques (Reichert et al., 1969).

Thyrotrophic activity of pure preparations remained after extensive degradation with papain; material of which 1·5 g. was obtained/kg. ox pituitary, was active at a dose of 25 μg. in the hypophysectomized rat. Thyrotrophin has a number of effects on thyroid tissue *in vitro*, including a prompt action on carbohydrate metabolism and on an ouabain-sensitive adenosine triphosphatase (Turkington, 1963). Mediation of these actions may proceed through cyclic adenosine-3′,5′-phosphate, as activation of adenyl cyclase in preparations from dog thyroid occurred promptly on addition of thyroid-stimulating hormone (Zor et al., 1969).

Posterior Lobe (Neurohypophysis)

Destruction of the neurohypophysis causes abnormalities which have been made good by extracts of specifically the posterior pituitary. Characterization and synthesis of pure substances (Table 16.1) which carry the activity of these extracts represents a major neurochemical achievement. A material regulating blood pressure had been extracted from the pituitary in a dialysable form, at the end of the last century. Its effects were not antagonized by agents which antagonized adrenaline, nor by denervation, and were enhanced by anaesthesia. Graduated membranes gave a good estimate of its molecular weight, and on chemical fractionation the pressor activity was found to be associated with antidiuretic action, also recognized in pituitary extracts. Identification and synthesis has shown the synthetic *vasopressin* (Fig. 16.2) to be active in quantities of less than 1 μg. in raising the blood pressure of small animals and in delaying their flow of urine. The compound thus plays a part in the important regulation of water and salt balance which is coordinated at the central nervous system and is disturbed in diabetes insipidus; this action of the hormone is at the kidney tubules. In bringing about this effect, vasopressin has been demonstrated to become attached to the kidney; it causes there an increased reabsorption of water. Cyclic adenosine 3′,5′-phosphate may mediate vasopressin action.

Vasopressin occurs at about 0·4 g./kg. in the posterior pituitary, comes into action quickly on injection to animals and is quickly inactivated. Plasma vasopressin in the rat shows a half-life of about 1 min.; in man, a half-life under normal conditions of about 5 min. may be greatly extended in association with over-hydration (see Ginsburg, 1968).

The property of contracting the uterus, also present in extracts of the posterior pituitary, was associated with material similar to vasopressin, but separable by solvents or electrophoresis. Again, chemical studies showed activity to lie in a peptide with nine amino acid residues, closely related to vasopressin but more basic. The *oxytocin* is active under appropriate conditions in doses of a fraction of a μg. in contracting the uterus, isolated or *in situ*. Ox posterior pituitary showed activity corresponding to about 0·5 g. oxytocin/kg.; the pure substance comes into effect quickly but briefly after being given parenterally. Structural requirements for action of oxytocin and vasopressin have been examined in detail (du Vigneaud; Rudinger: *Symposium*, 1964; Berde & Boissonnas, 1966).

The posterior pituitary has an especially high content of total peptides, which constitute some 3–4% of the dried gland as ordinarily prepared from the pig. About thirty different peptides have been characterized in extracts from it, apart from the compounds of known hormonal activity. Vasopressin and oxytocin each constitute about 0·4% of the dry weight, but are concluded to be secreted in association with a protein which forms 12% of the dry gland. On provoking secretion by keeping rats restricted in water intake for a month, vasopressin was lost from the posterior pituitary, together with a further 13% of the weight of the gland. The material lost was a particular non-lipid fraction, soluble in acidified 75% ethanol but insoluble in 85% ethanol (Ramachandran & Winnick, 1957; Albers & Brightman, 1959) and now identified as neurophysin (q.v.).

Involvement of the Hypothalamus in the Synthesis and Release of Pituitary Hormones

When the pituitary stalk is cut and the pituitary is prevented from reforming its association with the hypothalamus, pituitary secretions greatly diminish or cease. In the intact animal electrical stimulation of specific parts of the hypothalamus affects the secretions, as also do environmental and psychological factors, indicating connections through the hypothalamus to other parts of the brain. The following brief account notes some of the mechanisms involved, which are characteristically different in the anterior and posterior lobes of the pituitary.

Neurohypophysial Hormones: Synthesis

Linkage between the posterior pituitary and the hypothalamus has been investigated in considerable detail, in many species and by many techniques. The process of neurosecretion which it exemplifies gives an impressive demonstration of the versatility of the nerve cell (Scharrer & Scharrer, 1954; Dicker, 1961; De Robertis: *Symposium*, 1962; Sachs, 1970). In this instance cell bodies in the preoptic nucleus of the hypothalamus, possess axons which run, as the hypothalamic-hypophysial tract, mainly to the posterior pituitary or neurohypophysis where they end around blood vessels. Embryologically this is understandable as the neurohypophysis arises as an outgrowth from the floor of the third ventricle; some 100,000 neurones are involved in this way in the neurohypophysis of the dog. Extracts of certain hypothalamic areas and of the pituitary stalk show the presence of posterior pituitary hormones. Microscopical techniques show material of particular staining properties and common to the different parts of the cells in the hypothalamus, the pituitary stalk, and the neurohypophysis. When the stalk is constricted, microscopy and hormone assay show the material to accumulate in a fashion suggesting that it normally moves down the stalk to the pituitary. It has occasionally been seen outside the nerve endings and in the blood vessels leaving the pituitary. In the pituitary the stainable material is seen to be depleted by stimuli which release the hormones.

The posterior pituitary thus appears to act as a centre at which occurs storage and release of substances whose synthesis has commenced at the hypothalamus. The net synthesis of vasopressin in the experiments just described is relatively small; the hypothalamus plus pituitary of the dogs were estimated to contain about 5–50 μg. and to form it at about 0·01 μg./hr. Isotopic labelling methods show vasopressin and neurophysins both to originate in a region of the hypothalamus with the adjacent median eminence (Sachs, 1963, 1970; Fawcett et al., 1968). ^{35}S-Cysteine or ^{3}H-tyrosine were administered to dogs by infusion of the third cerebral ventricle, so that they arrived at this region but not at the pituitary itself. After 4–6 hr., both soluble and particulate proteins of the hypothalamus were extensively labelled, but those of the pituitary were not. Several days later, however, the pituitary contained much of a highly labelled protein shown by chemical characteristics and by immune reactions to be neurophysin. Movement of ^{35}S, introduced as ^{35}S-cysteine to the supraoptic nucleus of the rat, has been followed during 0·1–6 days after its administration (Nörstrom & Sjöstrand, 1971). Protein containing ^{35}S arrived at the posterior pituitary and was concluded to be a neurophysin component, travelling by axonal transport in the hypothalamic-hypophysial tract.

The hypothalamic vasopressin formed during intraventricular infusion of the ^{35}S-cysteine was itself labelled more extensively than the general hypothalamic protein: especially highly labelled was the vasopressin of large granules, which was at 30 times the specific radioactivity of associated protein. In the neurosecretory granules the vasopressin specific radioactivity was one-third that of the large granules. Presumably, therefore, this large-granule fraction represented the synthetic region and the neurosecretory granules, which acquired the vasopressin while still in the hypothalamic-median eminence region, were specialized for the storage and transport of vasopressin and possibly for its release. Similar relationships appear to hold for oxytocin, with a chemically distinct neurophysin and in different cells of the hypothalamus, though these matters have not been as extensively studied.

An intermediate in vasopressin synthesis was suggested by the above experiments and confirmed by examining tissues from the hypothalamic-median eminence region during in vitro incubation (Takabatake & Sachs, 1964; Sachs, 1970). Appearance of the infused amino acids in vasopressin commenced after about 1·5 hr. infusion. Hypothalamic tissues removed at 1·5 hr. and incubated in vitro, produced isotopically-labelled vasopressin even in the presence of puromycin. Both in vivo and in vitro, puromycin was shown to inhibit the production of newly-labelled vasopressin when it was present during an initial hour. Formation of the hormone may thus occur by the initial synthesis of a larger molecule, and subsequent split to yield the peptide hormones; an initially covalent link with a neurophysin has been envisaged (Sachs, 1970; Uttenthal & Hope, 1970).

Neurohypophysial Hormones: Release

The mode of release of the neurohypophysial hormones, like other aspects of the initiation of neural activity, is only partly understood; but pituitary secretion has specific chemical control. The normal stimulus for secretion of vasopressin is presumably the osmotic pressure of the blood; emotional stimuli also can inhibit urine flow in a matter of minutes. Vasopressin measured by antidiuretic properties has been found to be released by electrical stimulation of certain of the nuclei from which the hypothalamic-hypophysial tract originates, and recording electrodes in these positions can detect changes in cell-firing when hypertonic saline is injected to the carotid of rabbits. There is indeed remarkably sensitive response of the hypothalamus to small changes in osmotic pressure (Cross & Green, 1959; Dicker, 1961; Ginsburg, 1968). Thus release of vasopressin by very varied stimuli appears normally to operate through the hypothalamus. A similar interplay of emotional and physiological stimuli can occur in the release of the other major hormone of the posterior pituitary, oxytocin, as shown in its end effects on the uterus or on milk ejection.

Localized electrical stimulation within the hypothalamus of cats, and measurement of oxytocin and vasopressin in their jugular venous blood, has shown the two hormones to be susceptible to independent release (Bisset et al., 1963, 1970; see Haldar, 1970). Excitation of the supraoptic nucleus appeared to be most associated with release of vasopressin, and of the paraventricular nucleus, with oxytocin. This was shown in rats by stimulation through stereotaxically-placed electrodes and measurement of hormonal concentrations in jugular blood, and of frequencies of cell-firing (Dyball & Koizumi, 1969). Acetylcholine can cause release of vasopressin and this appears to depend on the hypothalamic centres concerned, being cholinergic.

In neurons of the hypothalamic-hypophysial tract of the toad, the terminal regions from which the hormones are discharged have been observed electron-microscopically to contain not only the granules which carry the hormones, but also small vesicles. The vesicles represent a population distinct from other organelles but resembling the synaptic vesicles of neurons of the cerebral cortex which contain acetylcholine (Chapters 12 and 14). Intravenous acetylcholine can cause antidiuresis by discharge of vasopressin, and the hypothalamic nuclei from which the hypothalamic-hypophysial tract originates, contain choline acetylase; the neurohypophysis contains little (see Dicker, 1961). In the cerebral cortex, nerve-firing is concluded to liberate the vesicle contents through the terminal membrane to the synaptic cleft; conceivably in the terminals of the posterior pituitary, an associated liberation can occur of the contents of the granules (Gerschenfeld et al., 1960; De Robertis, 1964). Liberation of vasopressin from the isolated pituitary of rats can be caused by electrical stimulation and by 50 mM-K^+ in incubating fluids provided these also contain Ca^{2+} (Douglas & Poisner, 1964). Cell depolarization with Ca^{2+} entry is considered to be involved.

Requirements for Ca^{2+} in vasopressin liberation parallels its requirement in discharge of catecholamine-containing granules (q.v.) and Ca^{2+} may be needed generally in neurosecretion; it is involved also in secretion of enzymes (Schramm, 1967). A further common factor is involvement of ATP. With suspensions of neurosecretory granules from cattle posterior pituitaries, ATP at about 0·5 mM accelerated the liberation of vasopressin (Poisner & Douglas, 1968). The granules contained an ATPase and a phosphoenolpyruvate ATP-regenerating system was more effective than ATP alone. The granules themselves contained little ATP: 1 μmole/g. protein, or one-twentieth of the molar content of vasopressin. The release of vasopressin was accompanied by liberation of much protein, presumably neurophysin, in constant ratio to the hormone. Concomitant release of neurophysin and hormone occurs also *in vivo* and suggests the granule contents to be secreted as a whole.

Anterior Pituitary: Releasing Factors

Relationships between the anterior pituitary and the hypothalamus are characteristically different (Guillemin, 1964; Harris & Donovan, 1966; Martini *et al.*, 1968; Schally *et al.*, 1968; James & Landon, 1968; Meites, 1970). This part of the pituitary, the adenohypophysis, arises embryologically from non-neural tissue and a variety of techniques has shown its main link with the hypothalamus to be by blood vessels and not by nerve fibres. A system of portal vessels runs from the hypothalamus by the median eminence of the tuber cinereum and the pituitary stalk to the anterior pituitary. On its interruption, anterior pituitary secretions cease. If in transplanted pituitary tissue the portal vessels are replaced by another blood supply, secretions are not restored. Presumably, therefore, specific substances are transmitted from the hypothalamus. They appear to be diffusible and thus the passage of the protein hormones themselves (Table 16.1) is probably contraindicated, though several of the hormones of the anterior pituitary have been detected in extracts from the hypothalamus. Extraction of the hypothalamus has however, yielded materials which appear to cause the release of several of the pituitary hormones. To establish this unequivocally *in vivo* has not proved easy; relevant experiments can be noted only briefly here, with special mention of those which concern cerebral interactions in experimentally simplified systems. Thus cultured pituitary and hypothalamic tissues, and examination of these parts of the brain *in vitro* in saline-based solutions, have contributed to defining the interactions involved.

In tissue cultures of the pituitary, hypothalamic extracts were effective in causing the release of adrenocorticotrophic hormone; their action was not reproduced by adrenaline, serotonin or a number of other known substances (Guillemin: *Symposium*, 1956). Some activity was shown by vasopressin, but other peptides in the extracts proved more active and were fractionated and characterized as α- and β-*corticotrophin-releasing factors*. Pituitary extracts also have been fractionated to yield an α-corticotrophin-releasing factor. The hypothalamic factor from large-scale extractions has been obtained in a rechromatographed form active in rats at 1 μg. and below (Schally *et al.*, 1962, 1968). Corticotrophin-releasing factor in dispersions of median eminence tissue from the rat was found on differential and density gradient centrifugation to be associated with fractions containing nerve terminals (Mulder, 1969). Hypotonic treatment of the terminal fraction altered these properties and suggested the factor to be attached to granules within the terminals.

The *thyrotrophin-releasing factor*, TRF, has been characterized as responsible for specific effects of hypothalamic extracts *in vivo* and on pituitary fragments *in vitro*. The extracts, made by dilute acid from sheep hypothalamus and puri-

fied by adsorption, greatly increased the release of thyrotrophic hormone from
the pituitary tissue to an incubating fluid. The active material was non-dialysable and could be inactivated by heat or by proteolytic enzymes. No thyrotrophic hormone was liberated by oxytocin or vasopressin, nor by preparations
which released other hormones from the anterior pituitary. An earlier belief
that, in some species *in vivo*, vasopressin liberated thyrotrophic hormone has
been shown to be due, rather, to vasopressin acting on the thyroid itself
(Garcia *et al.*, 1964; Guillemin *et al.*, 1963; Harris *et al.*, 1964). The hypothala-
mic-releasing factor is thus of considerable specificity; it has the properties of
a peptide.

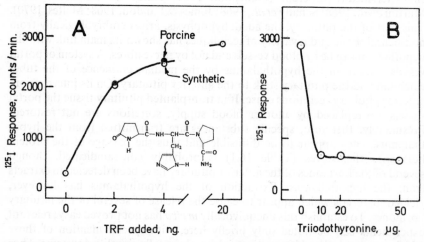

FIG. 16.3. Response of isolated pituitaries to thyrotrophin-releasing factor, TRF: structure,
    above (Bowers *et al.*, 1970; Burgus *et al.*, 1970).
   A. Rat anterior pituitary glands in bicarbonate glucose salines were incubated for 2 hr.
with fresh saline each 30 min., and then for a 1 hr. experimental period in salines with or
without TRF. The latter solutions were taken for a bioassay in pretreated mice, measuring
the increase in ^{125}I in the blood of groups of mice with and without the solutions being
assayed.
   B. In experiments conducted as those of A, 20 ng. of TRF were present in all salines during the 1 hr. incubation, together with the quantities stated of triiodothyronine.

Isolation and identification of TRF by two groups of investigators (Bowers
et al., 1970; Burgus *et al.*, 1970) involved its extraction from the hypothalamic
tissue of over 10^5 pigs and sheep, and showed that from the two sources the
product was identical. The few mg. of purified products from each species,
on hydrolysis yielded glutamic acid, histidine and proline in equimolar
amounts, and were active in mice assays in quantities of only 1–10 ng. The
molecular size of the factor approximated that of a tripeptide, and mass
spectroscopy gave data from which the structure was deduced. Also, of eight
synthetic compounds based on peptides of the three amino acids isolated, one
only was active: the pyroglutamylhistidylproline amide of Fig. 16.3. Its
relatively simple structure amazed and delighted; the peptide lacking the
terminal proline amide and the internal glutamyl amide was almost inactive.
The synthetic compound was identical in activity with that isolated from pigs

or sheep. Also, like natural TRF the synthetic compound was susceptible to inhibition of its activity by triiodothyronine. This inhibition (Fig. 16.3) can be seen as related to the control of thyroid function by feedback inhibition at the pituitary. However, although the TRF is a simple molecule sufficiently similar to triiodothyronine for competition to be envisaged, their interaction appears to be more complicated. Thus the inhibition of TRF action by triiodothyronine is prevented by cycloheximide or by actinomycin D (Schally et al., 1968).

The *growth-hormone releasing factor* also has been characterized in extracts from the hypothalamus and median eminence of cattle (Schally et al., 1968; Schofield, 1967). Gel exclusion techniques suggest a molecular weight of about 2,500 and chemically it appears to be a peptide, inactivated by proteolytic enzymes. Crude hypothalamic extracts and also the purified preparations of the factor stimulated release of growth hormone from isolated pituitary tissues during incubation in chemically-defined media. The release was shown from incubated rat pituitary by assays *in vivo*, and from slices of ox pituitary by immunochemical methods. Purified preparations of the factor acted at 5 ng./ incubated pituitary, and were capable of releasing 100–400 times their own weight of growth hormone. They also augmented the total amount of growth hormone in the tissue plus incubating fluid; inhibition of this increase by actinomycin D confirmed that synthesis as well as release was being affected by the factor.

Release of the *luteinizing hormone*, as observed by stimulation of ovulation (Campbell et al., 1964; McCann & Ramirez, 1964; Schally et al., 1968) has also been found to be controlled by humoural factors. In rabbits, the normal stimuli for ovulation are sensory, associated with coition. Electrical or mechanical stimulation of the hypothalamus but not of the pituitary will also cause ovulation, and by localized stimulation particular hypothalamic areas near the median eminence were shown to be involved. Material obtained by acid extraction from the median eminence of the ox, was then found to stimulate secretion of the luteinizing hormone when injected by slow infusion to the anterior pituitary. Its effects were observed by measuring the frequency of ovulation in rabbits and also by the diminution in ovarian ascorbic acid which is caused by the luteinizing hormone. By the latter method median-eminence extracts were found to act on intravenous injection. By both methods, extracts of the cerebral cortex were without activity and extracts from elsewhere in the hypothalamus were less active than those from the median eminence. Again, the active material proved to be distinct from several known agents and probably to be a polypeptide-like material, susceptible to some proteolytic enzymes and relatively heat-stable. Action of 20 ng. of purified preparations was demonstrated with incubated pituitary tissues, and resulted in release of up to 50 times this quantity of luteinizing hormone.

Release of the *follicle-stimulating hormone* is augmented by material extracted from tissues of the median eminence. Lesions in specific hypothalamic regions prove to interfere differentially with the different releasing factors, and the median eminence appears to include in its functions the ability to act as a storage site for the various releasing factors synthesized in the hypothalamus (Martini et al., 1968; Schally, 1968).

Metabolism of the Hypothalamus; Sensitivity to Specific Chemicals

Metabolic study of the hypothalamus, apart from its intrinsic interest, represents one way of finding how the hypothalamus influences pituitary secretion. Such influence is part of complex self-regulating systems which are central to the subject of neuroendocrinology; a few aspects only can be noted here.

Hypothalamic tissues show active carbohydrate metabolism: in glucose salines respiratory rates of some 85 μmoles O_2/g. tissue/hr. and glycolytic rates of 20 μmoles lactate formed/g. hr. have been found, with the utilization of an approximately equivalent amount of glucose (Roberts & Keller, 1955). After procedures liberating the pituitary hormones, respiratory rates increased both in hypothalamic and in anterior pituitary tissues.

In the brain of rats frozen *in situ* (see Chapter 3), hypothalamic areas were found to contain labile phosphates with the properties of creatine phosphate and adenosine triphosphate, in quantities corresponding to a total of about 10 μmoles P/g. tissue. Hypothalamic tissues from normal and hungry rats were found to differ in their incorporation of isotopic phosphate to these fractions; this was suggested as part of the mechanism regulating food intake from the hypothalamus (Larsson, 1954). Phosphatases, glycosidases (Robins *et al.*, 1968) cholinesterases, and monoamine oxidase have been found active in the hypothalamus; certain of these enzymes will be noted as related to the high content of their physiologically active substrates which also occur in the hypo-thalamus and were described in Chapter 14. Monoamine oxidase in hypothal-amic areas of female rats has been found to undergo cyclic changes in activity in association with the animals' oestrus cycle (Kamberi & Kobayashi, 1970). The median eminence showed especially high oxidase activity; inhibitors of monoamine oxidase can block ovulation. A number of peptidases occur in the hypothalamus; some of them are capable of degrading pituitary hormones (see Marks, 1968).

It is to be emphasized that the hypothalamus plays a large part in regulating metabolic events not only through the pituitary but also by impulse-trans-mission in nerve-tracts to other parts of the body: for in the hypothalamus are grouped centres concerned with the control of food intake, of intestinal motion and of body temperature. These centres often have specific chemical aspects in their functioning even though this is largely by nerve fibres, as has been richly exemplified by the chemotherapeutic development of drugs which can modify their functioning (see Chapters 14, 15; McIlwain, 1957; Efron, 1968).

Both neuronal and chemical factors are evident also in communication from the rest of the body to the hypothalamus. The hypothalamus is sensitive to the thyroid, gonadal and adrenal hormones whose liberation through the pituitary it promotes. Thus increased blood levels of oestrogens from the ovary depress the secretion of gonadotrophins from the pituitary. This occurs also on injecting oestrogens, when the ovary atrophies. Part of the mechanism concerned has been demonstrated using ³H-oestradiol. This became attached to tissue con-stituents in dispersions and extracts of rat hypothalamus. About 1 nmole oestradiol/mg. protein was so bound; the amount diminished when animals were pre-treated *in vivo* with non-labelled oestradiol (Eisenfeld, 1969; Ginsburg *et al.*, 1970). Also, administration of adrenal steroids decreases their secretion from the adrenal cortex, which atrophies. Moreover, these results require intact connections between hypothalamus and pituitary, so that the hypothalamus would appear to contain areas sensitive, directly or indirectly, to the adrenal hormone (see Harris, 1955; Bogdanove, 1964).

Control of the functioning of peripheral organs from the pituitary thus includes the hypothalamus in its regulatory cycle. There is indeed evidence for two types of regulatory cycle by which the brain responds to circulating hormonal factors, depending on whether the factor concerned is a peripheral or a pituitary secretion. Modification of pituitary secretions by the steroids, as just outlined, represents a 'long' feedback mechanism, and their modification by circulating adrenocorticotrophic hormone, a "short" feedback mechanism (see Martini *et al.*, 1968; Ganong & Martini, 1969). There is thus reproduced here, at the level of interaction between organs, the phenomena of sensitivity of a system to specific chemical products of its own activity. The main energy-yielding reactions of the brain were described in Chapters 5 and 6 as similarly sensitive to the products of energy-utilizing reactions and here the regulation involved response by a subcellular particle to change in level of phosphates or phosphate-acceptors in the cell. In this case, and with the pituitary-hypothalamic interconnections just described, the chemical sensitivity contributes to producing homeostasis or, when change is induced, a buffered and coordinated sequence of changes. This prompts consideration of the subjects which follow.

The Speed of Chemical Change in the Brain

In spite of the widespread effects of the brain, it performs in a physical sense relatively little external work. Neurosecretion from the hypothalamus or pituitary or in forming the cerebrospinal fluid accounts for very little of the exchange in material taking place in the brain; its external chemical work is a very small fraction of that performed by the kidney or mammary gland. Its external electrical work is also an extremely small part of the 12 cal./g. hr. made available by the cerebral metabolism of glucose. Rather, the brain impresses by the way in which its output, hormonally or in nerve impulses, is guided by certain selected events of the many which occurred in the history of an animal or of its species.

This organized output is interrupted by a few seconds' intermission in material supply from the bloodstream and ceases after a minute or so. Part of the 12 cal./g. hr. is thus expended in maintaining cerebral structure and readiness to react. Considering largely the cerebral nerve cells, there are at least three aspects to such maintenance. Probably the greater energy requirements are expended in keeping the differential distribution in sodium and potassium ions on which the electrical action potential depends. A further part must be utilized in the metabolism of substances concerned with synaptic transmission and other interactions between cells. Thirdly, the metabolic machinery of the cell itself requires renewal, as may be judged by the turnover of ribonucleic acid and protein and the supply of materials from cell nucleus to cytoplasm.

A special aspect of the renewal of cell structure becomes evident when it is recalled that neurons of the central nervous system have little ability to regenerate after damage and yet the central nervous system constitutes in higher organisms the major means of adaptation and learning. An event of a fraction of a second can affect behaviour for a decade; a major part of cerebral activities involves the integration of processes which differ greatly in their speed. How widely different in rate are different cerebral processes is indicated in Table 16.2. The rise or fall of potential occurring during transmission of a nerve impulse may occupy only a thousand-millionth of the time of slower, adaptive processes.

Intermediate in rate between these extremes come many of the processes of intermediary metabolism described earlier. These give to all cerebral processes their means of continuance. They are described in the table as occupying a few seconds because in such a period the total cerebral content of oxygen, hexoses,

Table 16.2

Rates of cerebral processes

Time-scale of process (seconds)	Description	Relevant controlling factors
10^{-4} to 10^{-3}	Rise and fall of action potential	Ion concentration and membrane potential
1 to 10	Intermediary metabolism (Table 16.3)	Concentrations of enzymes and metabolites
10^3 to 10^5	Growth and adaptation	Turnover of enzymes and structural components

or labile phosphates can undergo reaction. Barcroft (1934) commented, regarding the brain, that it was remarkable that a substance so necessary as oxygen should be stored to so slight an extent. At *A*, Table 16.3, are collected data showing that the brain holds equally little reserve of other of its major metabolites. Section *B* of the table shows other cerebral constituents to undergo comparably rapid reaction when judged in this way.

In these examples the quantities of cerebral substances reacting in unit time may differ considerably, being very small in the case of acetylcholine. By contrast, the fraction of the cerebral content which reacts per second shows much less variation. It is natural to query whether some technical limitation tends to bring about this result. One second is near the limit for observation of chemical change by ordinary means. However, much of the data has independent support from measurements over much longer periods.

The rates quoted in Section *A* of the table concern the whole brain, electrically stimulated in intact animals, and are supported by data obtained by other means. There is no reason for thinking them unrepresentative of changes occurring briefly when a given area comes to activity in normal animals. Certain similarities in rate arise because these substances react together, but the tissue content of the materials is not conditioned stoichiometrically. Rather, it is a characteristic of cerebral metabolic make-up that 5–25% of several of its constituents can react per second. In other tissues the content in many materials of the table and the rates of corresponding reactions can have very different values from those in the brain. The cerebral values must be judged to have some relation to the organization of activities in the brain.

Respiration of the brain and its oxygen content are not, however, unusual in comparison with values found in other organs of the body. The respiratory rate of kidney, liver, heart muscle and brain do not differ more than two- or three-fold. Considering for a moment cardiac function: the respiratory rate of heart muscle, the size of the heart, and the volume of blood which can be supplied through vessels of a given length and fineness are all interdependent. So also it would be anticipated are the respiratory rate of the brain, its size,

Table 16.3

The speed of some chemical changes in the brain

Substance	Cerebral content (nmoles/g.)	Maximum rate of change observed in the brain (nmoles/g. sec.)	Proportion of cerebral content reacting per second (%)
Section A			
Oxygen	300	40	13
Glucose	1,000	100	10
Glycogen (as hexose)	5,500	200	4
Lactic acid	2,000	120	6
Phosphocreatine	3,000	600	20
Adenosine triphosphate	2,600	700	27
Section B			
Nicotinamide-adenine dinucleotide	400	60	15
Ammonia	160	125	75
Acetylcholine	7	1	14

The sources of data are given in earlier chapters.

the fineness and number of its fibres and dendritic connections, and the maximum frequency of their firing at a given action potential without exhaustion. Cerebral apparatus with a variety of different properties can be conceived by reciprocal variation among such characteristics. With a more slowly responding brain or one in which the effect of incoming signals was more limited, the same quantity of reserve materials would give longer activity before exhaustion.

Reverting to how cerebral processes very different in rate can interact, this undoubtedly occurs in many ways. Processes of intermediate rate have been observed in the brain both electrically and metabolically. Many changes are slower in rate than those of Table 16.3. The changes of potential seen in the electroencephalogram occupy from a fiftieth of a second to a second and processes of these rates have been seen also with micro-electrodes in individual cells of the brain. However, the slower processes of learning or adaptation appear to involve a type of structural change. Much which is learned can survive the cessation of electrical activity in the brain. Possibly the structural change is at the fine terminals of neurons or in some balance of reaction rates which is expressed as a change in threshold. It will be noted from Chapter 14 that the brain can respond to particular visual signals by alteration in the metabolism of pineal melatonin. This adaptation proceeds by routes which are familiar in lower organisms and which involve controlling the production of the enzyme catalysing a critical stage of melatonin synthesis.

A further aspect of the speed of chemical change in the brain may be relevant to the question of how the effects of brief activity are prolonged. Maximal activity in the whole or a part of the central nervous system can be intermittent only; after a brief period of activity it must await restoring processes. Moreover, the restoring processes are markedly slower than the processes which accompany activity. Thus an appreciable proportion of cerebral phosphocreatine can be broken down by a few electrical pulses; its resynthesis takes place at only one-tenth of the rate of its breakdown. Restoration is even slower in the case of glycogen. An alteration of level occurring in 5 sec. may take about an hour to be restored. It thus extends the effect of a brief change nearly a thousand-fold and links the last two categories of Table 16.2. Moreover, during the period following activity the parts of the brain affected are chemically different from parts not affected.

These observations are again relevant to the small reserve which the brain holds of the metabolites listed in Table 16.3. Glycogen and possibly phosphocreatine are in a sense storage products. If their cerebral content were to be doubled or trebled this need not involve much change in other metabolites, but would presumably give longer survival to the brain when it was working maximally or when its blood supply momentarily failed. Muscle, also called on for intermittent intense activity contains some five or ten times the cerebral quantities of these substances. Moreover, at an earlier stage of development, parts of the brain also contain quantities of glycogen different from those in the adult. The cerebral cortex increases in glycogen content as it comes to functional activity; at the same time the glycogen of the medulla decreases. The cerebral content of glycogen is thus in a sense adjustable and a concentration, which at first sight appears low, may carry some compensating advantage. Thus it is to be noted that, other factors being equal, with larger reserves longer or more intense stimulation would be necessary to bring about the same proportional change in glycogen or phosphocreatine.

An advantage conferred by the presence of relatively small quantities of some critical cerebral reactants may thus be greater responsiveness to external change. An obvious disadvantage of such paucity of reactants is the likelihood of their exhaustion. In this situation an additional virtue can be seen in the neurosecretory granules or vesicles: a limited quantity of material can be released, act and be removed while ample supplies remain for subsequent occasions. The materials in such granules, it may be noted, are usually cerebral products, and not compounds supplied directly by the bloodstream. Of essential metabolites so supplied there is often little cerebral reserve. Moreover, sensitive hormonal regulation and response to the internal environment also presuppose rapid blood flow; with the substrates comes some measure of control of their utilization. Whether for these or other reasons cerebral functioning, in spite of its less material aspects, is the major bodily activity most dependent on continuous material supplies.

REFERENCES

ACHER, R. (1966). In Harris & Donovan (1966), **3**, p. 269.
ADELSON, J. W. (1971). *Nature, Lond.* **229**, 321.
ALBERS, R. W. & BRIGHTMAN, M. W. (1959). *J. Neurochem.* **3**, 269.
BARCROFT, J. (1934). Features in the Architecture of Physiological Function. Cambridge: University Press.
BARER, R., HELLER, H. & LEDERIS, K. (1963). *Proc. Roy. Soc. B.* **158**, 388.
BARONDES, S. H. (1962). *J. biol. Chem.* **237**, 204.
BERDE, B. (1968). (Ed.). Neurohypophysial Hormones and similar Peptides. Berlin: Springer.
BERDE, B. & BOISSONNAS, R. A. (1966). In Harris & Donovan (1966), p. 624.
BISSET, G. W., CLARK, B. J. & HALDAR, J. (1970). *J. Physiol.* **206**, 711.
BISSET, G. W., HILTON, S. M. & POISNER, A. M. (1963). *J. Physiol.* **169**, 40P.
BOGDANOVE, E. M. (1964). *Vitamins and Hormones,* **22**, 205.
BOWERS, C. Y., SCHALLY, A. V., ERZMANN, F., BOLER, J. & FOLKERS, K. (1970). *Endocrinology,* **86**, 1143.
BURGUS, R., DUNN, T. F., DESIDERIO, D., WARD, D. N., VALE, W. & GUILLEMIN, R. (1970). *Nature, Lond.* **226**, 321.
CAMPBELL, H. J., FEUER, G. & HARRIS, G. W. (1964). *J. Physiol.* **170**, 474.
CLEMENS, M. J. & KORNER, A. (1969). *Biochem. J.* **113**, 10P.
Colloquium (1960). Ciba Foundation Colloquia on Endocrinology. **13**. Ed. Wolstenholme & O'Connor. London: Churchill.
CROSS, B. A. & GREEN, J. D. (1959). *J. Physiol.* **148**, 554.
DEAN, C. R. & HOPE, D. B. (1968). *Biochem. J.* **106**, 565.
DE ROBERTIS, E. (1964). Histophysiology of Synapses and Neurosecretion. Oxford: Pergamon.
DICKER, S. E. (1961). *J. Pharm. Pharmacol.* **13**, 449.
DOUGLAS, W. W. & POISNER, A. M. (1964). *J. Physiol.* **172**, 1.
DURAISWAMI, S., MCSHAN, W. H. & MEYER, R. K. (1964). *Biochim. Biophys. Acta,* **86**, 156.
DYBALL, R. E. J. & KOIZUMI, K. (1969). *J. Physiol.* **201**, 711.
EFRON, D. H. (1968) (Ed.). Psychopharmacology. Washington: U.S. Govt.
EISENFELD, A. J. (1969). *Nature, Lond.* **224**, 1203.
ELLIS, S. (1960). *J. biol. Chem.* **235**, 1694.
ELLIS, S. & PERRY, M. (1966). *J. biol. Chem.* **241**, 3679.
EVANS, H. M., SPARKS, L. L. & DIXON, J. S. (1966). In Harris & Donovan (1966), **1**, p. 317.
FAWCETT, C. P., POWELL, A. E. & SACHS, H. (1968). *Endocrinol.* **83**, 1299.
FURTH, A. J. & HOPE, D. B. (1970). *Biochem. J.* **116**, 545.
GALA, R. R. & REECE, R. P. (1963). *Proc. Soc. exp. Biol. N.Y.* **114**, 422.
GANONG, W. F. & MARTINI, L. (1969) (Ed.). Frontiers in Neuroendocrinology. Oxford: University Press.
GARCIA, J., HARRIS, G. W. & SCHINDLER, W. J. (1964). *J. Physiol.* **170**, 487.
GERSCHENFELD, H. M., TRAMEZZANI, J. & DE ROBERTIS, E. (1960). *Endocrinol.* **66**, 741.
GINSBURG, M. (1968). In Berde (1968).
GINSBURG, M. & THOMAS, P. J. (1969). *J. Physiol.* **201**, 181.
GINSBURG, M., MARRIOTT, J. & THOMAS, P. J. (1970). *J. Physiol.* **209**, 39P.
GUILLEMIN, R. (1964). *Rec. Progr. Horm. Res.* **20**, 89.
GUILLEMIN, R., YAMAZAKI, E., GARD, D. A., JUTISZ, M. & SAKIZ, E. (1963). *Endocrinol.* **73**, 564.
HALDAR, J. (1970). *J. Physiol.* **206**, 723.
HARRIS, G. W. (1955). Neural Control of the Pituitary Gland. London: Arnold.

HARRIS, G. W. & DONOVAN, B. T. (1966) (Eds.). The Pituitary Gland. Berkeley:
        Univ. Calif. Press.
HARRIS, G. W., LEVINE, S. & SCHINDLER, W. J. (1964). *J. Physiol.* **170**, 516.
HARRIS, J. I. (1959). *Biochem. J.* **71**, 451.
HOLLENBERG, M. D. & HOPE, D. B. (1968). *Biochem. J.* **106**, 557.
HYMER, W. C. & McSHAN, W. H. (1963). *J. cell. Biol.* **17**, 67.
JACOBOWITZ, D., MARKS, B. H. & VERNIKOS-DANELLIS, J. (1963). *Endocrinol.* **72**, 592.
JAMES, V. H. T. & LANDON, J. (1968). *Mem. Soc. Endocrinol.* **17**.
KAMBERI, I. A. & KOBAYASHI, Y. (1970). *J. Neurochem.* **17**, 261.
KORNER, A. (1964). *Biochem. J.* **92**, 449.
LaBELLA, F. S., VIVIAN, S. & BINDLER, E. (1967). *Biochem. Pharmacol.* **16**, 1126.
LARSSON, S. (1954). *Acta Physiol. Scand.* **32**, supp. 115.
LEE, T. H., LERNER, A. D. & BUETTNER-JANUSH, V. (1961). *J. biol. Chem.* **236**, 2970.
LEVINE, R. (1966) (Ed.). *Proc. Assoc. Res. nerv. ment. Dis.* **43**.
LEWIS, U. J. (1963). *J. biol. Chem.* **238**, 3330, 3336.
LI, C. H. (1956, 1957). *Advances in Protein Chemistry*, **11**, 101; **12**, 270.
LI, C. H., LIN, W. K. & DIXON, K. S. (1966). *J. Amer. Chem. Soc.* **88**, 2050.
LOWRY, P. J. & CHADWICK, A. (1970). *Nature, Lond.* **226**, 219.
MARKS, N. (1968). *Internat. Rev. Neurobiol.* **11**, 57.
MARTINI, L., FRASCHINI, F. & MOTTA, M. (1968). *Rec. Progr. Horm. Res.*, **24**, 439.
McCANN, S. M. & RAMIREZ, D. V. (1964). *Rec. Progr. Horm. Res.* **20**, 131.
McDONALD, J., LEIBACH, F. H., GRINDELAND, R. E. & ELLIS, S. (1968*a*). *J. biol.
        Chem.* **243**, 4143.
McDONALD, J. K., REILLY, T. J., ZEITMAN, B. B. & ELLIS, S. (1968*b*). *J. biol. Chem.*
        243, 2028.
McILWAIN, H. (1957). Chemotherapy and the Central Nervous System. London:
        Churchill.
MEITES, J. (1970). Edit.: Hypophysiotropic Hormones of the Hypothalamus.
        Baltimore: Williams & Wilkins.
MELCHIOR, J. B. & HILKER, D. M. (1955). *J. biol. Chem.* **212**, 187.
MULDER, A. H. (1969). *Second Meeting Internat. Neurochem. Soc.*, p. 300. Milan,
        Tamburini.
NIALL, H. D. (1971). *Nature new Biol.* **230**, 91.
NORSTRÖM, A. & SJÖSTRAND, J. (1971). *J. Neurochem.* **18**, 29.
PARDOE, A. U. & WEATHERALL, M. (1955). *J. Physiol.* **127**, 201.
PARMAR, S. S., SUTTER, M. C. & NICKERSON, M. (1961). *Canad. J. Biochem. Physiol.*
        39, 1335.
POISNER, A. M. & DOUGLAS, W. W. (1968). *Mol. Pharmacol.* **4**, 531.
RAMACHANDRAN, L. K. & WINNICK, T. (1957). *Biochim. Biophys. Acta*, **23**, 533.
RAUCH, R., HOLLENBERG, M. D. & HOPE, D. B. (1969). *Biochem. J.* **115**, 473.
REISS, M. (1970). *Handb. Neurochem.* **4**, 463.
REICHERT, L. E., RASCO, M. A., WARD, D. N., NISWENDER, G. D. & MIDGLEY, A. R.
        (1969). *J. biol. Chem.* **244**, 5110.
ROBERTS, S. & KELLER, M. R. (1955). *Endocrinology*, **57**, 64.
ROBINS, E., HIRSCH, H. E. & EMMONS, S. S. (1968). *J. biol. Chem.* **243**, 4247, 4253.
RUDMAN, D., MALKIN, M. F., BROWN, S. J., GARCIA, L. A. & ABEL, L. L. (1964).
        J. Lipid Res. **5**, 39.
SACHS, H. (1960, 1963). *J. Neurochem.* **5**, 300; **10**, 289, 299.
SACHS, H. (1970). *Handb. Neurochem.* **4**, 373.
SCHALLY, A. V., ARIMURA, A., BOWERS, C. Y., KASTIN, A. J., SAWANO, S. & REDDING,
        T. W. (1968). *Rec. Progr. Horm. Res.* **24**, 497.
SCHALLY, A. V., LIPSCOMB, H. S. & GUILLEMIN, R. (1962). *Endocrinol.* **71**, 164.
SCHARRER, E. & SCHARRER, B. (1954). *Rec. Progr. Horm. Res.* **10**, 183.
SCHOFIELD, J. G. (1967). *Biochem. J.* **103**, 331.
SCHRAMM, M. (1967). *Ann. Rev. Biochem.* **36**, 307.
SKOSEY, J. L. (1970). *J. biol. Chem.* **245**, 510.
SMITH, M. W. & SACHS, H. (1961). *Biochem. J.* **79**, 663.
Symposium (1956). Hypothalamic-Hypophysial Relationships. Ed. W. S. Fields,
        R. Guillemin & C. A. Carton. Springfield: Thomas.

Symposium (1962). Neurosecretion. *Mem. Soc. Endocrinol.* **12**. Ed. Heller & Clark. London: Academic Press.

Symposium (1964). *Internat. Union Biochem.* **32**, 97.

TAKABATAKE, Y. & SACHS, H. (1964). *Endocrinology,* **75**, 934.

TURKINGTON, R. W. (1963). *J. biol. Chem.* **238**, 3463.

UTTENTHAL, L. O. & HOPE, D. B. (1970). *Biochem. J.* **116**, 899.

DU VIGNEAUD, V. (1955). Symposium on Peptide Chemistry. London: Chemical Society.

WEINSTEIN, H., MALAMED, S. & SACHS, H. (1961). *Biochim. Biophys. Acta,* **50**, 386.

WOOL, I. G., SCHARFF, R. & MAGNES, N. (1961). *Amer. J. Physiol.* **201**, 547.

WUU, T. C. & SAFFRAN, M. (1969). *J. biol. Chem.* **244**, 482.

ZIEGLER, D. M. & MELCHIOR, J. B. (1956). *J. biol. Chem.* **222**, 721, 731.

ZOR, U., KANEKO, T., LOWE, I. P., BLOOM, G. & FIELD, J. B. (1969). *J. biol. Chem.* **244**, 5189.

ZOR, U., KANEKO, T., SCHNEIDER, H. P. G., McCANN, S. M. & FIELD, J. B. (1970). *J. biol. Chem.* **245**, 2883.

Author Index

578 AUTHOR INDEX

584 AUTHOR INDEX

Subject Index

20